SEX, AGING, & DEATH
IN A MEDIEVAL
MEDICAL COMPENDIUM

VOLUME TWO

TABLE OF CONTENTS
(VOLUME TWO)

-11-

THE SICKNESS OF WOMEN

Monica H. Green and Linne R. Mooney

The text that opens the second major section of Trinity R.14.52 seems, at first glance, an anomaly. A lengthy treatise on gynecology and obstetrics, *Sickness of Women* claims to have been composed so "that oo womman may help another in hir sikenes and nat discure hir privitees to . . . vncurteys men." The intended audience, it is implied, is women. Why embed a text for female readers in this massive scientific and medical codex that we know was created for male users? We shall argue that, despite the prologue's formulaic audience claim (which is identical in all four extant copies of the text), *Sickness of Women* was included in Trinity R.14.52 not because it was meant to be used by women, but because it was of interest to the codex's (male) compilers, who correctly assessed that the text had always been meant for male as well as female readers. To be sure, *Sickness of Women* includes major sections on how to handle childbirth and other conditions that would, in the fifteenth century, normatively have been treated by female practitioners. Yet the text also includes extended passages in Latin and in other respects was only inadequately crafted to address a female audience. For latinate male readers, in contrast, the text could readily serve either clinical needs of attending female patients or intellectual concerns to understand the processes of generation. Both the content of *Sickness of Women* and its codicological placement here in the Trinity manuscript parallel uses that were made of gynecological literature throughout later medieval Europe.

Genesis of the Text

The text of *Sickness of Women* found in Trinity R.14.52, fols. 107r–135v, is the second redaction of a Middle English translation of the gynecological and obstetrical chapters from Gilbertus Anglicus's Latin *Compendium medicine.*[1] Gilbertus lived in the early part of the thirteenth century and seems to have studied at both Salerno and Montpellier. His *Compendium medicine*, composed ca. 1240, is a very long general encyclopedia of medical practice. It is arranged in the common *a capite ad calcem* format and consists of seven books. Gilbertus's *Compendium* quickly became a widely adopted textbook of medicine; exemplars show that it was "mass-produced" by the *pecia* system as early as the late thirteenth century in Paris.[2] A selective English translation of the *Compendium* was made early in the fifteenth century and proved to be widely influential.[3]

---

[1] One manuscript of each of the two versions of *Sickness of Women* was transcribed in the early 1980s, though in neither case did the editors correctly identify the text's Latin source or its relation to the other version. See Rowland 1981, an edition of Version 2 of *Sickness* based on London, BL, Sloane MS 2463; and Hallaert 1982, an edition of Version 1 of *Sickness* based on the Yale University manuscript. For important corrections to these editions, see Stannard and Voigts 1982 and Alonso Almeida and Rodríguez Alvarez 1996 [2000]. Alonso Almeida re-edited the Yale manuscript in his 1997 thesis; he plans to publish a revised edition.

As will be shown in what follows, the Trinity copy of *Sickness of Women 2* was almost certainly copied from Sloane 2463, the manuscript published by Rowland, or a very close relative of it. The Trinity copy is therefore not a novel witness to the text. Rather than being redundant of Rowland's edition, however, an edition of the Trinity text is merited, we believe, in order to correct the inaccuracies of that edition, to present fuller background information on the text's genesis and sources, and to set the text more securely into the material and probable social contexts of its use. The following analysis of the two versions of *Sickness* expands upon arguments that originally appeared in Green 1992 (citations of work by Green in this chapter refer to the writings of co-author Monica H. Green). *Pace* Rowland, *Sickness of Women 2* is by no means the "first" English gynecological handbook; at least four other texts (including, of course, *Sickness 1*) antedate it by several decades.

[2] A total of 27 extant manuscripts of Gilbert's Latin *Compendium* have now been identified. In addition to the lists in Getz 1991; Keiser 1994; and Sharpe 2001, 144, add: Cambrai, Bibliothèque municipale, MS 909 (808), s. xiv; Florence, Biblioteca Medicea-Laurenziana, Ashburnham MS 148 (*olim* 222; 154), s. xiv, fols. 5r–212v; Munich, Bayerische Staatsbibliothek, Clm 28187, s. xiv, fols. 1v–201r; New Haven (Connecticut), Yale University, Medical School Library, Cushing-Whitney MS 19, s. xiii ex./xiv in. (France), fols. 1r–178rb; Paris, BN, MSS lat. 6955, s. xiv, and lat. 16194, s. xiv; and Warsaw, Biblioteka Narodowa, MS III.8069, s. xiii ex./xiv in. Lost copies are attested from Cambridge, King's College; Cambridge, King's Hall; Cambridge, Peterhouse; Durham; the Austin Canons at Leicester; Oxford University, copy given by Duke Humphrey; Oxford, All Souls College; Ramsey; and Titchfield. See Sharpe 2001; Clarke 2002, 298, 332, 516, and 551. For the influence of Gilbertus's work, see G. Keil 1994; Riha 1994; Murano 2001.

[3] For lists of manuscripts, see Getz 1991, lxix–lxxii; Keiser 1998, 3834; and eVK, Author Index, s.n. Gilbert of England.

Sickness of Women, we believe, originated out of this translation of the full Latin *Compendium*.[4] In her 1991 edition of a later fifteenth-century manuscript of the Middle English *Compendium*, Faye Getz noted the appearance of *Sickness* within several manuscripts of the English *Compendium*.[5] These manuscripts often had further similarities, such as the regular inclusion of brief English texts on hematoscopy, scarifying, and cupping. Getz did not, however, recognize that *Sickness of Women* was drawn from Gilbertus and so did not pursue a stylistic analysis to confirm whether or not a single translator was responsible for the whole Middle English *Compendium*. Although the matter remains to be determined more definitively by complete collation of the more than two dozen extant manuscripts of the English Gilbertus,[6] on the basis of our own preliminary collation of select passages of the Latin *Compendium* and the Middle English *Sickness*, we find that *Sickness of Women* reflects many of the same translation and editing characteristics as the Middle English *Compendium* and so may well have originated from the hand of the same translator.

This first redaction of *Sickness of Women* (Version 1) translated fifteen of Gilbertus's twenty-two chapters on women's diseases from book 7 of the Latin *Compendium medicine*. (Omitted were Gilbertus's chapters on vaginal constrictives, impediments to conception, the generation of the embryo, signs of conception, urine of pregnant women, swelling of the legs, and

---

[4] *Sickness 1* already appears within the ME *Compendium* in the two earliest mss: Glasgow, University Library, Hunter MS 307 (U.7.1.), s. xv[1]; and London, Society of Antiquaries, MS 338, s. xv[1]. Moreover, in London, BL, Royal MS 18.a.vi, s. xv, *Sickness* still bears the "tail end" of the *Compendium*, i.e., two additional sections on phlebotomy and scarifying, respectively, followed by the same address to the reader found in the three fullest *Compendium* manuscripts: Hunter 307; London, BL, Sloane MS 3486, s. xv med.; and Oxford, Bodleian Library, Bodley MS 178 (SC 2073), s. xv[2]. In the Bodley manuscript, this passage reads "and yf eny man beholde it, and fynd eny thyng that displesith him lett him not repreve it, but lett him take suche a labour in hond ayen and let him be well avised, that he be not Repreved. ffor this in my masteris tyme and myne I have Well preved and cured and helid many a pacient, thanked be god of his grace sendyng to that is the heighest, and the best, leeche" (fol. 151v).

[5] Getz believed these were copies of the text edited by Rowland (i.e., *Sickness of Women 2*), rather than *Sickness 1*. As Keiser has noted (1994, 227–28), Getz's base manuscript (London, Wellcome Library, MS 537) is a much abbreviated and modified copy of the ME *Compendium*. Although valuable as a witness to the kinds of manipulations the text underwent in its later history (Getz demonstrates, for example, the consistent deletion of matters having to do with women and children from the Wellcome copy), the Wellcome manuscript is of little use in determining the original form of the full translation of Gilbertus's *Compendium*.

[6] Keiser (1994, 228) stresses that this work will have to be done in conjunction with a study of the Latin exemplars that the translator might have used.

breast cancer.)[7] With respect to the translator of the major portion of the Latin *Compendium*, George Keiser has noted that he displays a rather free hand, making frequent abbreviations, rearrangements, and, occasionally, amplifications of Gilbertus's long text. These same features can be found in the gynecological section. The result is a concise yet fluent and comprehensive English text.[8] *Sickness of Women 1* enjoyed a very healthy circulation in fifteenth-century England. It is found attached to the Middle English Gilbertus in six manuscripts, while in six further manuscripts it circulates independently of the full *Compendium*. These twelve manuscripts of *Sickness 1* make it the single most popular Middle English gynecological text known to us.[9]

The text of *Sickness of Women* presented here is a later redaction (Version 2).[10] This substantially rearranged and amplified version was, we

---

[7] See Green 1992, 74–75, for Gilbertus's chapters vis-à-vis Hallaert's edition of *Sickness of Women 1*. For our comparisons of the ME *Compendium* with its Latin source, we have employed the Latin printed edition (*Compendium medicine Gilberti Anglici tam morborum universalium quam particularium nondum medicis sed et cyrurgis utilissimum;* Lyons, 1510), where the chapters are unnumbered, and compared this in turn with one of the oldest extant manuscripts, Brugge, Openbare Bibliotheek, MS 469 (an. 1271). In the printed edition, twenty-one of the rubricated chapters in Book VII are gynecological and obstetrical. Correctly, a twenty-second chapter, *De impedimento conceptionis* (fols. 300vb–302va), should be separated off from *De sophisticatione uulue* (fol. 300ra–vb).

[8] As noted by Green (1992, 73), "the translator [of *Sickness 1*] took many liberties with his or her Latin source. Many chapters are drastically abbreviated; most discussions of diagnosis by urines are omitted, as are many individual ingredients, especially compound medicines. Despite the abbreviations, the translator usually caught the gist of Gilbertus's theoretical discussions, rendering them into simple but accurate English."

[9] In addition to the eleven manuscripts described in Green 1992, 78–81, add now London, BL, Harley MS 2375, s. xv, fols. 19r–29r. This is a complete copy of *Sickness 1* (with other selected passages from the ME *Compendium*) and not, as indicated in Green 1992, 74 n. 51, a "fragment." While the so-called *Trotula* treatises on women's medicine were translated more frequently (a total of five independent renditions have been identified), none of them had the circulation enjoyed by *Sickness 1*. The most popular *Trotula* translation is extant in five manuscripts. See Green 1997a and Barratt 2001.

[10] We have not attempted a full collation of all the copies of *Sickness of Women 1*, which would be necessary to pinpoint a probable exemplar on which the second redaction was based. In order to give some sense of the development of the text, we have, for the convenience of the reader, cited comparisons with Hallaert's edition of *Sickness 1* from the Yale manuscript. However, since it is clear that the redactor of *Sickness 2* was using a fuller rendition of the text than that found in the Yale manuscript, we have collated Hallaert's edition (**H**) with a much earlier copy, London, Society of Antiquaries, MS 338, s. xv[1], fols. 76v–85v (**A**), and cited significant variants accordingly.

believe, produced sometime around the middle of the fifteenth century. Of the four known copies, London, BL, Sloane MS 249 (fols. 180v–205v) seems to be the earliest, though it is unlikely to be the author's holograph.[11] London, Royal College of Surgeons, MS 129 (fols. 1r–45v) and BL, Sloane MS 2463 (fols. 194r–232r) are roughly contemporaneous with each other, both being produced just after mid-century. The fourth manuscript is our present codex, Trinity R.14.52. Our collation suggests that it may be a direct copy of Sloane 2463 or, at the very least, that it was made from a very closely related exemplar.[12]

Version 2 of *Sickness of Women* has three principal, striking changes from its predecessor. First, this redactor rearranged the original text of the Middle English *Sickness*, retaining all of its component material but laying out the chapters in a different order. This reordering brings the text somewhat back into alignment with the topical headings listed in *Sickness 1*'s original preface.[13] Second, this redactor interpolated major new sections of text.[14] Some of these are clipped wholesale out of other works. The extended discussion of fetal malpresentations comes from a late antique gynecological text by Muscio, while the brief section on swelling of the legs during pregnancy seems to be translated directly from Gilbertus's Latin

---

[11] Note that this was misdated to the sixteenth century by Green 1992, 81. Correctly, it should be dated near the middle of the fifteenth century. On errors in Sloane 249 that suggest that its scribe was copying off another exemplar, see Textual Notes to lines 240, 279, 458, 639, 806–807, and 881 (*inter alia*) and Explanatory Notes 25, 52, 64, 78, and 89.

[12] Although Trinity R.14.52 has numerous unique (and usually erroneous) readings—see, for example, Textual Notes to lines 116, 140, 165, 190–191, etc.—it otherwise agrees (often exactly) with Sloane 2463. In addition to readings the two copies share uniquely (see, for example, Textual Notes to lines 19, 548, 1256), the Trinity copy reproduces (as rubricated text) all but one of the marginal annotations found in Sloane 2463. (See Textual Notes to lines 250, 257, 283, 325, 331, 346, 412, 420, 620, 630, 897 and Textual Note to lines 375–376 for the omitted marginal note.) The Hammond scribe (or the scribe of his exemplar) also seems to have been prompted by corrections in Sloane 2463 to omit the recipe for staunching the flux on fol. 113r (see Explanatory Note 22), which in the other copies of *Sickness 2* was unwittingly duplicated. In no case does Trinity R.14.52 share readings solely with Royal College of Surgeons 129 or Sloane 249.

[13] The revised order is more typical of that found in the gynecological sections of most major medical compendia. See the discussion of chapter ordering below.

[14] In the edition, we have flagged all passages newly added by the *Sickness 2* redactor with paired double and single daggers.

Compendium.[15] Most of the other new sections are strings of additional remedies added at the end of the original sections, many of which may come from
the redactor's own practice. For example, after the end of the long *Sickness
1* account of menstrual retention (chap. 1), the redactor adds "a worshipful sirup" good for ladies and nuns, a laxative, a medicated pillow on which
the woman should sit while in a steambath, and a plaster that can be used
either as a fetal expulsive, an emetic, or a laxative (lines 236–292 below).
The redactor has a propensity for enumerating these new remedies: six
"needfull things" for uterine prolapse, three things to cast out the dead
child, sixteen manners of unnatural childbirth.[16] In order to make this new
material seem as congruous as possible, the redactor added another layer
of cross-references on top of the infrastructure already put in place by the
translator/redactor of *Sickness 1.* For example, in the first chapter (on menstrual retention), the *Sickness 2* compiler adds a cross-reference to a recipe
for musk oil which, s/he says, can be found in the later chapter on uterine
suffocation. Sure enough, in chapter 3 an extended description of musk
oil's preparation and multiple uses is appended to the original section on
uterine suffocation from *Sickness 1.*[17] Moreover, this redactor seems to have
had a particular fondness for certain preparations: a troche of myrrh credited to the Persian physician Rhazes, for example, is mentioned five times.[18]
The frequency of cross-referencing and approbations of efficacy give every
indication that the redactor was him/herself a practitioner with extensive
clinical experience, one who intended the text to be used in similar therapeutic contexts.[19] The redactor's third and final layer of intervention was

---

[15] On Muscio, see below; on the excerpt from Gilbertus, see Explanatory Note 76.
We have not yet identified the source for the new chapter on uterine mole, though
we suspect that it, too, derives from an earlier text.

[16] Actually, even these enumerations are inexact: there are eight additional treatments for uterine prolapse, not six; and four things to cast out the dead child, not
three. The sixteen manners of unnatural childbirth replicate the divisions in the
redactor's source, Muscio's *Gynaecia.*

[17] On the musk oil, compare chap. 1 (lines 268–269) with chap. 3 (lines 635–
676). In all, we have identified twenty cross-references, twelve of which replicate
(or modify) cross-references in *Sickness 1,* and eight of which occur in and refer to
material added by the redactor of *Sickness 2.* See especially Explanatory Notes 11,
13, and 44.

[18] A troche (ME *trociske*) is a kind of round, flat lozenge meant to be slowly dissolved in the mouth. For the troche of myrrh, see Explanatory Notes 13, 33, 53,
63, 71, and 84.

[19] On the addition of approbations of efficacy, see C. Jones 1998.

the addition of a prologue at the head of the text, stating his/her intentions in writing. No hint is given that the work is not completely novel.

Audiences, Explicit and Implicit

The text resulting from this complex process of rearrangement and interpolation is very intriguing, but it is also a very peculiar work that seems to want to fulfill multiple functions and address multiple potential readers. On the one hand, the sentiment of the prologue "that oo womman may help another in hir sikenes," i.e., the idea that the text was meant to be used directly by women, seems to be supported by the greater adaptation of *Sickness 2* to what must have been the medical needs of contemporary Englishwomen.[20] The detailed instructions on how the midwife should correct and extract the malpresented fetus, together with the extraordinary number of fetal expulsives, show the redactor's intense concern to aid women in childbirth—a physical trial that posed no small risk for fifteenth-century women of childbearing age.[21] In one of the novel additions to the text, the redactor makes clear that her/his concern for the parturient is paramount: "for whan the womman is fieble and the chield may nat come oute, than it is better that the chield be slayne than the moder of the chield die" (lines 679–681).[22]

But this concern with the constant risks of childbirth does not necessarily mean that the text was intended specifically for the use of midwives. Thus

---

[20] Although the reference in chap. 10 (line 1289) to "a riche womman" is original to *Sickness 1*, as is the concern in chap. 5 (line 839) for the cost of medicaments, the redactor of *Sickness 2* him/herself evinces a certain class consciousness in proferring remedies, on the one hand, "for ladies and for nonnes and other also that bien delicate" (chap. 1, lines 237–238) and, on the other hand, for poor women (chap. 7, line 987). Regarding the assumption that religious women in particular are delicate, see the late fourteenth-century *Nature of Women* in Green 1992, 86; and Barratt 2001, lines 119–121. For general background on childbirth in late medieval England, see Rawcliffe 2003.

[21] Grauer (1991) presents archeological evidence from a cemetery in York showing that the childbearing years (esp. ages 25–35) were indeed the highest period of differential mortality for women in medieval England.

[22] See also the preparation in chap. 10, added onto the end of the translation from Muscio, "For to delivere a womman of a child and *for to sle it if it may nat be brought furth*" (lines 1247–1248, emphasis added). This concern is not unique to the author of *Sickness 2*. Surveying a variety of English texts, Stoertz (1996) finds more recipes to expel the dead fetus than for delivering a live one. A similar concern with expelling the dead fetus can be found in an andrological and gynecological treatise in Oxford, Bodleian Library, Bodley MS 483, fols. 112v–114v.

far, individual women who identify themselves (or are identified) as midwives (*obstetrices*) have only infrequently been found in contemporary archival
records,[23] and at the moment we can say little about the potential audience
of literate midwives that might have existed in fifteenth-century England for
a specialized book on obstetrics. We suspect that the obstetrical information
that did appear in medical texts such as this was often read to midwives or
communicated to them through other indirect means,[24] and it may well have
been such a scenario of transmission that this author envisaged.

---

[23] See the evidence cited in Green 1994, 334, and Rawcliffe 1995, 199. Other midwives identified more recently include one "Matillis Medewif" who was practicing
in York in 1327 (see Parker 1929, 170); one Maud Swaneslone who was called to
act as "midewyf" at the birth of John de Worthe, in the village of Little Horstede,
Sussex, some twenty-one or more years before 1377 (*MED*, s.v. *mid-wif; Calendar of
Inquisitions Post Mortem [48-51 Edw. III]* 1952:342 [p. 341]); and three listed in the
poll taxes recently edited by Fenwick (1998): Matilda Kembere and Marg[ery?]
Josy in Reading (41) and Felicia Tracy in Canterbury (430). (Our thanks to Peter
Biller for confirming the York citation, to Jeremy Goldberg for alerting us to the
poll taxes as a resource, and to Professor Fenwick for searching her computer files
for midwives in vol. 1 and identifying the one in Canterbury.) More midwives will
no doubt be located as publication of the Poll Taxes nears completion. Bennett
(1994, 57) has identified one in the Poll Tax of Southwark, and she has alerted
us (personal communication, June 2003) to a record of money paid "for men-
deng of the medwyffes pew" in the churchwardens' accounts for 1530–31 at a parish church in Southwark (London Metropolitan Archives, P92/SAV/13). Looking
solely for formal occupational labels has its own limitations, of course, especially
when researching female practitioners; see Green 1994.

No evidence has yet been found either that English midwives organized among
themselves or that they (or their knowledge) were officially regulated during this
period. Formal licensing of midwives is not attested in England until the early sixteenth century; see Evenden 2000, 25. For the situation in France (where a form of
episcopal licensing was instituted by the early fourteenth century), see Taglia 2001.
Even in the absence of licensing, it is conceivable that some literate, specialist midwives did exist in fifteenth-century England and that some of them may have used
Sickness of Women or similar texts in their training and practice. Archival research
on these issues is badly needed.

[24] For example, in her study of Glasgow, University Library, Hunter MS 117, C.
Jones (1998) has found within a general compendium of medical recipes a sec-
tion of obstetrical remedies headed "Medicine to the art of a midwyf." Obstetri-
cal remedies can be found scattered throughout English medical manuscripts (cf.
Stoertz 1996 and eVK, Subject Index, s.v. Gynecology and Obstetrics). For some
Latin obstetrical instructions (drawn from Muscio) called "A proscesse for women
that ben in trauel of childryn and how the mydwyffe shal do helpe," see Oxford,
Bodleian Library, Bodley MS 591 (SC 2363), fols. 107v–109r.

If not midwives, then for whom does this author believe s/he is writing? The gestures in the prologue to a general lay female audience may be sincere as far as they go, but we believe they reflect more the author's allusions to another text on women's medicine already in circulation than his/ her own clear conception of how to construct a medical text for an audience of women. *Sickness 2* has several important parallels with a late fourteenth- or early fifteenth-century Middle English gynecological text called *The Knowing of Woman's Kind in Childing* which was likewise addressed to a female audience. While it is clear that *Sickness* owes no direct textual debt to *Knowing*—not a single passage is borrowed verbatim from the earlier text nor did the *Sickness 2* author employ the same sources as his/her predecessor—their structural similarities are unlikely to have been merely coincidental.

    Knowing fused an Old French translation of the *Liber de sinthomatibus mulierum* (one of the so-called *Trotula* texts) with at least two different Latin texts that offered additional treatments for gynecological and obstetrical conditions (Green 1996a; Green 1997a; Barratt 2001). In the same manner, *Sickness 2* starts with a pre-existing gynecological text (in this case the already-Englished Gilbertus Anglicus, *Sickness of Women 1*) and then goes on to incorporate additional material. Most notable in both *Knowing* and *Sickness 2* is the extended obstetrical information that derives from the late antique gynecological text of Muscio. Whereas the author of *Knowing* had employed a strictly textual adaptation of Muscio's work (the *Non omnes quidem*), the redactor of *Sickness 2* employs a different spin-off from Muscio's *Gynaecia*, a series of fetus-in-utero diagrams with brief accompanying text that offered instructions on how to manage malpresented fetuses.[25] (See

---

[25] On the *Non omnes quidem* and the independently circulating fetus-in-utero figures from Muscio, see Hanson and Green 1994. The only extant English copies that have both the fetus-in-utero figures and the accompanying text are Oxford, Bodleian Library, Ashmole MS 399, ca. 1292 (which has only ten of the usual sixteen or seventeen figures); and Stockholm, Kungliga Biblioteket, MS X.118, ca. 1425–1435, a scroll manuscript in which the figures (here fifteen in number) accompany a copy of John Arderne's *De arte phisicale et de cirurgia*. An English manuscript containing the figures without the accompanying text is Oxford, Bodleian Library, MS Laud Misc. 724, ca. 1400 (England, perhaps London), where they are found following a series of surgical images. Cf. Pansier 1909 for the text and illustrations in a contemporary Italian manuscript. Trinity R.14.52 is the only one of the four extant copies of *Sickness 2* to omit these figures, though the blank spaces on fols. 124v–126r show that they were meant to be included. For reproductions of several of the images from Sloane 2463, see P. M. Jones 1998a, 39.

plates 3a–3d.) The two texts differ, as well, in the kinds of other sources they draw on. Whereas none of *Knowing's* sources could be considered "cutting edge" by the end of the fourteenth century,[26] *Sickness 2* employs works still actively circulating in university milieux: Avicenna's *Canon*, Bernard de Gordon's *Lilium medicine*, and Rhazes' *Liber ad Almansorem*.[27] The author of *Sickness 2* also incorporated notes on cures that came to his/her attention from practitioners and laywomen in London and the vicinity.[28] *Knowing*, in contrast, has no such specific contemporary features.

Just as striking as the structural similarities these two texts share are their rhetorical similarities. Compare the rhetoric of the Prologue to *Sickness 2* with the opening of *Knowing* (parallel passages have been highlighted in bold text; important novelties in *Sickness* are italicized):

---

[26] On the sources of *Knowing* (the most recent of which seems to have been the thirteenth-century Old French translation of the *Liber de sinthomatibus mulierum*), see Green 1997a, 84–85. Barratt provides full identification of the source material in her 2001 edition.

[27] The only "old" text is the excerpted material from the twelfth-century *Trotula* ensemble (lines 1743-1820) which, as we note below, we believe to be a later appendage to the text.

[28] The references to (apparently) contemporary practices or practitioners are as follows:

1) a remedy taught by "the Priour of Beremondesey"—chap. 2 (340–341)

2) remedy "*probatum est* in Chepa, London"—chap. 2 (402–403)

3) remedy "proeved at Cicestre on Barons wif"—chap. 2 (408)

4) a bath for menstrual retention "proved in Essex"—chap. 2 (474)

5) "a womman in London . . . had this idropesy"—chap. 6 (938)

6) a pessary for *mola*, "hoc Augustinus"—chap. 11 (1420); see Explanatory Note 70.

7) cure of a woman with *mola matricis*—chap. 11 (1427–1431)

8) a plaster for swelling of the testicles "secundum magistrum Ricardum Mersh"—chap. 18 (1679–1680)

9) a remedy for vomiting and lack of appetite, "Probatum est de Lightfoote Gardener"—chap. 18 (1712)

These are not necessarily all new empirical practices. The remedy said to have been proved in Cheapside, for example, comes directly from *Sickness 1*; only the approbation is new in *Sickness 2*. The crediting of a "stuphe" near the end of chap. 18 to "Edmond Priest" (1729) is not the work of the original redactor of *Sickness 2*, but may originate in a marginal note in Sloane 2463; see Explanatory Note 85.

Knowing of Woman's Kind

**And for as moche as whomen
ben more febull & colde be
nature þan men been & have
grete travell in chyldynge, þer
fall oftyn to hem mo diuerse
sykenes than to men, and namly
to þe membrys þat ben longyng
to gendryng.**

**Wherfore in þe worschyp of
oure Lady & of all sayntys I
thynke to do myn ententyffe
bysynes for-to drav oute of
Latyn in-to Englysch dyuerse
causis of here maladyes, the
synes þat þey schall knov hem
by & þe curys helpyng to hem.**
. . . And be-cause whomen of
oure tonge cvnne bettyre rede
& vndyrstande þys langage þan
eny oþer **& euery whoman let-
tyrde [may] rede hit to oþer
vnlettyrd & help hem & con-
ceyle hem in here maledyes
with-owtyn schevynge here
dysese to man, I have þys
drawyn & wryttyn in Englysch.**
And yf hit fall any man to rede hit,
I pray hym & scharge hym in ovre
Lady be-halue **þat he rede hit not
in no dyspyte ne sclavndure of no
woman** ne for no cause but for þe
hele & helpe of hem, dredyng þat
vengavns myht fall to hym as hit
hath do to oþer þat have schevyd
here preuytees in sclavndyr of hem,
vndyrstondynge in certeyne **þat
þey have no oþer euylys þat nov be
a-lyue than thoo women hade þat
nov be seyntys in hevyn.**[29]

Sickness of Women

**For as moche as ther bien many wym-
men that han many diuers maladies and
sikenessis nygh to the deth** *and they also
bien shameful to shewen and to tellen their
grevaunces to any wight,* **therfor I shal
sumdel write to their maladie remedy,
prayeng to God [and to blessid moder
Marie ful of grace] to sende me grace
triewly to write to the pleasaunce of
God and to al wymmens helpyng;** for
charite axith this that every man shuld
travaile for helpyng of his brethern and
sustren after the grace of God that he
hath vnderfong. **And though wymmen
have divers evils and many grete grevaunces mo than al men knowen of, as I
saide,** *hem shamen for drede of reprevyng in
tymes comyng and of discuryng of vncurteys
men that loven wymmen but for their lustis
and for their foul likyng;* and if wymmen
bien in disease, **suche men han hem in
dispite** and thynken nat how moche disease wymmen han or tha[t] thei han
brought hem furth in-to this world.
**And therfor in helpyng of wymmen I
wil write of wymmen privy sikenes the
helpyng of, that oo womman may help
another in hir sikenes and nat discure
hir privitees to suche vncurteys men.**
But neuertheles whosumever he be that
[dispisith] a womman for hir sikenes
that **she hath of the ordynaunce of God,**
he doeth a grete synne, for he dispisith
nat al only hem but God that sendith
hem suche sikenes for their best; and
therfor no man shuld dispise other for
the disease that God sendith hym, but
to have compassioun of hym and releve
hym if he myght.

---

[29] Oxford, Bodleian Library, Douce MS 37 (SC 21611), s. xv in., fols. 1r–2r; ed. Barratt 2001, lines 12–31.

Both texts begin by emphasizing the plurality and the severity of women's diseases.[30] *Sickness* then goes on to problematize women's shame over their diseases as the principal barrier to proper care.[31] In fact, *Sickness* immediately repeats this pairing of the severity of women's diseases with the problem of shame and fear of reproach. In the latter passage, the author stresses that women fear punishment in the future for revealing their diseases (thereby compromising their honor?). They also fear immediate abuse by "vncurteys men" who "loven wymmen but for their lustis and for their foul likyng." *Knowing* and *Sickness* then reconverge in explaining how they expect their text to function: they both are meant to be used by women directly so that they can help themselves and other women, thereby avoiding any need to disclose their diseases to men. Both texts, moreover, charge men not to slander or despise women for their sicknesses and remind them that women's diseases are no different from those suffered by women who are now saints in heaven (*Knowing*) or that these sicknesses are sent directly by God (*Sickness*).

It seems quite likely, then, that the author of *Sickness 2* was aware of the existence and the rhetorical posture of *Knowing* even if s/he didn't employ it as a direct model. Both texts see male involvement with women's diseases as potentially threatening to women, and both claim to wish to empower women to "help one another" by reading (and using) their text, thereby allowing them to bypass any dependence on males. We will return in a moment to the suitability of *Sickness 2* for women's use. The question here is what role men were now expected to play in women's healthcare, specifically with respect to access to and use of these texts. Whereas *Knowing* imposes a strong injunction on potential male readers—in effect threatening them with damnation if they misuse the information gained from the text—*Sickness* more mildly reminds the (potentially hostile or prurient) male reader that despising anyone for her or his diseases is sinful and that he should instead have compassion for sick women.[32] There is in *Sickness of Women 2*, therefore, no injunction *tout court* against men reading the text,

---

[30] *Knowing* actually begins with a prior passage (drawn directly from the Old French *Liber de sinthomatibus mulierum*) explaining how the differentiation of the two sexes is part of God's master plan for continually repopulating the earth. Note, too, that *Knowing* emphasizes the severity of women's diseases in comparison to men's, whereas in *Sickness* no such comparisons are employed.

[31] This is a very old topos in medieval gynecological literature (see Green 2000a), making it all the more significant that *Knowing* had omitted the passage on women's shame when it translated the Old French *Liber de sinthomatibus mulierum*.

[32] For continental parallels of this issue of slander, see Green 1998. On medicine as an act of charity, see Getz 1990a.

nor even a presumption (as there is in *Knowing*) that the male reader is not within the normative or "approved" intended audience.

The redactor's belief that men would also be using this text helps explain the many internal ambiguities within the text of *Sickness of Women*. As already noted, *Sickness 2*, ostensibly a "women's version" of the text, reflects an active and interventionist appropriation of the Gilbertus gynecology. Be that as it may, there are some notable adaptations that were not made. Unlike the two female-addressed English translations of the *Trotula* (*Knowing* and the late fifteenth- or early sixteenth-century *Book Made by a Woman Named Rota*), *Sickness of Women 2* includes no second-person addresses directly aimed at female readers.[33] Those second-person forms that do appear here (e.g., the constant imperative forms "take," "make," "mix" in recipes) could be taken as "generic" addresses. The text could be used without "translation" as easily by a male practitioner providing care to female patients as by a female practitioner doing the same. Although one London woman's self-cure is recounted at length, self-treatment does not generally seem to be assumed. There is a clear expectation that the reader would be doing all his/her own preparation of medications (which would entail ready access to apothecaries' weights and measures as well as other equipment).[34] The extraordinary range of *materia medica* employed likewise makes use of the text by "amateurs" seem rather farfetched. Moreover, it should be stressed that the obstetrical information, as much as every other part of the text, could also be used directly by male readers without "translation." All the obstetrical passages either describe "hands off" therapies—potions to be administered, baths to be prepared, etc.—or they give

---

[33] There are two intriguing scribal slips in *Sickness 2*. The first is in chap. 1 (line 198). Whereas in the other three copies of *Sickness 2* the instruction had been given to "put [a suppository] in the prevy membre," the Trinity scribe wrote "put in *thi* prevy membre." A second error, which may go back to *Sickness 1*, is in chap. 15 on wounds of the uterus: "And if *thi* veynes bien broken . . . " (line 1506); cf. **H**, line 656, "if þy veynes ben broke" vs. **A** (fol. 84r), "þe veynes." Beyond these, there are no direct addresses to a presumed female reader in *Sickness 2* except for generic second-person imperatives. Aside from a brief linguistic comment in lines 46–47, first-person plural forms are found only in the Muscio section (lines 1148–1246) and, at the end of the text, in the selections from the *De curis mulierum* (lines 1743–1793), which was written by a female author apparently for a female audience. These are literal translations of the Latin texts and do not reflect the translator's own experience in manually assisting at birth or correcting prolapsed uteruses, nor, necessarily, anything about the audience expectations of *Sickness 2*.

[34] In the *Book of Rota*, in contrast, which is clearly addressed to women, the author repeatedly advises his/her readers to go to apothecaries to obtain the medicines prescribed.

instructions *to the midwife* (or "a prevy womman"), a third party presumed
not to be the direct reader of the text.[35] (Again, it is worth stressing that all
of chapter 10 up through the sixteenth malpresentation, including the illustrations, comes from a pre-existing Latin text and not from any immediate
observation on the part of the author.) There is nothing in the text that
gives fresh clinical advice on handling childbirth in the active, hands-on
way midwives and female attendants must have done on a daily basis.

Similarly, it is necessary to explain the considerable presence of Latin
in a text ostensibly addressed to women. We think it possible that in its
first draft the text ended after the section on swelling of the feet, right
before the beginning of a long, eclectic string of Latin recipes (lines 1576–
1713) where the exclusive focus on female conditions evaporates: emmena-
gogues are followed by anaphrodisiacs for men (where we find second-person addresses to the male reader!), induration of the uterus gives way to
kidney and bladder disorders and swelling of the (male) testicles,[36] conditions of the breasts are followed by remedies for the plague, eye disease,
and vomiting, a prognostic test to determine if a patient will live or die,
and then more remedies for vomiting. The text then reverts to English and
its original focus on women, although this section, too, is clearly an afterthought not integrated into the text as a whole.[37] In Sloane 249 (the earliest of the extant manuscripts of *Sickness 2*), before the beginning of the

---

[35] All but one of the references to midwives derive either from *Sickness 1* (lines 741,
1261, and 1449), Muscio's *Gynaecia* (the series of references in lines 1148–1246),
or the *Trotula* (line 1744). The one new reference comes in chap. 3 (line 635): the
midwife is to anoint the patient's vagina with musk oil as a treatment for uterine
suffocation. The *Sickness 2* redactor is also responsible for the two references to "a
prevy womman" (lines 995 and 1514).

[36] The female gonads were identified in medieval medicine as "testicles" as well, but
it is clear in this passage that the male organs are being referred to.

[37] This section consists of selections on uterine prolapse and infertility translated
from the Latin *Trotula* (see Explanatory Note 86), followed by recipes for bladder
stones and palsy. The *Trotula* passages have no correspondence with any of the
other five known ME translations of the *Trotula* and are probably, like the Muscio
excerpts in chap. 10, the work of the redactor himself. Notable in the *Trotula* section is the consistent use of the term "marice" or "marys" to refer to the uterus in
Sloane 249, the earliest copy of *Sickness 2*; "moder," which is the normative term in
the rest of *Sickness of Women 2*, is not used. In fact, of the thirty-two instances where
we find "marice" in chaps. 1–17 of Sloane 249, twenty-four are in passages newly
added by the *Sickness 2* redactor. This contrast in vocabulary is muted here in Trinity R.14.52 because of alterations made by the Hammond scribe or his exemplar
(see n. 69 below).

long Latin section, there is a mark of closure followed by a blank line, suggesting that this was indeed the original end of the text.[38] This still does not explain, of course, the presence of the Latin passages within chapters 1–17. Perhaps the redactor believed that women's encounters with Latin in their psalters would have been enough to get them through the brief phrases slipped into many of the new recipes (e.g., *teranda & conficiatur . . .* and *cum succo* plantayne *in quo lapis ematicis fuerit fricatus,* lines 359, 377–378). This author does not, after all, make an explicit claim in her/his prologue that women could only read English (indeed, s/he says nothing at all about choice of language), and the "average" literate woman's command of Latin is something we can only speculate about at the moment.[39] Nevertheless, it is striking how far this redactor has moved away from the English base text of *Sickness 1,* where there are virtually no Latin phrases at all. Like most English medical books in the fifteenth century, *Sickness of Women 2* could only be fully usable by a reader with Latin (Voigts 1996). It is as if the redactor, him/herself comfortable with code-switching between Latin and English, forgets that the text's declared audience may not have this same facility in Latin.[40] Indeed, we believe several marks of university learning—the frequent reversion into Latin, the references to Avicenna, Bernard de Gordon, and Rhazes—betray the redactor's masculine identity.[41] The redactor clearly had extensive experience aiding women in both their gynecological and obstetrical afflictions (the latter in so far as he could provide a whole range of potions, plasters, and pessaries to expel the child and the afterbirth or to remedy a prolapsed uterus). And there is every reason to

---

[38] Cf. the similar mark on fol. 180v of Sloane 249, between *Sickness 2* and the religious text that precedes it, a list of masses to be said for delivery from all evils "thurgh the grace of seynt Susanne." (See n. 53 below.) This mark appears nowhere else in fols. 180r–204v of Sloane 249 (originally an independent pamphlet). Significant shifts in script suggest that some of the recipes at the end of the text were added at different times by the same hand.

[39] For a review of scholarship on women's literacy, see Green 2000b.

[40] For example, at the end of the newly added obstetrical material from Muscio in chap. 10, but before returning to the original *Sickness 1* material on problems in delivery, the redactor adds three new recipes to deliver a dead child (or even kill a living one if need be). There is no obvious reason why the third of these recipes should be in Latin while the first two are in English. This redactor is also clearly as comfortable with the Latin names of *materia medica* as with English forms.

[41] Again, comparison with *Knowing* is helpful. This earlier author (who was probably also male, but less invested in university learning) adds an unusual amount of general background information on anatomy and physiology. Aside from single references to "Dame Fabina Prycyll" (**D** 719), "Dame Cliopatre" (**D** 726), and an unnamed woman of Salerno (**D** 685), there is no name-dropping whatsoever.

believe that the redactor took it as his own responsibility "to have compassion of [women] and releve [them] if he might" (lines 23–24). Yet it is the midwife or, in two cases, "a prevy womman" who performs the most intimate manual procedures on the female patient. This author's gynecology and obstetrics is entirely "hands off," and he writes as if his readers will stand in the same distanced position from the female patient's body. Neither midwives nor female patients, apparently, are construed as the direct audience of this text.

An Unfinished Text

While the redactor may have simply been thoughtless in his code-switching and failure to adopt an address to female readers, a number of other peculiarities and incongruities in *Sickness 2* make it likely that the text as we have it is nothing more than a rough draft. We have already noted the marked break in the earliest manuscript, Sloane 249, between chapters 1–17 and the rather chaotic Latin and English section at the end of the text. Yet even within chapters 1–17 we can see both order and disorder. As noted above, the redactor rearranged the chapters of *Sickness 1* as he compiled his new text. As it is now structured, the text moves from menstrual difficulties (too much or too little), to uterine conditions (suffocation, prolapse, wind, dropsy, excoriation, tumors, and aching), to obstetrical conditions (particularly extraction of the malpresented or dead fetus), uterine mole, expulsion of the afterbirth, mechanisms to promote conception, excessive lochial flow, lesions and cancers of the uterus, and swelling of the legs during pregnancy. Up through this point of the text, therefore, the redactor has more or less followed a "natural history" of women's conditions.

Despite this logical reordering, the redactor did not correctly number the newly ordered chapters nor did he emend what he construed as a table of contents following the Preface to reflect either the text's full contents or its new order.[42] The gaps or errors in enumerating the sections of *Sickness 2* come exactly at the points where the redactor interrupts the order of his source. In Table 1, we compare the chapter divisions of *Sickness 1* (SW1) and *Sickness 2* (SW2).[43] The redactor begins easily enough by presenting *Sickness 1*, chapter 1, as his own chapter 1. Then he jumps to *Sickness 1*, chap-

---

[42] In *Sickness of Women 1*, this list was presented not as a table of contents of chapters, but as an unnumbered prose recitation of the various types of women's diseases. It was nevertheless construed as a table of contents (i.e., numbered and arranged in line-by-line fashion) by the *Sickness 2* redactor. See Explanatory Note 4.

[43] This analysis of the chapter arrangement is based on a collation of all four extant manuscripts of *Sickness 2*. As we note below, only the Trinity scribe attempted some correction of the misnumbering, though even he did not rectify all the gaps.

ter 4, followed immediately by 5, 6, and 7. But then for what should be the new chapter 6, the redactor jumps back to *Sickness 1*, chapter 2; here, in this section on dropsy of the uterus, we find neither a rubric nor a chapter number in any of the four copies of *Sickness 2*. The redactor regains focus and numbers chapters 7, 8, 9, and 10 correctly (corresponding to *Sickness 1*, chaps. 3, 8, 11 and 12, respectively). The redactor then includes a completely new section, on the uterine mole, to which no chapter number is assigned.[44] The next chapter on removal of the afterbirth (corresponding to *Sickness 1*, chap. 13) is labelled "the 11. chapiter," with "the 12. Chapiter" (a new section on fertility enhancers) followed by "chapter 13" on excessive lochial flow (*Sickness 1*, chap. 14). (The Trinity scribe, in contrast to his predecessors, recognized the section on uterine mole as a separate chapter and, although he did not number it, he corrected the numbering of subsequent chapters.) The next three chapters—on, respectively, uterine tumors (equals *Sickness 1*, chap. 9), uterine cancer (equals *Sickness 1*, chap. 10), and edema of the legs (a new addition)—are not numbered at all in any of the four extant manuscripts, nor is the long random Latin-English section at the end numbered. One would think that, at the very least, the redactor could have corrected this numbering and revised the table of contents (itself drawn directly from *Sickness 1*) to correctly reflect the contents of this new text on which he clearly has labored so intensely.

TABLE 1

corrected chap. no.	chap. no. in SW2 Contents (fol.107v)	chap. no. within Trinity text	chap. title in Trinity text	chap. order in SW1
1	first	first	the stoppyng of their bloode	1
2	secunde	secunde	to moche flowyng of bloode	4
3	thridde	thrid	the suffocacioun of the matrice	5
4	iiij	iiii	the precipitacioun of the moder[45]	6
5	—	v	the wynde of the matrice	7
6	vij	[unnumbered]	[the chapter on dropsy is untitled in the text; in the text's Table of Contents, it is referred to as "the swellyng of the matrice"][46]	2

(*continued on next page*)

[44] This and the chapter on uterine cancer are the only chapter headings that use Latin instead of English.

[45] In the table of contents within the text of *Sickness 2*, a ninth chapter is listed with the subject "goyng out of the matrice bynethfurth." In the text itself, however, there is no separate chapter on uterine prolapse besides chap. 4.

[46] In the general Contents List at the beginning of the codex (fol. II verso), instead of providing a title, the scribe repeats verbatim the opening eleven words of the chapter.

TABLE 1 (continued)

corrected chap. no.	chap. no. in SW2 Contents (fol.107v)	chap. no. within Trinity text	chap. title in Trinity text	chap. order in SW1
7	v	vij	rawnesse that whan the matrice semyth flayne	3
8	vj	viij	of aposteme of the matrice	8
9	x	ix	of akyng of the matrice	11
10	viij	x	the grevaunce that wymmen han in beryng of theire children	12
11	—	[unnumbered]	De mola matricis	—
12	x	xii	of the secundyne	13
13	—	xiij	to make a womman able to conceive chield	—
14	—	xiiij	of bledyng over-moche after that she hath had hir chield	14
15	—	[unnumbered]	[the chapter on "wounds in the matrice" is untitled in the text][47]	9
16	—	[unnumbered]	De cancris & de vlceribus matricis	10
17	—	[unnumbered]	ffor swellyng of wymmens legges whan thei bien with chield	—
18	—	[unnumbered]	Ad restringendum cohitum[48]	—
19	—	[unnumbered]	It happith of dyuers wymmen grete greuaunce in travailynge of chield	—
20	—	[unnumbered]	A goode medicine for the stone proved triewe and a medicine for the palesye	—

The curious section near the end of the text, *Ad mulieres tantum* ("For women especially," lines 1714–1725), suggests that the redactor himself found this now substantial text somewhat hard to navigate: this list reads as if it were the author's own quick reference notes back to what he views as the main features of the text, perhaps meant to be used as emergency measures in cases of "suffocation" or other crises.[49] Aside from the first direc-

---

[47] This chapter goes unrecognized in the general Contents List at the beginning of the codex.

[48] We have adopted these last three chapter divisions and titles from the Hammond scribe's Contents List at the beginning of the codex (fols. II verso and III recto). They do not, of course, actually convey the miscellaneous contents of the final five leaves of the text.

[49] In Sloane 249, Royal College of Surgeons 129, and Sloane 2463, each entry of this itemized list is placed on a separate line. The Hammond scribe, in contrast, condensed it into a single paragraph in **T**, making it difficult to read quickly.

tive to perform phlebotomy and administer fumigations (written in Latin), all the instructions refer back to the redactor's own additions: a potage, a drink, a pillow, a bath, etc. Here again we see his signature habit of offering enumerated lists, which by their mnemonic function would support his ability to intervene quickly and effectively as a practitioner in women's health conditions.

Perhaps if he had had more time, the redactor would have couched the entire text in a more "woman-friendly" second person, as had the author of *Knowing of Woman's Kind* and as would the later author of the *Book of Rota*. Perhaps if he had had more time he would have translated all the Latin passages into English.[50] Surely if he had had more time he would have corrected the chapter numbering and the Table of Contents. As it was, even though *Sickness of Women 2* includes material that unquestionably addresses the pressing contemporary medical needs of English women, the text itself is not written in a way that readily encourages women's use of the text. At the same time, there is nothing that excludes or even necessarily discourages use by males. *Sickness of Women 2* is, if anything, more a testament to the redactor's own practice of gynecology and obstetrics—and thus to gynecology and obstetrics viewed from a male perspective—than a work that could easily be used by women, whether laywomen or midwives, who had access to nothing beyond the most rudimentary education. Hence we should not be surprised that the text could be absorbed *with no adaptation whatsoever* into codices prepared, in all likelihood, for the primary if not exclusive use of male readers.

Female and Male Users of the Text

The four extant manuscripts of *Sickness of Women 2* suggest two different paths along which the text might circulate. On the one hand, it seems likely that despite its clumsy adaptation to the needs or competencies of female readers, *Sickness 2* did in fact pass occasionally through women's hands. As noted by Green in 1992, the "women's versions" of several late medieval gynecological texts—that is, texts implicitly or explicitly claiming a female

---

[50] Whether the redactor himself was responsible for rendering the Muscio section into English as well as the *Trotula* section at the end (see n. 37 above) is unclear. No other ME translation of Muscio is known, aside from the material embedded in the *Knowing of Woman's Kind*, which comes from a different version of Muscio's text. Given the *Sickness 2* redactor's tendency to lapse into Latin, however, the consistent use of only English in the Muscio and *Trotula* passages is notable.

audience—often circulated in small codices or pamphlets in which they were either the only text or the main text accompanied by one or two minor additions (e.g., miscellaneous recipes, an herbal, etc.). This characteristic is true, for example, of three out of the five extant manuscripts of *The Knowing of Woman's Kind*.[51] An isolated codicological context also characterizes one of the two extant copies of the fifth translation of the *Trotula*, the female-addressed *Book of Rota* mentioned earlier, which was produced perhaps in the late fifteenth or early sixteenth century.[52] In the earliest extant manuscript of *Sickness 2*, Sloane MS 249, *Sickness 2* is the main text, preceded only by directions for saying a week-long series of votive masses "in remembraunce" and "thurgh the grace of seynt Susanne" in order to be delivered from all diseases and misfortunes of life.[53] RCS 129 likewise reflects the codicological character of the early manuscripts of the woman-directed *Trotula* translations: a moderately-sized (220 x 153 mm) volume, it contains a beautifully illuminated copy of *Sickness 2* followed by a single recipe for *aqua vitae*. Neither of these two manuscripts of *Sickness 2* nor those of the female-addressed versions of the *Trotula* bear any *ex-libris* marks to confirm female ownership.[54] Nevertheless, a survey of all currently known medical manuscripts that were owned by medieval women (admittedly, not a massive corpus) indicates that more often than not these tended to be small collections or pamphlets. Sloane 249 and RCS 129 thus conform codicologically to patterns common to medical books owned by women.[55]

---

[51] Barratt notes (2001, 4–5) that two of these independently circulating copies of *Knowing* have passing statements that may indicate preparation for a particular woman. See also Green 2000b, 32–37, on gynecological texts in other vernacular traditions.

[52] On *Trotula* Eng5 (*The Book Made by a Woman Named Rota*), see Green 1997a, 88–89. In 1544, the *Book of Rota* was adapted by the physician and alchemist Robert Green of Welby for his own use; aside from an inadvertent slip at the end of the text, he removes all of the second-person addresses to the female reader. On Robert Green and his books, see Pereira 1999, 354.

[53] This brief text (ed. in Green 2003) includes reference to "perell . . . in geysyne" (i.e., childbed) as one of the calamities from which an individual can be delivered. Although there is nothing else gender-specific in the text ("dethe . . . yn bataill" probably being more of a threat to men), the dedication of the series of Masses to "seynte Susanne" may allude to the image of the biblical Susanna as a model for innocent but aggrieved women (cf. "The Pistil of Swete Susan," ed. Peck 1991; available at http://www.lib.rochester.edu/camelot/teams/susanfrm.htm). Our thanks to Tess Tavormina for bringing this possible correlation to our attention.

[54] Sloane 249 was apparently owned and annotated in the sixteenth century by John Wotton, M.D., whose alphabetized collection of medical receipts and disease definitions is now bound with the manuscript.

In contrast, Sloane 2463 and our present manuscript show a dramatic shift in codicological context. The complete contents of Sloane 2463, a quite "deluxe" manuscript composed as a single unit, are as follows:[56]

fols. 2r–51v: Guy de Chauliac, *Lantern of Physicians* (= *Chirurgia Magna* interpolated with Henri de Mondeville)

fols. 53r–151v: *Book of Operations* or *Curation of Wounds* (a surgical text based on Henri de Mondeville and Guy de Chauliac)

fols. 151v–152v: miscellaneous recipes

fols. 153v–188v: *Antidotary* (a formal collection of medical recipes, grouped according to their physiological function rather than by symptom or disease)

fols. 188v–193v: *Proper Medicines and Divers Members* (a series of recipes)

fols. 194r–232r: *Sickness of Women* 2

Sloane 2463's texts are highly technical with equal focus on the theoretical and the practical elements of surgery and adjuvant pharmacy; in other words, this is not the sort of material one would consider "self-help." We need not be surprised by the incorporation of a gynecological and obstetrical text into such a professional surgical (and probably male) context, however.[57] First of all, male ownership of both Latin and vernacular

---

[55] Green (2000b) includes comprehensive lists of female book owners as well as medical texts addressed to or commissioned by women.

[56] The eVK numbers are, respectively: Guy de Chauliac, *Chirurgia* (Wallner Version 4; eVK 2005); *Book of Operations* (eVK 2196 and 7160); miscellaneous recipes (eVK 4923); *Antidotary* (eVK 7232 and 7158); *Proper Medicines and Divers Members* (eVK 3805); *Sickness of Women 2* (eVK 1956, 7249, and 8201). The minimal gynecological content of these other texts (such as the anatomy in Guy de Chauliac) would be complemented, not duplicated, by *Sickness of Women 2*.

[57] Sloane 2463, whose original owner(s) are unknown, would later be owned in the sixteenth century by Richard Ferris, sergeant surgeon to Queen Elizabeth and master of the Barbers' and Surgeons' Company; it was subsequently owned by John Feld. Its content (not to mention its quite deluxe physical character) suggests creation for a professional medical practitioner, probably a surgeon. Linda Voigts (personal communication with M. Green, 22 August 1995) has noted Sloane 2463's strong parallels with a group of other surgical manuscripts of the fifteenth century. Most closely related to Sloane 2463 is Sloane 3486 (s. xv med.), which includes a copy of *Sickness of Women 1* within the context of the whole ME Gilbertus compendium plus three of the four surgical texts found in Sloane 2463.

gynecological material is as amply documented in England as it is on the
Continent throughout the medieval period.[58] Second, we should remember that the *source* of most of the material in *Sickness* was the male-authored
Compendium medicine of Gilbertus Anglicus, and transposition into the vernacular does not seem to have radically altered the text's audience.[59] When
the gynecological section was split off from the *Compendium* and circulated
independently, it tended to circulate within codices of more "lay" character,
i.e., with texts (like dietaries, recipe collections, brief astrological and prognostic texts) that could conceivably be used by educated people to assist
in their own health maintenance. No male owners of the latter volumes
have yet been confirmed for the fifteenth century, but, as already noted by
Green in 1992, the addition of the reader address "Sirs" at the head of one
of these copies reaffirms to its male readers that they are officially "autho-
rized" to read this text.[60] Third, other sorts of evidence attest to male practice on women. The fifteenth-century practitioner, Thomas Fayreford, for
example, is known from his clinical records to have treated at least twelve
women for gynecological complaints (P. M. Jones 1998b), while a York priest
who was censured in 1424 for making "incisions of wounds and women's
breasts" seems to have been criticized for performing surgery rather than
practicing on women *per se*. It is his status as a priest, not his identity as a

---

[58] On male owners of the *Trotula*, see Green 1996b; Green 1997a, passim. No female
owners of the work, whether in Latin or the vernaculars, have thus far been documented prior to the sixteenth century. On owners of German gynecological texts,
see Kruse 1996; Green 1997b.

[59] The fifteenth-century barber-surgeon Richard Dod of London is the only identifiable owner of the Gilbertus *Compendium* containing *Sickness 1* (BL, Sloane 5).
This is probably the same Richard Dod who owned San Marino (California), Huntington Library, MS HM 505, a copy of Henry Daniel's *Liber uricrisiarum* (Hanna
1994, 192), and may well be the same one from the London parish of St. Andrew,
Holborn, who was involved in a court case on 31 August 1460 (Jenks 1985, 224). A
certain Thomas Betrisden is credited with the compilation of Sloane 3486, another
copy of *Sickness 1* where it appears within the Gilbertus *Compendium*. Codicological characteristics of most other copies of *Sickness 1* make it likely that their owners
would similarly have been professional practitioners. On the ownership of Glasgow,
University Library, Hunter MS 509 (V.8.12), which lacks the gynecological section,
see Keiser 1994, 229–30.

[60] Longleat House (Warminster, Wiltshire), Longleat MS 174, s. xv[2], fols. 107r–115v.
On this manuscript and its probable ownership by a sequence of individuals with
lay and professional interests in science and medicine, see Harris 2001. Two copies where *Sickness 1* is still embedded in the full ME Gilbertus likewise have this
address. See Green 1992, 58.

man, that renders the interaction problematic.[61] The decision of the compiler or commissioner of Sloane 2463 to include *Sickness 2* in a surgical compilation may thus reflect the regular engagement of men with matters of women's health in fifteenth-century England.

The incorporation of *Sickness of Women 2* into Trinity R.14.52, on the other hand, may have had less to do with immediate concerns about gynecological or obstetrical practice than with a desire to have theoretical information on the processes of conception and birth. As the other essays and texts within this present volume make clear, Trinity R.14.52 displays a pronounced concern with questions of generation, longevity, and general issues of human physiology. It is in no way unique in this focus. Interest in generation was increasing throughout Europe from the thirteenth century on, both in academic circles and on the margins of university culture, and the juxtaposition of such texts as the pseudo-Galenic *De spermate*, Constantine the African's *De coitu*, and tracts on the elements and astrology alongside seemingly "practical" gynecology had, in fact, become quite common throughout Europe by the fifteenth century (Green 1998; Green 2000a). These interests in generation might lead to manipulation of pre-existing texts, as can be seen in the copy of *Sickness of Women 1* in Oxford, Bodleian Library, Lyell MS 36, s. xv[2] (Green 1992; Hanna 1997). Here, a compiler has inserted new material on uterine anatomy (including the theory of seven cells, now changed to nine cells), the placenta (the *secondyne*), and then a list of five principal causes of miscarriage. He then rearranged the chapter order, here beginning with Chapter 13 on the afterbirth. Due to the loss of at least three leaves in this section of the manuscript, we cannot know the text's full extent, but it is striking that it incorporates some material in common with (but not deriving from) *Sickness 2*.[62] The bulk of this new material revolves around three topics: pregnancy tests, ways to determine the sex of the child, and assistance in birth. After another lost leaf, we find

---

[61] York, Borthwick Institute for Historical Research, Dean and Chapter Act Books, vol. 1, fol. 69r; our thanks to Mr. P. M. Stell for bringing this fascinating document to our attention. In the seventeenth century, it was normative for uncomplicated childbirth to be attended by midwives, though equally normative for male surgeons to be summoned when an impacted fetus needed to be surgically extracted; see Evenden 2000. The earlier history of midwife-surgeon relations in England has not yet been surveyed, though we believe it likely that a similar gender division of labor existed. Hence, it would be quite reasonable to expect that surgeons would be as interested in obstetrical material as physicians (who treated internal disorders by diet or drugs) would be in gynecological material. On the circulation of gynecological texts among fourteenth- and fifteenth-century French surgeons, see Green 1998, 165–66 and 174.

[62] For example, the last four recipes appended to the end of Chapter 5 in *Sickness 2* (lines 863–890) also appear, but in different order, in Lyell 36, fol. 149r.

an acephalous text on the nature of the seed.[63] Later bound with a copy of the pseudo-Aristotelian *Secretum secretorum*, the manuscript appears to have been associated with scholars at Magdalen College, Oxford.

If the compiler or commissioner of Trinity R.14.52 did indeed seek out Sloane 2463 as his exemplar (see n. 12 above), this would suggest his connections with professional medical practitioners in London. The compiler of Trinity R.14.52 takes the male appropriation in a slightly different direction, moving the text out of a strictly clinical context into one characterized by interests in generation and measures that the head of a bourgeois household should take to ensure that his women were safely delivered of his heirs. Did the women of the Cook or de Vale households read this text? Perhaps. But if they did so, it was probably despite, rather than because of, the intentions that motivated the compiler of Trinity R.14.52 to incorporate *Sickness of Women 2* into this massive collection of late medieval English scientific and medical learning.

Later Use and Annotation of the Text

It may be the initially non-clinical interest in this text that accounts for the paucity of annotations by the Hammond scribe and, apparently, the complete lack of any by the manuscript's original owner(s). As noted earlier, the Hammond scribe's marginal additions to this text consist solely of the repetition of a handful of glossings he found in Sloane 2463 or a closely related manuscript.[64] Given the professional therapeutic context of *Sickness 2* in Sloane 2463, it is not surprising that these notes merely highlight specific therapeutic preparations. Moreover, the Hammond scribe did little to improve the text (especially the often difficult sections in Latin); on the contrary, his is in many respects the most corrupt of the four extant copies, which is not surprising since he may have had little or no expertise in copying medical texts.[65] His itemized description of the contents of *Sickness 2* in the codex's Contents List (fols. II verso to III recto) does nothing more than give chapter titles or the opening passages of the chapters. If the commissioners of the manuscript had particular interpretive goals in mind for *Sickness of Women* beyond a generic interest in fertility and generation, they gave no indication of this to the scribe.

More expansive and interpretive are the glosses added by the **"principal annotator,"** a late fifteenth- to early sixteenth-century hand that also

---

[63] This text was not noted in any previous description of the manuscript. It appears on fol. 150r–v.

[64] These notes are often but not always preceded by a red or rose paraph.

[65] As noted by Mooney above (chap. 3), none of the other known manuscripts by the Hammond scribe contains medical texts.

added texts and marginal headings at many other points in the manuscript, considered by some scholars to belong to the writer of the Bampton (*alias* Brampton) ownership note at the end of the volume (Gross 1996, 110–12 n. 68; Pahta, chap. 1 above). In *Sickness 2*, this principal annotator seems to have added marginal notes in two or more circumstances: first to provide headings for major ailments, such as "Ded Child" or "þe Flux," and types of remedies, like "Suppositorie," "A precius drynke," "A plaster"; and another set of notes, less carefully written and more random, noting symptoms, like "vrynes Fatt," "vryne discolurd," or "watery & thyn Flowres." Since these annotations are written at different times, the size of script and color of ink varies. This scribe also seems to be responsible for the symbol that looks like double-crossed "H," sometimes with a macron over it, which in fact represents an upper case "N," for "Nota." The symbol sometimes accompanies notes of the major ailments written by this hand, sometimes follows such notes beside the text where remedies for them are described, and is sometimes an integral element of the note (for example, *N[ota] bene & probatum* in the margin of fol. 124r).[66] As noted by Pahta (chap. 1 above), these annotations are primarily navigational: they help the reader find specific passages on points of interest in the text. These are *clinical* interests, not theoretical ones. Apparently, this text is being used by B(r)ampton (or whoever this annotator was) as a resource for treating female patients.[67]

Most of the later annotators seem to have brought similar clinical interests to the text, suggesting that the text retained practical utility as a gynecological and obstetrical resource well into the sixteenth century when, despite the publication of a large number of gynecological and obstetrical treatises on the continent, in English only one printed text was available.[68] These later annotators can be identified as follows:

A **second annotator**, writing in a more upright hand, and without yellow wash, has added "planetis" to the margin on fol. 107r. The only explanation we can imagine for this obscure note is that this was

---

[66] Most of the annotations by this hand have initials touched with yellow, as are initials in the text: the yellow wash may have been added to both text and annotations at some period after the original text was copied.

[67] None of the annotators is interested in the section on male anaphrodisiacs. Only the principal annotator adds a comment here, the illogical "consevyng Child" (see Textual Note to line 1642). Perhaps a negative adverb is missing?

[68] This was Eucharius Rösslin's *The Byrth of Mankynde*, which was translated from the Latin *De partu hominis* by Richard Jonas in 1540 and reprinted numerous times. Interestingly, Sloane MS 249 was marked up by a sixteenth-century hand with "modernized" forms, almost as if it were being prepared for publication. To our knowledge, however, none of the ten ME gynecological texts circulating in the fifteenth century ever made the transition into print.

somehow meant to signal the association of matters of birth with the several astrological texts found later in the manuscript. Cf. Oxford, Bodleian Library, Lyell MS 36, s. xv², which reflects a similar appropriation of *Sickness of Women 1* into a scientific miscellany (see Green 1992).

The fact that the remaining annotations are brief, and that many of them are written in hands of the late fifteenth or early sixteenth century, like those of the principal annotator, make all identifications of different fifteenth- and sixteenth-century annotators tentative.

A **third annotator**, who may be writing much later, adds "Not" for "*Nota*" a number of times in the margins, in grey-brown ink and fine-tipped pen: fols. 108v, 109r, 112r, 134v. His/her interests focus on symptoms of menstrual retention, the cure of excessive menstrual bleeding effected by the Prior of Bermondsey, and the diagnosis of sterility.

A **fourth annotator**, writing in rusty-colored ink, added notes or "N" for "*Nota*" in the late fifteenth or sixteenth century: fols. 110v, 115v, 117r, 119r, 119v, 121v, 124v, 129r, 130v (three notes), 131r, 134v (two). These at times also appear to be the work of the principal annotator.

A **fifth annotator**, writing in grey ink without yellow wash, may be the principal annotator writing later in life: this hand appears somewhat shaky at times, that is, he seems to have less control over his handwriting. Examples of this hand are "to late blod is good" on fol. 109v, "lete her blod" on fol. 112r, "and lettithe blod" on fol. 112v, and "hertis horne brent" on fol. 113r; also perhaps the larger "Suffocacio" on fol. 114v. These annotations show a clear interest in letting blood.

A **sixth annotator**, writing in the late fifteenth or sixteenth century and using grey ink, adds "per magistro heryson" to a note on fol. 108v.

A **seventh annotator**, of uncertain date, adds an upper case "H," similar to the "N" for "*Nota*" elsewhere in the manuscript, to the margin on fol. 109r.

An **eighth annotator**, writing in grey ink in the late fifteenth or sixteenth century, added "proved per certe" to a note by the principal annotator on fol. 112r; this hand may also be responsible for other non-yellow-washed grey additions to notes, as "In wemen" added to the note "Hete" on fol. 111v and "flowers" added to notes on fols. 111v and 114r, "for wemen" on fol. 115v, "In wemen" added to the notes on fol. 120r, etc., notes in grey ink such as "Stanchyng of blod" on fol. 113v, and the repetition of "Cold humors" in the margin of fol. 117r.

A **ninth annotator**, writing in brown ink with small and upright script, adds "for her pottage" to fol. 112r and "In pottage" to fol. 113r; both have initials yellow-washed and may be written by the principal annotator, writing later.

A **tenth annotator**, perhaps sixteenth century, writing with grey ink, adds "To Conceive" above principal annotator's note "To Consaue" on fol. 134v.

An **eleventh annotator**, writing much later, in very small print, adds "frankincense" and "Hiparici minoris" to the right margin of fol. 117v.

A **twelfth annotator**, writing much later, in grey-brown ink, adds "resta bouis" in the right margin of fol. 113v, and appends "alias Ætites invenitur in nido Aquilæ" to the previous note on fol. 127v.

Editorial Practice

The following edition of *Sickness of Women 2* reflects the readings of TCC R.14.52, fols. 107r–135v (**T**). In all cases where the reading of **T** seemed questionable or unclear, we have collated the text with the three other extant copies of *Sickness 2*: London, BL, Sloane MS 249, fols. 180v–205v (**S1**); Sloane MS 2463, fols. 194r–232r (**S2**); and Royal College of Surgeons, MS 129, fols. 1r–45v (**Rs**). In cases where we have determined that **T**'s reading is in error (and so removed it to the apparatus), the corrected reading (in square brackets) usually reflects the consensus of the other three manuscripts, converted to **T**'s spelling; occasionally we correct **T** on the basis of **S2** alone. In the few cases where we have inserted a hypothetical, emended reading (again using square brackets), we record all four manuscripts' readings in the apparatus. Simple corrections of minor, obvious spelling errors of only one or two letters are indicated with square brackets in the text, but not included in the textual notes. Orthographic variants have not been noted unless they are important to resolving the sense.[69] In

---

[69] One vocabulary change that the Hammond scribe made regularly (assuming this was not already present in his exemplar) was to change almost all occurrences of "moder" (i.e., the uterus) to "matrice." This change is particularly intriguing since, as has already been noted, the Hammond scribe was not skilled with medical vocabulary. His attempt to use "matrice" (almost) consistently to refer to the uterus, reserving "moder" for the pregnant or parturient woman herself, may reflect a greater distinction among some English speakers, at least in London, between the two terms. If there was such a trend toward distinction, however, it did not hold: a sixteenth-century owner of Sloane 249, the earliest copy of *Sickness 2*, "updated" his copy merely by changing "moder" to "mother" and adding the missing "t" to "marys/marice." Both "mother" and "matrice" would continue to be used to refer to the uterus well into the 19th century whereas "maris" died out after the 15th century (*OED*, "maris"; "matrice"; and "mother" n.[1], sense II). In 1544 in his copy of an English version of the *Trotula*, Robert Green of Welby ascribed the latter usage to ignorant women: "the matrice, the wyche þat women for the lake of knoleg calle ther maris" (Glasgow, Glasgow University Library, Hunter MS 403 [V.3.1], an. 1544, p. 363). See Explanatory Notes 34, 49, 57, and 58.

general, then, variant readings are cited only to help clarify readings in **T**; they are not exhaustive and do not pretend to reflect a full history of the development of the text.

We have expanded all standard abbreviations silently, with the exception of pharmaceutical symbols and abbreviations, which we preserve, as follows: *Rx* = Take (*Recipe*); *lb.* and *li.* = pound (*liber, libra*); *s.* = half (*semis*); *m.* = handful (*manipulus*); ℥ = ounce; ʒ = dram; ℈ = scruple; *ana* = '(the same amount) of each.'[70] We have indicated the relatively few marginalia by the original scribe in bold text within angle brackets; rubricated words and phrases within the text are also given in bold (the scribe uses a display script for these rubricated passages, but not for his marginalia). The extensive marginal annotations made by later hands are recorded in the Textual Notes, keyed to the most closely related word or phrase in the nearby text and identified in almost all cases by means of the numbers assigned to the annotators in the preceding section of this Headnote. Paragraph division, punctuation, and capitalization of the text are editorial and we have omitted the frequent paraph symbols found in the manuscript, many of which are excessive and distracting. Our principal intervention has been to signal those sections that were newly added by the *Sickness 2* redactor, through the use of paired double and single daggers (†† / †) at the beginning and end of each such section.

In the Explanatory Notes, we have compared certain readings in *Sickness 2* to Hallaert's edition of *Sickness 1* from New Haven, Yale University,

---

[70] The pharmaceutical measures in *Sickness of Women 2* are the standard ones, whose ratios are often described in short lists added to medical manuscripts, such as BL, Additional MS 30338, fol. 11r–v (also ed. in Hall and Nicholas 1929, 35):

> Forte rede & vndyrstonde þe wrytyng þat comeþ here-after & suche oþer wrytynge as leches wryteþ in makynge of here medicynes, wheþer it be in Englysh oþer in Latyn, þow shalt vndirstonde þat a pound is þys y-wryte, *lj. j*; & half a pound thus, *lj. dj.*; oþer þus, *lj. s.* [*s* with curved line through it]; & a quartroun of a pound is þus y-wryte, *quart. lj.* An vnce ys þe twelfeþe part of a pound & is þus y-wryte, ℥ *j*; & half an vnce þus, ℥ *dj.*; oþer þus ℥ *s.* A dragme is þe eyghteþe part of an vnce & is þus y-wryte ʒ*j*; half a dragme ys þus y-wryten ʒ *dj.*; | oþer þus ʒ *s.* A scripule ys þe þridde part of a dragme & is þus y-wryte ℈, & an half scripule þus ʒ *dj.*, oþer þus, ℈ *s.* A scrypule weyeth a peny & a dragme þre pans, & an vnce two schillynges, & a quatroun of a pound sixe shyllynges, & half a pound twelf schyllynges & a pound foure & twenty shyllynges. An hanful is þus y-wryte *m. j*; half an hondful þus *m. dj.*; oþer þus *m.* ℈ *j*; oþer þus, *m. s.* & þus þey beþ wreton in Latyn bokes.

For similar texts, see eVK, under the subject "Weights and Measures" (61 hits in Middle English).

Medical Library, MS 47 (s. xv²), fols. 60r–71v (**H**), and we have checked these readings in turn against an earlier manuscript, London, Society of Antiquaries, MS 338 (s. xv¹), fols. 76v–85v (**A**). This comparison proves that **A** does in fact present a tradition closer to that which the *Sickness 2* redactor was using. (Other copies of this tradition include London, BL, Royal 18.A.VI, Sloane 5, and Sloane 3486. In the Society of Antiquaries copy, as well as these other three manuscripts, *Sickness 1* is found with the full Gilbertus *Compendium* or, in the case of the Royal manuscript, a remnant of it, whereas in the Yale manuscript *Sickness 1* is found independently.) We leave for other scholars the important task of establishing the full textual tradition of *Sickness 1* and its relation to the Latin tradition of Gilbert's *Compendium*.

As moche as ther bien many wymmen that ben many
dyuers maladies and sikenesses nygh to the deth and they
also bien oshamful to oshewen and to tellen ther greuaunces
to any wight therfor I shal symdelwrite to then maladie tyme
by prayeng to god . . . .
to sende me grace treuly to write to the plesaunce of god and to
al wymmens helpyng for charite ayeth this that euery man
shuld trauaile for helpyng of his brethern and sustren after
the grace of god that he hath vndersong . and though wymmen
haue diuers euils and many grete greuaunces mo then al men
knowen of . as god knith hem shamen for drede of reprouyng in tymes
comyng and of dispisyng of vncurteys men that louen wymmen but for ther lustes and for ther foul likyng and if wymmen
bien in disease suche men han hem in dispite and thynken nat how
moche disease wymmen han or then ther han brought hem forth
in to the world . and therfor in helpyng of wymmen I wil write
of wymmen by silenet . the helpyng of . that oo womman
may help anothier in hir sikenes and nat discuer hir cortesies
to suche vncorteys men . but neuertheles whoso muche be
that displesith a womman for hir silenet that she hith of the
ordynaunce of god he doeth a grete synne for he dispiseth nat
aloonly hem . but god that sendith hem suche sikenes for them
best . and therfor noman shuld despise othir for the disease that
god sendith hym . but to haue compassion of hym and releue
hym as he myghte

Ther for yee shul vnderstonde that wymmen han lasse hete
in ther bodies then men han and more moistenes for de-
fante of hete that shuld dry ther moistenes and ther humours
but natheles of bledyng to make ther bodies clene and hole
from sikenes and ther han suche purgacions from the tyme of
xij wynter age in to the age of . l. wynter. but natheles
sum wymmen haue it lenger as they that bien of high complexioun and bien norysshed with hote metis and with hote
drynkes and liuen in moche rest and ther haue this purgacioun
in euery moneth ones but er be wymmen that bien with

Plate 1. *The Sickness of Women 2*, Prologue. Cambridge, Trinity College, MS R.14.52, fol. 107r. By permission of the Master and Fellows of Trinity College, Cambridge.

THE SICKNESS OF WOMEN

[fol. 107r]

††For as moche as ther bien many wymmen that han many diuers
maladies and sikenessis nygh to the deth and they also bien shameful
to shewen and to tellen their grevaunces to any wight, therfor I shal
sumdel write to their maladie remedy, prayeng to God and to his
5 blessid moder Marie ful of grace[1] to sende me grace triewly to write
to the pleasaunce of God and to al wymmens helpyng; for charite
axith this, that every man shuld travaile for helpyng of his brethern
and sustren after the grace of God that he hath vnderfong. And
though wymmen have divers evils and many grete grevaunces mo
10 than al men knowen of, as I saide, hem shamen for drede of reprevyng in tymes comyng and of discuryng of vncurteys men that loven
wymmen but for their lustis and for their foul likyng; and if wymmen bien in disease, suche men han hem in dispite and thynken
nat how moche disease wymmen han or than thei han brought hem
15 furth into this world.

And therfor in helpyng of wymmen I wil write of wymmen prevy
sikenes the helpyng of, that oo womman may help another in hir sikenes
and nat discure hir privitees to suche vncurteys men. But neuertheles whosumever he be that [dispisith] a womman for hir sikencs that
20 she hath of the ordynaunce of God, he doeth a grete synne, for he
dispisith nat al-only hem but God that sendith hem suche sikenes for
their best; and therfor no man shuld dispise other for the disease that
God sendith hym, but to have compassioun of hym and releve hym if
he myght.†

25 Therfor yee shul vnderstonde that wymmen han lasse hete in their
bodies than men han, and more moistenes for defaute of hete that
shuld dry their moistenes and their humours; but natheles of bledyng[2]
to make their bodies cleene and hole from sikenes, and thei han suche
purgacions from the tyme of xij winter age into the age of l wynter.[3] But

---

4–5. and to his blessid moder Marie ful of grace] *canc.* T, *eras. of almost one full
line between* Praying to god *and* ful of grace S2, & to his blessefull moder marie
full of grace S1, & to hys blessyd [ ] modyr marie full of grace Rs

17. womman] *marg. ann. 2:* planetis

19. dispisith] S1Rs displeasith TS2

30 natheles sum wymmen have it lenger, as thei that bien of high complexioun and bien norisshed with hote metis and with hote drynkes and
liven in moche rest. And thei have this purgacioun in every moneth
oones but it be wymmen that bien with **[fol. 107v]** chield or ellis wymmen that bien of dry complexioun and trauail moche; for wymmen
35 after thei bien with chield til they bien [delivered] they ne have nat this
purgacioun, for the chield in hir wombe is norisshed with the bloode
that thei shuld be purged of. And if thei have purgacioun in this tyme,
it is a token that þe chield refusith that bloode, and than that chield
is fal into sum sikenes or it wil die in his moder wombe. Wymmen that
40 bien of high complexioun and faren wele and liven in moche ease han
this purgacioun ofter than oones in a moneth; and this bloode that
passith from wymmen in tyme of their purgacioun cometh out of the
veynes that bien in the matrice ††that is clepid the moder and norice
to the chieldren right conceived in hem.† Þe matrice is a skynne that
45 the child is enclosed in his moder wombe and many of the sikenessis that wymmen han comen of the greuaunces of this moder that we
clepen the matrice.

¶ The[4] first is stoppyng of the bloode that thei shuld have in their purgacioun and be purged, as I have saide.
50 ¶ The secunde is to moche flowyng of suche bloode and in vntyme, and
that sikenes fieblith wymmen ful moche.
¶ The thridde sikenes is suffocacioun of the matrice.
¶ The iiij is precipitacioun of the matrice.
¶ The v is whan the matrice is fled from withynfurth.
55 ¶ The vj is whan ther is aposteme of the matrice.
¶ The vij is the swellyng of the matrice.
¶ The viij is of traualyng that wymmen han in þe chieldyng and the
harde grevaunces that thei han or thei bien delivered.
¶ The ix is goyng out of the matrice bynethfurth.
60 ¶ The x is witholdyng of the secundyne and ache of þe matrice.

**The first chapitre of this booke is of the stoppyng of
their bloode that thei shuld have in their purgacioun.**
Wytholdyng of this bloode that thei mown nat have þeir purgacioun-
is in due tymes comen in dyuers maners and of dyvers encheasons,
65 as of hete other of colde of the matrice, other of hete or of cold of

---

35. delivered] S2S1, *om.* T, *illegible* Rs
48. The first] *marg. ann. 3?:* n[ota]

the humours that bien enclosed withinfurth in the matrice, other of
grete drynes of hir complexioun, **[fol. 108r]** other of moche wakyng,
other of grete anger, other of moche sorowe, other of moche fastyng.
Signes and tokenes general of thiese sikenessis bien thiese: ache and
70 dolour with greuaunces and hevynessis from the navil dounward to
their prevy membre and ache of their raynes and of their rige-bone
and of their forhede and of their necke and of their eyen, and infectioun of þe bries, that is to say, chaungyng of their colour into another
coloure than thei shuld have; also hevynes aboute the mowth of þeir
75 stomac and ache aboute the shulder bladis both bifore and bihynde,
and hevynes of their thighes and their [hippis] and their hondis and
of their legges. And thei han otherwhile an vnskilful appetite to metis
that bien nat accordyng to hem, as to ete colis, ryndes, or shellis; and
their facis bien evil colourd, and otherwhile thei wexen wannyssh in
80 their visages. And oþerwhile in this tyme thei han wil to cumpany
with men, and so thei don and bryng furth chieldren that bien mesels
or have sum other suche foul sikenessis. And long witholdyng of this
bloode maken wymmen otherwhile to falle into a dropesy, oþerwhiles
makith hem to have the emerawdis, otherwhiles it grevith the herte
85 and the lunges and makith hem to have the cardiacle, and otherwhiles
it affraieth the herte so moche that it makith hem to fallen doun in
a swoun as though thei hadden þe fallyng evil and thei liggen in that
sikenes a day or two as though thei wern dede. ††And otherwhiles thei
han scotayne with grete stonyeng in the brayne and whan that al thyng
90 tournyth vp-so-doun.[5]†

And if this witholdyng [be for] the sikenesse of the bloode in the
matrice, that the bloode may nat flowe in due tymes as it shuld, their
vrynes wil be otherwhile as rede as bloode; and in tyme that thei shul
shewen and in tyme that she shuld have their purgacioun, it wil be
95 derke and the veynes wiln be ful of bloode and the colour of their bries,
that is to say, of their chaungyng, than wil be of cliere rede.

But [if] this withholdyng be of another humour that is hote and
drie and is clepid coler, than thei feelen brynnyng and prikyng of heete
withynfurth and their vryne is of high colour and fattye; and in tyme of

---

67. of hir complexioun other of moche wakyng] of her complexion other of
moche wakyng oþer of moche thenkyng S2S1Rs
76. hippis] S2S1Rs, lippis T
91. be for] S2S1Rs, bifore T
93. rede] *marg. ann. 1:* Vrynes Ruge
97. if] S2S1Rs, of T
99. high colour] *marg. ann. 1:* Vren high Colured

100 their purgacioun a iij or a iiij **[fol. 108v]** daies whan thei gon to prevy,
that thei bien delivered of a colerik matier that is as it were a brond.
And their bryes bien of swart rede colour. And if this witholdyng be
of cold and a moist humour that is clepid fleame, the vryne is fat and
discoloured; and in tyme of their purgacioun, whan thei gon to prevy,
105 thei bien delivered of a flewmatik matier that is white and thikke. And
their bries bien of fieble colour and swellith sumwhat.[6] But if witholdyng be of a cold dry humour that is in their veynes and is clepid malencoly, thei feelen moche hevynes benethfurth and their vryne is discoloured and thynne and hath in it smale gravel, otherwhiles of the colour
110 as it were asshen and otherwhile the vryne is blac and fat and therin be
litel blake motis and derke; and in tyme of their purgacioun if thei delivere hem of any thyng it is but litel in quantite. And wymmen that bien
istoppid contynuauly, their vryne is medled with litel smale thynges as
blac as coles; otherwhiles it is white and thikke and derk as mylke; oth-
115 erwhiles it is white and thynne and white sqwamous matier hangyng in
the vryne, other smale bodies blac imedled [with þe] vryne.

The[r] bien corrupt humours in þe matrice without the veynes in
the holownes of the matrice, and thei letten wymmen of their purgacioun. And iij humours ther bien that bien wont to be in the matrice,
120 as fleame, coler, and malencoly. The tokens of fleame bien thiese: thei
feelen moche moistnes, and thei han no likyng to medle with men,
and thei feele hevynes and cold from the navil dounward, and whan
they han their purgacioun thei bien delivered of moche fleame wiþ the
bloode that thei bien ipurged of. And their vryne is white or moche
125 drawyng to white; and if suche humours be resolved into wynde, thei
flee vp to the herte and to the lunges and make the womman flee into a
cardiacle. But if ther be moche malencoly in the matrice, thei han litel
likyng to medle with men, and whan thei don so ther passith but litel
matier from hem, and thei feelen moche cold and hevynes bineth their
130 navil, and thei feelen as it were a cold wynde mevyng in the matrice.
And in the tyme of their purgacioun thei bien delivere of litil matier

---

103. vryne is fat] *marg. ann. 1:* Vrynes Fatt

108–109. discoloured] *marg. ann. 1:* Vryne discolurd

114. blac as coles] *marg. ann. 1:* Vryne with small blak thynges

116. with þe] S2S1Rs whiche T

117. Ther] S2S1Rs, Their T

120. fleame (2)] *marg. ann. 1:* Tokens of Fleame; *marg. ann. 3:* Not[a]

125. drawyng to white] *marg. ann. 1:* Vryne blank; *marg. ann. 6 or ann. 1 writing later:* per Magistro Herysone

and that is [medled] with malencoly that is of swart yalow **[fol. 109r]**
colour, and the mowth of the matrice (that is to say, hir prevy membre)
is astonyed and hath but litel feelyng ne but litel likyng though thei
135 medle with men. And their vryne is otherwhile swart yalow and fatty
and otherwhile it is of fieble colour, and if ther be moche coler in the
matrice, thei feelen hete therin, ache and prikyng and hardnesse, and
thei bien hote aboute the mowth of the matrice and han grete desire
and likyng to company with men; and so thei delivere hem of matier,
140 but þe [mater] is but a litel in quantite. And in tyme of their purgacioun, if thei bien delivered of any bloode, it is but litel and of a rede
swart colour.

    Cura. For to help wymmen of this sikenes ther bien many dyuers
medicynes, as bloode letyng in oþer placis to delivere hem of bloode
145 that thei mown nat be ipurged of, and that is profitable lest thei falle
into a cardiacle other into a dropesy. And profitable bledynges bien
at the vaynes of þe grete toes, and to be igarced on the legge beneth
the sparlier both bifore and behynde, and to be cupped beneth the
teatis and also beneth the raynes behynde. Also stuphes bien profit-
150 able to hem, imade of herbis that wil and mown open the vaynes of the
matrice, that the bloode may have the rather his issue.

    And if thei bien stopped thurgh coler, that is to say, thurgh an
humour that is hote and drie, make a stewe of herbis that bien openyng, as of pollipodie levis, ivy, savyne, [mader,] origanum, rosemary,
155 comyn, lorel levis, affodil, fenel, mugwede, calamynt, isope, puliole,
nept, and suche other; and late hir sitte on an holow stoole over thiese
herbis whan thei bien weele isoden and hote, and sithen lete hir drynke
a draught of wyne that mugwede and pollipodie bien soden in. And
otherwhiles make hir right sory and otherwhiles right wroth and other-
160 whiles right mery, and late hir vse hote sauces and kene, as garlik and

---

132. medled] S2S1, mellyd Rs, *om.* T

133. prevy membre] *marg. ann. 3:* Not[a]

135. swart yalow] *marg. ann. 1:* Vren swart yellowe

136. colour] *marg. ann. 7:* N[ota]

140. mater] S2S1Rs, water T

143. For to help wymmen] *marg. ann. 1:* To Helpe Wemen; N[ota]

154. pollipodie levis] pollipodie lorell leves S2S1Rs   mader] madir S2 (*at be-*
ginning of line), S1Rs, *om.* T

155. lorel levis] *om.* S2S1Rs

157. lete hir drynke] *marg. ann. 1:* A drynk

159. make] maker T, *perh. in anticipation of foll.* hir

peper and mustard and crasses and suche other, and lete bathe hir in
the bathis imade of suche herbis as I spak of right now;[7] and late hir
walke moche and travaile wele and ete wele and drynke wele, and than
thei shuln sone be purged of their blode. And aboute that tyme of the
165 mone that thei shuln [have] their purga- **[fol. 109v]** cioun, if thei have
non, late hem bleede a goode quantite of bloode at hir grete too and
another day at hir other grete too; and everiche wike oones lete hir
vsen to bien ibathed in suche herbis as I spak of rather, and she may be
holp though hir sikenesse have dured hir long tyme.
170   But if thiese greuaunces bien of cold, first yeve hir this medicyne
to make the matier that grewith hir the more able to passe lightly away
from hir: Take raddish of fenel, percely, dawke, and [merche], the rootes of thiese and nat the levis, and than take the levis of mugwede, of
savyne, of calamynt, of origanum (if thow hast nat al thiese herbis, take
175 thoo that thow maist have) and seeth hem in vynegre for-to thei bien
wele isoden, and than clense it and cast to the vynegre half so moche
hony as the vynegre is and lete hem two buyle toguyder a while over
the fuyre, and sithen whan it is cold lete hir vsen therof a ij daies or
iij. But medil it with water that raddissh and madder haþ bien soden
180 in and after that late stue hir and bath hir with suche herbis as I saide
rather, and after that this is soden late hir drynke a draught of wyne
that savyne other mugwede is soden in and medle that wyne with water
that polipodie is soden in. And if thei have no purgacioun, late hem
bleede a goode quantite of bloode, as I saide afore.[8]
185   **Suppositorie**. Suppositories bien convenient medicynes for thiese
sikenessis, and thei shuln be put in wymmens prevy membres as men
putten suppositories in a mannes fundament for to purgen his wombe.
But thiese suppositories that bien ordeyned for wymmen shuld be
bounde with a threde aboute oon of hir thighes lest thei wern drawe
190 al into the matrice. And it is profitable to vse suche suppositories a iiij
or a v [daies] bifore the tyme of the moneth that thei shuld have their
purgacioun and thei mown the lightloker bien ipurged. One supposi-

---

165. have] S2S1Rs, *om.* T
170. bien of cold] *marg. ann. 1:* of Colde, *with marg. pointer*
172, merche] S2Rs, m'che S1, wrye T
182. savyne other mugwede] *foll. by* other madir S2S1Rs
184. of bloode] *marg. ann. 5:* to lat blod is good
185. Suppositories] *marg. ann. 1:* Suppositoris; N[ota]
190–191. a iiij or a v daies] a foure dayes other a fyve S2, a iiij or a v tymes [dayes S1Rs] T
192–193. One suppositorie] *marg. ann. 1:* Suppositorie

torie is this: take triacle diatesseron ʒ *s.*, and of cokle flour as moche, and as moche of myrre, and stamp hem toguyder with booles galle that

195 savyne or rewe is rotened within; than make it up with coton and therof make a suppositorie as **[fol. 110r]** grete as thi litel fynger and put it in hir prevy membre. But anoynte it first with cleene hony and oile toguyder and straw theron powder of scanomy and put in thi prevy membre;[9] thus myght a man do with the roote of lupines, that is moche better.

200 Another suppositorie: take the roote of smalache, the mounte-naunce of thy fynger, al grene and larde it wiþ the roote of peletir of Spayne and sithen put that roote in th'erth ageyn a fourtenyght or a iij wikes and than take it vp and wipe it cleene and put into hir prevy membre al a day and al a nyght. And afterward take it oute and anoynte

205 it with oile of lorel other with mete oile and put it in eftsones and lete it ligge til she have hir purgacioun, for though ther were a ded chield in hir wombe, it wold bryng it out; and the same vertue hath the roote of attory and also best is the rootis of vynes, if it be dight in the same wise. But or than she vnderfange this suppositorie, thow shalt seeth saveyne

210 and f[u]rsis, puliol roial, lorel levis in water and lete the womman sit therin a goode while afterwarde, and sithen lete hir wasshe hir prevy membre †† as deepe as she may reche inwarde and thus doo a goode while† with water; †† than do drie hir with a cloth and put in that sup-positorie of apium or of *acarus vt supra.*†

215 Another suppositorie: take the flour of cokel and medle it with hony and with coton and make a suppository therof. Another is this: take peleter of Spayne ʒ 3, of litel peleter as moche, cokel floure ʒ 1, of *diagredij* ʒ 7; put al thiese into a litel lynnen bagge that thy fynger wil in and lete hir put it in as deepe as she may so that she may pul it out

220 lightliche, for it wold make hir have a purgacioun anon. If hir wombe be sore of suche suppository, lete anoynte within with oile of roses or of violet or with mete oile or with fressh buttur that is nat salted.

Other medicynes ther bien the whiche if a womman drynk hem, thei wiln make hir to have a purgacioun either deliver hir of a ded

225 chield if þer be any in hir, as bawme precious idrunke and the juce of

---

198. thi] þe S2S1Rs

199. lupines] *marg. ann. 1:* [id est] gret Morrell, *with marg. marker*

203–204. put into hir prevy membre] *marg. ann. 1:* Suppositorie

206. ded chield] *marg. ann. 1:* a ded Child; N[ota])

210. fursis] S2S1, farsis T

215. Another suppositorie] *marg. ann. 1:* Suppositorie; N[ota]; S2 *has same rubric marg. note by its main scribe at this point.*

225. bawme precious idrunke] *marg. ann. 1:* A precius Drynk; N[ota]

isope other of diptayne and of leeke and of toun-cres ipoudred **[fol. 110v]** and idrunke. But if this sikenes come of anger oþer of sorowe, lete make hir myrry and yeve hir comfortable metis and drynkes and lete hir vsen to bathen otherwhiles. And if it be of moche fastyng other
230 of moche wakyng, lete diete hir moche with goode metis and drynkes that mown make hir to have goode bloode, and lete hir make hir mery and gladde and leve the hevynes of hir hevy thoughtes.

Goode electuaries for thise sikenessis bien thiese: theodoricon ipericon, theodoricon anacardi, and trifera magna, [panchristum],
235 and diaspermaton is the best of theym.

†† Also a worshipful sirup that myghtily bryngith furth the corrupt bloode from the matrice and this sirup is for ladies and for nonnes and other also that bien delicate. Take rootis of litel mader, knowholme, sperage rootis and þe roote of *ciperi ana* quartern *s.*, of mugwede, of
240 saveyne, [nept], valerian, calamynt, puliol *ana m.* 1, herbe baume *m.* 2, the seede of ceremountayne ʒ 1, spikenarde ʒ *s.*, miced, liquorice, reisouns and their stones piked oute *ana* ʒ 1, cleene hony *lb. s.*, þe floures and the levis grene of rosemary, floures of sticados arabike *ana* ʒ 1, of lof sugre quartern ʒ; make a syrub iclarified *lb.* 1 *s.* and yeve to
245 the womman two ounces therof and other two of the decoccioun of rede chiches, other do therto *lb.* iiij fyne clarre other of fyne pyment and do to the sirup and medle hem wele toguyder and yeve hir therof erly and late, at every tyme ʒ 6 and yeve hir ʒ 2 of benedicte in hir potage, and make hir potage therof.
250 **<laxatief>** Take fenel levis, avence, borage, violet, watercresses, stanmariche, isop, saverey, mercury, malues, chervoile *ana* ʒ 2 and make wortis and lete hir ete at oon messe with benedicta ʒ 1 and at another messe more isoden with benedicta ʒ 1 and it is easy. And if thow yeve hir drynk of it cliere made with the sirup a grete draught and

---

226. toun-cres ipoudred] tounkers & þe seed of *(end. of line* S2) tounkers ypou- derd S2S1Rs *(possible eye-skip at page break in* T*)*

233. Goode electuaries] *marg. ann. 4, using rusty ink:* Electuaris*;* S2 *has same ru- bric marg. note by main scribe at this point*

234. panchristum] pax^m S2, panx^m S1Rs, papillum T

237. for ladies and for nonnes] *marg. ann 8:* Ladyes & Nonnes

238. Take] *marg. ann. 1, writing at later time:* Suppositure

240. nept] next TS2S1Rs

241. miced] misid S1

242. cleene hony lb. s.] *follows* floures of sticados arabice ana ʒ i S2S1Rs

250. laxatief] TS2 *(marg.),* om. S1Rs

255 it shal purgen both the matrice and also the body esily; and withoute
penaunce to do this in a clos chamber from cold and from aire.

<Pelowe> Also to make a pelow that the womman shuld sitte on[10]
þe whiles thei bien in the stuphe for to mollifie harde retencions and
to nesshen the weyes of the matrice is this made: take mug- **[fol. 111r]**
260 wede and savory *ana* [*m.* 2], and the levis of pastinake, the levis of costy,
of malues, mershe-malowe, lynseede, fenygreke, of doder, of hemp
seede, lavender seede, of ceremountayne *ana* ʒ 2, percely seede, fenel
seede, anise, anete, *asori, dauci ana* ʒ *s.*, floures of camamyl, floures of
eleryn, of rosemaryn, of bothe sticados *ana* ʒ 2, al to bete hem in a
265 morter and put hem into a poket litel, to the quantite of a span breede
and in length. Whan this bag is fulfilled, lete the womman sitte theron
in the bath, and whan she cometh out of the bath, late anoynte hir
with oile myscelyn, the whiche is wretyn in þe chapitre of suffocacioun
herafterwarde.[11] And yeve hir to drynke electuary emagoge[12] ʒ 2 with
270 wyne that archimisie is soden in, or panchristum with me[t]he, and
late bryng hir in a bedde right easily made, and than yeve hir a suppository provocatief.

Also take ysope, rootis of gladen, of savayne, of rewe, of savery *ana*
ʒ 4, of diptayne, of nept, of fenel seede, of anyse seede *ana* ʒ 2, with
275 wyne of Gascoyne *li.* 1 and *s.*, of cleene rennyng water *li.* 1, of myre ʒ;
and bray thi seedis and stampe thyn herbis and þe myrre right smal
and lete seeth hem a while and lete it stonde til it be cold; clense it as
moche as she may drynke at ones bi þe morow. Also yeve it with trosikes
of deliveryng of chield, that bien writen in the chapiter of *mola matri-*
280 *cis*[13] with other medicynes and plasters there iwriten; and this medicyne
both bryngeth furth ded chield and quike, wherever it be in the wommans wombe, and that soone.

<Emplastrum> Also this emplaster solutief, if it be laide on a wommans share, it deliverith a ded chield other of any other beeste therin

---

257. Pelowe] TS2 (*marg.*), *om.* S1Rs

260. m. 2] m ij S2S1Rs, *om.* T   of costy] of costy (*end of line*) of costy T

263. dauci ana] *foll. by* al to bete hem in a morter, *canc.* T

270. methe] meche T

271–272. suppository provocatief] *marg. ann. 1:* Suppositorie

274. of (4)] *foll. by* fe *canc.* T

279. deliveryng of chield] *marg. ann. 1:* Delyueryng of Child

279–280. mola matricis] mala matricis S1Rs

283. Emplastrum] TS2 (*marg.*), *om.* S1Rs

284. ded chield] *marg. ann. 1:* Ded Child

285 ibredde;¹⁴ and if [it] be laide on the stomac it makith a womman to
[spewe]; and if it be laide on þe wombe it makith hir to go to prevy.
Rx electuary 2 *elebori nigri ana* ʒ 4, *lactice* ʒ 3, ciclamie, *interioris* [*colloquintide*], *succi titinmale ana* ʒ 6, *cocanidij* ʒ 2, *terbentyni* ʒ 4, *mel quod sufficit*; but I forsoþ do to thiese medicynes in the stide of hony galbanum
290 *li. s.* whan it shal do it [to] deliver a womman from hir chield; and if I
shal make a laxatief,¹⁵ put therto May butter that is fressh with a goode
quantite of bolis galle.†

**The secunde chapiter is of [fol. 111v] to moche flowyng of
bloode of vntyme and this sikenes fiebliþ moche wymmen.**

295 To moche flowyng of bloode at this membre cometh in many maners,
as of grete plente of bloode that is in the womman, other it is of the
sikenes of the bloode þat thurgh his keneship pressith veynes, other it is
of the subtilite of the bloode that swetith oute thurgh the smale poores
of þe veynes and so flowith oute, other for the bloode is vndefied and
300 rennyng and thynne as water, other it is of fieblenes of the womman
that may nat witholde the bloode within hir, other it is of sum brekyng
of sum veyne that is in the prevy membre, other there nygh. If it be in
the first maner,¹⁶ thei bleeden and thei feelen heete and smertyng in
their prevy membre and they bien delivered of to litel bloode; anon
305 that cometh swiftly furth oute and other it is blac or yalow as safron or
of the colour of fuyre, and than thei han otherwhile their gomes iclove
and their neither lippis of their mowth, and thei feelen smertyng and
akyng and prikyng aboute their teatis. And but if it be in the thridde
maner, the bloode cometh softly a litel and a litel and that is thynne
310 and cliere. And if it is of heete, he shal fynde¹⁷ heete withynfurth and
other tokenes of heete withynfurth and withoute. And if it is of the iiij
maner, the bloode is watery and thynne and she hath evil defieng both
in hir stomac and in hir wombe, and she feelith hurlyng of wyndes
vp and doun in hir wombe. And if it be in the v maner, thow myght

---

285. it (1)] S2S1Rs, *om.* T

286. spewe] S2S1Rs, speke T

287–288. colloquintide] colloquindide Rs, colloquinitide TS2

290. to] S2S1Rs, *om.* T

303. heete] *marg. ann. (prob. ann. 1 writing at later time):* hete; *marg. ann. 8:* in
wemen

310. cliere. And] *marg. ann. 1:* N[ota]

312. watery and thynne] *marg. ann. 1:* watery & thyn, *with* Flowres *added poss.
by same hand at a later time*

315 knowe it bi the fieblenes of the womman body; and the bloode that
passith from hir it cometh fiebliche and contynuauly and in his goyng
it makith non angwissh ne greuaunce. And if it be in the vj maner, the
bloode cometh contynual and with greuaunce, and otherwhile it hath
his kyndely colour and otherwhiles it hath nat, but cometh out cor-
320 rupt in maner of quetor. And wher that ever this sikenes cometh and
in what maner, thow shalt nat sodainly stoppe it, the bloode of his flowyng ne no maner of flux, but if a man other a womman[18] be the more
ifiebled therby, for than men **[fol. 112r]** shuln ceasen it as men may
and ellis nat.

325   **<of moche bloode> Cura:** And if there come grete plente of bloode,
lete drien hir with metis and drynkes[19] that gendren but litel bloode, as
fruyte and herbis, and lete hir bleede at the veyne of hir arme and to
be cupped vnder her teatis and aboute hir raynes and hir liendis and
to be garced on hir legges to withdrawe the bloode awaywardis from
330 the matrice.

    <Suppository> A powder: Take *psidia, ypoquistides, acasia, coloph*[*on*]*ia*
and make therof suppositories, or medle al this with anyse or planteyne and emplaster it aboute both bifore on the matrice and behynde
evene agenst it.

335   Other medicynes also þat bien goode to staunche the bloody flux,
††as take a grete roote of *enula campana li. s.* & ʒ 6, of cleene water a
galoun and an half, and seeth hem toguyder to a potel and than clense
it and put therto half a *lb.* of white sugre and seeth it eftsoones a litel
and lete it keele; and lete hir drynke therof erly and late, and it shal
340 staunche withyn iiij daies. This medicyne [taught] the Priour of Beremondesey to a womman that was ny ded on the flux of hir matrice; and
to amende hir stomac he lete take two handful of the myddil rynde of
the brome and lete it seeth in iij potels of cliere water to a potel, clense

---

316. fiebliche] *marg. ann. 1:* Febeliche
322. flux] *marg. ann. 1:* Flux
325. of moche bloode] TS2 (*marg.*), *om.* S1Rs
331. Suppository] TS2 (*marg.*), *om.* S1Rs   colophonia] S2S1Rs, colophia T
332. with anyse or] with þe jus of S2S1Rs
335. flux] *marg. ann. 1:* Flux
337. half and] *marg. ann. 1:* N[ota]
340. taught] S2S1, staungchyd Rs, *om.* T
341. flux of hir matrice] *marg. ann. 1:* To moche Blood; *marg. ann. 8:* proved
per certe
342. to amende hir stomac] *marg. ann. 3:* Not[a]

and put therto half a pownde of white sugre and lete it seeth eftsones
345 and yeve hir to drynke.†

    <of sharpnes> But if this flux come of a leinnes or of a sharpnes
of the bloode, lete hir bleede a litel on the arme and sithen lete hir
drynke a litel rubarbe ʒ 2, sene ʒ 2, wiþ the juce coct and borage and
fenel *ana* ʒ 6, to make hir bloode cleene; and sithen lete hir drynke the
350 juce of mynte and of popie and of pla[n]tayne clarified and scomed,
and that wil staunche the bleedyng; and if thow do therto the juce of
daisy and the powder of gallis that men make ynk of, it wil sowde and
hele the veynes that bien broken thurgh sharpenes of þat bloode; and
lete hir vse hockes, beetis, and violetis and plantayne in hir potage to
355 abate the keenes of the bloode; and lete hir vse purslane, letuse, mynte,
plantayne, sorel, and roses in medycynes to make the flux to cease.

    Also lete hir vse confery and daisie *ana* dragma 1. Rx *gallie*, san-
dragon, bole, ††*corallis* **[fol. 112v]** *albi* and *rubie, manne, masticis ana* ʒ 2,
conserue rosarum ʒ 2, *zucari albi* ʒ 5, *teranda & conficiantur* and lete hir vse
360 this electuarie with þe juce of plantayne or moleyne; or ellis take the
same powder and† seeth it in rayne water and make a pissarie and so
mynistre hir with; this wil sowden the veynes that bien broken.

    Also take ceruse, almaundis, muscillage of *psilij ana* ʒ 1 & *s.*, lete
wete a weke therin and put in hir prevy membre in maner of a sup-
365 pository. Also a plaster made of muscillage of psilium and of lynsede
ipowdred, of dragaunce ilaide on hir share: it is profitable for hir grevaunces.

    Also take the powder of psilium ibrend and egipsium ibrend and
bole and sandragoun, psidie, acornys of okes, balaustia or in stide of
370 it the oken ryndes and simphite and sumac *ana* ʒ 2 & *s.*, camphore ʒ 1
s.; powder al thiese toguyder and temper it with the white of eyren and
make ij emplasters therof, oon to ligge on the share, another to ligge
on the raynes.

    And this maladie cometh of the succide of the bloode,[20] lete hir
375 vse comfortable electuaries, and namly if a womman be of fieble com-

---

346. of sharpnes] TS2 (*marg.*), *om.* S1Rs

347. lete hir bleede] *marg. ann. 5:* lete her blod

351. staunche the bleedyng] *marg. ann. 8:* stancheyng of blood

354. in hir potage] *marg. ann. 9 (or poss. ann. 1 writing at later time):* for her pottage (*cf.* in pottage *note on fol. 113v*)

361. pissarie] *marg. ann. 1 writing at a later time:* A pyssary

364–365. suppository] *marg. ann. 1:* Suppository

365. Also a plaster] *marg. ann. 1:* A plaster

375–376. fieble complexioun] *marg. ann. 1 writing at later time:* Febull complex-
cion; *marg. ann. by main scribe in* S2: Of sugite of bloode, *om.* (*exceptionally*) T

plexioun, ††*athanasie* ʒ 2, *zuccari atri* ʒ 5, *albi rosarum* ʒ s., *diatoniden,
diacodion, gallie mustice ana* ꝺ 12 & *s.*, *zucari atri* ʒ 5 *cum succo* plantayne
in quo lapis ematicis fuerit fricatus;† and lete diete hir with metis that wil
make hir bloode thikke, as with almaunde mylke and rise made with
380 almaunde mylke and furmente. Also menge therwith gotes mylke, for
that is ful profitable for this sikenes, for it makith þe bloode thicke and
sowdith the veynes that bien broken and lettith þe bloode of his flowyng.
   But for to make it right profitable, take cleene stones that han long
385 leyn in cleene rennyng water and heete hem wele in the fuyre and sithen
quenche hem in þe mylke of almaundis, in the mylke of a gote that is
fedde wiþ goode herbis or with cowes mylke, and thei shuln consume
the watrynes of the mylke; and lete hir vse goode moton and goode
hennes that bien wele flesshed and litel fatte; and among al thyng-
390 es that men vsen, rise and whete thickith moche a manncs bloode and
wurtis made of arage and of beetis þat makith the bloode thynne. And
lete hir vse *zuccarum rosarum* and *dia-* **[fol. 113r]** *papauer* and thiese
thicken: lete hir vse whan she goeth to bedde and erly whan she aris-
eth. Than take mum[i]e, *olibani*, mastik, and þe hertis horn ibrent til it
395 be white, and of cveriche of thiese liche moche, and powder hem and
tempre hem with the juce of mynt othcr of plantayne or of mugwede
and make hem of þe quantite of a beane and lete hir vse ij or iij at oon
tyme. And if thow take the mawe of a sowkyng hare or of a sowkyng
calf and do brenne it into powder and medle it with the powder afor-
400 saide with pellis forsaide, thei wiln be moche the bettir. Also take hertis hornes wele ibrend ʒ s., ot ey-shellis ʒ 3, powder al thiese 3 toguyder

---

376. zuccari atri ʒ 5] *foll. by* cum succo planteyn, *canc.*   zuccari atri ʒ 5 albi
rosarum ʒ s.] succre albi rosarum ʒ semis S2S1

377. mustice ana ꝺ] *the scruple sigle here is, exceptionally, in the form of a capital* S,
similar to the abbreviation for scilicet *on fol. 133v. Confusion over the sigle used here
is shared by the other MSS: in S2, this same measure indicated by a badly drawn cres-
cent that looks like an s; in S1 by an s over which a 16th-century annotator has drawn
the* ꝺ *sigle; and in Rs by an s*

382. lettith þe bloode] *marg. ann. 5:* and lettithe blod

384. stones] *marg. ann. 1:* Stones; N[ota]

394. mumie] mumne *(extra minim)* T   hertis horn] *foll. by* with the juce of
mynt other of plantayne or of mugwede, *canc. (apparently an eye-skip corr. by the
scribe himself)* T

399. brenne it into powder] *marg. ann. 1:* A powder

400–401. hertis hornes wele ibrend] *marg. ann. 5, or poss. ann. 1 writing later:*
hertis horne brent

and lete hir vsen it in potage, in sawce, and in drynke: ††*probatum est*
in Chepa, London.²¹†

Another: take lynseede al hole and sethe it in sheepis mylke other
405 gotes mylke and lete hir ete it, other femygreke, that is moche better. ††Take þe rootis of dragaunce ʒ 5, the levis of mersh ʒ 3, powder
thiese toguydre and drynke it with goode ale, and she shal be hole:
this was proeved at Cicestre on Barons wif that was nygh ded on this
maladie.†²²

410   Another: also the juce of mugwede idrunke other the herbe emplastred is goode to staunche þe flux.

<fieblenes of complexioun> And if this sikenes comyth of fieblenes
of a wommans complexioun, lete hir vse comfortable metis and drynkes
and *zuccarum rosarum* and diapapaure and the oile of myntis iclarified
415 and cast therto a litel quantite of suger to make it swete.

Another: take encense, mynte, sandragon, mastic, violet, and storax *rubie ana* ʒ 6, powder al thiese toguyder with the juce of plantayne
and with vynegre and plaster both bifore and behynde, that is to [say]
on hir share and on hir raynes.

420   <of brekyng of veynes> And if it come of brekyng of veynes, the
aforsaide suppositories and electuaries²³ bien goode for hem. And
other medicynes ther bien ful goode that staunchen the bloody flux
and thei bien goode for this sikenes; and to take a fat eele and lay hym
al quike on the colis and late the womman stonde therover and lete the
425 smoke come into hir prevy membre or into a mannes fundament if he
have the flux and in the same maner do with colophony.

---

402. in potage] *marg. ann. 9, or poss. ann. 1 writing later; certainly by the same hand
as wrote* for her pottage *on fol. 112r:* in pottage

404–409. take lynseede al hole . . . on this maladie] *In* S2S1Rs, *but not in* T, *this
recipe is repeated. In* S2, *the repetition is dotted for expunction and crossed out in red,
as if at the time of rubrication by the scribe. See Explanatory Note 22.*

408. Cicestre] Suscester Rs, Surcester S2S1

411. flux] *marg. ann. 1:* Flux

412. fieblenes of complexioun] TS2 (*marg.*), *om.* S1Rs   sikenes] modicy
sikenes T

416. Another] *marg. ann. 1:* Medicynes

417. the juce of plantayne] *marg. ann. 1, writing later:* þe Iuyse of planteyn

418. that is to say] .i. S2S1Rs, that is to (*end of line*) T

420. of brekyng of veynes] TS2 (*marg.*), *om.* S1Rs; *marg. ann. 1, writing later:*
Brekyng of veynes, stanchyng blod

422. staunchen the bloody flux] *marg. ann. 1, writing later:* For stanchyng þe
flux

A profitable bath for **[fol. 113v]** this sikenes and also for the flux:
take a goode quantite of vryne with water[24] and the v part therof stronge
vynegre and seth therin the rynde of the blac plomtre and of an apen-
430 ers tre and of a chestayne tree and of an oke, of roses, of plantayne, of
confery, þe rynde of assh, daisie, ribwort, mynt, acornes of an oke, penthaphilon, smolent isode allon in rede wyne, and plastred bifore and
behynde shal staunche bi his owne myght. But seeth al thiese thynges
in water til the water be blac and thikke and lete wrappe þe man or the
435 womman in a sheete and sitte in that bath, and lete vse rosted metis
and brede of whete and made with the juce of plantayne and mylfoile.

Lete ete partriches irosted other hennes rosted with wex and lete hir
vse to drynk water of rosis and of plantayne, other ellis reyne water, other
ellis water that mastik is soden in, other wyne medled with water.

440   ††Or ellis take water of roses ʒ 10, masticis ʒ 2, galange ʒ 1 & *s.*,
ʒ 1 & ꝫ, macon, cucube, nardi, cinamon *ana* ʒ 1, *rose puluerizantur* and
put al tho into oo pot of g[la]se with the water of *rosarum zuccarum* ʒ 2,
stop it and lete it seeth in water an houre. This water idrunke is goode
for al maner of sikenes of the herte in a cold case and for the cardiacle
445 and for swounyng and for the flux that comyth of cold.†

Also take a quike turtil and brenne hir al quike with the fethers
and take ʒ 1 of mumie and as moche of sandragon and bren hem wele
therwith in an erthen pot and lete hir vse that powder in sauce, in
potage, and in drynke.

450   ††Also make powder of hertis hornes ibrent and of ey-shellis ibrent
ana ʒ 10 and drynke of this powder 2 drames at ones with the juce
of planteyne other goode meane ale þat is nat myghti, and she shal
staunche.

Also take bole armoniac, caruie seede *ana* ʒ 3, zinziber ʒ 1, coral
455 fyne and rede ʒ 1, make powder and gyve it hir and it staunch[ith].

---

427. bath] *marg. ann. 1, writing later*: A bathe   flux] *marg. ann. 1:* Flux;
N[ota]

428. vryne] Iren S2S1Rs   vryne with water] *marg. ann. 1, writing later*: N[ota]
dyuers waters for to stope þe Fluxe

437. partriches . . . hennes rosted] *marg. ann. 1:* metis

440. take water] *marg. ann. 1:* Flux

442. glase] galse T

443. water (2)] *marg. ann. 1:* wateris

448. in an erthen pot] *foll. by* al to poudre S2S1Rs

452–453. and she shal staunche] *marg. ann. 8*: Stanchyng of blod

454. Also take] *marg. ann. 1:* Flux

455. it staunchith] S2S1Rs, it staunche T

A goode medicyne for thiese fluxes made: take galingale, canel *ana*
ʒ 2, coral rede and white *ana* ʒ 3, sandragon, [bole] armoniak *ana* ʒ 2
& *s.*, gumme arabik, mirtil, *coliandri infusi i*[*n papaueris*] *albi & nigri,*
acasie, liquorice ana ʒ *s.*, make powder herof and yeve it hir with the juce
460   of pervynke or of plantayne: make powder herof or of turmentil or of
rost bones or of molen.

Also take *ypoquistidos, acasia, lapis ematiste* [**fol. 114r**] *ana* ʒ 1, make
powder and drynke it with the juse of roses or ellis with rose water or
powder of anathasia ʒ 3 idrunke with the juce of sloue; or ellis a pissa-
465   rie made of juce of sloue with þe newe powder of anathasia and that is
icast into hir prevy membre: it staunchith it if it be curable.

Also take bole fyne with the juce of plantayne and make a suppository with coton and put into the membre: it helpith moche.

Also powder of the flour of rise or of pomegarnad, that is to say,
470   balaustie, with the juce of sanguynarie; and so ipissaried it is right profitable. Or ellis menge turmentil, moleyn, rost bones, *pervinca, virge pasto-*
ris, and seeth al thiese in tanners woose that is clepid [amonge hem] the
first bech. And whan they bie al isoden, lete the womman sitte therin vp
to the navil also long as she may endure, for this is proved in Essex.

475   Also powder of coral that is fyne and right rede and idrunke, it
staunchith al the fluxes; also maces and safron toguyder staunchith it.

Also take vitriole brent or vnbrent ʒ 1 and juce of plantayne ʒ 7
with the stone of ematiste ʒ 1 and cast it into prevy membre and it
staunchith.

480   Also if hir thynke that it brennyth that comeþ from hir at the prevy
membre, take than the muscillage of psilium, of the muscillage of the
seedis of quynces and of the gumme of *draganti ana* ʒ 1, of wommans

---

457. bole] S2S1Rs, *om.* T

458. in papaueris] i pᵃuis TS2S1Rs (*cf. common abbrev.* pa[pa]u[er]is, *attested on*
fol. 114v, and the common occurrence of white and black [albi & nigri] *poppy in med-*
ical recipes)

461. rost bones] *marg. ann. 12:* resta bouis

466. it staunchith . . . curable] *marg. ann. 1:* For to muche Blod, *plus later add.:*
.i. Flowres

467–468. suppository] *marg. ann. 1:* Suppositorie

469. flour of rise or of pomegarnad] flowre of Ryse of pondgarnardys S2Rs,
flour rys of pomegarnardes S1

472. amonge hem] S2S1Rs, and menge T

474. endure] *marg. ann. 1:* A speciall medicyn

476–477. staunchith it. Also] *marg. ann. 1:* Flux

478–479. it staunchith] *marg. ann. 1:* Stanchyng þe flixe; N[ota]

482. draganti] draganti albi S2S1Rs

mylke ʒ 6, cast it into prevy membre and this medicyne helith and
staunchith al bloode that cometh thurgh hote causes.

485   Also another precious medicyne is this: take saundres, the rede
and the white, spodie, sumac, myrtil *ana* ʒ 2, *acasie* ʒ 3, *ypoquistides* ʒ 3,
juce of plantayne, juce of rede roses or the water of roses *ana* quater 3,
barly mele as it sufficith; make a plaster of al thiese materials first ipowdred and that plaster shal be nesshe sumdel.

490   Also another precious plaster is this, whan the bloode is colerik:
take the juce of plantayne *li.* 1, water of roses a quarteron, of vynegre ʒ
s., of rede coral, of cacabre, of *lapis amatiste*, of bole armoniac, of myrtil, of acornes cuppes, of *olibani ana* ʒ 2, of *terre sigillate* ʒ s., al thiese
ipowdred and herof make to emplasters, oon afore vnder the navil and
495 another laide to behynde on the raynes.

    Also the vtmoste is bath made of water þat alum of plume is soden
in, for it is expert; and Avicen techith it in **[fol. 114v]** the 2 chapitre
[of bothor].²⁵

    Also vnderstande if the matier be right colerik, it is nede that it
500 be purged with medicynes that purgen colre, as thus: Take of *myra-*
bolans citryn ʒ 1, *reubarbium* ʒ s., *puluerizantur* and put therto *diapapa-*
ueris ʒ 3, [*electuarij*] *de succo rosarum* ʒ 1, and medle hem toguyder with
the [pulpe] of *cassia fistula* as it sufficith to the forsaide, and drynke ʒ
3 of white whay that borage was soden in, and whan it is don bi iij or
505 iiij daies, than yeve hir ever bitwene *zuccarum rosarum* ʒ 2, powder of
anathasie newliche made ʒ 1, white *zuccarum cassatyne* ʒ 6 idraven toguyder: drynke this with the juce aforsaide. And if it staunche with non of
thiese medicynes, do sette bloode boxes on his teatis with fuyre and but
thiese sufficen God [that is] medicyne and non but he.†

510 **The thrid chapiter is of the suffocacioun of the matrice.**
Suffocacioun of the matrice is whan a wommans herte and hir lunges
bien ithrust toguyder bi the matrice that a womman semeth ded save
bi hir brethyng, and sum clepen it a cardiacle for it is greuaunce of the

---

485. another precious medicyne] *marg. ann.* 1: A precius medisyn

490. plaster] *marg. ann. 1* A plastere

498. of bothor] of bothe S2S1Rs, above T

500. purgen colre] *marg. ann.* 1: A gud Medicyn to purge Coller

502. electuarij] electi (*lacking mark of suspension*) T

503. pulpe] S2S1Rs, oulie T

503–504. drynke ʒ 3] drynk ʒ iij (iiij S2Rs) S2S1Rs, drynke it ʒ 3 T

509. that is] is S2, this T

512. a womman semeth ded] *marg. ann.* 1: A Woman to seme ded

herte. For whan ther cometh a corrupt smoke from the matrice and
515 goeth vp to the hede—oþerwhile bi the rige-bon into hir hynder partie of the hede, otherwhile bi the brest into the former partie of the
hede—and for the brayne of wymmen is more myghti than their herte,
therfor that smoke may nat abide in the hede but smytith doun into the
herte and grevith the herte ful moche and makith the herte to closen
520 hym toguyder more than he shuld do bi kynde. And in this evil, wymmen fallen doun to the grounde as though thei had the fallyng evil and
liggen so in a swoune, and this acces endurith otherwhiles ij daies or iij.
And þis sikenes cometh of dyvers encheasouns, as of witholdyng of the
bloode that thei shuld bien purged of, other of sum corrupt humours
525 and venymous that bien in the matrice. As men bien delivered of seede
that passith from their stones that bien bi her yerde, and also men
fallen into dyuers sikenesses for witholdyng of their seede withyn hem,
right so doeth wymmen; but whan wymmen han this sikenes, or than
they fallen adoun, þei feelen moche ache and greuaunce from their
530 navil dounvard and they bowen their hede doun to their knees for **[fol.
115r]** greuaunce and witholden their wombe and clippen it harde toguyder with their handis and maken other men oþerwhiles to thristen their
wombe toguyder and thei holden their teth toguyder and sithen thei
fallen doun to grounde as though they wern ded, and other thei beten
535 the erth with their handes for þe grete grevaunce that thei han.

And if this grevaunce come of þe forsaide witholdyng of bloode,
men shal best knowe bi the pacientis tellyng, for she may best witen
whether she [were] purged of hir bloode as she shuld be other nay. But
if it is of corrupt humours that bien in the matrice, that may be in ij
540 maners, as of hote humours other of cold. If the humours bien hote,
she feelith prikyng and brennyng in the depnes of the matrice and
therof bien resolued hote smokes that bien disparpled þurgh al the
body and makith hir to have an vnkynde hete, in maner of a fever, in
the body. But if the humours bien cold, than haþ she moche hevynes

---

515. to the hede oþerwhile] *marg. ann.* 5, *or possibly ann.* 1 *writing later:* Suffocacio
527. seede withyn hem] *marg. ann.* 1: N[ota]; Sed of men
530. navil dounvard and they] *foll. by* feelen their hede dynne, *canc.* T
533. teth toguyder] *marg. ann.* 1: N[ota]; Wemen
535. with their handes] with her hondes and with her fete S2S1Rs
538. were] S2S1Rs, *om.* T
541. prikyng and brennyng] *marg. ann.* 1: Prykkyng & Brannyng
544–545. hevynes in . . . hir matrice] *marg. ann.* 1: hevynes in þe matrice

545 in the depnes of hir matrice and therof is resolued a cold smoke that
smytith vp to the hede bi the rige-bon and bi the stomac also, and she
feelith otherwhiles grete greuaunce aboute the spleene in the lift side;
but if it be of corrupt seede [as I saide] bifore,[26] than the [grevaunce is]
withouten thiese forsaide tokenes. But nevertheles the matrice seemyth
550 replete of suche moystnes.

Cura huius: for to help wymmen of this sikenes it is nedeful to
purge the matrice of bloode, if it is in the first maner, [or of the corrupt humours that bien in þe matrice if it is in þe ij maner] other in the
thridde maner. Natheles if it come in the thridde maner, it is profitable
555 to haue cumpany with man; but this is to vndirstande in lawful cumpanyng, as with their husbondes and with non other, for in certayne it
were bettir for a man or for a womman to have the grettest sikenes of
the body the whiles thei liven than to be helid thurgh a deede of lechery other any other deede agenst Goddis hestis;[27] and so bi that is saide
560 biforc, in the chapiter of witholdyng of bloode,[28] thei mown be iholpen.
Natheles that tyme that wymmen han accesse of þis sikenes, thei mown
receive no strong medicynes to purgen hem, but it be strong wymmen
that bien of strong complexioun. And therof whan thei bien in their
accesses, medle oile of baie and **[fol. 115v]** oile of roses toguyder, of
565 both iliche moche, and therwith anoynt their armes and hir handis, hir
legges and hir feete, and lete settc a bloode glas with fuyre on hir share
without chaungyng; and lete hir smel stynkyng thynges that stynken
horribely and foule, as fcltes ibrent, other houndes her, other gotis her,
other hors bones ibrent and sithen iquenchid, other hertis horn, other
570 old shone, other fethers brent, other a weeke wet in oile and itende and
sithen iquenched, other a wullen clew, other a quike cole so smokyng:
lete hir take that smoke.

Other take the powder of castory and galbanum resolued in vynegre and as moche of brymston, *psilij,* peusadanum and [put] therto a
575 peny weight of petrolion and lete cast al thiese on the coles so þat the
smoke mowe to hir nose and in at hir mowth.

---

548. as I saide] S1Rs, *om.* TS2   grevaunce is] S2S1Rs, grevaunces T

552–553. or of the corrupt humours that bien in þe matrice if it is in þe ij man-
er] S2S1Rs, *om.* T

562. medicynes] *marg. ann. 1*: Medicyns

564. oile (2)] *marg. ann. 1*: Oyles; N[ota]

567. stynkyng thynges] *marg. ann. 1*: To Smell Stynkyng Thynges

573. Other take] *marg. ann. 1*: A good medycyn

574. psilij] p(er)silij S2S1Rs   put] S2S1Rs, that T

††Other take oile comune *li.* 2, floures and levis of rosemary, nept, calamynt, *pulegij*, [t]ym, origanum, isope, savoray, lorer levis, shavyng of cipres *ana* ʒ & *s.*, clowes, *calami aromatici, ciperi, macis ana* ʒ 2, *mirre* ʒ
580 1, *vini albi aromatici li. s. coquantur* and seeth hem til the wyne be consumed and than clense it, &c.†

And from the navil donward to hir prevy membre lete anoynt hir with wele smellyng thynges and swete, as oynementis and oiles; and make hir a fumygacioun binethfurth and draw the matier from þe
585 herte donward; and suche thynges that bien goode [herefore] is *gallia muscata*, muske, exilocassie, aumber, frankencens, *storax liquida, calamus aromaticus, lignum aloes*, bawme, and suche other thynges that han a sweete savour. And also in þe tyme of hir accesse, lete bynde hir legges and hir thies toguyder and frote warm the soolis of hir feete with
590 vynegre and salt. And make hir a fumygacioun binethfurth of swete smellyng thynges so that the smoke ne the savour come nat vp to hir nose, but lete hir smelle *asafetida* and other stynkyng þinges, as I saide bifore;[29] and make hir to sneese with the powder of castory, of pepir, of euforby, of pyretrum [*ana*] ƺ *s.* cast into hir nose. Other in tyme of hir
595 acces, yeve hir triacle ʒ 1 and anoynt the mowthe of the matrice with wele smellyng [oynementes].

A goode fumygacioun to waken hir in þe tyme **[fol. 116r]** of hir acces: take a peusadanum ʒ 7, of galbanum ʒ 12, of cost also moche, of pepir 11 graynes, and a litel bawme tho that may be made into powder.
600 Powder hem but resolue galbanum in vynegre and cast it on the coles and lete hir hange hir nose over the smoke. And al thiese medicynes shal be don in þe tyme of hir acces whan she is fallen doun to grounde; but bifore and after thow myght gyven medicynes to make hir to have hir purgacioun, as it is saide bifore.

605 And if the humours be of cold that makith hir to have that grevaunce, lete bathen hir in a bath of hote erbis; and whan she comyth outwarde of the bath, yeve hir a draught of wyne that comyn and gyngier

578. tym] thym S1, thyn S2Rs, pym T

580. and] id est S2S1Rs

582. lete anoynt hir] *marg. ann. 1:* Oyntment *with* for wemen *added by the eighth annotator, in grey-brown ink*

585. herefore] S2, here afore T

588. And also] *marg. ann. 4, using rusty-colored* ink: A speciall Medesyn

589. warm] wel S2S1Rs

594. ana] S2, a li. T

596. oynementes] S2, vynetrentes T

598. take] *marg. ann. 1:* Medycyn

bien soden in. But if it be of corrupt seede, lete hir eftsoones be garced
beneth the sparlyuer both behynde and bifore; and lete hir bleede also
610 atte the veyne vnder þe ancle and at hir grete toes. And lete bray in a
morter of bras loveache, wormode, isope, and sote, and sithen seeth
hem in water and plaster it bifore [fro] the mowth of the stomac to hir
prevy membre, and also moche behynde on hir bak, also on hir sides.
Sote also isoden and iplastred in the same [wise] without any other
615 þing helpith, other wormode bi hymsilf helpith hem in oonys liggyng
to hem though men do no more.

Also take *sal-gemme, sal-[nitri]*, powder and distemper hem with
vynegre and wiþ salt water and wete a wike of coton therin and put it
in hir prevy membre and it wil deliver hir of that corrupt seede.

620 **<metis þat encreasith sperme>** And be thei ware of metis that
encreasiþ seede both in a man and in a womman, and suche metis bien
yolkes of eyren and fressh flessh and namliche of swyne, of cokkis, of
sparowis, partriches, quaile, and brawne of a bore and þe stones of
beestis, as of bores, of boles, of wulfis principaly, and the mary and the
625 fatnes and the brayne of beestis, prunes, datis, almaundis, figges, notis,
pastinakes, rapes fried with hony and oile of [benen] and peson, and
strong swete wyne and satournous, and goode wyne that is myghti and
swete, both white and rede, and mete also and moche rest and sleepe
and likyng in bathis; also that thei dwel nat long in bathis.

630 **[fol. 116v] <to wast sperme>** But lete vse suche thynges that wastith
sperme and consumeth seede, as fastyng and wakyng; isope, rewe and
comyn that thurgh their heete consumen the seede; and other thynges þat menvsen the seede, as colde herbis, as *agnus castus*, water lilies,
and suche other.

635 ††Also if the mydwif wete hir handis in oile of puliol and in oile
mushilyng *ana* ʒ 3 medeled toguyders and than anoynt the orifice of

---

609. bleede] *marg. ann. 1:* Blood
612. fro] S2S1Rs, *om.* T
614. wise] S2S1Rs, *om.* T
617. nitri] S2S1Rs, viter T
620. metis þat encreasith sperme] TS2 (*marg.*), *om.* S1Rs
621. encreasiþ] corruptith *canc.;* encreasiþ *in marg., marked for ins.; foll. by
main scribe's marg. note (see prec. Textual Note)*   suche metis bien] *marg. ann. 1:*
Sperme þat incresythe by metes & drynkes
626. benen] S2S1, benes Rs, beven T
630. to wast sperme] TS2 (*marg.*), *om.* S1Rs
633. menvsen] men vsen T, menusith S2Rs, meunseith S1
635. mydwif] *marg. ann. 1:* Midwyf

hir prevy membre, it shuld make tikelyng in the matrice, and for she
wil come dounward with swete smellyng thynges.[30]
  Now to [m]ake oile muschilyng thow shalt do thus: take ij galons
640 and an half of goode mete oile þat is right swete and put therto a *lb.*
of puliol roial, of rosemary, of cost, of camamyl, lavender, of bawme,
of wooderof, of isope, savorey, and shavyng of cipres *ana li. s.*, of calamynt, of fetherfoy, of fenel, of wormode, of sauge, of rewe, of origanum,
of sothernwoode, of Seynt John (that is to say, herbe John) worte *ana*
645 ʒ 12. Wash hem first in water and seeth hem in maluesyn and grynde
hem and put hem in the oile aforsaide and put therto of þat wyne a
quart; and so lete the herbis rote in the oile with the maluesy a ix daies
or ellis more if thow myghtest; than anon do seeth al thiese in a double
glas over the fuyre and lete hem seth right wele til thei bien nygh con-
650 sumed, than clense it thurgh a faire newe canvas that is wide threded.
And whan this is clensed, make this powder: Rx *lignum aloes*, maces,
*carpobalsami, xilobalsami, calamy aromatici, nardi, cip[r]i, masticis, croci,
gariofili, mirre, galange, castore, cipressi ana* ʒ 5, [*calami*] *aromatici, storacis*, calmynt *ana* ʒ 5 & *s.*, *musci boni*, camphore, and thy muske and than
655 medle hem with oile ʒ 2 and of camphore ʒ 6, ambre ϶ 2; grynde this
camphory and thi muske and than medle hem with oile ʒ 2, but al the
oþer save thiese 3 (*id est*, camphore, muske, and storax) shal nat be put
into the oile til the spices be grounden and soden in þat oile in a glasen
vessel. And whan it [is] nygh cold put in the storax, but whan it is right
660 colde put in the camphore and muske and the ambre and do it vp, for
it is never the worse though it stonde on the [l]eis.[31]
  For this oile is goode for al maner of sike- **[fol. 117r]** nes that cometh,
namly of cold and specialy for the suffo[ca]cioun of the matrice; if it be
anoynted therwith withynfurþ or ellis coton iwete therin and vnderput,
665 it provokith the matrice and comfortith it. Also this oile is for þe cold-
nes of the stomac if it be anoynted therwith; and also for þe fevers tercian and quartan other cotidian that comen thurgh fleame natural if

---

639. make] take TS2S1Rs   oile muschilyng] *marg. ann. 1:* Medycyn Riall
653. castore cipressi] rasure cipressi S2S1Rs   calami] S2S1Rs, calamum T
654–657. musci boni . . . save thiese 3] musci boni camphore ʒ .vj. ambris ϶ .ij.
grynd thy (thyn Rs) camphore & than medle hem with oyle ʒ .ij. But all the to-
ther saue these thre S2S1Rs
659. is] S2S1Rs, *om.* T
661. leis] seis TS2S1Rs. *See Explanatory Note 31.*
663. suffocacioun] suffo- (*end of line*) cioun T
667. quartan other cotidian] *marg. ann. 1:* iiij^tien Feuer iij^cian cotidian

the pacient be anoynted therwith. And this oile, afore the [hour] of
his acces, anoynte wele his rige-bon, it [fornemeþe] the quakyng of the
670 feveres and moche more; if the pacient drynke ther[of] ℥ 1 with goode
fyne maluesyne ℥ 4 a ij houres afore his acces, it shal make that his acces
shal nat come. This oile is goode agenst colde palasie, cold rewmes, if
[the nape] of the neck be anoynted therwith; also this oile doeth away
al maner of aches that comen thurgh cold if thei bien anoynted ther-
675 with; also for al maner of colde gowtis it is goode to anoynt therwith
and colde dropesies and al suche other.

Also the rote of yres: vnderput it into the matrice other subfumed
with yres, makeþ hir to lessen hir chi[eld], for yres rotis bien hote and
drie and han vertu to open and to hete and to consume and wast; for
680 whan the womman is fieble and the chield may nat come oute, than it
is better that the chield be slayne than the moder of the chield die. And
also it bryngeth furth the ded chield mervously and the sccundync and
menstruat with his subfumygate.³² Or ellis takc *li. s.* of his rotis and of
savayne ℥ *s.* and seth hem in white wyne and do therto powder of pau-
685 lyni ℥ 12, hony ℥ 1, of that decoccioun quartern 1, bolis galle ℥ 1, and
make a pissary and yeve trocissis of murs³³ ℥ 2 with this decoccioun: Rx
ameos, woderof, percely seede, bawme, carui, anete, iris, mugwed *ana* ℥
1, white wyne *li.* 3; seeth hem, þan grynde saverey, isope, woderof, diptayne *ana* ℥ 1, temper it vp with ℥ 4 of the decoccioun.†

690 **The iiij chapiter is of the precipitacioun of the moder.**³⁴
The precipitacioun of the matrice is another sikenes whan the matrice
fallith from hir kyndely place. And that may be in ij maners: other asidc
or ellis donwarde. **[fol. 117v]** If it fallith aside, men may it knowe bi the

---

668. therwith. And this oile] with this oyle S2S1Rs   hour] houre S2, oure
S1Rs, hony T

669. fornemeþe] S2S1Rs, for the ne meye T

670. therof] S2, ther T

672. cold rewmes] *marg. ann. 1, using grey-brown ink*: Cold Humours; *marg. ann.
8:* Cold Humours

673. the nape] the nede S2S1Rs, ther neede T; *in S2 there is a supralineal correction by the main hand of* nede *to* nape

678. chield] chide T

682. ded chield] *marg. ann. 1:* Ded Child

683. his (1)] hit S2S1, hyt Rs

691. precipitacioun of the matrice] *marg. ann. 4, using rusty-colored ink*: precipitacioun of þe moder

692. place] *foll. by* into anoþer place S2S1Rs

greuaunce of the side; dounwarde, it may falle in ij maners: othe al oute
695 of the wombe or ellis nat fully out. If it fal nat fulliche out, they feelen
moche grevaunce above the share and aboute þe raynes; and if it go al
aboute, the wymmen may seene that hirsilf. This sikenes cometh oft of
witholdyng of bloode þat wymmen shuld have bien purged of, or ellis
of corrupt humours þat bien in the matrice that makith hir to fallen
700 adoun or aside, other the matrice fallith adoun out at the wombe for the
palasy þat the matrice hath caught thurgh cold in long sittyng on colde
stones or suche other wey, other thurgh longe abidyng in a colde bath,
other for moche drynkyng of colde water. And whan þe matrice hath
this palasy, she fallith doun out at the wombe withoute grevaunce, oth-
705 erwhiles the matrice fallith out for greuaunce that a womman [hath]
in beryng of chielde. And if this greuaunce com of witholdyng of hir
bloode other of corrupt humours þat bien in the matrice that thristeth
hir out of hir place, whether that thei bien hote or cold, thow myghtest
knowe bi the tokenes þat wern itold in the next chapiter;[35] and than the
710 sikenes is helid if the matrice be purged of the bloode that is wiþholden
or of the corrupt humours that bien withyn hir, as it was told bifore.

But if it come of the palasy of þe matrice, lete hir vse oximel that
was told bifore.[36] And afterwarde gyve hir *theodoricon empericon*; aftir-
ward on the thridde day make hir a stuphe of calamynt, of origanum,
715 of lavender, of sauge, of cressis, of prymeroses, of confery, and of rewe;
and whan she cometh from the stuphe, yeve hir triacle with wyne that
sauge is soden in; and þe next daie after, lete hir bleede at the veyne
vnder þe ancle. And make hir an oyntement of clotes and oile of notes
and wex ifried toguyder and iwrongen thurgh a cloth and sithen cast
720 theron powder of encence and mastik and with this anoynt hir from
the navil donward both bihynde and bifore.

Item, the oile of *ipie minoris* drunken with wyne clarre twies on
a day wil drawen vp the matrice; other ellis medle the juce of clotes
and **[fol. 118r]** *agrippa* toguydres over the fuyre and therwith anoynte
725 hir behynde and before from the navil dounward and ther above ley

---

694. of the side] *marg. ann. 1:* In the syde

704. grevaunce] *foll. by* oþer ache S2S1Rs

705. hath] S2S1Rs , *om.* T

713. theodoricon empericon] *marg. ann. 1:* Medicyn

720. encence] *marg. ann. 11, a much later hand writing very small print:* frankincense

722. oile of ipie minoris] jus of ipie minoris S2S1Rs; *marg. ann. 1:* Oyle of ipie;
marg. ann. 11, a much later hand writing very small print: Hiparici minoris

723. drawen] r *written over* a

the wull of a sheepe that is ishore vnwasshen; other anoynte hir above
the share and aboute the raynes with hote hony and theron strawe
the powder of mastik and of encens and of hertis hornes ibrent and of
coloph[on]ie, oþer of piche and the powder of cresses, and sithen hele
730 hir with asshis on that anoyntyng both bifore and behynde. And þe
same medicynes bien goode if it come for cause of cold humours that
bien withyn the matrice.

But if it come of hote humours, gyve a lectuary *de sucro rosarum* and
after that make hir a stuphe of cold herbis; and after lete hir bleede
735 at the vayne vnder the ancle and anoynt hir with cold oynementis and
with cold oiles. Other take as moche of hony as of oile and cast powder
of comyn to hem and seeþ hem toguyder, and afterwarde wete therin
wul of a sheepe that is nat wasshen other a blac felt and ley it from the
navil dounward and sumwhat above.

740 But if the matrice fal doun out of the wombe benethfurth at the
prevy membre, if it be whan she hath born chield, lete the mydwif put
it in ageyn with hir hande, but anoynte she hir hande first with oile and
sithen make hir a fumygacioun benethfurth of maythes other of drie
oxdirt cast on the coles, and lete hir smel wele savourde thynges.

745 Other if the matrice wil nat lightly be put in ageyn, seeth coost and
wormode and mugwede in water and do the womman in the water the
whiles it is warme vp to þe teatis and lete hir sitte therin a goode while.
Afterward whan she is come out of the wate[r], lete put the matrice
softly in ageyn and heve hir feete and hir legges hier than hir hede,
750 liggyng so ix houres of the day, that the matrice may go into hir kyndely place. And whan the matrice is in, take the powder of thiese thynges:
of galle muste, of notemuges, of spikenard, of clowes, and powder hem
all toguyder and temper þat powder with oile of puliol and do that into
a smal lynen bagge of smal and of soft cloth, and make it of the shappe
755 of [fol. 118v] an evenlong balle after the shappe of an egge and put
that balle into the prevy membre and lete the matrice that she falle nat
out ageynwarde and bynde it with a swetheles aboute hir raynes that it
fal nat out ageyn.

But or thow bynde the swetheles, make a plaster aboute hir raynes
760 of the powder of ker-seede and of bay and of lorel, of comyn and of

---

729. colophonie] S2S1Rs , colophie T

731. humours] *foll. by* gyve hir a lectuary, *canc.*

741. whan she hath born chield] *marg. ann. 1:* a sp[ec]iall medicin for a woman new delyuered

759. plaster] *marg. ann. 1:* Plaster

wield myntis; hette in a vessel over the fuyre and sithen medle it with
hony and lete hem ligge thus ix daies; and in þe meane tyme lete hir
dieten hir with metis and with drynkes that she have no neede to go
oft-sithes to the prevy chambre ne to mak water.[37]

765   Otherwhiles sum wymmen han so grete penaunce in beryng of a
chield that the skyn that is betwixt the ij prevy membres brekith ato
and al is an [hole] and so the matrice fallith over and out therat and
wexith harde. To help wymmen of this myschief, first seeth butter and
wyne toguyder half an houre and al warme lete legge it to þe matrice
770 and softly tawen it with that wyne a goode while to make the matrice
nesshe; and sithen put it in softly ageyne and sowe toguyder that peece
that is tobroken with a silken threde with a quarel nedil in iij placis or
in iiij, and sithen do p[i]cche on a soft lynnen cloth and ley it to the
prevy member and the stenche of that piche shal make hir to drawe
775 inwarde to hir owne place. Afterwarde make powder of the rote of
confery and of canel, and straw that in the sore for-to it be hole; and
lete hir liggen, as I saide rather, a vij or a ix daies and lete hir ete and
drynke in that while but litel, and kepe hem wele from cold and from
metis and drynkes that myght make hir to any cowgh.

780   And for to kepe wymmen from this myschief in that tyme that
thei trauailen of chield, lete make a rounde thyng of the shappe of an
egge of smal lynnen cloth and put it in hir fundament [& euery tyme
of chield & euery suche tyme lete þrist þat balle in hir fundament] and
that shal have the skyn hole from brekyng.[38]

785   ††But in the precipitacioun of the matrice vi thynges bien nedeful.
The first is ventusyng and that in iij stides: The first is a litel vnder
the navil, but **Lilie** seith[39] that it shuld be don on the teatis, and on
either half the sides of the **[fol. 119r]** womman, and that is don for the
matrice shuld arise vp into hir owne stide ageyn.

---

767. hole] S2S1Rs, hote T   over and] *om.* S2S1Rs

768. To help wymmen] *marg. ann. 1:* A medicyn Riall For wemen

769–770. legge it to þe matrice and softly tawen it] legge it to þe moder & softely handel þe moder & softely tawen it S2S1Rs

773. picche] pacche T; *marg. ann. (a much later hand, writing small):* pitche, *corresponding to* pacche *in text, underlined by (this?) later hand*

780. And for to kepe wymmen] *marg. ann. 1:* N[ota]

782–783. & euery tyme of chield & euery suche tyme lete þrist þat balle in hir
fundament] S2S1Rs; *om.* T

785. precipitacioun] *marg. ann. 1:* precipitacioun

788. the (2)] *catchword by main scribe:* womman

790　　The secunde thyng is subfumygacioun and that is with an instrument that is clepid *emboton* and it is made thus: take a litel erthen pot,
the whiche the womman shal sitte on a siege with an hole on that siege,
and in that litel pot shal fuyre of coles be put in and that is shitte
aboute with clothis. But *embotus*, [*id est*] a litel pipe, shal be on that oon
795　end of that potte and þe womman shuld nyme the smoke bi that instrument so that the instrument shal entre into that prevy membre of the
womman and the powder shal be put into the colis vnder the womman.
Take turmentil, acasie, the rotes of bistorte, *serepinum ana* ʒ 3, psidie,
balaustie *ana* ʒ 2 & *s.*, *galange, nucis cipressi, foliorum galbani*, myrte *ana* ʒ
800　5; make powder. Cause is whi, this powder is made of stynkyng spices
and stiptik, [f]or stynke makith the matrice to arise into hir place; but
be ware that non of that stynche come to the wommans nose, but she
shal hold sum thyng that is of swete smel at hir nose. And this shal be
don the whiles that the ventusyng buystes bien on the wombe.
805　　And **Avicen** 3ᶜ:⁴⁰ a bath is goode in thiese needis. Take rede rose
levis ʒ 2, myrte, the rotis of moleyn *ana m.* 2, turmentil, rotis of [bis-
torte], antere, mastik, olibany *ana* ʒ 4, asafetida ʒ 4, mugwede drie,
lauendre drie *ana* ʒ 2; bete al thiese in a morter and put hem in a poket
and seeth it in a litel raspaice, and this bagge be it draynt in the bath
810　wiþ smythes water, and this is goode for it is made of stynkyng and of
stiptik thynges.
　　Also the iiij askith to have an oynement to anoynt with the mowth
of the privitees and the parties of hir reynes and is this: take a *li.* of
myrtil, oile of lilie, oile of mastik *ana* ʒ 6, asafetida, rotis of bistorte,
815　turmentil *ana* ʒ 3, *cere* ʒ 3.
　　Þe 5 also suppository is made thus: Rx assafetida ʒ 1, *masticis,
olibani*, seedis of myrtil, *galange, nucis cipressi ana* ʒ 1; make powder and
temper it vp with myrtil and make a suppository.

---

794. id est] S2S1Rs, in T　　oon] ouer S2S1Rs

797. vnder the womman] *marg. ann. 1:* Medecyn for Wemen

798. psidie] persidie S2S1Rs

801. for] S2S1Rs, stor T

805. And Avicen 3ᶜ] And saith Avicen 3º also S2S1Rs　　a bath] *marg. ann. 1:*
A bathe

806–807. bistorte] bistorte Rs, historte TS2S1

813–814. a li. of myrtil] olei myrtil S2S1Rs

814. oile of lilie oile of mastik] *marg. ann. 1:* Oiles; of myrtill a*dded by ann. 4,
using rusty-colored ink*

The vj is that a plaster be ordeyned on the prevy membre lest the
820 matrice falle ageyn, and that plaster shal be þe quantite of a pawme
of the hande and may be made thus: take mastik ℥ 4, *olibani* ℥ *s.*, *nucis*
cipressi, gallarum, myrtil *ana* ℥ 1, **[fol. 119v]** psidie, balaustie *ana s.*, terbentyne ℥ 1; make powder of al tho that may be made powder and tem-
per it vp with oile of rosis and make therof an emplaster and in breede
825 of vj fyngres mele, in length of viij or ix fynger mele, and make the
plaster thynne.

Also make the womman to spewe moche, for it is on of the best þat
may be don therto; also nyme heede that al maner stynkyng thynges in
this cause shuln bien put benethfurth and al maner of swete smellyng
830 thynges to the nose in this cause.†

The v chapitre is of the wynde of the matrice.
Moche wynde ther is also in the matrice that growith in wymen ful moche
and that cometh otherwhile from without, otherwhile from within, that
makith the matrice to ake and to swelle. And the tokenes of suche bien
835 swellyng and moche hurlyng and noise withynfurth and gnawyng of
þe wynde withyn the matrice. And for this sikenes, hem is goode to
vsen electuaries that wil consumen and distroien wyndes. And suche
electuaries bien diaciminum, dianisum, diaspermaton; and other þinges
of light cost[41] wil distroie suche wyndes, as comyn, anete, anise, fenel
840 seede, carui, *apij,* loveache, cres-seede, peritory both emplastred without and within.

Also in maner of medicyne a plaster made of comyn and of soote
soden toguyder in water: wasshe hir wombe therwith wele doun to the

---

820. plaster] *marg. ann. 1:* Plastere
822. gallarum] galange S1 (*glossed as* gallaronni *by a 16th-c. annotator*)   psi-
die] persidie S2S1Rs
825. fynger] r *written over* s, *poss. intended as* fyngers
826. plaster] *marg. ann. 1:* Plastere
828. stynkyng thynges] *marg. ann. 1:* Stynkyng thynges
832. Moche wynde . . . in the matrice] *marg. ann. 1:* Muche wynd; in þe Matrice *added by ann. 4, using rusty-colored ink*   growith in wymen] grevith wom-
en S2S1Rs
834. suche] suche wynde S2S1Rs
838. electuaries] *marg. ann. 1:* lectuaries
839. as comyn] *marg. ann. 1:* Medicyne
842. plaster] *marg. ann. 1:* Plaster

prevy membre; and also laide to the wombe hote is right profitable
845 agenst the wynde over [all.

Oþer] lete hir bath hir in water wher hockis and peritory bien
soden in and wassh wele hir wombe with the herbis. And whan she
cometh out of the bath, lete hir have a plaster of peritory al warme as
she may suffre and ley it to hir bely. Other lete seeth savayne and rapis
850 in watir and with that water wasshe hir wombe wele downe to the prevy
membre, and this also is profitable.

Other medicynes ther bien that bien goode for stiches and for
wyndes in a mannes body and in his guttis bien goode for this sikenes,
as a plaster made of culver dirt soden in wyne other the wyne idrunke.
855 Other take hote sheepes dirt and stamp it in a morter with gotes mylke
and afterwarde lete cast therto a litel quantite of piche and seeth hem
wele to- **[fol. 120r]** guyder and sithen plaster it vp in a pece of lethir and
ley it warme to the wombe; other take the erth that is tofore a beestis mangier that is totrode with the beestis feete and beperisshed, and
860 heete that erth wele agenst the fuyre and ley it there-as the grevaunce
is, and make hir to absteyne hir from metis þat bien wyndy, as bien
pesen and beanes and fecches and rawe fruytes and rawe herbis.

††Also for the wynde in the matrice, take powder of comyn, of
anete, of galangale, of zedewale, of carui *ana* ʒ 3, spikenard, canel,
865 cokil *ana* ʒ 1, castory ʒ s., hony ʒ 3, terbentyne ʒ 1: make a suppositorie
of al thiese thynges aforsaide and put it into the prevy membre and it
shal consume al maner of wyndes and foule retenciounis of þe matrice
and al stynches. Also levis of nettil igrounde and vnderput, anon it
makith fallyng wymmen to risen holl. Also ivy grounde and soden with
870 the grece of hennes or of gandres and hote laide bifore and behynde,
anon it helith. Also nettil seede with wyne drunke fordoeth swellyng
of wynde. Also doeþ 15 graynes of piony in wyne and drunke: fordoth
suffocacioun of the matrice and helpith that sorowe. Also drastis of oile
ihet and with oile put to fordoeth al the swellyng of the matrice. Also so

---

845–846. all. Oþer] S2S1Rs, *om.* T

848. plaster] *marg. ann. 1:* Plastere

852. stiches] *marg. ann. 1:* Stiches

858. that is] that is that is T

863. wynde in the matrice] *marg. ann. 1:* Wynd; In Wemen *added later, poss. by* ann. 1

865. make a suppositorie] *marg. ann. 1:* Medycine

868. Also levis . . . vnderput] *marg. ann. 1:* N[ota]

874. swellyng] *marg. ann. 1:* Swellyng

875 doeth terbentyne, so doeth fomentacioun *origani* and p[essa]ried, and
so doeth savayne and so do b[i]tter almaundis iclensed and grounde
and put in: bryngeth furth al [inster]⁴² and al the corrupt humours of
the body. And so doeth aristologia with hony and put in. Also myrre
idrunke with the juce of archimesie doeth merveilous. So doeth saturey
880 put in: bryngeth furth ded chield.⁴³

  Of to moche flux: make a suppository of gotis dunge with the juce
of sanguinary and put vnder; staunchiþ al bloody flux. So doeth a bath
of plantayne, of the myddil ryndes of an oke, *virga pastoris*, sanguinarie,
and suche other. Ipericon idrunke staunchith flux of the wombe.

885   For the woo after the birth: take yolkis of eyren soden in water and
grounde *cera & oleo & succo archimesie et cimino* powdred and make an
emplaster bifore and behynde and anon the penaunce shal cease.

  And also if she have fevors, take oynons soden in water and grounde
with **[fol. 120v]** yolkes of eyren soden in water with oile and powder of
890 comyn and make an emplaster.†

[The vi chapitre]
A dropesie of the matrice cometh otherwhiles of witholdyng of bloode
that a womman shuld be purged of, and than she may nought be helid
but she be purged of that bloode. Otherwhiles it comyth of wynde and
895 of fleamatik humours that bien in the matrice, and than a womman
swellith with this dropesie as though she were with chielde.

  <Tokenes of chield> And ther bien many dyvers tokenes to knowe
oon from another, for this swellyng cometh sodainly, the other dropesies don nat so; this swellyng comeþ otherwhiles and otherwhiles vanys-
900 shith away, but th'ooþer abidith alway to a woman be delivered of a
chield. This walkith from place to place, and th'oother don nat so. Also

---

875. pessaried] S1Rs, pressaried S2, pressoried T
876. bitter] S2S1Rs, better T
877. inster] S2Rs; inste S1; *om.* T. *See Explanatory Note 42.*
880. ded chield] *marg. ann. 1:* Ded Child
881. gotis] gosty gotis TS2S1Rs
882. bloody flux] *marg. ann. 1:* flux
884. flux of the wombe] *marg. ann. 1:* flux of þe wombe
887. emplaster] *marg. ann. 1:* Plastere
891. The vi chapitre] *blank line* S2S1Rs, *partial blank line* T
892. dropesie of the matrice] *marg. ann. 1:* Dropecy of þe Matrice
897. Tokenes of chield] TS2 (*marg.*), *om.* S1Rs; *marg. ann. 1:* N[ota]
898. swellyng] *marg. ann. 1:* Swellynges
901. walkith] *marg. drawing of pointing hand added by ?some later hand, and in the text, underlining of* this walkith from place to place

this hath vncertayne moevyng, but th'oother moeven certainly and at
certayne tymes both in the day and also in the nyght. But the idropesie
of the matrice moevyng and stiryng is oft-sithes bi nyght and sielden
905 bi day.

Also in dropesie of the matrice, the chekes bien nessh and soft
and fiebliche colourd, but wymmen with chield bien otherwhiles wele
icoloured and their chekis hard. And ther is a grete difference also
betwene the dropesie of the matrice and the wyndynesse of the matrice,
910 for wyndes wil lightly vanyssh away, the dropesy wil nat so. Also wyndes
bien otherwhile in that oon side of the matrice and otherwhile in that
other side, but idropesie occupieth al the matrice. Also wyndes bien
evermore withyn the matrice and they may be without grete fieblenes
of the matrice, that it ne is nat myghty to defie the fleamatike humours
915 that bien withyn hir and she may nat put hem away from her.

Cura. For to help the matrice of this sikenes, it behovith that the
matrice be purged of the humours that bien withyn hir and that hath
be tolde here biforne,[44] both in the precipitacioun of the matrice and
also in witholdyng of the bloode. Natheles make hir a stuphe of tyme,
920 of calamynt, of origanum, of saverey, of lavendre, of rewe, of puliol roial
and mountayne, of mugwede, of lorel levis and the croppes of henbane,
of comyn, **[fol. 121r]** carui, of sm[a]lache, loveache, chervoile, percely,
stanmarche, of everiche an handful; lete seeth hem in water and do stuphe hir in þat seeþing of tho herbis also long as she may; and whan she
925 goeth out of the stuphe, ley the herbis to the matrice.

A goode suppositorie to purge the matrice of suche fleamatik
humours: take þe flour of cokil and medle it with hony and oile and
make it sadde as past is that brede is made of, and wynde it in a soft lynnen cloth and put it in hir prevy membre, but tie it a yerde aboute hir
930 thies lest the matrice drawe it in al to hir, and lete it lye ther al a nyght
and lenger if it be neede. ††But first make a plaster of leekis grounde
and fried in hir owne juce and ley it from hir navil dounward to hir
prevy membre and over it; on the morow,† if the matrice smert withynfurth of the sharpnes of the cokil, anoynt it with oile of rosis other of

---

906. dropesie] *marg. ann. 1:* Dropesi
907. wymmen with chield] *marg. ann. 1:* Wemen with Child
910. wyndes] *marg. ann. 1:* Wyndes
916. Cura] *marg. ann. 1:* Medecynes
922. smalache] smallache S2S1, smalage Rs, smlache T
926. suppositorie] *marg. ann. 1:* Suppositorie
929. a yerde] with a threde S2S1Rs
931. plaster] *marg. ann. 1:* Plastere

935 violet [and with þe muscillage of dragantum made with þe juce of vio-
let] and with the white of an ey and medle hem toguyder and anoynt
the place therwith til it be hole.

††And ther was a womman in London and had this idropesy and
she was holden vncurable thurgh al the lechis in that Citie of London,
940 but the womman toke and made hir wortis with thiese herbis þurgh hir
owne wit: she toke cresses an handful, of sowth thistil and southistils
of the fen, of wielde sauge, of percely, of betayne, of mylfoile, of gooldis, of everiche the vj part of an handful, and made hir wortis and ete
herof al grene as moche as ever she myght susteyne and kept hir from al
945 drynkes save from thiese wortis, that she ete of hem agenst nyght ix or
x tymes in the day in stide of drynk. And she must algatis [drynk], she
drank this tysan: she toke a dissh ful of barly, of wormode, of rotis of
stanmarche, of percely, anise seede, of fenel, of goldes, ambrose, sowthistil, and of scarliol *ana li.* 1 and seeþ al thiese in iij galons of cliere water
950 til the halfuendel was consumed away, and herof she drank erly and
late. And she lete garcen hir legges overal agenst the fuyre and after
she laide to hir legges levis of clotis, and so she had after þat wrapped
hir legges in the clote levis and it drowe out al þat myschief. And she
bathed hir prevy membre with the juce of **[fol. 121v]** puliol roial and
955 with origanum and mugwede with a pipe, and þeron was a bladder and
she lete powre the juces into hir wombe bi hir prevy membre. And she
made a plaster of diptayne, of isope, of saverey, and leide it to hir prevy
shap withoutefurth and this plaster brought furth hir prevy termes,
and with thiese medicynes she was made hole. The brede that she ete
960 was this: a pecke of beane mele and dide do knede it with vynegre and
lete bake it and ete of that brede in hir potage abovesaide; and she
wissh hir body aboute the liver with the juce of elfhame.†

The vij chapiter is of rawnesse that whan the matrice semyth flayne.
The matrice semyth oft flayne and raw as a thyng that were forscalded,
965 that is whan kene coleryk humours chaffith and brenneth aboute the

---

935–936. and with . . . þe juce of violet] S2S1Rs; *om.* T

939. vncurable] incurable S2S1Rs   Citie] towne S2S1Rs

940. wortis] *marg. ann. 1:* Wortis

946. And] & yf S2S1Rs   drynk] S2S1Rs, *om. (at end of line)* T

947. tysan] *marg. ann. 1:* Tyssan

950. was] was was T

957. plaster] *marg. ann. 1:* Plastere

959. brede] *marg. ann. 1:* Bred

964. flayne and raw] *marg. ann. 1:* Rawnes & Flayn within þe Matrice

matrice withynfurth; and þe signes and the tokenes herof bien brennyng and prikyng withinfurth, and otherwhiles the matrice is forblayned
and scabbed wiþinfurth of suche humours and than she shal feele
moche ichyng withynfurth.

970   **Cura.** To hele theym of this greuaunce, lete purgen hem with the
electuary of *succo rosarum* and sithen lete make hir a stuphe of colde
herbis and afterwarde lete hir bleede on the vayne vnder the ancle
withynfurth of the foote. And afterwarde lete tempre licium with kow
mylke and cast it into the matrice with a pissarie, as men don purge a
975 mannes wombe with a glister thurgh his fundament and lete cast it in at
oon tyme the quantite of a *li.*, and lete hir vse this the thridde day that
I vnderstonde from thre daies to thre daies for-to she be hole. Anoþer
powder: take of the seede of white popie and gumme arabik and dragance and spodie *ana* ʒ 1, powder hem with rayne water and make
980 rounde ballis of hem and whan it nedith, medle hem with cow mylke
and late vnderfonge therwith of a pissarie at hir prevy membre. Also
anoynt it withynfurth with the mary of a calf other with fressh butter
other with sum other such fresh thynge. And in clensyng of the matrice
for corrupt humours, be ware ther come no violent thyng in hir, lest
985 thow make the womman barayne forever, but vse thiese thynges in pissaries **[fol. 122r]** that maken comfort to the matrice.

        ††And if the womman be poore, than seeth moleyne and the barke
of sloue trees in tan-water and whan thei bien wele soden, lete hir sitte
therin vp to the navil and whan þat she is wery, reise hir from that
990 bath and make hir this smokyng: take rose levis, clowes, frankencense,
myrre *ana* ʒ 1 and bruse hem toguyder and whan al this is do, than
cast that powder on smale coles, and lete hir sitte a while therover; or
ellis take mastik ʒ 1, bole armoniak, *terra sigillata*, wormeton, powder
of oke tree that no lyme comyth nygh, sandragon *ana* ʒ 1, *litargij aurei* ʒ
995 2: powder al thiese right smal and lete a prevy womman cast it þer that
the rawnesse is, and this powder shal hele it, &c.†

966–967. brennyng and prikyng] *marg. ann. 1:* Burnyng & prikkyng

967. and prikyng withinfurth] and prikkinges & smertinges withynforth S2S1,
& smertyng & prykyng withynforth Rs

970. Cura] *marg. ann. 1:* Cura

977–978. Anoþer powder] *marg. ann. 1:* Powder

983. clensyng of the matrice] *marg. ann. 1:* Clensyng; of women *added by ann.
4, using rusty-colored ink*

986. maken comfort to the matrice] mowe comfort þe moder S2S1Rs

996. powder] *marg. ann. 1:* A powdere

The viij chapiter is of aposteme of the matrice that is ful sore.
Apostem of the matrice cometh in dyvers parties of the matrice, and
otherwhile in the mowth of the matrice and otherwhile in the most
1000 inner partie of the matrice. If it be clene in the depnes of the matrice,
she feelith ache from the mydrif to the prevy membre, and hir sides
swellen and thei han greuaunce to brethen and to drawe wynde also;
but the grettest greuaunce that thei han is aboute their share and their
raynes. And þis empostem cometh otherwhile of hote humours and
1005 otherwhiles of cold. If it is of bloode, ther is ache and prikyng ther as
the matier of the apostem is engendred toguyder[45] and thei han contynuauly an contynual fever but nat to strong; and the veynes of the legges
swellen, hir vryne is cliere rede and otherwhiles dym rede, and a maner
of swart rede above vnder the sercle. If it be of coler, that is an hote
1010 humour and drye, she hath thiese forsaide tokenes, but thei bien more
violent than bien bloody tokenes, ††the vryne is moche thynne, ful
citryne, the pownce right swift, the maladie in the right side for þe gal
wher is dominioun stant.† If it is a cold humour and a moiste, she feelith both grevaunce and hevynes in the matrice and hir vryne is troubly
1015 and fiebly coulourd and of the colour of asshen vnder the sercle.[46] If it be
of malencoly, that is a cold humour and a drie, she hath moche hevynes
in the matrice and the vaynes of hir legges bien of swart yalow colour
of lede,[47] and thei fallen in an easy fever. But **[fol. 122v]** whan ther is
apostem in the matrice and the vryne is white and thynne, that is a fie-
1020 ble signe. For to help of that sikenes: first lete hym bleede at the veyne
vnder the ancle, and afterward in the firste bigynnyng of th'empostem,
thow must vse colde plasters that bien repercussyves to dryve the mat-
iers ageynward, as, make a plaster of the inmost pillyng of hemp and
of the juce of pety morel warmed and lay that to th'emposteme a twies

---

998. Apostem of the matrice] *marg. ann. 1:* Apostem in þe Matrice
998–1000. parties of the matrice . . . partie of the matrice] parties of the moder other whyles in þe innermest (nyghness Rs) partye of the moder & oþerwhiles in the mouthe of the moder S2S1Rs
1006. engendred toguyder] genderd togedre S2S1Rs
1008. rede (1)] *marg. ann. 1:* Vren Red
1012. citryne] *marg. ann. 1:* vren Sitrine
1015. asshen] *marg. ann. 1:* vren lik ashen
1019. white] *marg. ann. 1:* vren white
1020. signe] *marg. ann. 1:* Apostume   bleede] *marg. ann. 1:* Bledyng
1022. colde plasters] *marg. ann. 1:* Cold plastures
1024. lay that to th'emposteme] *marg. ann. 1:* Cura

1025 or a thries and remoeve it in the day; also anoynt the wombe ageyn
th'emposteme with oile of roses other of violet. And if th'empostem
be of heete oþer of hote humours, lete hir ete cold herbis, as pertulake, letuze, and endyve and suche other and drynk the water that is
distilled of suche herbis. Afterward than whan th'emposteme is fully
1030 waxen, make emplaster to make it to wex and to ripe and nesshe to
breke, as is a plaster that is made of whete mele soden in oile other
in fressh butter and a litel water; other make a plaster of mele of lynseede other of fenygreke medeled with lye, but lete nat that lye be to
stronge, other medle suche strong lye with barly mele and make therof
1035 a plaster. ††Other take oile comune, soure dough, fressh butter other
gre[c]e, juce of mersh *ana* ʒ 2, lyneseede, fenygreke *ana* ʒ 1 & *s*., bismalow isperate ʒ 3, water of snailes ʒ *s*.; seeth al thiese toguyder. *Probatum est.*†

But if th'emposteme come of cold humours, gyve hir the suripe that
1040 is made of fenel rotes, of perccly and of mersh with their seedis and of
dauke and of carui, raddissh, *enula campana, zuccara* water and hony as
moche as nedith. And in the begynnyng also of this empostym, make
hir emplastres of origanum, of isope, of centory, of rue, and of celidoyne *ana* ʒ 1 soden in wyne other in water and lay to al warme. After
1045 whan the apostem is ful woxen, make emplasters to make th'empostem
ripe. Oon is this: take whete mele and oile of olive and hony and make
therof a plaster. Another: make a plaster of snailes soden in hony with
whete mele other with mclc made of lynseede; other make a plaster of
the rotis of affadil stamped and reisons and figges that bien drie soden
1050 with wyne, hony, and oile; [oþer make a plaster of soure dough soden
in oile, oþer a plaster of rewe soden with wyne & with oile], other of fenel
seede other of mersh other of rewe istamped and soden in oile. And lete
anoynte hir with hote oynementis, as with **[fol. 123r]** dewte and with
marciaton. Other thynges ther bien ful goode to make th'emposteme
1055 ripe, as the gres of hennes and of ganders and the mary of an hert other

---

1025. remoeve it in the day] remove it aday S1Rs, remeue a day S2

1028. drynk the water] *marg. ann. 1:* Waters to be dronk & Cold waters

1031. plaster] *marg. ann. 1:* A plastere

1036. grece] grete T

1037–1038. Probatum est] *marg. ann. 1:* Probatum est

1045. apostem] *marg. ann. 1:* postum   emplasters] *marg. ann. 1:* A plastere

1046. olive and hony] violet & hony S2S1Rs

1050–1051. oþer make a plaster of soure dough soden in oile oþer a plaster of
rewe soden with wyne & with oile] S2S1Rs; *om.* T

of a calf and rede wex and oile of roses and wommans mylke and the white of an ey: þei bien goode to plaster withouten and bien profitable also to be resceived withynfurth a pissory at the prevy membre.

1060 And whan th'empostem is tobroken, thow shalt knowe it bi the quitour and the corrupcioun that cometh away therfrom: take than meth and warme it ʒ 12, and do therto ʒ 7 of clene hony, and lete hir receive therof the quantite of ʒ 16 þurʒ a pissary to make the matrice clene; other take th'oother medicynes that weren itold in the next chapitre.[48]

The ix chapitre is of akyng of the matrice.

1065 Ache of the matrice cometh other of a ded born chield þat is born rather than his tyme, wherfor the moder[49] hath a grete likyng and a grete comfort of the chield that is wiþin hir, and whan she lesith it, she makith a kyndly mornyng and sorowyng, right as a cow doeth whan she hath lost hir calf; and that sorowyng is ache of the matrice. And other-
1070 while the matrice akith for cold, and otherwhile for heete, but that is but sielden. If it be of cold, ther is ache and prickyng in the lift side and other tokens that hat[h] bien told before;[50] and herfor take puliol roial, origanum, lorel levis, calamynt, and hockes and seth hem in water and in wyne, and therwith wassh hir wombe from the navil dounward to
1075 hir prevy membre; sithen take clowes, spikenard, notemuges, galingale and make hir a fumygacioun bynethfurth. ††Or ellis take myrre, olibanum, origanum, calamynt, cipresse, anyse and make fumigacioun; take laudanum for fumygacioun.† Other thynges also that I have told here-biforne bien goode for the ache of the matrice, whether it be of
1080 cold other of heete.[51]

But for the ache of þe matrice that cometh afterward that a womman hath born a chield, take rewe and mugwede and wormode *ana m.* 1, camphory ʒ 2, stampe hem and powder the camphory and seeth hem in oile of puliol and heete it wele agenst the fuyre and wrap it in a cloth
1085 **[fol. 123v]** from the navil dounward.

1058. pissory] *marg. ann. 1:* A pissarij

1061. 12] xxij S2S1Rs

1065–1066. ded born chield . . . his tyme] *marg. ann. 1:* Childeren borne or theyre Tyme & is Dede

1076. fumygacioun] *marg. ann. 1:* Fumygacioun

1079. ache of the matrice] *marg. ann. 1:* Ache in þe Matrice

1082. hath born a chield] *marg. ann. 1:* Aftere a womman be delyuerd

Also for ache that cometh of hardenesse of the matrice, take saxifrage and groundeswilly and of old caule and mugwede and hockis
and betayne and seeth hem wele in water and lete the womman sitte
in that water vp to the teatis; and whan she cometh out therof, make
1090 a plaster of hockes, of wormode, and of camphory stamped toguyder
with oile of puliol other of lorel and seeth hem on the fuyre and ley it
on the matrice. For the same, take the levis of the herbe þat is clepid
bawme *m.* 1, wormode, hockes *ana m. s.*, grynde hem with a litel white
wyne and oile de baye and hete it and ley it on, as is beforesaide. Other-
1095 whiles whan the womman is delivered of chield, the matrice walkith in
the wombe from oon place to another and akith, for also moche as she
is sodainly empted of the chield and made hir ful before. And for this
sikenesse take the croppis of ellern and stamp hem and wryng out the
juce, and ther with eyren and with whete mele make hir thynne cakes
1100 and frye hem so in fressh grese and that shall cease the ache. And gyve
hir warme wyne to drynke that comyn was soden in.

**††If thow wilt knowe wele and triewly whether a womman
be with chield other nat withouten lookyng of hir water.**[52]
Iff a womman be with chield, take hir to drynke meth whan she shal
1105 go to bedde, and if she have moche woo in hir wombe, it is a signe that
she is with chield. Also if the troscisses of the myrre, as Rasis [saith],[53]
with water that *juniperij* is soden in and after that thei bien idronke, if
she be with retencioun of hi[r] [floures] than is there right grete sorow
folowyng, and also thei casten out a ded chield and the cause is for the
1110 trocisses maken subtile and vi|sc|ous matier. Also thei open and thei
beten the matrice, and also thei strengthen the vertu expulsief and

---

1086. hardenesse of the matrice] *marg. ann. 1:* Ache of hardnesse of þe Matrice

1086–1087. take saxifrage] *marg. ann. 1:* Cura

1090. plaster] *marg. ann. 1:* A plastere

1093. 1] ii S2S1Rs

1095–1096. walkith in the wombe] *marg. ann. 1:* A walkyng in A womanis
wombe after she be deliuerd

1097–1098. for this sikenesse] *marg. ann. 1:* Cura

1104. Iff a womman be with chield] *marg. ann. 1:* To know yf A woman be with
child

1105. go] wende S2S1Rs

1106. saith] S2S1Rs, seeth T

1108. floures] S2S1Rs, figures T

1110. viscous] S2S1Rs, vicious T

therfor þei bien goode. Also the thynges that shal casten oute a ded
chield fro the matrice, thei must be myghtier than thoo that helpen to
have easy birth.[54] The thynges that helpen to have furth a ded chield
1115   from the matrice bien iij thynges: the first is galbanum **[fol. 124r]** ʒ 2,
resolued in gotis mylke that the womman may vse easily a 2 ʒ of the
mylke other 3.

The secunde [is] to make a suppository thus: Rx [*elleboris*] *nigri*,
stafisacre, *aristolochia rotunda*, [bothon], morien, *granorum lauriole, pulpe*
1120   *coloquintide, gummi aromatici ana* ʒ 2, *fel bouis* ʒ 1, make powder (saue of
gummi aromatici); resolue y[t] in iuce arthemesie with the whiche medle
al thiese powders and make a suppository; or ellis with more *fel bouis*
and of the iuce of arthemesie make a pissarie with a litel oile.

Also a plaster that castith out a ded chield from the matrice; oon
1125   therof is this: take galbanum *li. s.*, temper it with the iuce of mugwede
and ley it in a lether in quantite of a pawme and ij fyngres more in
length, in breede of a litel pawme, and ley it vnder the navil toward
the prevy membre. Another, take the iuce of rewe *li. s.*, myrre powdred ʒ 4, powder of colloquintide ʒ 3, and encorpore hem toguyder in
1130   a nessh manere, make a plaster and warme ley it to vnder the navil on
the wombe.

Also to have easy birþ of the chield, take ʒ 6 of barke of *cassy fistule*
and drynke it wiþ wyne other with the broth of rede chiches. Another,
take asorie, castory *ana* ʒ 2, subtily powderd, and yeve it with decoc-
1135   cioun of rede chiches.

The iij is as Avicen saith:[55] take myrre, castory, *storacis*, calamynt
ana ʒ *s.*, inward barke of canel ichosen, savayne *ana* ʒ *s.*, make powder
and gyve it hir whan she travailith of chielde with a litel hony and it helpith moche to delivere the chield and the secundyne.

1140   Anoþer thyng is necessarie, that is that hir knees bien bounden
to hir navil and that she be put in a short place; and than gyve hir
vomytis for it helpith moche. Also take egremoyne with his rotis and
ley the rotis toward the matrice and whan she chieldith do it awey lest

---

1112–1113. casten oute a ded chield] *marg. ann. 1:* To cast out a ded Childe

1118. is] S2S1Rs, *om.* T   suppository] *marg. ann. 1:* Supositorie   elleboris]
ell'is Rs, oll'is S1S2, all'is T

1119. bothon] bothor S2S1Rs, bother T

1121. yt] it S2S1Rs, ye T

1123. pissarie] *marg. ann. 1:* A pissarie

1124. a plaster that . . . ded chield] *marg. ann. 1:* A plastere to be delyuerd of
A ded Child

1142. vomytis] *marg. ann. 1:* vomytis   Also take egremoyne] *marg. ann. 1:* Cura

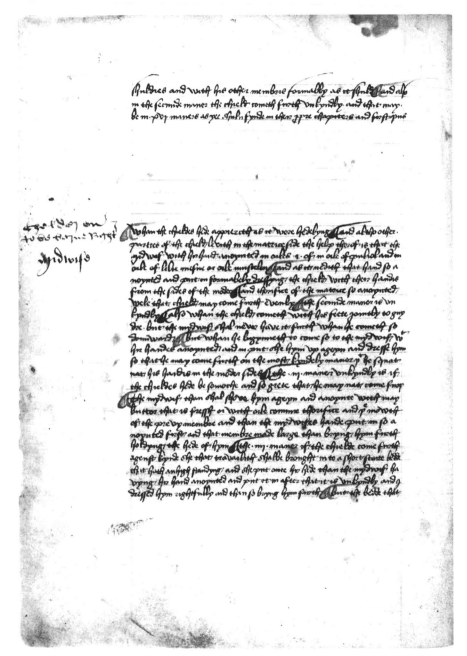

Plate 2. *The Sickness of Women 2*, chap. 10: Fetal presentation types 1-4, with blank space left for fetus-in-utero drawings (compare drawings in British Library, Sloane MS 249, plate 3a below). Cambridge, Trinity College, MS R.14.52, fol. 124v. By permission of the Master and Fellows of Trinity College, Cambridge.

the matrice folowe. And this experyment, tellen al þe doctours, if God
1145 wil it helpith moche to have chield.†

**The x chapitre is of the grevaunce that wymmen han
in beryng of theire chieldren.**[56]

††Greuaunces that wymmen han in beryng of their chieldren cometh
in ij maners, that is to say, kyndely and vnkyndely. Whan it is kyndely,
1150 the chield cometh furth withyn a xx throwes or withyn a xij throwes
and the chield cometh furth as it shulde, first the hede and sithen the
necke and with the armes and þe **[fol. 124v]** shuldres and with his
other membris formably as it shuld. And also in the secunde maner the
chield cometh furth vnkyndly and that may be in xvj maners, as yee
1155 shuln fynde in their propre chapiters and first þus:

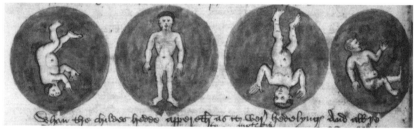

Plate 3a. Fetus-in-utero illustrations for *The Sickness of Women 2*, chap. 10 (figures 1-4), from London, British Library, Sloane MS 249, fol. 196v. By permission of The British Library. Cf. blank space left in TCC R.14.52, fol. 124v
(plate 2 above).

Whan the chieldes hede appierith, as it were hedelyng, and al tho
other parties of the chield levith in the matrice side, the help therof is
that the midwif with hir hand anoynted in oiles, *id est*, in oile of puliol
and in oile of lilie mesue or oile muscelon and, as it nedith, that hand
1160 so anoynted and put in formabely, dressyng the chield with their handis from the sides of the moder[57] and th'orifice of the matrice so anoynted wele that chield may come furth evenly.

1145. chield] *marg. ann. 1:* To haue Child; N[ota] bene & probatum

1150. withyn a xx throwes . . . xij throwes] within a xx[ti] throwes or withyn tho
twenty S2S1Rs

1151. furth] in fourme S2S1Rs

1155. þus] *followed by nine lines left blank for illustration*

1156. hedelyng] *marg. note, poss. ann. 4, using rusty-brown colored ink, and writing
with a shaky hand:* Chelderen to be borne right

1158. midwif] *marg. ann. 1:* Midwife

1159. in] S2S1Rs, of in T   mesue] TS2S1, mefue Rs

The secunde maner is vnkyndely: also whan the chield cometh
with his feete jointly toguydre, but the mydwif shal never have it furth
1165 whan he cometh so dounward; but whan he bigynneth to come so to,
the mydwif with hir handes anoynted and in, put she hym vp ageyn and
dresse hym so that he may come furth on the most kyndely maner þat
he squat nat his handis in the moder sides.[58]

The iij maner vnkyndly is if the chieldes hede be so moche and
1170 so grete that he may nat come furþ; the mydwif than shal shove hym
ageyn and anoynte with May butter that is fressh or with oile comune
th'orifice, [*id est,*] þe mowth of the prevy membre and than the mydwifes hande put in so anoynted first, and that membre made large,
than bryng hym furth holdyng the hede of hym.

1175 The iiij maner if the chielde come furth agenst kynde, she that travailith shal be brought into a short st[r]aite bedde that hath an high
standyng and she put oute hir hede. Than the mydwif havyng hir hand
anoynted and put it in after that it is vnkyndly, and idressed hym right-
fully and than so bryng hym furth; but the bedde that **[fol. 125r]** the
1180 womman shal ligge in shal be made harde.

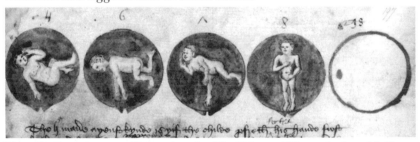

Plate 3b. Fetus-in-utero illustrations for *The Sickness of Women 2*, chap. 10 (figures 5-8), from London, British Library, Sloane MS 249, fol. 197r. By permission of The British Library. Cf. blank space left in TCC R.14.52, fol. 125r. (The
handwritten number "238" in the upper right corner refers to an earlier folia-
tion of the manuscript and has nothing to do with the numbered images.)

The v maner agenst kynde is if the chield profre his hande first
furth and his hede be turned ageyn and the mowth of that prevy membre be straite or shitte; than with [that] constreyneng of þe handes of
the mydwif, that thilke way be larged and that the chieldis hande be
1185 put in ageyn that the chield be nat slayne thurgh the mydwifes defaute;

1172. id est] i. S2S1Rs, and T
1176. straite] S2S1Rs, staite T
1180. harde] *foll. by eight lines left blank for illustration*
1181. The v maner agenst kynde] *marg. ann. 1:* Byrthe of A child
1183. that] S2S1Rs, than T

we comaunde the mydwif hand put in, dressyng the chieldis shulder to
be put bakwardes and hir handis rightly dressid to hir sides; and than
the hede of the chielde take, than so [lete] bryng hym furth.

1190 The vj maner agenst kynde is if the chielde profre furth his both
handis with his ij shuldres and sittyng his ij handis that j on that oon side
and that other on that other side, and the hede is turned bakward into
the side ageynward: the mydwif with hir hande shal put hym ageyn, as we
saide in the next chapiter, that is, she shal dresse his handis to his sides
and take the chieldes hede and easily bryng hym furth. If he have a litel
1195 hede and his handis if he cast first outwarde, þe mydwif shal ordeyne
that the hede may com to the mowth of the prevy membre, and so bi hir
handis she shal bryng hym furth bi the grace of God.

The vij is if the chielde cast furth first his right foote: the mydwif shal never bryng hym furth so, but she shal first sette hir fyngres
1200 and put it vp ageynward; and after that she shal put in hir hand and
amende that with that other foote so correct hem both toguydres,
if it may be, and his handis to his sides and his feete so as thei shuld
bien, and so bryng hym furth.

[The viij is if the chielde put furth] both the feete and that other
1205 dele of the chielde left in þe body bowyng, as we saide first: the mydwif with hir hande isho- **[fol. 125v]** ven in and she busily dressyng the
chield and so bryng hym furth, as I saide aboven.

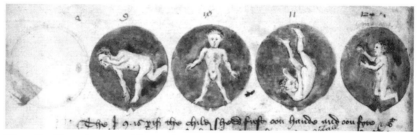

Plate 3c. Fetus-in-utero illustrations for *The Sickness of Women 2*, chap. 10 (figures 9-12) from London, British Library, Sloane MS 249, fol. 197v. By permission of The British Library. Cf. blank space left in TCC R.14.52, fol. 125v.

The ix is if the chielde shewe first oon hand and oo foote and with
that other hand he hilith his face: the mydwif settyng hir fyngres of hir
1210 oon hand in the grynde of the womman that travailith and with that

---

1188. lete] S2S1Rs, but T

1204. The viij is if the chielde put furth] S2S1Rs, *om.* T

1207. aboven] *foll. by nine lines left blank for illustration*

1208. The ix is if] *marg. ann. 1:* Byrthe of Childere

other hand put it vp ageyn, as we han saide aforn, and so bryng hym
furth if thow maist.

The x is if þe chield shewe first furth his feete departyng and his
oon hand bitwene his feete and his [hede] hangyng backward: the myd-
1215 wif, with hir hand put in, correctyng the chield and leyeng his oon
hand bi his other downe bi his sides and mendyng his hede in the best
maner and the feete rightly dressed, and than the mydwif bryngyng
hym furth.

The xj is [if] the chieldes necke come first forward; than the myd-
1220 wif hir hand put in and shove hym vp ageyn bi the shuldres, highing
lift the child and so to the orificium bryng hym downe and so bryng
hym furth.

The xij is if the chield shewe first furth his knees bowid: than the
mydwif shal put hym vp ageyn bakward, and the handis of the mydwif
1225 sette oon in hir g[r]yndes, and than hir other hand anoynted and put
in and so amendyng so the knees, and hym take bi the shuldres and so
bakward softly bryng hym furth; and so whan his feete bien amended
puttyng hym vpward vnto he be right as he shuld be, and than bryng
hym furth bi the grace of God, and the mydwif be connyng.

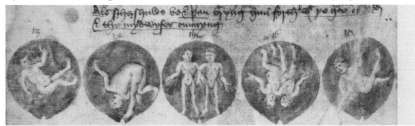

Plate 3d. Fetus-in-utero illustrations for *The Sickness of Women 2*, chap. 10 (figures 13-17), from London, British Library, Sloane MS 249, fol. 197v. By permission of The British Library. Cf. blank space left in TCC R.14.52, fol. 126r (plate
4 below). On the disordered sequence of the images, see Explanatory Note 56.

1230   **[fol. 126r]** The xiij is if the chield shewe first furth his thies and
his comyng furth so ersely: than the mydwif, with hir handes put in
ageyn bi the feete, she shal bryng hym to the orifice and evene have
hym furth.

1214. hede] S2S1Rs, feete T
1219. if] S2S1Rs, of T
1225. oon] ouer oþer S2S1Rs
1229. connyng] *foll. by three lines left blank at bottom of fol. 125v; nine lines left blank
at top of fol. 126r for illustration*
1230. The xiij is if] *marg. ann. 1:* byrthe of Childere

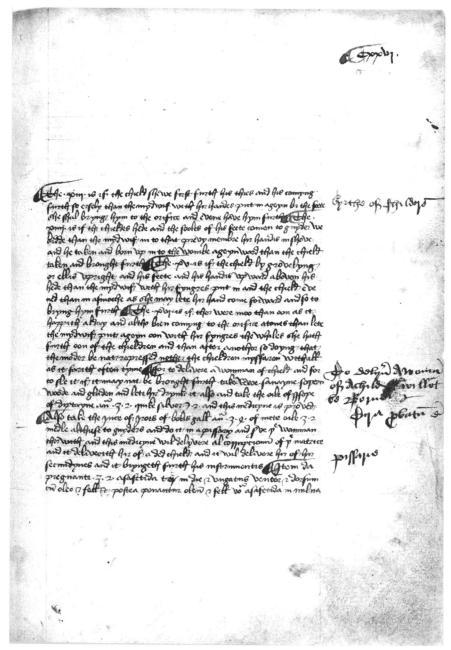

Plate 4. *The Sickness of Women 2*, chap. 10: Fetal presentation types 13-16, with blank space left for fetus-in-utero drawings (compare drawings in British Library, Sloane MS 249, plate 3d above), followed by medical receipts. Cambridge, Trinity College, MS R.14.52, fol. 126r. By permission of the Master and Fellows of Trinity College, Cambridge.

The xiiij is if the chieldes hede and the sooles of his feete comen
1235 toguyder: we bidde than the mydwif into that prevy membre hir handis in shove and [hym] taken and born vp into the wombe ageynward,
than the chield taken and brought furth.

The xv is if the chield ly grovelyng or ellis vpright and his feete and
his handis vpward aboven his hede: than the mydwif with hir fyngres
1240 put in and the chield evened, than in as moche as she may lete hir hand
come forward and so to bryng hym furth.

The xvj is if ther were moo than oon, as it happith alday, and al tho
bien comyng to the orifice at ones: than lete the mydwif put ageyn oon
with hir fyngres the whiles she hath furth oon of the chieldren, and
1245 than after another, so doyng that the moder be nat repressed nother
the chieldren mysfaren withall, as it farith often tyme.

For to delivere a womman of chield and for to sle it if it may nat
be brought furth: take rewe, sauayne, soþernwoode and gladen and
lete hir drynke it; [and also] take the oile of isope, of diptayne *ana* ʒ
1250 2, quike-silver ว 2. And this medicyne is proved. Also, take the juce of
iroes, of bolis gall *ana* ʒ 4, of mete oile ʒ 2, medle al thiese toguyders
and do it in a pissary and serve þe womman therwith; and this medicyne wil delyvere al corrupcioun of þe matrice and it deliverith hir of
a ded chield and it wil delivere hir of hir secundynes and it bryngeth
1255 furth his [menstrues]. *Item, da pregnanti* ʒ 2 *asafetida ter in die &* [*vngantur*] *venter & dorsum cum oleo & fell, & postea ponantur oleum & fell* [*bouis*]
asafetida in uulua [fol. 126v] *cum pluma.*†

And the greuaunce that wymmen han in beryng of chieldren
cometh otherwhiles of the greuaunce of the chield, and that may be for
1260 the child is wele woxen in his moder wombe tofor þat she hath caught
the dropesy; and this the mydwif may wele knowe and the womman

---

1236. hym] Rs, he TS2S1

1237. taken] *foll. by* by þe hede S2S1Rs

1240. hir hand] þe hede S2S1Rs

1247–1248. For to delivere . . . brought furth] *marg. ann. 1:* To Delyuer A Woman of A child þat will [n]ot be Borne

1249. and also] S2S1Rs, also and T   oile] juse S2S1Rs

1250. proved] *marg. ann. 1:* Cura probatum

1252. pissary] *marg. ann. 1:* Pissarie

1255. menstrues] S2S1Rs, instrumentis T

1255–1256. vngantur] vngatus TS2S1Rs

1256. bouis] bovis S1Rs, vocatur TS2

1257. uulua] uuluis S2

1261. dropesy] *marg. ann. 1:* Dropesy

also. And otherwhiles it cometh thurgh the fieblenesse of the matrice,[59]
that she is nat myghti to put out the chielde from hir; and this may be
in ij maners, as for grete sikenes that þe womman hath had and that
1265 hath fiebled hir moche, or for grete thought of the womman and if
she conceived [in] the first of the xij yeeris.[60] Oþerwhiles [it] cometh
of the stoppyng of the matrice, and that may be in ij maners, as of
fa[t]nes that stoppeth the mowth of the matrice and that witholdith
the blode that she shal bien purged of or that þei bien [con]ceived; or
1270 otherwhiles it cometh for the chield is ded in his moder wombe. And
tokenes ther bien: oon is this, that thei feele no stiryng nor moevyng
of the chield withynfurth; another is the secunde day of hir travalyng
hir mowth stynketh; and another is that thei feelen grete ache and
greuaunce aboute hir navil; another is dissolucioun of hir face and of
1275 al hir body; another is that thei desiren thynges þat bien contrarious
to hem; another is they han moche wacche and litel sleepe; another is
that thei han grete penaunce to make water and to go to þe prevy, and
also that thei han grete penaunce aboute the share; and if the chield
[comeþ] nat outward as he shuld, the mydwif may helpen weele inowgh
1280 without any other medicynes, ††as I have here-afore told.†[61]
    But if the greuaunce be of any of thiese iij that I have rehersed,[62]
make hir a bath of hockis, of fenygreke, of lynseede or wormoode,
of sothernwoode and of peritory, of fenel and of mugwort soden in
water and lete hir bathe therin a goode while; and whan she cometh
1285 furth oute of the bath, lete anoynt hir from the navil dounward to the
prevy membre with butter and with [dewte] and with aragon, bifore

1266. in] S2S1Rs, and T   it] S2S1Rs, *om.* T
1268. fatnes] fatnesse S2S1, fastnes T
1269. conceived] conceyued S2S1Rs, received T
1271. tokenes ther bien] *marg. ann. 1:* A ded Child in þe moders wombe to be
knowen; N[ota]
1276–1277. is that thei han grete penaunce] *The scribe of S2 originally omitted a
line of text here, probably due to eye-skip between one* penaunce *and the other; but he
discovered his mistake in proofreading and inserted the missing text in the lower margin
with a rubric sign similar to upper-case* I *inserted both where the text is missing and before the marginal note:* to make water & to go to priuy And also þat þei haue gret
penaunce. *Note that in S1 the first* penaunce *is followed only by* to ma *at the end of
a line, and the second* penaunce *occurs at the end of the following line; such a placement would have invited eye-skip by the copyist of S2 if S2 was copied from S1. In Rs,
the clause,* another is that thei desiren thynges that bien contrarious to hem *follows* sleepe.
1279. comeþ] S2S1Rs, *om.* T
1282. bath] *marg. ann. 1:* A bathe
1286. dewte] deawte S2S1, doawte Rs, draket T

and bihynde also. And sithen make hir a fumygacioun beneþfurth of
spikenard ʒ 1 & *s.* and of the rootis of cost ʒ 1. And also whan she is
come out of the bath, if she be a riche womman, yeve hir ʒ 1 of opi-
1290 balsamy with warm wyne; if she be a poore womman, seethe the rotes
of cost and of mugwede in wyne and do therto ʒ 2 [**fol. 127r**] of bolis
gall and lete hir drynk it whan she comyth out of the bath. Other temper borax ʒ 2 with wyne and yeve hir that to drynke. †† Other yeve hir
the juce of diptayne, isope *ana* ʒ 3, argent vief ʒ *s.* and this wil cast out
1295 the chield quike or ded, and better and if it be yeven with a trosciscy
of myrre after Rasis ordynaunce:[63] take of myrre ʒ 2, *lupinis* ʒ 2 & *s.*,
of rewe levis dried with wielde mynte, of puliol *id est* woderof,[64] of sermyny, of asafetida, serapin, *opopanicum, galbanum, gummi aromatici ana*
ʒ 8, of fyne maluesy as it nedith: make ballis as it were table men of the
1300 weight of ʒ 2 everiche of hym weieng; yeve hir oon of hem with decoccioun of *juniperij* in wyne, for thiese bien goode for hevy birthes and
for to bryng furth the secondynes, and distroieth *molam matricis.*[65] If
thiese may nat be hadde,† make a plaster of mugwede soden in water
and emplaster þe womman therwith from the navil to the prevy mem-
1305 bre, for it makith a womman soone to be delivered of hir chield if it
[be] quike other dede in hir wombe and it drawith out the secundyne;
but lete it nat ligge ful longe, for it wil drawe oute the matrice also.

    ††A noble precious powder for wymmen that bien in travailyng of
chield and for after throwes: take ʒ 3 of the scalis of *cassia fistula,* ʒ 1 of
1310 isope: powder al thiese in feere and yeve it the womman with þe juce
of veruayne. Iwarmed and idrunke it makith hir soone to be delivered
and it drawith oute the secundyne; also it makith a womman that is
stopped soone to be delivered bi the purgacioun of hir bloode.†

    Also ciclamen istrawed vnder the womman whiles she is in travail-
1315 yng it makith hir soone to be delivered; the juce of veruayne doeth also
idronk. Other lete hir drynke an eyshel-ful ful of the juce of leeke other

---

1287. fumygacioun] *marg. ann. 1:* Fumygacioun

1294–1295. cast out . . . quike or ded] *marg. ann. 1:* To cast out a ded Child

1297–1298. sermyny] sermini S2, cermini Rs, cerminis S1

1299. table men] table meyne S2Rs, tabille meyne S1

1302. secondynes] *marg. ann. 1:* Secondynes

1304. emplaster] *marg. ann. 1:* plastere

1306. be] S2S1Rs, *om.* T   drawith out the secundyne] *marg. ann. 1:* Cura

1308–1309. travailyng of chield . . . after throwes] *marg. ann. 1:* quyk or ded child to be delyuerd

1309. cassia fistula] cassie fistula & an ounce of saueray S2S1Rs

1310. powder] *marg. ann. 1:* A precius powdere for wemen in þer travelyng

1315–1316. veruayne . . . i-dronk] *marg. ann. 1:* verven dronken

of diptayne. Hockis also [haven] a grete myght to delivere a womman
of chield, and so hath the water of mannes leer that he hath wasshen
in his handis.[66]

1320   Tokens whan a womman shal be delivered of chield bien grete stir-
ynges and moevynges in hir wombe, and otherwhile al the wombe
moevith vp to the stomac, and makith a womman to have grete wil
to cast; and she hath moche hevynesse aboute the navil and than the
chield stirith fast to passen from his moder: than lete hir stoppe hir
1325 nosethrilles that the spirites may go doun to the matrice and comforten
hir and hir birthen; and lete [fol. 127v] guyrden hir with a guyrdel of
an hertis skynne; and if she swoune lete put swete smellyng thynges
at hir nose and lete frote þe soolis of hir feete and the pawmes of hir
handis with keene bitynge thynges, as with vynegre and salt. Bawme,
1330 *id est, opobalsami,* imade in maner of a suppository makith a womman
to be delivered of chield and it drawith out the secundyne also, but it
makith hir bareyne evermore after; and the juce of rewe and mugwede
makeþ a womman soone to be delivered of chield though it be ded in
hire wombe; and it is profitable to make hem to sneese with powder of
1335 peper and of castorie and cast it in hir nose; and the juce of this saturey idrunke maketh a womman soone to be delivered of chield and
if the herbe be plasterd to hir wombe it makith the chield com out,
quike or ded.

A precious stone that hight isopus[67] hath a grete vertu to help wym-
1340 men that thei were delivered of chield. Also don [yeven] a womman
that hath a ded chield in hir wombe the mylke of a bicche medled with
hony and make a plaster of wormode and bynde it to hir lift hippe; also
wommans mylke and oile toguyder idrunke makith a womman to be
delivered of chielde.[68] ††Also *Rx sauine, gladiolarum, id est, yris, abrotani,*
1345 *rute, diptani, isopi, saturey ana ʒ s., bene terantur cum vino optimo albo ʒ 3,*
et bibatur & cito liberabitur.†

1317. Hockis also haven] S1Rs, hockis also sauayne also TS2
1317–1318. to delivere a womman of chield] *marg. ann. 1:* A drynk to delyuer
A woman of her child
1320. shal be delivered] *marg. ann. 1:* Tokyns of here delyuere
1326–1327. guyrdel of an hertis skynne] *marg. ann. 1:* A Gyrdell of an hertis
Skynne
1331. to be delivered of chield] *marg. ann. 1:* To delyuer A woman of her Chyld
1333. ded] *marg. ann. 1:* A ded Child
1339. isopus] isapis S2S1Rs; *marg. ann. 1:* A precius stone called isopus, *foll. by*
marg. ann. 12: alias Ætites invenitur in nido Aquilæ
1340. don yeven] done yeven S2S1, don the ston on (ston *canc.*) T, take Rs
1342. plaster of wormode] *marg. ann. 1:* A plastere for A womman with Child

††[xi] *De mola matricis*[69]

Mola matricis is in ij maners: on maner is mola whan it is a wiked nature and than it is a fleshly lump the whiche a litel and a litel encreasith and
1350 wexith in the matrice, as it were in likenes of a chielde verily conceived, in the which is encheasound and caused as the moder vnderstondith of the wommans owne seede moche witholden in the matrice with lack-yng of mannes doyng; for if it were of a mannes seede that it were nat myghti that it shuld have lif thurgh reason of the whiche thyng the
1355 vertu natural and þe heete natural of the matrice, thei maken ther a fleshly lump without lif.

Another is cleped mola nat trewe and that is in ij maners: oon is that is engendred of wynde, a litel and a litel gadred in the matrice encheasounyng therin grete wyndenes; the signe of it is if the matrice
1360 be touched it makith a sowne, as it were in a tympanyt, and in suche a dropesy that is engendred and igadred thurgh [fol. 128r] wynde. Another maner is mola that is nat veray, the whiche is engendred thurgh foul roten humours and grete and [tough] to dissoluen in the matrice, and ther is foule grete humours maken grete [swellyng], as it were another
1365 maner of idropesy that is cleped alchitees. And thiese ij maners of molis is al oon cure. And also I have saide mola wexeth in the matrice as it were a chield quike and moevith, but nat so swiftly; but it moevith dedly and sielden and it castith out wynde otherwhiles from the matrice and otherwhiles lumpes of flessh.
1370 Cure of this maladie is right hard and long or it be do: first make hir a bath of herbis into þe whiche the womman shal wende first to soften hir bones and hir joyntes. Take al the malowes, fenygreke, herbe bawme, primerol, lilies, camamyl, wormode, calamynt, sothernwoode, *polipodij*, braunche v[r]syne, violet, peritory, fenel levis, and lynseede
1375 and make therof a stuphe. And whan the womman hath seten therin long inowgh, than in hir comyng out yeve hir 2 ʒ of this trociscy [Rasis]

1347. De mola matricis] *unnumbered in all mss*

1348. Mola matricis] *marg. ann. 1:* Mola matricis

1350. in likenes of a chielde] *marg. ann. 1:* A woman to seme with Child & is not

1357. mola] *marg. ann. 1:* Mola

1359. signe] *marg. ann. 1:* Signum bonum

1363. tough] tough S2Rs, togh S1, though T   to] *foll. by* defoulen, *canc.* T

1364. swellyng] S2S1Rs, sore styng T

1366-1367. as it were a chield quike] *marg. ann. 1:* Mola like A quyk child

1370. Cure] *marg. ann. 1:* Cura

1374. vrsyne] S2, vesyne T

1376. Rasis] S2S1Rs, cast T

with the juce of rewe and of nept and anoynt hir navil dounward: *dial-tea, oleo liliorum*, May butter that is fressh and do wrappe al hir body al about with an hoote double sheete; than make hir a fumygacioun
1380 of spikenard and of comyn and of costy. Whan that is don, lete anoynt hir privite withynfurth thus: take bolis gall ʒ 6, oile 2 ʒ, medle hem toguyders and make an oynement and do therto ʒ 1 *euforbij*, the juce of savayne ʒ 2, peleter of Spayne ʒ 1, scamone ʒ 4, rotis of diptayne ʒ 1: make powder of al thiese, put it in a bolis galle and medle hem toguyd-
1385 er wele and with a long fether anoynt hir withyn also depe as thow may and put in inowgh and lete hir ligge so hir hede lowe and hir taile ende high; and if she worthe owhere iholpen this wil shewe sum doyng, for this medicyne wil delivere though ther were a chield quike or ded.

Another maner trocisces bien thiese: Rx *asafetida* ʒ 10 & *grana* 16,
1390 *gummy aramatici, galbani, serapini, opopan[acis], agarici, foliorum cene, lupiny, castory, olei benedicti ana* ʒ 2 & s., *boracis* ʒ 2, *bdellij* ʒ 1, *buccarum lauriis, pionearum, polipodij, nuchij ceresorum, seminis petrosilij, juniperij, feniculi, aristologie rotunde &* [*longe, xilobalsami, carpobalsami*], *cassie liggnij, ciperij, genciane, centaurie, rute, macis, cucube,* sawine, iris, achory,
1395 asarie, nept, calamynt, *diptani, reub[arbi],* [*nar*]*dy, squinanti, origani, croci, carui,* **[fol. 128v]** anise, *rubie maiorum ana granorum* 25, *succi rute, mel, vini aromatici ana* quartern 1, *coquantur*—[*id est,* seeth]—the juce of rewe, the wyne and of hony a litel. Than ley *asa, gummi aromatici, galbanum, serapinum, & borax* and ley al thiese infuse al nyght and a day;
1400 on the morow seth hem ageyn and than clense hem thurgh a cloth and seeth that is so clensed til the juce of that rue and the wyne be consumed; than al þe spices and the gummes ipowdred and so [put] therto and make of the weight of ʒ 2 everiche, [yeve] oon balle in mola, as I saide bifore.
1405   And also make a suppository of ʒ 1 of thiese ballis: farine, stafisacre, of euforbie, of peleter of Spayne, scamony *ana* ʒ 1, bolis gall ʒ

1387. worthe owhere iholpen] TS2, worthe euer yholpyn S1, wyll euer be helpen Rs

1388. quike or ded] *marg. ann. 1:* A ded Child

1390. opopanacis] opopan (*without suspension mark*) T

1393. longe xilobalsami carpobalsami] lon. xiloba. carpobal. S1, lon. xilob' carpol' S2, lon. xilob' cappol' Rs, lonylob' carpol T

1395. reubarbi] S2Rs, reubarbii S1, reubia T   nardy] nardi S2S1Rs, vidy T

1397–1398. id est seeth the juce of rewe] S2S1Rs, or the juce of rewe seeth T

1402. put] S2S1Rs, that T

1403. yeve] yif S2S1, yf Rs, if T

1. Make a litel bagge of lynnen cloth that is wele overwered and make a suppository, for it wil both bryng furth ded chield if any ther be and it bryngith furth the secundyne and the bloode and it bryngith furth
1410 lumpes of the mola; but yit yeve hir to drynk a bal with þe juce of dip- tayne, of savoray *ana* ʒ 2, quike-siluer ɘ *s.*: this is oon of þe best that if a womman travaile of chielde and it be ded to deliver hir therof.

Also anothe[r] pissary is take the juce of wormode, of mugwede, of pulliol, of diptayne, of origani, of saverey, of sauayne *ana* ʒ 2, bolis gall
1415 ʒ 32, of peleter, of gladen, of lauriol, of oile, of cleene hony *ana* ʒ *s.*; medle al thiese toguyder and with an instrument put it into hir wombe bi the prevy membre with a litel powder of euforbie and a litel of *elle- boris albi ana* ʒ 2, for this pissary distroieth al maner of molis of the matrice and bryngeth furth with grete violence; and though a womman
1420 were stopped iiij or v yeere, it wil do his dever, *hoc Augustinus.*[70]

But first whan the womman is comen oute of þe bath aforsaide, first after that she is anoynted and than wrapped in a sheete and the ballis aforsaide, thow shalt make hir to sneese, and whan she is thus iserved, thow shalt teene hir and make hir anangred; and than thow
1425 shalt make hir aferde and whan thow hast thus idon, thow shalt yeve hir a pissarie aforsaide or the suppository also in *mola matricis.*

Ther was a womman and she was delyvered bi the wyndyng of ij towailes aboute hir myddil and ij stikkes: that on was bounde on that on side of þe womman and that other on that other side of hir til the
1430 wombe of hir was made right smal; and the womman had right fayre [fol. 129r] chieldren yit therafter.

Or ellis yeve hir trocisces of myrre [that] **Rasis** makith in his booke of *Almosorum*[71] the whiche bien thiese: take mirre ʒ 3, *lupinis* ʒ 5, levis of drie rewe, of wielde mynt, of woderove, mader, ameos, asafetida, *sera-*
1435 *pium,* opopanak, galbany, *gummi aromatici ana* ʒ 2: make trocisces with goode wyne *romanici:* yeve ʒ 2 of hem with decocioun of duratief seedis and of savayne, mader and of saverey *ana* ʒ 2, etc.†

The xij chapiter is of the secundyne that is witholdyng in womman after chielde beryng.

1408. ded chield] *marg. ann. 1:* Ded Child bonum est

1413. pissary] *marg. ann. 1:* A pissarie

1416. put] cast S2S1Rs

1419–1420. though a womman were stopped] *marg. ann. 1:* To make A Wom- an have here Flowres

1432. trocisces] *marg. ann. 1:* Trosisces   that] S1Rs, þa S2, and as T   Rasis] *marg. ann. 1:* Rasis

1436. romanici] ro[man]ici TS2, poiᵃe (?) Rs, roᵃia S1

1440 Secundyne is a litel skyn that goth aboute the chielde while he is in
his moder wombe, right as ther is an inner skyn that goth aboute a
noote kernel; and otherwhiles a womman is delivered of that secundyne whan she is delivered of hir chield; and otherwhiles she is delivered of hir chield and the secundyne levith stille behynde withyn hir
1445 for the grete fieblenes of hir matrice. And that may come of moche fastyng other of grete anger, wrath, other smytyng, other sum long flux of
the wombe [þe whiche thynges sleeth a chield in his moder wombe];
but than the moder deliverith hir of the chield but the secundyne levith stil withyn the matrice, and the mydwif shuld anoynt hir handis
1450 and with hir nailes pul out þe secundyne if she mowe. And if she mow
nat, bore holes in a stoole and lete hir sitte theron and make a fumygacioun vnderneth of þe hornes of a gote and of the clawes of hir feete,
so that the smoke smyte vp right to hir prevy membre; other ellis take
salt other asshen of a vyne ibrent and temper hem with water and yeve
1455 hir to drynke.

Also make hir a bath of wormode and of hockis, calamynt, fenygreke,
origani, and make hir sitte in that bath vp to the navil; and whan she
cometh oute of that bath anoynt hir from the navil dounward with fressh
butter and with oile of baie and aragon and [with dewte] and with the
1460 same anoynte hir sides and hir bak aboute hir raynes. Also take the juce
of percely and of leeke and medil hem with puliol and yeve h[ir] to
drynke, other the juce of borage, and that wil draw out the secundyne.
††*Et sic require in suffocacione menstruorum.*[72]†

††The xiij chapiter is to make a womman able to
1465 **conceive chield if God wil.**

1440. Secundyne] *marg. ann. 1:* Secundyne

1445–1446. moche fastyng] *marg. ann. 1:* Moche Fastyng

1447. þe whiche thynges sleeth a chield in his moder wombe] S2S1Rs; *om.* T

1448. secundyne] *marg. ann. 1:* Secundyne

1449. mydwif] *marg. ann. 1:* Midwif

1451–1452. fumygacioun] *marg. ann. 1:* A Fumygacioun

1454. a vyne] a uyne S2S1, a nyght Rs

1456. bath] *marg. ann. 1:* A bathe   hockis] *foll. by* and holyhokkis S2S1Rs

1459. with dewte] S2S1Rs, w'drawe T

1461. hir] hyr Rs, hym T, hem S2, them S1

1462. secundyne] *marg. ann. 1:* Secundyne

1464. xiij] 12 S2S1Rs

1464–1465. able to conceive chield] *marg. ann. 4, using rusty-colored ink:* Abull
to conseue child

First if she be replete of hir menstrues, do clense hir with medicynes *in retencione menstruorum, et in suffocacione men-* **[fol. 129v]** *struorum* with bathes and stuphes. Other take calamynt, nept, saveray, fenel, peritory, isope, mugwede, rewe, wormode, anyse, comyn, rosemaryn, tym, puliol
1470 roial, mountaign origanum *ana m.* 1, wyne a galoun, water 6 galouns and seeth hem; or yef hir to ete this medicyne: take powder of cloves ℥ 3, 4 yelkis of raw egges and medle þe powder and the yolkes toguyders and bake it on a hote stone and yeve it the womman fastyng 4 daies without drynk a goode while after it is eten. Also for a man or for a wom-
1475 man, make an emplaster of iiij yolkis of raw egges, of powder of cloves ℥ s., of safron ℥ 1: first anoynt with hote oile of rosen on the mowth of the stomac and straw theron sum of the powder and make a plaster and ley it to.†

The xiiij chapiter is of bledyng overmoche after
1480 **that she hath had hir chield.**
The wymmen that bleeden otherwhiles to moche after that þei han born their children and that maken hem ful fieble: but thow ne shalt in this case yeven hir no medicynes that bien comfortatif nother bathis nother strong strictories, but other medicynes, as it was told afore in
1485 the chapiter [of to moche flowyng of bloode:[73] lete hir bleede vnder the ancle on that oon foote and another day vnder that other ancle] and yeve hir than other medicynes, as it was saide here before, as we shuld have yeven hir medicynes that were told in the chapiter of witholdyng of bloode. And sum wymmen han corrupt matier as quetir passyng awey
1490 from hem, and otherwhiles suche matier passith from hem in stide of bloode, and otherwhiles with the bloode that the bloode thei shuld bien purged of.

And if thei bien old wymmen other wymmen that bie bareyn, it nedith nat to yeve hem medicynes therof. If thei be yong wymmen, lete

---

1466. First] *marg. ann. 1:* A woman to conseue A child

1468. Other take] *marg. ann. 1:* Cura

1471. powder] *marg. ann. 1:* Powdere

1475. emplaster] *marg. ann. 1:* A plastere

1479. xiiij] 13 S2S1Rs

1481. bleeden] *marg. ann. 1:* Bledyng

1484. other medicynes] *marg. ann. 1:* Cura

1485–1486. of to moche flowing . . . vnder that other ancle] S2S1Rs, on that oon foote and another day vnder the ancle of to moche flowyng of bloode lete hir bleede vnder the ancle T

1494. yong wymmen] *marg. ann. 1:* yong wemen

1494–1495. lete seeth] *marg. ann. 1:* Cura

1495 seeth kerslokis other turmentil and v-levid gras other skirwhittes[74] in
wyne, and lete hir sitte over the smoke therof, that it may come to hir
prevy membre; oþer take puliol and make powder therof and put it in
a bagge so brode and so long that it wil overhille both prevy membris
of the womman, and al warme ley it to thilke membris and bynd it fast
1500 that it fal nat away.

[xv Woundis of the matrice]

Woundis of the matrice bien ihelid with the juce of **[fol. 130r]** plantayne and of salatry and with the white of an eg and the juce of purslane ††*ana* ℥ 6, *gummi draganti, gummi arabici ana* ℥ 6; *infundantur* and
1505 it wil be like a muscillage worthy and goode to keele and to hele.† And
if [the] veynes bien broken,[75] thei shuln bien heled with the juce of centory and with bole and with sandragan and with seedis of myrtils and
with the rounde aristologium and with suche other medicynes. ††Also
take this for a principal medicyne for al maner woundes in this place,
1510 if it come of moche heete, as comonly it doeth, more than of cold: take
of *gummi arabici* and *gummi draganti* whit ℥ 6 and infuse it in ij vncis
of water of roses and a ℥ of oile of myrtils with powder of mastik and
olibani ana ℈ 6; and al thiese shuln be made in oon confeccioun as in
maner of an oynement. And lete a prevy womman ley ther the sore is
1515 this medicyne aforsaide, nowght only to woundis of this place but also
in al other placis and to chynes and cliftes in the lippis of the mowth.

Another medicyne for the same: take gumme arabic, *draganti* ℥ 4,
borace ℥ 2, camphory, bole, alcamy, *sanguis draconis ana* ℥ 1, *masticis*,
myrtils, ceruse, *olibani*, litarge *ana* ℥ s., *olei bodegaryni* ℥ 4, *aqua rosarum*
1520 ℥ 8: lai þe *gummi draganti* and the borage in the rose water infuse a day
and a nyght til thei bien al relinted, than clense hem thurgh a shire
cloth til thei bien brought al cleene thurgh; than al tho other spices
made into subtil powder and imedled with the oile aforsaide and with

---

1501. xv Woundis of the matrice] *om* TS2S1Rs

1502. Woundis] *marg. ann. 1:* Woundes

1502–1503. plantayne] *marg. ann. 1:* Cura

1506. the veynes] þe veynes Rs, thi veynes T, thy vynes S1, þy wynes S2

1509. principal medicyne] *marg. ann. 1:* A speciall Medicyn for hete or cold

1515. woundis of this place] *marg. ann. 1:* Woundes in A woman

1517. medicyne] *marg. ann. 1:* Cura; N[ota]

1518. alcamy] alcamie S2, alcanne S1Rs

this muscillage til thei bien right wele incorporate and put to vse whan
1525 it nedith. This medicyne is goode for al maner cankers, cankretis, hote
woundis, *horispilatus, id est,* wield fuyres, feluns, carbuncles, mormals of
colre adust, and al suche other. If the woundes come thurgh cold, take
the muscillage of the fenygreke ȝ 4, of sarcocol, infuse in decoccioun of
camomyl, spikenard, *masticis,* myrre, cynamun, castory *ana* ℈ 1, right sub-
1530 tily made into powder: medle hem toguyder with wommans mylke and
with the juce of plantayne *ana* ȝ 2 and *s.*; whan thei bien wele imedled,
do it to the malady in the prevy membre, for this medicyne fordoeth al
the maladies of that place, if it be curable with medicynes.†

[fol. 130v]
[xvi] De cancris & de vlceribus matricis.
1535 Cancryng and festres of the matrice comen of old woundes of the matrice
that wore nat wele helid, but that maner of sikenes we wil spcke but litil
of, for phisiciens sayn that cancres that bien hidde, it is bctter that thei
bien vncurid than cured or heled. But natheles this oynement is goode
þerfor and for icchyng also and blaynes that bien in the matrice: take
1540 a goorde that is ripe and pare hym without and clense hym also of that
that is withyn hym. And after than stamp hym right smal and than sette
it in a potte on the fuyre with oile of roses and wex and sheepis talow.
And whan thei bien wele soden, cast therto powder of mastic and of
olibanum and lete theym buyle wele toguyder, and sithen thurgh a cloth
1545 clense and therwith anoynt hem withynfurth. And this other oynement
is goode also for brennyng and for scaldyng; but whan suche a sore is
anoynted therwith, ley ther-above ivy levis soden in wyne.
††A sowdyng medicyne for al maner cancres mater; take this med-
icyne for al: first take rootes of rede dockes *li. s.,* rotes of yris *li.* 1, seeth
1550 thiese rotis in cliere water 3 quartes and a quart of white wyne; seeth
hem til a potel and put therto a litel hony, as ȝ 6, with the white of

---

1525–1527. cankers . . . suche other] *marg. ann. 1:* Cankers Felouns, wildfyre
& mony other

1526. feluns] TS2, felonus Rs, folous S1

1527. take] *marg. ann. 1:* N[ota]

1534. xvi] *unnumbered* TS2S1Rs

1535. Cancryng and festres of the matrice] *marg. ann. 1:* Cancres & festers in
A woman

1538. this oynement] *marg. ann. 1:* An oyntment

1548. A sowdyng medicyne] *marg. ann. 1:* A medicyne; N[ota] *in rusty-colored
ink*

eyren 16 and clarifie it and wasshe the prevy membre therwith right
wele. Take coton right wele itosed and put that coton easily into a lynnen
poket, than wete that poket with that coton and esily it shal be clensed
1555 and do awey the filth therfrom. Than make þis plaster: take gumme
draganti albi, gummi of arabie *ana* ʒ 2, ley hem infuse in water of roses
til thei bien right soft; than take [a]lso aloes, washe of ceruse, iwasshe
of frankencence, of sandragan *ana* ʒ 2, of litarge of gold ʒ 1, wex ʒ 2,
of oile of roses ʒ 6, and make a brasen morter right hote and put therto
1560 the wex and with the muscillage of *draganti* and of þe gumme of arabie
and medle hem toguyder right wele and lete hem sumdel keele. Than
put in the oile of roses with the powders and medle hem right wele
toguyder. And whan thei bien right wele incorporat and is right cold,
put therto camphory **[fol. 131r]** with a litel more oile of roses iground
1565 and herof make prevy medicynes, for it is right goode.†

††**[xvij] For swellyng of wymmens legges whan thei bien with chield.**[76]
Wymmen whan thei bien with chield their legges wiln swelle. Than take
that lieth in the smethis trough vnder his gryndyng stone and drie it
and make powder of it and dissolue it with vynegre and anoynt ther-
1570 with that place that swellith so. Oþer lei it theron in maner of a plaster;
other take the floure of beane mele and medle it with vynegre and with
oile and lay it on the swellyng; or anoynt it with blac sope and sithen
lay a plaster theron of eldren levis fried bi hymsilf in a panne without
any other liquor; and the same medicynes bien goode for swellyng of a
1575 mannes feete or legges that jorneyen bi the wey.
      Ad menstruenda provocanda Rx percely rotis, fenel *ana m.* 1, of isope
levis, saueray, *betonice, foliorum lauri,* roscmary, lavender *ana m. s.*, nept
m. 3, *diptani, rute, arthemisie ana* ʒ 3 *& s., carui, polipodij* ʒ 4, *vini albi
lagenam vnam, toncis & coctis* [ad] *medietatem collatis & iterum coctis cum*
1580 *croco* ʒ *1, gariofili* ʒ *2, granorum paradisi* ʒ *s., m[e]llis* ʒ *6, fillicie fetide.* Rx

---

1553. a] *ins. above line*
1555. plaster] *marg. ann. 1:* Plastere; N[ota] *in rusty-colored ink*
1557. also] 'a' *conjectural, covered by dropped ink* T
1564. camphory] *catchword by main scribe:* with a litel
1566. xvij] *unnumbered* TS2S1Rs   swellyng of wymmens legges] *marg. ann. 1:*
Swellyng of legges
1567. Than take] *marg. ann. 1:* Cura
1569. anoynt] S2, *foll. by* it T
1574. goode for swellyng] *marg. ann. 1:* For Swellyng; N[ota] *in rusty-colored ink*
1579. ad medietatem] S2, & medietatem T
1580. mellis] mollis T

terebenti albi granosi, colloquintida, cuscutem, aloe [*citrini*], *zinziberi, epithemi ana* ℥ *2, sene* ℥ *2, ellebori albi et nigri, croci, piretri, seminis cicute, seminis anisi, ameos, carui, cinapij & nastarcij ana* ℥ *s., reubarbij, serapium, galbani, opoponacis, bdellij, asafetida ana* ℥ *2 & s., mirre* electuarie, *olei bene-*
1585 *dicti ana* ℥ *2, sarcocolle, castorie, diagredij, euforbij, esule, ligni aloes, centauree, sticados ana* ℥ *1, agarici* ℥ *2; fiant pillule cum succo porry dosis* ℥ *2 & s., cum decoccione supradictis.*

    Emplastrum. Rx *malbarum m. 2, millefolij, feniculi, ebuli ana m. 1, foliorum porry m. 3, scindantur minutissime & terantur & frixantur cum pauca*
1590 *aqua & fiat emplastrum circum circa totum ventrem vsque ad vuluam.*

    Fomentacio. Rx *radicis iris quartern 1, anisi* ℥ *1, rose marini, calamynti, isopi, saturei, origani ana* ℥ *1 & coquantur tam in vino* [*quam*] *in aqua & ponantur herbe in sacculo & post fomentacionem ponatur sacculus ad vuluam.*

1595   *Ad molam matricis & ad fetum mortuum:* Rx *seminis porri, apij, mirre, spikenardi, calamynti, squinanti, corticis cassie fistule ana* ℥ *2, anisi; fiat puluis & recipiatur mane non exitu a balneo, cum aqua & vino, melle, decoccionis saturie, isopi, diptani, rubie* [**fol. 131v**] *maioris, nepite, iris, solsequij, abrotani ana m. 1.*

1600   *Item secundum Rasim:*[77] Rx *as*[*e*], *aristologie rotunde & longe ana* ℥ *6, mirre, agarici, nardi ana* ℥ *3, fiant trocisci ponderis vnius* ℥ *3, cum decoccione juniperij, & sunt forte educentes embrionem.* Rx *achori, asari,* [*amomi seminis,*] *atriplicis,* [*maratri*] *ana* ℥ *1 & grana 18,* [*anisi*] ℥ *2, aristologie longi, arthemesie, cassie ligni ana* ℥ *2,* ℈ *2, & grana 2, centaurea* [*minor*] ℥ *1,* ℈
1605 *1 & granum 1, centaurie maioris* ℥ *2, dauci, ellebori nigri* ℥ *1, folie lauri* ℥ *1 & s., grana 9, liquericie* ℥ *4, lupinorum* ℥, *melancij* ℥ *2, mirre* ℥ *6,* ℈ *2 & grana 3, tirobi* ℥ *3, stepceree* ℥ *6, macedonisi, piretri* ℥ *2,* ℈ *2, grana* [*2*], *piperis nigri* ℥ *5,* ℈ *1, grana 2, ciperi* ℥ *1, seminis rute* ℥ *2,* ℈ *2, grana 2, spikenardi* ℥ *2 et grana 2, apij, sauine* ℥ *1, smirinis, id est classa* ℥ *2, squinanti* ℥

1581. aloe citrini zinziberi] aloe ci. zz. S2S1, aloeci zz Rs, aloe a zz T

1588. Emplastrum] *marg. ann. 1:* Emplastrum

1591. Fomentacio] *marg. ann. 1:* fomentere

1592. quam] quanto TS2S1Rs

1600. ase] S2S1Rs, asi T; *marg. ann. 1:* Cura

1602–1603. amomi seminis atriplicis] S2S1Rs, arancuse a triplicis T

1603. maratri] S2S1Rs, marcitri T   anisi] S2S1Rs, ana T

1604. centaurea minor] centauria iiij^{or} S1, centauria iiij RsS2, centaurea 4^{or} T (*confusion of four minims of* mi *with numeral* iiij)

1605. dauci] dauci cretici ℥ 2 S2S1Rs

1607. tirobi] cirobi S2S1Rs   2 (3)] ii S2S1Rs, *om.* T

1609. smirinis] smirnis S1

1610   *1, ꝺ 2, xilobalsami ʒ 1, ꝺ 2 & grana [2], pulegij pionearum mundatur ʒ 1,*
ꝺ 1, gariofili ʒ 2, radicis caparis, cinamoni ana ʒ 3, mel quod sufficit, dosis ʒ
4 cum succo nepito.

    Antidotum [emagogum antedictum,[78] *id est, quod datum emagogum], id*
est, sanguinem menstrualem ducens vsque ad multas mulierum passiones &
1615 *matricem que non vsu purgantur quia mirabiliter purgat, scilicet menstruales*
et fetum mortuum in vtero occidit & extrahit & post partum ad sanitatem pro-
ducit, petram in vesica frangit et expellit, vrinam movet, stranguriam sanat,
epatis eufraxim emendit splenis sclirosim et omnia intranea, & magnam vtili-
tatem prestat ad istam indignacionem facit. Sanat eos qui cibum non continent,
1620 *fleuma fortiter educit, & eos curat qui colicam paciuntur. Neufraticis prodest;*
homo autem qui vsus fuerit sanitatem optinebit. Cum nil forcius mulieribus
inuenitur que illis sunt vtilia; propter quod cauendum est paci[enti]bus emo-
roydas aut fluxum matricis aut dissinteriam. Emoroydas prouocat; vias tocius
corporis aperit & fetum mortuum & secundinam extrahit & vesicam purgat,
1625 *stomachum calefacit, vomitum compescit, ventositatem consumit.*

[xviii: *Ad restringendum cohitum*]

    Ad restringendum cohitum. Rx olei ʒ 4, camphore ʒ 3; pul[ueriza]ta
camphor[a] & ministrantur & vnge renes & castitatem seruabit. Item, si quis
comedit florem salicis vel populi omnem ardorem libidinis in eo refriger[ab]it
1630 *[b]ene hoc longo vsu. Item, veruena portata vel potata non sinit virgam erigi*
donec deponatur & si sub ceruicali posueris non potest erigi virga **[fol. 132r]**
7 diebus, quod si probari volueris da gallo mixtam cum furfure & super gal-
linas non ascendet. Item, herba columbina in testic[ul]is extinguit libidinem.
Item, inunge corrigiam aliquam cum succo veruene & porta ad carnem & eris
1635 *effeminatus; & si qua tetigerit erit ineptus ad talia quia cor tangen[ti]s emol-*
lit. Item, lapis sulpicis portat[us in] sinistra manu erectionem virge tollit. Item,

---

1610. 2 (3)] *om.* T

1613. Antidotum emagogum antedictum id est quod datum emagogum] Antidotum E mag' antedictum .i. quam datum emagodum S2S1, Antidotum .4.ʳ
mag' antidoto .i. quadratum emagodum T

1615. mirabiliter purgat] *marg. ann.. 1:* A purgacioun riall

1618. epatis eufraxim] operatis eufraxim S2S1Rs

1622. pacientibus] pacibus *without suspension mark*

1627–1628. puluerizata camphora] pulᵗᵃ camph' S2S1Rs, pulta camphore T

1629. refrigerabit] S2S1Rs, refrigerit abit T

1630. bene] bene S1S2, vene T, vn' Rs

1633. testiculis] S2S1Rs, testicis T

1635. tangentis] S2S1Rs, tangens T

1636. sulpicis] TS2, salpicis S1Rs   portatus in] S2S1Rs, portata & T

testiculi galli cum sanguine suo suppositi lectum coitum iacenti in eo vigitant.
Item, semen lactuse exsiccat sperma & cedat desiderium coitus & pollucionem.
Item, lapis tophasius[79] *generat castitatem & reprimit venerem. Item, succus jus-*
1640 *quimani testiculos invnge calorem & t[u]m[o]cionem & libidinem extinguit.*
Item, lapis ambree portatus dat castitatem. Item, semen salicis su[m]ptum libi-
dinem extinguit. Item, eruce, rute, & agni casti siccentur & puluerizentur &
simul comedentur tollent polluciones.

De duricia *matricis* *et eius asperitate. Fomentum aque decocciones malue*
1645 *vel alte[e] duriciem tollit. Item, [axungia] anceris & succus porri misce &*
vngantur collum matricis post menstrua contracta; matricem relaxat. Item, lol-
lium, mirram, thus album & coctum simul in vino vel aqua & fumigetur vel
vngatur clausa[m] matricem aperit & ad conceptum disponit. Isaac.[80] *Item,*
radix [elleboris] elixata & fomentata omnem dolorem tollit. Item, emplastrum
1650 *ex nepta ante & retro prius terificata apositum educit matricem. Item, vinum*
decoccionis origani prouocat menstrua. Rx [olei] li. 1, coloquintide ℥ 1, succum
rute ℥ 3, absinthij, pulegij ana ℥ 1, et coquantur, &c.

De *ictaricia* *vrina. Paris cum succo marubij bibita curat. Item, succus*
vrtice rubie cum seruicia bibita. Item, rasura emboris bibita curat effitus. Item,
1655 *crocus dissolutus in aqua & potatus sanat statim. Succus camamil datus potui*
epatis febribus cum aqua calida mire prodest. Item, succus solatri cura[t] itteri-
ciam. Item, aqua pilosella bibita vel vinum decoccionis statim sanat.

De lapide: succus arthemesie multus & bibitus curat lapidem & frangit.
Item, betonica cum mulsa & pipere data potui tollit dolorem & lapidem renum
1660 *& vesice excludit. Item, cortex lauri & eius bacce calculos frangit & expellit.*

Ad *stranguriam* *&* *impedimentum* *vrine. Fimus bouinus cum melle cale-*
[fol. 132v] *factis & apponitus multum valet. Item, pili leporis vsti & bibiti*
statim facit mingere. Item, mingat paciens 3 diebus super vrticas maiores con-

---

1640. tumocionem] S2, tmcionem *without suspension mark* T

1642. extinguit] *marg. ann. in grey-brown ink, with shaky hand, poss. ann. 1 writ-ing later:* consevyng Child

1645. altee] S2S1Rs, altes T   axungia] S1Rs, aux[ungi]a S2, auxia T

1648. clausam] clausa TS2S1Rs

1649. elleboris] S2S1Rs, elbe T   dolorem tollit] *foll. by* Item succi neptis clys-terium prouocat S2S1Rs

1651. olei] S2S1, ollei T

1652. ℥ 1] ℥ ij S2S1Rs

1653. De ictaricia vrina] *marg. ann. in grey-brown ink, with shaky hand, poss. ann. 1 writing later:* Ictericia vrina   Paris] Pacis S2S1Rs

1654. effitus] effit' S2, effic' Rs, effij S1

1656. curat] S2S1Rs, cura T

1662. apponitus] appositus S2S1Rs (*and so passim below*)

tinuis & exsicca & sic liberatur. Item, galbanum appositum super ventrem sub
1665 *vmbilico statim minget. Item, radix rafan[i] in vino albo infusas rotulas 10 tri-*
tas per noctem, & mane collatas statim minget. Item, radix pentafilon li. 1 s.,
turmentil ℥ 6, terantur & cum ptisana cocta & bibita statim curat stranguriam
ex calore. Item, vesica capree vsta & bibita. Item, sotulares porcin[a]s vstas &
bibitas curat. Item, aduelune assate valeant [contra] distillaciones vrine &
1670 *amigdale comeste. Item, folia agni casti posita in lecto soluit ardorem vrine pro-*
prietate sua & non racionem.[81]

   De inflacione testiculorum. Farina fabarum cum succo ebuli & oleo com-
muni & apponita statim tollit inflacionem & tumorem. Si virga inflatur cera
℥ 2 cum oleo communi ℥ 5 & herbe portulace [trite] et commixte soluit tumor-
1675 *em. Item, farinam ordij in [mulsa] cocta vel vin[o] alb[o] & emplastra tumor-*
em tollit. Item, folia jusquimani li. 1, folia malue li. s. cocta in aqua & trite
& frixate in melle & vino albo tollit tumorem. Item, Rx foliorum maluarum
m. 3, foliorum absinthij m. 2, ebuli m. 1, coquantur in aquis & illa expressa
& herbis tritis & cum melle frixatis cum forma emplastri apponatur secundum
1680 *magistrum Ricardum Mersh.*[82]

De t[u]more mamillie pro multitudine lactis.

   Fiat descensium ex bolo ℥ 1, oleo rosarum ℥ 3, aceti & succo solatri appo-
nito. Item, farine fabarum cum albedine ouorum quod sufficit. Item, radix cal-
lium, menta, farina fabarum, cunam apponita quia singula lac dissoluunt.
1685 *Item, stercus hominis combustus vlcera cancrosa & quasi insanabilia sanat, &*
portat politricum super se semper quod certissime sanat cancrum. Item, stercus
caprinum cum melle distemperatum fistulam & cancrum interficit & omnem
[spurciciam] aufert. Item, folia jusquimani coct[a] & trit[a] cum vitellis coctis
ouorum & oleo rosarum & apponentur. Item, bardanis cocti sub cineribus cum
1690 *[axungia] & melle apponitis sanat putridas mamillas & vlcera. Item, fimus*
murum cum aqua invnctus duriciem vberum & dolorem ac tumorem soluit.
Item, sanguis leporis cum eius co- **[fol. 133r]** *agulo facit concipere bibitus.*

1665. rafani] S2S1Rs, rafan T   10] x S2S1, quod (?) Rs

1668. porcinas] porcinos TS2S1

1669. valeant] valeant (vᵃnt S1) S1T, vnt² RsS2   contra] S2S1Rs, quater T

1674. trite] *corr. in marg. by main scribe with ins. mark in line*

1675. mulsa] multa TS2S1, pulta Rs   vino albo] S2S1Rs, vini albi T

1679–1680. secundum magistrum Ricardum Mersh] *in marg.* S2, *om.* S1Rs

1681. tumore] timore T   pro multitudine lactis] *marg. ann. 1:* To muche Milke

1686. super se semper] super se semper super se S2S1

1688. spurciciam] inspurciciam T   cocta & trita] S1, cocti & triti T

1690. axungia] aux[ungi]a S2, auxa T

Ad pestilenciam: *Rx mirre, pimpernel, fumeterre ana ʒ 12, boli bibitus ʒ 6, rute ʒ 15, diptani, [tormentillis] ana ʒ 6, ligni aloe, sandalis, rubie, pulegij,*
1695 *origani, aristologie rotunde, [baccarum] laure ana ʒ 10, genciane ʒ 6, puluerizentur.*

    Pro omni egritudine oculorum: *Rx 80 testitudinis in numero & feniculi m. 12, coquantur in aqu[e] lagena s.* **Contra vomitum:** *Rx seminis acedule, coste, berberis, coralli rubij & albi, ossis de corde cerui, psidij, sandalo-*
1700 *rum, olibani, tormentillis ana ʒ 3, cumini infusi, anisi vst[i], mente, rubie, galange, ligni aloe, gariofulli, amomi, croci, macis, nardi, carui, zedoarie, cucube, croci, macis, amomi interioris, cinamomi, zinziberi, allij ana ʒ 1, granarum paradisi, piperis longi & nigri, rosarum rubearum ana ʒ 4, subtilissime puluerizentur zuccari albi li. 1, ciconiorum ʒ 12, aque rosarum ʒ*
1705 *6, & fiat electuarium; [ingue in modum] dia[c]itonicem, id est, confeccio [cit]oniorum.*

    Probacio vite: *Rx foliorum jusquimani, foliorum rute terantur & fiat emplastrum ad timpora ad frontem. Si dormit, saluus erit; si non, [non].*

    [Contra vomitum.] *Rx [chinarum] macedoni[c]orum, salgie, rubie, cerfolij, ipie minoris ana ʒ 3, terantur & bibantur cum zona potu, id est, serui-*
1710 *cie ʒ 3, hoc tribus diebus mane videlicet contra vomitum & [fastidium] tollit*

1693. Ad pestilenciam] *in ordinary script, not display script* T

1694. tormentillis] Rs, tormelle TS2S1

1695. baccarum] S1, vaccarum TS2Rs

1697. egritudine oculorum] *marg. ann. in grey-brown ink, poss. ann. 1 writing later:* Ie sight *plus ann. 1's* N[ota]   testitudinis] testudinis S2S1

1698. aque] aqua TS2   Contra vomitum] *marg. ann. in grey-brown ink, poss. ann. 1 writing later:* contra vomitum

1700. vsti] S2S1Rs, vste T

1701. amomi croci] amomi interioris cinamoni zinziberi albi ana ʒ 1 granarum paradisi amomi croci S2S1Rs

1702–1703. cucube croci macis amomi interioris cinamoni zinziberi albi ana ʒ 1 granarum paradisi piperis] cucube piperis S2S1Rs

1705. ingue in modum diacitonicem] S2S1Rs, inguem modicum dianitonicem T

1706. citoniorum] S2S1Rs, siconiorum T

1707. Probacio vite] *marg. ann. in grey-brown ink, poss. ann. 1 writing later:* probacio vite

1708. non] *om.* TS2S1Rs

1709. Contra vomitum] *om.* TS2S1Rs   chinarum] S2, china ʒ 3 (terantur & bibantur *canc.*) T (*incomplete corr. of eyeskip error*)   macedonicorum] S2S1Rs, macedoniorum T

1711. fastidium] fastigium TS2S1Rs

& dat appetitum comedenti, &c. Probatum est de Lightfoote Gardener[83] *quem vxor sua vocat pater, super quem Gardener probatum erat.*

Ad mulieres tantum:[84] *Fiat fleobotomia sub cauillis cum fumigacione radi-*
1715 *cis yris.* First ther must be made to hir a potage, as it is writen in *retencione menstruorum.* 2. After that she must have hir drynke, as it is writen in *suffocacione menstruorum.* The thrid, she must have a pelow that she must sit on in the bath, writen in *suffocacione menstruorum.* The iiij, she must have hir bath, as it is writen in *suffocacione menstruorum.* The 5, she must have
1720 an vnguent for hir lymmes, as it is writen in *suffocacione menstruorum.* The vi, she must have suppositories, as it is writen in *mola matricis.* The vij, she must have pissaries, as it is writen in *mola.* The viij, she must have emp[l]astres for hir wombe, as it is writen in chieldyng in the birth. The ix, she must have anoyntyng to bryng furth. The x, she **[fol. 133v]** must
1725 have trocisces of mirre with their decoctions of duretik.

For brekyng: take rosemary, rede myntis, lorel levis *ana* ʒ 3 & *s.*, clowes ʒ *s.*; seeth al thiese in rede wyne 3 quartis, of zucre roset ʒ 3 and clense it.

A stuphe secundum Edmond Priest:[85] take of mugwort, wormode,
1730 and nept, origanum, peritory, puliol montayne, rewe, of eche iliche moche; buyle hem wele al toguyder in water and make a stuphe.

A drynke: take also wyne that comyn and percely rotis, [&] mugwort, rotes of persenepe of the fielde and rotis of gladyn boiled in with hony a saucerfull clarified.

1735 **Another drynke**: take mugwort, diptayne, sauayne, Inglissh mader, piony, of eche iliche moche and stamp hem and buyle hem in osey wyne or bastard and put therto clarified hony and drynk it oft with powder of jeate. A plaster: take levis of marygoolde, chikemete, perito-rie and stamp hem with the seedis of gromel and of columbyne, with
1740 xij pepercornes; make a plaster and drynke of the herbis.

1714. Ad mulieres] *marg. ann. 1:* A speciall medicyne; For wemen *added in paler brown ink, prob. by the same hand, writing later*

1729. A stuphe] *marg. ann. 1:* A stuphe   secundum Edmond Priest] *in marg.* S2, *om.* S1Rs

1732. A drynke] *marg. ann. 1:* A drynk   &] S2S1Rs, of T

1738. A plaster] *marg. ann. 1:* A plastere

1740. herbis] *foll. by* A plaster, *rubricated and in display script:* TS2S1Rs

**[xix: It happith of dyuers wymmen grete greuaunce
in travailynge of chield]**[86]

Dyvers tymes it hapith of dyvers wymmen a myscheuous grevaunce in
travailyng of chield for defaute of goode mydwifes, and that greuaunce
1745 kepen prevy and it nedith for to be holpen. To sum wymmen happith
this greuans that the peritoneon brekith, that ther is but oon issue
for both voidaunces; and of thiese wymmen oft tymes cometh out the
matrice for the wey is made so large in hir trauailyng and so the matrice
wexith harde and wil nat be sette ageyn in hir owne place but if it be
1750 holpen with medicyne. And þe help must be in this maner: take goode
wyne and make it hote and put butter in that wyne that be fressh and
nat salt, and with the wyne softly wipe the matrice often tymes til it wex
souple and soft, and than esily put it into the membre ther it shuld be.
And after that sowe the breche of the peritoneon[87] in iij placis or iiij
1755 with a duble silken thrcdc. Than put a lynnen clowte into the membre
after the quantite of thc membre (*scilicet, vulue*). And after that lyne it
above with tarre and that shal make the matrice withdrawe and so sitte
fast for the stynkyng of the tarre and þan shal **[fol. 134r]** the breche
be helid and closed with powder of confery and of pety consowde and
1760 of canel. And ley the pacient in hir bedde vpright, so that hir feete lie
hier than hir hede, and lete hir ly so ix daies, and so without remoev-
yng from thens to hir nedis, and make hir ete liquite meatis mesurably
in that season and drynke also. And aftcr ix daies bien passed make
hir arise and mesurably lete hir keepe hirsilf from trauaile or busynes
1765 and she must kepe hir from bathis and from al metis that bien evil to
defien and from hevy metis and from al suche metis as wil engendre
the cough. Also it is for to wite that ther must be put into hir ars hole a
towaile made of lynnen cloth to stoppe that th'egestion go nat oute but
whan tyme of voidaunces bien in the ix daies aforsaide.[88]

1741–1742. It happith . . . of chield] *Title taken from Contents List at beginning of
T, fol. II verso.*

1743–1744. grevaunce in travailyng] *marg. ann. 1:* Wemen in þer Travelyng

1747. of] S2S1Rs, oft T   thiese wymmen] *marg. ann. in brown ink, prob. ann. 1
writing later:* For wemen; *marg. ann.. 1:* N[ota] this

1750. take] *marg. ann. 1:* Cura

1750–1751. goode wyne] good why3t wyne S2S1Rs

1752. wipe] moist S2S1Rs

1767. into hir ars hole] *marg. ann. in pale brown ink, prob. by ann. 1 writing later:*
For wemen, *foll. by* Secretes, *written at another time in grey ink*

1770   Ther bien also other wymmen in the whiche oft tymes their matrice
wil come downe and sum tyme arise for sum cause. And it bien suche
wymmen that mow nat konne suffre a mannes yerde for the gretnes
þerof, and sumtyme thei bien constreyned to suffre, wil they nil they.
To suche wymmen we put the medicyne aforsaide of the lynnen clowte
1775 and moist it with hote oile of puliol or muscelyn and we put it into the
membre (*id est*, vulua), and we bynde it therto til the matrice be setelid,
and the wymmen bien forboden metis that shuld maken hem to cowgh,
and drynke also.

Also it is to wite that the comyng out of the matrice of an old wom-
1780 man is vncurable, and also in a yong womman if it come out with moche
bloode and so haþ bien long tyme duryng. But that hath nat long tyme
dured may be holpen thus: at the begynnyng we muste moist the matrice
with the water of malowes that the holy-hocke was soden in; and after
that we anoynte the membre (*scilicet*, vulua) with aragon and the share
1785 also; and also with marciaton and oile of puliol and so we put in ageyn
the matrice. And [t]han we make þe womman sitte on a siege wele
closed with clothis, and than vnder the siege with hote coles and we put
on þe **[fol. 134v]** coles stynkyng thynges, as clowtis of wul and her, and
stynkyng herbis, as hemlocks and suche other; and so shal the matrice
1790 abide in hir place. And whan the matrice is thus in, we make a plastre and ley on the share of mastik, of frankencense, of bole armoniac
and sandragon and picche medled toguyder and that kepith it evermore stil.

If so be a womman desire to conceyve of a man that she wold con-
1795 ceyve of, it must first be wist [if] she be able to have hir desire, that is,

---

1774. To suche wymmen] *marg. ann. 1, very pale ink*: N[ota]

1775. and moist it] with þe tarre. And yf we haue no tarre, we take a lynnen
clout & moysten it S2S1Rs

1776. id est] scilicet S2S1Rs

1777. metis] m *written over* l *or* b T   cowgh] *marg. ann. 1*: Coghyngis

1779. comyng] c *written over what appears to be first stroke of* w *or* v T

1782. at the begynnyng] *marg. ann. 1*: N[ota] this

1783. of malowes that the holy-hocke] þat malowes & þe holyhok S2S1Rs

1785. and also] S2S1Rs, and also a womman T

1786. than] S2S1Rs, whan T

1788. coles] *marg. words and letters (pen trials?) in later hand at top of fol. 134v*: Jan;
Marke e (*with two superscript strokes?*); e?

1795. if she] yf she S2, yf þey S1Rs, is she T

for to witen if any defaute be in any of oon of hem both. Thus it may be wist: take ij litel pottis, as it were mustard pottes, and in eche of the pottis put whete branne and put of þat mannes vryne in that oon pot and of the wommans vryne in that other pot, and so lete the pottis stonde
1800 ix daies or more. And if case be that the man be nat able, thow shalt fynde after the ix daies wormes in the vryne and foule stynkyng; and if the defaute be in the womman, thow shalt fynde the same proef. And if the wormes appiere nat in nother vryne, thurgh medicynes þei mown bien amended and have their desire with the grace of God, as thus:
1805 Take the stones of a bore and drie hem in a potte closed with a co"> covercle wele luted or pasted aboute the jointours that non eyre come out; than sette it in an ovyn and whan thei bien dried, make powder therof and lete the womman drynk therof after that she is purged of hir floures.[89] And than lete hir go to man and she shal conceive with the grace of
1810 God; but she must drynke that powder with wyne.

Also if she desire to conceive a man chield, than she must take the matrice of an hare and the kunt and drie it in the forsaide maner and powder it and drynke the powder therof with wyne. And if the womman desire a femal chield,[90] lete hir drye the stones of an hare, and
1815 in th'end of hir floures make powder therof and drynk therof to bed-wardis and than go pley with hir make whan tyme is.

Another medicyne for wymmen that may nat conceive: take the stones and the liver of a pigge that is delivered of sow alon and make powder therof, and gyve the womman to drynke with wyne whan she
1820 goeth to bedde to hir make, and she shal conceive. Witnesse **Trotula**.[91]

1796. in any of oon of hem both] of one of hem or of bothe S2S1Rs; *marg. ann. 1:* To knowe þe man & woman whey they haue no Child & in whos defaute it is, *prec. by ann. 1's form of* N[ota] *in rusty-colored ink*

1798–1799. in that oon . . . that other pot] *marg. ann. 3:* Not[a]

1805. stones of a bore] *marg. ann. prob. by ann. 4, or ann. 1 writing later (with same form of 'N' for 'Nota'), using rusty-brown ink:* Stones of a bore; N[ota] bene

1806–1807. come out than sette it in an ovyn] come out ne yn in an ovene Rs, come oute in an ovene S2S1

1808. of hir floures] de floribus (*in display script*) S2S1Rs

1811. to conceive] *marg. ann. 10, writing somewhat later in grey ink, perhaps to clarify spelling of 'conceive' in the foll. note:* To conceive; *marg. ann. 1:* To consaue A Child

1814. a femal chield] *marg. ann. 4 or ann. 1 writing later, in rusty-colored ink:* N[ota]

1820. Trotula] *in display script* TS2S1Rs; *end of* Rs

[fol. 135r]

[xx: A goode medicyne for the stone proved triewe
and a medicyne for the palesye]

A goode medicyne for the stone proeved triewe. Take the seedis of
gromel, careway, percely, saxfrage, fenel, loveache, smalache, stan-
1825 marche, and cheri stones kernels, rotes of phelipendula of eche of thiese
iliche moche of weight; and make powder of it and drynk a sponeful at
ones of the powder in white wyne or in ale warmed first and last til she
be al hole; and if she vse it in potage it worchiþ the better. And if ye
have the colik put to the powder of baies of þe laurer half as moche in
1830 weight as of oon of the forsaide seedis. **Anoþer medicyne for the stone**.
Rx rotes of percely, rotes of fenel, rotes of smalache, rotes of radissh,
rotes of gromel, rotes of saxfrage, rotes of alisaunder, rotis of phelipendula of eche an handful; fenel seede, percely seede, smalache seede,
louache seede, carewey seede, gromel seede, saxfrage seede, kernels of
1835 chery stones, alisaunder seede of iche an ounce, a[n]amonie half an
vnce: bray al thiese a litel and buyle hem in iij potels of water to a potel
with easy fuyre, the vessel covered. And whan it is cold, streyne oute
the liquor and medle therwiþ iiij vncis of suger and buyle hem a while
toguyder, and than ther is a drynke of the whiche [vse] bi the morowe
1840 first, at nyght last, a goode draught mylke warme. Rx *benedicte* ʒ 1, *inte-*
rioris coloquintide ʒ *s., hermodactillis* ꝫ 2, *pul*[*ueris*] *d*[*omi*]*nici, diamargarit*
ana ꝫ *s.; fiant pelli cum aqua ardif vel spigeanil*. And this medicyne afore
writen is goode to dissolve the collik.

     A goode medicyne for þe palasie. First take primerols, wield sauge,
1845 strawbury levis, folefoote levis, of eche a goode handful and hak hem
right smal, and þan buyle hem: if it be for a man in a potel of barowes

---

1821–1822. A goode . . . the paleseye] *Title taken from Contents List at beginning*
of T, fol. II verso.

1823. stone] *marg. ann. 1:* Stone; *in later hand:* n[ota] ex[aminat]ur

1830. stone] *marg. ann. 1:* Stone; *in later hand:* n[ota] ex[aminat]ur

1833. handful] S1 *breaks off here due to loss of following leaf*

1835. anamonie] omamonie S2, amamonie T

1839. vse] S2, *om.* T *(in S2,* vse *occurs on the second of two lines ending in* whi- *or*
why-, *which may contribute to T's omission)*

1841. pulueris dominici] pul din^ci TS2

1842. spigeanil] spigeinill' S2 *(i.e.,* spigurnella)

1844. palasie] *marg. ann. 1:* Palasie; *in later hand:* n[ota] ex[aminat]ur

1845. strawbury levis] straweberiwise S2

grece, and if it be for a womman in a potel of sow gres. And buyle al
toguyder with a sookyng fuyre iiij or v houris at the lest and than lete it
stonde al nyght in the potte that it is buyled in, and in the mor[o]wtide
1850 heete it and drawe it thurgh a straynour; and kepe it in a close vessel, and it wil kepe itsilf vj or vij yeere goode inowgh. And ley the sike
agenst the fuyre nat to hote, and anoynte the sike therwith twies a day
ther he is diseased vpon the ioyntes.

A medicyne for the palasie. Take peleter of Spayne, herbe benet,
1855 anise, percely, galingale, clowes, notemuges, sauge, rewe, stanmarche,
macis, frenssh sene, the **[fol. 135v]** seede of a beest that is cald castory,
and long peper *ana* iliche moche an vnce if thow wilt, or ellis more or
lesse, and make hem al toguyder in a powder, and sarce hem cleene.
And ete of that powder half a sponeful in the potage afore mete and
1860 eche day duryng thi lif wassh thy nekke and thi handes and al the joyntes of thyn armes with aqua vite and eche third day drynke a sponeful
of aqua vite after thi mete.

For to make aqua vite aforsaide. First take ij galons of the strengest
wyne that thow maist gete and put it in a cleene vessel and put therto
1865 origanum and lauender and tyme, rosemary and sauge, wield sauge,
puliol mountayne, puliol roial, primerollis, cowslippes, carlokes, of
eche evene porcioun and powder of castory aforsaide *di. li.* and a potel
of grete mustard; and put al thiese in the wyne into a vessel and stil it
vp in ij stillatories and vse it as it is beforsaide.

1870 **A medicyne for the palasie that makith a man to tremble**. Take rede
fenel, percely, savayne, laurer levis, of eche an handful and an handful of white malues and another of raddissh and an handful of avons
and ij handful of prymerols and a handful of lavender and another of
isope and another of borage and another of croppes of rede netlis and
1875 ij handful of betayne and ij handful of hertis tung and ij of solsequium
and a handful of violet and another of waterkersen, and also moche of
sauge as haluendel thyn other herbis amounten the weight. And than
lete wassh hem right cleene and stampe hem and than do hem into
a newe erthen pot and do þerto a galoun of fyne rede wyne, and iij

---

1849. morowtide] S2, morwtide T
1854. palasie] *marg. ann. 1:* Palasie; *in later hand:* n[ota] ex[aminat]ur
1856. the] *signature(?) added to lower marg.:* Thomas Sandye (*or* Sandys?)
1862. aqua vite] *marg. ann. 1:* Aqua vite; *in later hand:* n[ota] ex[aminat]ur
1870. palasie] *marg. ann. 1:* palsye; *in later hand:* n[ota] ex[aminat]ur
1872. avons] avence S2

1880 potels of fyne spryngyng water, and do therto a potel of fyne lif hony
      that is buyled and wele iscomed and than seeth al thiese wele toguyd-
      ers til that thei come to a galoun, and than take it down of the fuyre
      and strayne it thurgh a straynour, and do it in a faire cleene vessel and
      cover it right wele and lete the sike vse of that drynke first and last, at
1885 even hote and at morow cold, til he be hole of þat malady.†

Explanatory Notes

[1] **and to his blessid moder Marie ful of grace:** This passage was presumably expunged during the Reformation.

[2] **but natheles of bledyng:** There is a lacuna here in all copies of *Sickness of Women 2*. In **H**, the passage reads: "but neuer þe lese kynde hathe ordeyned wymmen a purgacyoun of bledynge at certayn tymes" (lines 5–6); cf. **A**, fol. 76v.

[3] **from the tyme of xij . . . of l wynter:** For differing medieval views on the normal ages of menarche and menopause, see Green 1992, 85; Green 2001, 20–21.

[4] The list of ten topics (or eleven, if one distinguishes "witholdyng of the secundyne" from "ache of the matrice") here at the beginning of the text does not correspond to either the number or the ordering of the chapters within the text. There is no precise correspondence in the differently ordered *Sickness of Women 1* (cf. **H**, lines 24–32), either, since the list had been meant as a general summary of the kinds of diseases to which women were subject, not a table of contents *per se*. (In no copy of *Sickness 1* that we have examined is it even laid out in list form nor are the topics numbered.) Note that what is listed in the *Sickness 2* Table of Contents as a separate chap. ix, "goyng out of the matrice bynethfurth," is in the text actually part of chap. iiii, "precipitacioun of the moder." See Headnote, Table 1, above.

[5] **And otherwhiles thei han scotayne . . . tournyth vp-so-doun:** This passage is not found in **H** (cf. line 62), nor is there any corresponding passage in the Latin. There is, however, a chapter in the full ME Gilbertus *Compendium medicine* that mentions that one of the signs of "scotomy" caused by melancholy is menstrual retention; cf. **A**, fol. 9r.

[6] **their bries . . . and swellith sumwhat:** The term "bries/bryes" occurs four times in *Sickness 2*, all in this first chapter: lines 73, 95, 102, and 106. Rowland 1981, 63, understood the term to mean "waters" (and therefore, "urine") and so altered the word "swellith" here in line 106 to "smellith" (Rowland 1981, 64). However, examination of *Sickness of Women 1* as well as the Latin *Compendium medicine* shows that "brics/bryes" means "eyelid" and is a translation of the Latin *palpebre* (cf. Norri 1998, 322: *bries* 'eyelids; eyebrows; eyelashes'; and 338: *eyebryen* 'eyelids'). Nevertheless, the *Sickness 2* redactor himself seems to have been unclear what the term meant. In the second usage, the phrase in *Sickness 1* had read "& þe colour of þe bries of hir iren wolen be as cleer red" (**A** 77v; **H**, line 67, deletes *of þe bries*), translating the Latin *et purpureus calor* [correctly, *color*] *palpebrarum* (Gilbertus, *Compendium*, Lyons 1510, fol. 291rb). Although scribes of *Sickness 1* did not have trouble with the term *iren*, which seems to be an otherwise unattested plural form of *eie* (we find the more normative form *yeen* in **H**, lines 67, 72, and 76, for example; however, cf. Textual Note to line 428, where *iren* was used to mean "iron" in **S2S1Rs**), the *Sickness 2* redactor altered the phrase to read "the colours of herr bries .i. of her changyng, than woll be of a cler rede" (**S1** fol. 182r; cf. **T** lines 95–96). In so doing, he repeated

what he seems to have understood as a definition of *bries* from line 73 above, but which was in fact a clarification of what an *infection* of the *bries* was, not a definition of *bries* itself.

[7] **as I spak of right now:** This corresponds to the phrase "a boue sayde" in **H** (line 132).

[8] **late hem bleede . . . I saide afore:** This cross-reference is the same in **H** (line 153), not an addition of the redactor of *Sickness 2*.

[9] **and put in thi prevy membre:** All three other copies of *Sickness 2* instruct the reader to put it in "*the* prevy member." The change here in **T** seems to be simple scribal error, since no other passages explicitly address a self-medicating female reader. There is also a lacuna in *Sickness 2* here vis-à-vis *Sickness 1*, perhaps due to an eye-skip or perhaps simply to the *Sickness 2* redactor's desire to be more economical. Where *Sickness 2* has "But anoynte it first with cleene hony," **H** (and the other copies of *Sickness 1* that we have consulted) has "but a noynte it furst with þe juse of mercurye. Or elles take þe rote of hook, or of mader, and larde yt with scamonye and a noynte yt with hony, and put yt yn, or a noynte oon of the forsayde rotes with hony" (**H** 164–167).

[10] **a pelow that the womman shuld sitte on:** This medicated pillow seems to be a novel therapy. It has not yet been documented in any other medieval gynecological text.

[11] **oile myscelyn . . . in þe chapitre of suffocacioun herafterwarde:** This is the first original cross-reference added by the redactor of *Sickness of Women 2*. The recipe in question can be found in chap. 3 below.

[12] **And yeve hir to drynk electuary emagoge:** The compiler at this point does not identify what this hemagogic (bloodflow-inducing) electuary is. Yet later, in the long Latin section of the text (lines 1613–1625), we find an *Antidotum emagogum antedictum, id est, quod datum emagogum, id est, sanguinem menstrualem ducens.*

[13] **trosikes . . . in the chapiter of *mola matricis*:** A cross-reference by the *Sickness 2* redactor to the troche described in chap. 11 below. The error, "*mala matricis*," in **S1** is a further indication that that MS is not the author's holograph.

[14] **it deliverith . . . beeste therin ibredde:** In addition to the uterine mole, which was believed to be a lifeless lump of flesh (see chap. 11 below), there was also a notion current in some medieval medical texts that a monstrous creature could be conceived in the womb. In twelfth- and thirteenth-century texts, this was called by various terms such as *frater Lumbardorum* or *arpa*. (Our thanks to Mireille Ausecache for sharing with us her recent findings on this textual tradition.) See, for example, Rufinus's extended account from the late thirteenth century: "Theriac drunk with the juice of a leek expels the dead fetus, that is to say, the animal that is found in the wombs of the women of the Salernitans and the Apulians, which is marvelous to hear of and which induces a sort of stupor in the human mind. For this animal is most wondrous, and it is

affirmed for certain by learned Salernitans, that is, Alexander, master Maurus, and many other learned men, that those women who bear sons [have] midwives prepared with sticks held in their hands so that, when it first comes out, they immediately kill this *grapalus* and they take every precaution that when it exits from the vagina it not touch the ground, and they put something under it lest this happen, because, as the learned men say, if it touches the ground, the child coming forth after it will die immediately from leprosy." See Thorndike and Benjamin 1946, 317.

[15] **but I forsoþ do to thiese medicynes . . . and if I shal make a laxatief:** These are the only two passages where the redactor refers directly to his own clinical practice.

[16] **If it be in the first maner:** Following this phrase in **H** is the additional passage: "þe womannes veynes ar þen ful of blode in dyuersc places of hyre body, and if it be in þe secounde maner, when þey hafe þer floures, þat is to say when . . . " (lines 270–272). The several scribes of *Sickness 2* (and perhaps the redactor himself) seem to have compensated for the lacuna by interpreting "and other" two lines below as introducing "þe secounde maner." ("And" is capitalized in **S1**, fol. 185r, signaling that it starts a new sentence.)

[17] **And if it is of heete, he shal fynde:** In **H** (line 280), this had read, correctly, "sche." The masculine pronoun is found in all four copies of *Sickness 2*.

[18] **a man other a womman:** Bleeding hemorrhoids in men were often likened to the menstrual flux in women; see Green 2001, 215.

[19] **lete drien hir with metis and drynkes:** Instead of "drien," **H** (line 294) has "diete" (cf. **A**, fol. 80r). This conforms to the Latin, "Dieta sit pauci sanguinis generatiua" (Gilbertus, *Compendium*, Lyons 1510, fol. 295vb). Rather than being a simple transcriptional error, however, the reading here in *Sickness 2* (on which all four copies agree) may reflect a clinical understanding that an excess of blood does, indeed, need to be "dried" out.

[20] **succide of the bloode:** Instead of *succide* (which the *MED* documents only from this text, offering a hypothetical etymology from the Latin *sucidus*, "juicy"), **H** reads *sotelte* (line 320). Although the scribe of **S2** added the marginal note "Of sugite of bloode" (see Textual Note to lines 375–376), the Hammond scribe did not copy it here in **T**. This is the only case where he omitted one of **S2**'s marginalia.

[21] *probatum est* **in Chepa, London:** Note that it is only the assurance of efficacy that is new here in *Sickness 2*. The remedy itself is unchanged from its form in *Sickness 1*.

[22] **take lynseede al hole . . . on this maladie:** In **S1**, this recipe occurs first at the bottom of fol. 186v and again at the top of fol. 187r. The repetition of this error in **S2** and **Rs** supports our belief that **S1** (or a direct derivative from it) is the source of the other copies. As noted in our apparatus, the **S2** scribe recognized the repetition and marked it for expunction. The Hammond scribe,

copying (we believe) directly from **S2**, had the duplication flagged for him and so did not reproduce the error.

[23] **the aforsaide suppositories and electuaries:** This cross-reference is original to *Sickness 1* (cf. **H**, line 355).

[24] **a goode quantite of vryne with water**: In *Sickness 1*, this had read "a goode quantite of reyne water" (**A**, fol. 80v; **H**, line 361). (We have not been able to find an exact source for this passage in the Latin Gilbertus.) The transformation into "Iren with water" (**S2S1Rs**) seems to have originated with the redactor of *Sickness 2*, with the Hammond scribe reinterpreting it again as "vryne with water."

[25] **and Avicen techith it in the 2 chapitre of bothor:** In his *Canon*, Avicenna devoted two chapters to "hemorrhoids, *bothor,* and 'mulberry-like swellings' which appear in the uterus and vulva" (*De emorroydibus & bothor & moro que apparent in matrice & clauo*; *Canon* 3.21.4.20–21 [Venice 1507, fol. 377rb–va]). *Bothor* is the Arabic name for a kind of small pustule, often used for those occurring either in the eye or on the female genitalia; cf. Norri 1992, 306, and Trotter 1999, 35. Although Avicenna (at least in the printed edition) makes no explicit mention of baths made with alum (he says only that the woman should sit in "styptic baths" [*Et fiat vt sedeat in aquis stipticis*]), alum was considered one of the principal styptic substances, so the inference that our author has drawn is quite reasonable. Note that the error "of bothe" by the scribe of **S1** is yet another indication of his unfamiliarity with medical terminology (cf. Explanatory Notes 13, 52, 78, and 89).

[26] **but if it be of corrupt seede [as I saide] bifore:** Both **S1** and **Rs** preserve the fuller reading that was found in *Sickness 1*, "if it be of a corrupt sede as y sayde be fore" (**H** line 415; **A**, fol. 81v). The agreement of **S2** and **T** in this omission is further evidence of their commonality against **S1** and **Rs**.

[27] **for in certayne . . . deede agenst Goddis hestis:** Although this passage is not found in **H** (cf. line 422), it is found in other copies of *Sickness 1*; cf. **A**, fol. 81v.

[28] **in the chapiter of witholdyng of bloode:** This cross-reference is original to *Sickness 1* (cf. **H** line 423).

[29] **and other stynkyng þinges, as I saide bifore:** This cross-reference is also original to *Sickness 1* (cf. **H** lines 445–446).

[30] **Also if the mydwif . . . with swete smellyng thynges:** It is ironic that the redactor of *Sickness 2* has added this injunction that the midwife masturbate the woman suffering from uterine suffocation since it directly contradicts Gilbertus's own rejection of masturbation as a remedy. As he says, "Caueant a generantibus sperma neque audienda sunt mendosa delitamenta magistrorum qui docent digitorum fricationem et regularium in regulari vsu veneris hanc egritudinem remouere" (They should beware substances that generate sperm, nor ought the lying conceits be listened to of masters who teach that this sickness can be eliminated by rubbing with the fingers and regular sexual intercourse; *Compendium,* Lyons 1510, fols. 297vb–298ra. Compare the admonition against

non-marital sex in lines 555–559 above.) Be that as it may, therapeutic masturbation had been recommended for uterine suffocation by a variety of medical
writers since antiquity and the compiler of *Sickness 2* clearly had no problem
with it. Compare, for example, Rhazes in his *Liber ad Almansorem*: "Obstetri-
ci quoque precipiatur vt digitum oleo bene redolente inungat, et in circuitu
oris vulue dum est intus bene commoueat" (The midwife should be instructed
to anoint her finger with a redolent oil and to move it vigorously around the
mouth of the vagina; Rhazes 1497, fol. 50va). On sex as therapy more generally, see Cadden 1993, esp. chap. 6.

[31] **leis:** Although all four MSS agree in reading *seis* here, Rowland's suggested
emendation of *leis* (lees, dregs, precipitated matter; cf. *MED*, s.v. *lie*) seems reasonable, given the likely difficulty of keeping all the gums and spices dissolved
in the *oile myscelyn* as it cooled. The sense is that the oil is of medicinal benefit
("it is never the worse") even if the gums and spices settle to the bottom of the
vessel in which it is stored, so that the oil itself is "standing on the lees."

[32] **And also it bryngeth furth . . . with his subfumygate:** See Explanatory Note
72 below. On these views about the processes of birth and the need for obstetrical intervention, see Explanatory Notes 52, 54, and 59 below.

[33] **trocissis of murs:** On the troche of myrrh, see chap. 10, lines 1295-1302, below.

[34] **precipitacioun of the moder:** This is one of the few instances where the
Hammond scribe (or the scribe of his exemplar) failed to change "moder" (in
the sense of "uterus") to "matrice." Cf. Headnote, n. 37.

[35] **thow myghtest knowe bi the tokenes þat wern itold in the next chapiter:** In
H (lines 503–504), this reads "þou mayst knowe be tokennys to be in þe next
chaptere *be fore*" (emphasis added; cf. **A**, fol. 82v), that is, in the *previous* chapter on uterine suffocation. The following chapter, both here and in *Sickness 1*,
is on wind in the uterus, where there is no differentiation made between hot
or cold causes.

[36] **lete hir vse oximel that was told bifore:** There is, in fact, no other reference
to oximel in the text. In **H** (line 303) the passage reads similarly: *vse the oximell
be for sayde*. Although mention is made of oximel in the corresponding passage
of the Latin Gilbertus (*Si fiat ex paralisi, digeratur materia cum oximelle*; Lyons
1510, fol. 298rb), it seems that the cross-reference itself is the addition of the
English translator of the full Gilbertus *Compendium medicine*, where there are
multiple earlier references to oximel (cf. Getz 1991, 345, s.v. *oximel*), including
instructions on the preparation of its several different types (Getz 1991, 3–4).
It would seem, then, that it is to one of these earlier, non-gynecological chapters of the ME *Compendium* that the translator is referring. This offers further
proof that *Sickness of Women 1* originated as part of the complete translation of
Gilbertus and not as an independent text.

[37] **Other if the matrice . . . ne to mak water:** This discussion of uterine prolapse
(lines 745–764) derives, via Gilbertus, from Trota, *De curis mulierum*, ¶227. Cf.
Green 2001, 158–59.

[38] **Otherwhiles sum wymmen . . . hole from brekyng:** This passage on ano-vaginal fistula (lines 765–784) likewise derives, via Gilbertus, from Trota, in this case from *De curis mulierum,* ¶149; cf. Green 2001, 124–27. Compare this with the end of the text below, chap. 19 (lines 1743–1769), where the same section is translated anew. The fuller readings found in **S2, S1,** and **Rs** (see Textual Notes) correspond to the readings in **H** (lines 548–569).

[39] **but Lilie seith:** A reference to the *Lilium medicine* by Bernard de Gordon (d. 1308), a member of the medical faculty at Montpellier. In Book VII, cap. 13, *De casu et precipitatione matricis,* there is the following instruction: "Deinde si precipitatio est in altero uertebrorum, fiat uentosa in altero, et si fuerit casus fiat uentosa sine scarificatione subtus mammillas" (Then, if there is prolapse [of the uterus] on one side of the spine, let a cupping-glass be applied on the other side, and if it has fallen out, apply a cupping-glass without scarification under the breasts; Bernard de Gordon 1480, fol. 188vb). The English compiler obviously has not translated this exactly, and while there are certainly other similarities between this author's "six needful things" and Bernard's text, the correspondence is not precise.

[40] **And Avicen 3ᵉ:** The "3ᵉ" is not a reference to a part of Avicenna's *Canon,* but rather to the third of the six remedies for uterine prolapse being given in this section (cf. "The first," "The secunde thyng," and "Also the iiij" in lines 786, 790, and 812). Either our English author was working from a very different text of the *Canon* than was printed in 1507, or he was very creatively manipulating it. This third "nedeful thyng" and the latter part of the previous one both accord only slightly with the therapy for uterine prolapse found in *Canon* 3.21.4.7: "Et pone ventosam super radicem suminis eius, et super dorsum ipsius. Et fac eam odorare odores bonos valde vt ascendat matrix causa earum ad superiora. Et caue ne approximare ei facias aliquid fetidum, quare fugiat matrix ad inferiora. Cumque dies terna affuerit permuta lanam eius et pone eam lanam infusam in vino in quo decocta sunt myrtus & rosa & acatia & cortices granatorum & alia ab istis, tepido. Et embroca ex illo super sumem eius & ipsius pectinem & administra super eam linimenta facta ex sauich & facta ex herba que nascitur super lapides cum sunt in aqua & facit lubricare pedem, & facta ex lentibus cum stipticis. Hoc enim regimen quandoque sanat eam. Et fac eam sedere post illud in decoctione squinanti & myrtis & rosarum." (And place a cupping-glass upon the base of her breast, and upon her back. And make her smell especially good smells so that because of them the uterus rises upward. And beware lest you should cause anything bad-smelling to come near her, for that will cause the uterus to flee downward. And when the third day has come, change her woolen bandage [described earlier as a way to truss up the uterus] and place on her a woolen bandage infused with warm wine in which myrtle, rose, acacia, pomegranate bark [or rinds?] and other things like this have been infused. And poultice her with this upon her breast and pubic area, and place upon her liniments made of *savich* and made from the herb which grows upon rocks when they are in water, and have her foot rubbed, and [give her

food?] made from light things as well as styptic ones. For this regimen sometimes cures her. And make her sit afterward in a decoction of camel-grass and
myrtle and roses.)

[41] **and other þinges of light cost:** Although **H** has the reading "Also oþer þynges of leuys of coste" (**H** 577), **A**'s reading ("oþer þynges of liȝter cost," fol. 83r)
shows that some concern with the affordability of medicaments was already apparent in *Sickness 1.* The following list of medicaments, which have no correspondence in the Latin text, are the *Sickness 1* translator's own additions. See
also n. 20 of the Headnote.

[42] **inster:** Neither this word, found in **S1Rs**, nor the variant *inste* in **S2**, is recorded in the *MED.* If not an error, the word may be an otherwise unattested
derivative (perhaps a superlative?) of the adjective *inner(e)*, signifying the interior organs or products of the body.

[43] **fordoth . . . bryngeth . . . bryngeth:** The subjects of these verbs in lines 872–
880 should probably be read as an implied *it*, referring to the various herbs
that have these medicinal effects. Note that the herbs are named *before* their effects, a pattern that is somewhat obscured by the omitted subjects.

[44] **and that hath be tolde here biforne:** This cross-reference had appeared
here in *Sickness 1*, though in a different form. In **H** (lines 228–229), this had
read "and þat is tolde in þe precipitacyon of þe moder and with yn holdynge of
blode." In *Sickness 1*, of course, these two chapters *followed* the chapter on dropsy (see Headnote, Table 1). At least in this instance, the redactor of *Sickness 2* is
paying enough attention to his new chapter order to add the correct modifier
"biforne." Cf. Explanatory Note 48 below.

[45] **engendred toguyder:** We find nothing to support Rowland's emendation of
"gendred togedre" in **S2** to "gadered togedre" (1981, 114). The sense is clearly
that as the "matier" of the aposteme is produced (presumably pus, sanies, etc.),
ache and pricking sensations arise.

[46] **swart rede above vnder the sercle . . . vnder the sercle:** Both these references to "the sercle" (lines 1009, 1015) were original to *Sickness 1* (**H**, lines 608 and
611) and derive directly from the Latin of Gilbertus (*Compendium*, Lyons 1510,
fol. 298vb). Rowland (1981, 115) mistranslates "vnder the cercle" as "under the
opening of the anus." Correctly, "the sercle" is a technical term of uroscopy,
the uppermost of the conventional layers of urine in a uroscopy flask or "jordan" (*MED*, s.v. *cercle* [n.], sense 13). The fourteenth-century compiler/trans-
lator Henry Daniel defines the *circulus urine* thus: "þe 1st region of þe uryn,
circulus urine (þe cerkyl of þe uryn), is þe over party of þe uryn þat schewes
evermare þe disposicion of þe membris of þe lyf & of þare place" (Jasin 1983,
293). Cf. P. M. Jones 1998a, 45–46 and 54. For urine charts in color, see Murdoch 1984, 305–6; Rawcliffe 1995, pl. 5.

[47] **and the vaynes of hir legges bien of swart yalow colour of lede:** There is a
lacuna here in all copies of *Sickness 2*, apparently due to an eye-skip by the re-

dactor or already present in his exemplar. In **H**, the full passage reads: "And þe veynes of hire legges ben swart yeloo colour. And hire vryn also. And so some tyme þe vryn ys of þe coloure of leed . . . " (lines 612–614); cf. **A**, fol. 83v.

[48] **other take . . . in the next chapitre:** In **H** (line 652), this reads "in þe chapture of fleynge of þe moder," i.e., chap. 3 in *Sickness 1* but chap. 7 here in *Sickness 2*. Although the phrase "in the next chapitre" seems to direct the reader to the chapter that follows here, which is *Akynge of the matrice*, the word *next* may mean "immediately preceding" (see *MED*, s.vv. *next(e* adj., senses 1d and 3a, and *next(e* adv., sense 2b). The sixteenth-century annotator of **S1** (where the reading is the same as here in **T**) recognized the ambiguity and added the clarification "before" at the end of the sentence, thus directing the reader back to chap. 7.

[49] **wherfor the moder:** This is the second of four instances (cf. Explanatory Notes 34, 57, and 58) where the Hammond scribe (or his exemplar) retained the term "moder" instead of changing it to "matrice." Here, however, it is possible he understood that the woman was mourning (emotionally) rather than the uterus (physically). Cf. the Latin, "Delectatur enim multum matrix in amplexendo ipsum [*sc.* fetus] et retinendo" ("For the uterus delights very much in embracing and retaining the fetus": Gilbertus, *Compendium*, Lyons 1510, fol. 308ra).

[50] **other tokens that hath bien told before:** This cross-reference is original to *Sickness 1* (cf. **H** line 681) and goes back to Gilbertus's Latin text (Lyons 1510, fol. 308vb), though given the drastic abbreviation in the course of translation, it is not immediately obvious to where the reader is being referred.

[51] **Other thynges also that I have told . . . other of heete:** This passage, although found neither in **H** nor in the Latin *Compendium*, does occur in **A** (fol. 84v). The cross-reference seems to be a general recommendation to previously described therapies rather than to a specific passage.

[52] **If thow wilt knowe . . . withouten lookyng of hir water:** Despite the prominent heading, this new material added by the redactor of *Sickness 2* is probably not meant to be separated from the foregoing *Akyng of the matrice*. Only the first recipe here is a pregnancy diagnostic; the rest of the section is devoted to fetal expulsives. The rationale for these additions seems to come from the redactor's conviction, already articulated in chap. 4, that "whan the womman is fieble and the child may nat come oute, than it is better that the chield be slayne than the moder of the chield die" (lines 680–681). The first principal cause of "ache" listed here in chap. 9 is that which comes from a dead fetus that is not expelled. Clearly, the redactor is very concerned to offer lots of information about fetal expulsives (cf. new material added by the redactor in chaps. 1, 2, 5, 10, and 11), and the bulk of this new material here in chap. 9 (from *If thow wilt* to the beginning of chap. 10) is precisely on the topic of how to expel the fetus. The rubric, therefore, is misleading since the concern is not with pregnancy tests in general, but with the specific issue of determining if a woman is pregnant and there-

fore in need of a fetal expulsive. (See also Explanatory Note 89 below for another erroneous rubrication of what should have been regular text.)

⁵³ **Also if the troscisses of the myrre, as Rasis saith:** See Explanatory Note 63 below.

⁵⁴ **Also the thynges that shal casten oute a ded chield from the matrice, thei must be mightier than thoo that helpen to have easy birth:** The rationale behind this statement stems from the traditional belief that the fetus actively pushed itself out of the uterus during birth, the uterine contractions merely helping in that process. A dead child, of course, could contribute nothing to the birthing process, hence the need for stronger expulsives.

⁵⁵ **The iij is as Avicen saith:** Cf. the *confeccio bona valde* for easing delivery described in Avicenna, *Canon* 3.21.2.31, "De medicinis facilem efficientibus partum": "Confeccio bona valde de qua dicitur quod non equatur ei aliquid. Recipe myrrhe & castorei & storacis omnium ana aur .i. cinamomi sauine amborum ana aur. semis conficiantur cum melle cuius dosis sint duo aur. & melius est vt detur in potu cum vino" ("A very good medication, of which it is said that nothing is equal to it: Take myrrh and castoreum and storax, one aur. of each of them all; cinnamon and savin, half an aur. of both of them; let them be compounded with honey, of which the amount should be two aur. And it is better if it is given in a drink with wine": Venice 1507 ed., fol. 370va).

⁵⁶ **The x chapiter . . . of theire chieldren:** The long section that follows this heading, on ways to correct the malpresented fetus at birth, derives ultimately from the *Gynaecia* of the late antique writer Muscio, who was drawing in turn on the *Gynecology* of the early second-century Greek author Soranus; see Rose 1882, 84–89. The *Sickness 2* redactor makes use of two different adaptations of Muscio's Latin text. First are the obstetrical sections of an abbreviation known as *Non omnes quidem*, which had also been used by the author of the Middle English *Knowing of Woman's Kind* (Barratt 2001). Second is an independent adaptation of the illustrations of the different presentations of the fetus at birth, accompanied by the text that explained them. (Here in **T**, space was left for the illustrations but they were never added.) This synthesis of two different texts helps explain why *Sickness 2* has a sequence of seventeen fetal figures instead of the more common sixteen. As explained by the text, there is one "kyndely" fetal presentation at birth and sixteen "unkyndely" ones. *Sickness 2* actually deletes two images that were found in the normal sequence. The fifth and sixth births (respectively, two hands presenting or a small head presenting with both hands) are here fused into a single image, figure 6. It also omits both the text and the image of a complete horizontal breech position (figure 3 in the normal sequence).

Sickness 2 then adds in three new images. (1) The third image depicts a fetus with an overlarge head, a condition not mentioned by Muscio but added in the *Non omnes quidem* version of the text. (2) The fourth manner of birth, as described in the text, is not a presentation at all but general instructions on how to reposition the fetus; not surprisingly, the image of a half-sitting fetus that accompanies it is really just "filler." Both of these two additions were prompted by passages in the *Non omnes* version of the text. (3) The eleventh image, in contrast, and its accompanying text describing what to do "if the chieldes necke come first forward," seems to come from a unique tradition of the fetal images themselves, since we find the "neck presentation" only in one other manuscript, Paris, BN, MS lat. 7056. The final image, numbered 17, is not "new" but simply out of sequence; it should have appeared before the two sets of twins as an illustration of the fifteenth manner of birth.

Two further novelties in these obstetrical passages show the redactor's attention to clinical detail. First, the specification of the number of contractions it takes to expel the child (line 1150) has no known parallel in other medieval gynecological writing. Second, we find here explicit disagreement with the author of the Middle English *Knowing of Woman's Kind* over podalic extraction: whereas both Muscio and the *Knowing* author had recommended extraction by the feet if the child would not otherwise come out, our author explicitly condemns the procedure, saying "but the mydwif shal never have it furth whan he cometh so dounward" (lines 1164–1165).

[57] **from the sides of the moder:** This is another instance where "moder" should have been changed to "matrice." (Cf. Explanatory Notes 34 and 49 above.) Since it has already been explained that only the child's head has yet appeared, clearly the sense is that the midwife is to loosen the child from the sides of the *uterus*.

[58] **in the moder sides:** Again, "moder" should have been changed here to "matrice."

[59] **thurgh the fieblenesse of the matrice**: Although from our perspective it seems that the Hammond scribe should have retained the term "moder" here instead of changing it to "matrice," in fact he seems to understand that the uterus ("she"), not the woman herself, is lacking sufficient strength to expel the child. See Explanatory Note 52 above.

[60] **for grete thought of the womman and if she conceived in the first of the xij yeeris:** There is an error here that originated, apparently, in some copies of *Sickness of Women 1*. The Latin reads *Item [difficultas partus] ex debilitate matricis habet fieri sicut in iuuencule que in .xij. anno concipiunt* (Gilbertus, *Compendium*, Lyons 1510, fol. 306vb), which the translator of *Sickness 1* rendered as "As of sekenes þat þe woman haþe had, þat haþe febullye hire myche. Or elles for grete ȝonge of þe wommen as if sche conseyued in hir twelueþe ȝeer" (**A**, fol. 84v). **H** (line 714), however, as well as all four copies of *Sickness 2*, has the erroneous reading "grete þought," apparently due to a misreading of some form of *youth* (e.g., *ȝought, ȝouȝþ*, etc.) as *þought*. Rowland did not recognize the error of *ȝought/þought* and then compounded the confusion by mistranslating the latter part of the passage as "if this is the first time that she has conceived for twelve years" (134). As pointed out by Stannard and Voigts (1982, 424), the phrase should correctly be rendered "if she conceived before age twelve."

[61] **as I have here-afore told:** This phrase is not found in **H** or **A**. It shows the redactor of *Sickness 2* highlighting the lengthy obstetrical instructions he has inserted above.

[62] **But if the greuaunce be of any of thiese iij that I have rehersed:** In **H**, this clause read "But and þe greuaunce be of ony *oper* encheson" (lines 730–731, our emphasis; cf. **A**, fol. 85r). **S2, S1,** and **Rs** have an identical reading as **T**, save for the absence of the number "iij." Whether the change suggests early textual corruption or the *Sickness 2* redactor's own deliberate alteration is unclear.

[63] **with a trosciscy of myrre after Rasis ordynaunce:** Here, at last, is the full description of the troche of myrrh that the redactor has already alluded to three times before (see Explanatory Notes 13, 33, and 53 above). It is repeated in somewhat different form in chap. 11 below (Explanatory Note 71). In Rhazes' *Liber divisionum*, cap. XLIIII on *Medicine menstruorum et emoroidarum*, we have found the following recipe: "Confectio trocisci de mirra alleuians partum et prouocans menstrua: cinnamomi, mirre, ana ʒ ij. et semis, foliorum rute exiccatorum, calamenti, cordumeni [*sic*], pulegii, rubee, ase, serpini, opponacis ʒ ij. Fiant trocisci pondere ʒ ij. et detur in potu vnus cum decoctione sauine" (The confection of a troche of myrrh for alleviating [the pains of] birth and provoking the menses: [Take] two and a half drams each of cinnamon and myrrh; two drams [each] of dried leaves of rue, calamint, cardamom, pennyroyal, madder, asafetida, serapinum, and opoponax. Make troches in the weight of two drams and let one be given in a drink with a decoction of savin: Rhazes 1497, fol. 86rb). Note the discrepancies in the ingredients, which is hardly uncommon in medieval recipes. The term *sermyny* here, which is otherwise unattested, may be a corruption of *cinnamoni*.

[64] **puliol *id est* woderof :** "Puliol" (pennyroyal) and "woderof" (woodruff) are not synonyms (cf. Hunt 1989, 301, 315), which means that the ".i." (for *id est*) in all four copies of *Sickness 2* is in error. If we can assume the redactor was knowledgeable enough about herbs that he wouldn't make this kind of mistake, this error may suggest that **S1** is not the author's autograph.

[65] **and distroieth *molam matricis*:** On the uterine mole, see chap. 11 below.

[66] **Hockis also haven . . . wasshen in his handis:** Although not found in **H** (cf. line 752), this passage does appear in **A** (fol. 85r).

[67] **isopus:** A late marginal note to this passage draws a parallel between this stone and the stone called *aetites*, or the 'eagle-stone,' a hollow, geode-like stone said to be found in the nest of the eagle, as described by Pliny, *Historia naturalis* 10.4, 30.44, 36.39. See *OED*, s.v. *aetites*. The form *iaspis/iaspus* is found in both *Sickness 1* and the three other copies of *Sickness 2*. It translates the Latin *Iaspis optimam habet virtutem producendi fetum* in Gilbertus's original *Compendium* (Lyons 1510, fol. 307rb). The power of jasper to deliver a woman suffering a difficult labor is also attested in several Middle English lapidaries, and the *aetites* is said to aid in delivery and help prevent the loss of a child (Evans and Serjeantson 1933: jasper, 23, 43, 93, 121; *aetites*, 53, 66, 87, 126). **T**'s error here (which

confuses the herb hyssop with the stone jasper) is probably another sign of the Hammond scribe's general inexperience with medical texts. The late marginal annotator who suggests that jasper is the same as the *aetites*, though mistaken (the two stones were always recognized as distinct in the lapidaries), still may be making an understandable error since the use of the eagle-stone seems to have increased quite substantially after religious birthcharms were suppressed during the Reformation (our thanks to Mary Fissell for this information [personal communication]).

[68] **A precious stone . . . delivered of chielde:** Although not found in **H** (cf. line 771), this passage does appear in **A** (fol. 85v).

[69] *De mola matricis:* This entire chapter is a new addition of the *Sickness 2* redactor. We have not yet been able to identify its source, though we think it likely that it derives from a Latin text.

[70] *hoc Augustinus:* A manuscript of the late fourteenth or early fifteenth century contains an atelous medical treatise by 'Sir Austyn the leche' of which only four chapters survive, including a brief mention of excess humours in the uterus (*matrice*), of which the writer says he will treat in a later chapter: 'But for it is þing of myche priuyte. and also for ribaudis I schal reste at þis tyme to telle þerof. til I come into þe same mater þat I þenke to meue and to telle of / Of þis y nowe ceese' (fol. 53v); the manuscript, BL, Sloane MS 100, all written by a single hand, also includes many recipes for various ailments, but not one corresponding to this pessary, at least in what survives of the manuscript. In his *IMEP* volume on the Ashmole Collection, L. M. Eldredge lists six other manuscripts containing a text on the four humours and four elements related to portions of the text in Sloane 100 (1992, 13: Ashmole 342, Item 2), but none that we have examined so complete as Sloane 100, nor any others naming Sir Austin the Leech as author or compiler. The version in Ashmole 342, fols. 119r–126v, copies chapters 1–3 of Sloane 100, and so includes the reference to excess humours in the *matrice*, with the same deferral to later writing, right at the end of the text as it survives in that manuscript. Also, a clerk named Austyn put together a ME medical compilation for the London barber-surgeon Thomas Plawdon in the early fifteenth century, but examination of that text does not produce any parallel with the recipe attributed to "Augustinus" here. (Our thanks to Linda Voigts for allowing us to consult her microfilm of Plawdon's manuscript, Cambridge, Gonville and Caius College, MS 176/97.) Neither Talbot and Hammond nor Getz include Sir Austin the Leech in their lists of English medical practitioners.

[71] **Or ellis yeve hir trocisces of myrre that Rasis makith in his booke of** *Almosorum:* The following recipe repeats, in slightly different form, one already given above in chap. 10.

[72] *Et sic require in suffocacione menstruorum:* The use of the phrase *suffocacio menstruorum* here seems to reflect a curious confusion on the part of the redactor of *Sickness 2*. There is, it is true, an explicit reference to expelling the afterbirth in chap. 3 on uterine suffocation: "And also it [root of iris] bryngeth furth the

ded chield mervously and the secundyne and menstruat with his subfumy-gate" (lines 681–683). However, as is clear from the cross-references in the section *Ad mulieres tantum* near the end of the text (lines 1714–1725), the redactor understands *suffocacio menstruorum* not as an equivalent for *suffocacio matricis* (translated in chap. 3 as "suffocacioun of the matrice") but as the proper Latin term for "the stoppyng of their bloode that thei shuld have in their purgacioun" (chap. 1). We have discovered no other such confusion in medieval gynecological texts between *retentio menstruorum* and *suffocatio matricis*.

[73] **as it was told afore . . . flowyng of bloode:** Both this cross-reference and the one that follows ("medicynes that were told in the chapiter of witholdyng of bloode") are original to *Sickness 1* (**H** lines 800–801 and 805). There should, however, have been three cross-references here, the absence of the third one apparently being due to an eye-skip. Correctly, after "yeven hir medicynes," the passage should read: "before sayde. In case þat sche hafe no purgacyoun of blod after bering of childe, gif hire medycyns tolde in þe chaptre of with holdyng of blode" (**H** lines 803–805).

[74] **kerslokis other turmentil and v-levid gras other skirwhittes:** There is no mention in **H** (line 811) of turmentil or five-leaved grass (cf. **A**, fol. 85v), nor is there any in the Latin Gilbertus. The latter mentions only *eruca agrestis*, which is correctly translated in **H** as "karlokkes or skyrwyttes." Cf. Hunt 1989, s.vv. *eruca*; *quinquefolium*; and *tormentilla*. The phrase "other turmentil and v-levid gras" thus seems to be a misplaced interpolation.

[75] **And if [the] veynes bien broken:** On the unusual use of the second-person form in the variant readings, see the Headnote, n. 33.

[76] **For swellyng of wymmens legges whan thei bien with chield:** This brief passage (through "or legges that jorneyen bi the wey") is found in both Gilbertus Anglicus's *Compendium medicine* and one of Gilbertus's main sources, Roger de Baron's *Practica maior*. Aside from the omission of one final recipe *ad inflatione pedum ex dolore matricis* (which derives from Trota, *De curis mulierum* ¶215), the text as translated here corresponds better to Gilbertus's version than Roger's. Compare Roger, *Practica maior*, in *Cyrurgia Guidonis de Cauliaco, et Cyrurgia Bruni, Teodorici, Rolandi, Lanfranci, Rogerii, Bertapalie* (Venice, 1519), chap. 73, fol. 222va, with the Lyons 1510 edition of Gilbertus, fol. 309va–b. None of the copies of *Sickness 1* that we have thus far examined has this chapter, suggesting that it was not rendered into English at the same time as the other gynecological material. At the end of this chapter in **S1**, there is a mark of closure, then a blank line before the subsequent jumble of Latin and English recipes ensues.

[77] *Item secundum Rasim:* We have not yet been able to locate this remedy in any text of Rhazes.

[78] *Antidotum emagogum antedictum*: The scribal errors underlying this difficult passage are already found in the earliest manuscript, **S1** (see Textual Note to line 1613), which capitalizes the *E* of *emagogum* and then leaves a space before *mag*'. Rowland (1981, 156) interpreted *E mag*' in **S2** as *Edmund* [sic] *magistri*, apparently trying to connect this recipe with that attributed to Edmond Priest

below (line 1729; Rowland 1981, 164). We believe this "above-mentioned hemagogue" to be the "electuary emagoge" mentioned in chap. 1 above (line 269 and Explanatory Note 12).

[79] **tophasius:** On the chastity-preserving virtue of the topaz as recorded in medieval lapidaries, see the explanatory note to Chaucer's "Tale of Sir Thopas" 717 (Benson 1987, 918).

[80] **Isaac:** We have not been able to locate this passage in the works of Isaac Israeli.

[81] **folia agni casti . . . non racionem:** "The leaves of agnus castus placed in the bed relieve the burning of the urine by their nature and [do not relieve] the cause [of the burning or of the urine]."

[82] *secundum magistrum Ricardum Mersh:* No individual by the name Richard Mersh or Richard Marsh/March is noted in Talbot and Hammond or in Getz 1990b.

[83] *Probatum est de Lightfoote Gardener:* Unidentified. Like the other references to specific practitioners (see Headnote, n. 28), this is an addition by the redactor of *Sickness 2* and is found in all four MSS.

[84] *Ad mulieres tantum:* This passage seems to be a "quick reference" guide written by the redactor of *Sickness 2* himself so that he could quickly find the most important sections of the text. All refer to the redactor's own additions to *Sickness 1.* They are as follows:

1) "a potage as it is written in *retencione menstruorum*": chap. 1 (lines 236–249).

2) "hir drynke as it is written in *suffocatione menstruorum*": chap. 1 (lines 250–256). On the use of this term *suffocatio menstruorum,* see Explanatory Note 72 above.

3) "a pelow that she must sit on in the bath, writen in *suffocacione menstruorum*": chap. 1 (lines 257–266).

4) "hir bath as it is written in *suffocacione menstruorum*": chap. 1 (lines 266–267).

5) "an vnguent for hir lymmes as it is writen in *suffocacione menstruorum*": apparently a reference to "oile myscelyn" (i.e., *oleum musceleon*) first mentioned in chap. 1 (line 268) and fully described in chap. 3 on uterine suffocation (lines 639–676).

6) "suppositories as it is writen in *mola matricis*": chap. 11 (lines 1405–1410).

7) "pissaries as it is writen in *mola*": chap. 11 (lines 1413–1420).

8) "emplastres for hir wombe as it is writen in chieldyng in the birth": perhaps a reference to chap. 9, "Also a plaster that castith out a ded chield" (lines 1124–1131).

9) "anoyntyng to bryng furth": not identifiable.

10) "trocisces of mirre with their decoccions of duretik": these have been mentioned four times in the text. The reference here is probably to the complete description of their preparation in chap. 10, which is repeated in slightly different form at the end of chap. 11. See Explanatory Note 63 above.

[85] *secundum Edmond Priest:* Unidentified. This is the only one of the local references not found in **S1** or **Rs**. It seems to have originated as a marginal addition in **S2**, and was copied by the Hammond scribe as text rather than marginalia.

[86] **It happith of dyuers wymmen grete greuaunce in travailynge of chield:** The following seven sections seem to have been translated and appended as a group. (See the Headnote, n. 37.) Six of the seven derive from the *Trotula,* a compendium of twelfth-century texts of Salernitan origin. The first, on ano-vaginal fistula, corresponds to *De curis mulierum* ¶149; note that this same section had already appeared in chap. 4 on *Precipitacioun of the Moder* above, where it was drawn from Gilbertus Anglicus's Latin *Compendium medicine* which, in turn, had drawn on the *De curis mulierum.* The second section on uterine prolapse caused by forced sexual intercourse corresponds to *De curis mulierum* ¶150; cf. Green 2001, 126–27.

The third section, which distinguishes curable from incurable cases of uterine prolapse in old and young women, comes from an as yet unidentified source. Intriguingly, it maintains the same first-person plural forms as the previous section.

The following four sections on conception also come from the *Trotula,* in this case the *Liber de sinthomatibus mulierum,* ¶¶75, 75a, 76, and 77. Note the interesting misunderstanding in the translation of ¶76. The Latin was very clear that this whole recipe was intended *ut masculum concipiat.* The instructions were divided into two parts: the man is to consume the uterus and vagina of a female hare, while the woman is to consume the testicles of a male hare. The English translation assigns to the woman herself the consumption of the female hare's genitals, and then misinterprets the second part as a separate recipe on how to conceive a female child. Aside from one late antique Latin text, this is the only positive attempt at conceiving girls that we have found in a medieval gynecological text. See Green 2001, 220 n. 130.

[87] **the peritoneon brekith . . . breche of the peritoneon:** On usages of *peritoneon* for what in modern anatomy is called the *perineum* (the area between the vagina and the anus), see *MED,* s.v. *peritoneum.* See also Norri 1998, 382.

[88] **Also it is for to wite . . . in the ix daies aforsaide:** The last sentence of this paragraph shows either that the translator was working from a defective copy of the Latin *Trotula* or that he misunderstood the text. A crucial passage at the beginning of the sentence has not been translated. In its original form, the Latin passage had read: *Hoc etiam sciendum est qualiter eis in partu sit subueniendum. Paretur itaque pannus in modum pile oblonge et ponatur in ano ad hoc ut in*

quolibet conatu eiciendi puerum firmiter istud ano apponatur, ne fiat huiusmodi continuitatis dissolutio. ("It should also be known how they should be cared for in [subsequent] childbirth. Let there be prepared a cloth in the shape of an oblong ball, and let it be placed in the anus so that, in each attempt at pushing out the child, this is firmly pressed into the anus so that there not be [another] dissolution of continuity [of the flesh] of this kind.") In the version of the *Trotula* this translator was using (perhaps a copy of the transitional ensemble), the first sentence was dropped. The translator apparently didn't understand that this anal support was to be used only during subsequent childbirth and not, as it seems to be understood here, as a mechanism to prevent miscarriage. Cf. chap. 4 above, where the sense of the text was better preserved.

[89] **after that she is purged of hir floures:** The English-Latin phrase found in **S2S1Rs,** "after that she is purged *de floribus*," may well be the work of the *Sickness 2* redactor (it corresponds to the Latin in *Trotula,* ¶75a, "post purgationem menstruorum"). It is odd, however, that all three MSS incorrectly interpret the Latin *De floribus* as a heading and capitalize it.

[90] **And if the womman desire a femal chield:** On this misunderstanding of the Latin text of the *Trotula,* see Explanatory Note 86 above.

[91] **Witness Trotula:** This rubric shows that the redactor of *Sickness 2* was well aware of the source of the preceding recipes. It is not clear, however, that he meant to suggest that the whole text was a translation of the *Trotula;* indeed, it is not even clear that the highlighting of the name was intended. (See Explanatory Notes 52 and 89 above for other instances of incorrect rubrication.) Be that as it may, the scribe of **Rs,** where this section closes the text, understood the name to refer to the whole work, for he opens the text with the general title *Liber Trotularis.* None of the other three manuscripts of *Sickness of Women 2* includes that or any other title.

-12-

JOHN OF BURGUNDY: TREATISES ON PLAGUE

Lister M. Matheson

The Trinity manuscript contains three plague treatises in English that are all ultimately derived from a Latin work written by an author who names and describes himself as Master John of Burgundy ("*Johannes de Burgundia*"), otherwise known as "*cum barba*" ('with the beard'), citizen of Liège and practitioner of medicine.[1] The work is variously titled in its different manuscripts and versions, and I follow Brussels, Bibliothèque Royale, MS II.1413 and London, BL, Sloane MS 2320 in calling it *De epidemia*. John's original treatise was probably compiled in 1365, as a French translation of 1371 informs us;[2] its immediate stimulus was not the Black Death of 1347–1351 but the pandemic *pestis secunda* (or *pestis puerorum*) of 1361–1362, an outbreak of "plague" that was especially fatal among children and the landed gentry.[3] In the introduction to his treatise, John claims to have writ-

---

[1] Sudhoff 1912, 62, upper text, lines 1, 3; 63, lower text, lines 42–43; 69, line 260. See also Explanatory Note 10 below. For early attempts to identify John of Burgundy with John Mandeville, the author of the *Travels*, see D. W. Singer 1916, 161 and notes 1 and 2; Singer and Anderson 1950, 25–26. Modern scholarly skepticism about the true identity and biography of the latter makes such an identification unlikely; see Hanna 1984, 121–23; Higgins 1997, 260–64.

[2] D. W. Singer 1916, 212. The translation is found in Paris, BN, fonds français, nouv. acq. MS 4515 (earlier numbered 4516), written in 1371 by Raoul d'Orléans for Gervaise Crestien, the physician of Charles V of France; the manuscript also contains a French translation of Mandeville's *Travels*.

[3] Shrewsbury 1971, 126–30. On the medical ambiguity of medieval disease terms like *pestis*, see note 16 below.

ten two other works on the plague and he gives their incipits (lines 75–82 below), though they do not seem to have survived.

The original form of John's treatise was known in continental Europe, both in Latin and in rare French and Hebrew translations, but its circulation was limited (Matheson 2005). However, it achieved great popularity in England through several subsequent Latin and English versions—more or less in its own right (occasionally misattributed to some other author), in adaptations (often attributed to "John of Bordeaux"), and in other works as an unacknowledged source.[4] Such popularity, rather than his medical qualifications, probably accounts for the attribution in England of other works to John of Burgundy: the *Trotula* (in an English translation);[5] a *Practica physicalia* containing about 295 recipes in Oxford, Bodleian Library, Rawlinson MS D.251, fols. 72v–113r;[6] astrological and medical items appended to the *Governal of Health* in London, BL, Sloane MS 989, fols. 35v–126r, 127r–132v;[7] and an astrological tract translated by John Bolte in Oxford, Bodleian Library, Ashmole MS 340, fols. 45v–47r (now missing), 48r–54r.[8]

John of Burgundy, *De epidemia:* Long Version with Astrological Prologue

The first plague treatise in the Trinity manuscript begins at the top of folio 153v, without title but with a decorated initial capital letter and the second letter capitalized: "Bicause that al thynges here in erth, as wel þe elementis as thynges spryngen and compowned of the elementis, bien graunted and ladde bi the bodies tha[t] bien in the spieris or cerclis of the firmament . . . ." Further down the first page of the text there is a space, where the scribe breaks off in the middle of a line with the words "able to brenne right so nother," leaves the next three lines blank, and then recommences with a paraph and

---

[4] The Dominican friar John Moulton's adaptation, incorporated in *The Myrour or Glasse of Helthe* (first printed prior to 1531), is a good example of such appropriation and adaptation; see Keiser 2003, 292–318, 323–24.

[5] "Iohn of Burgwen," in one (s. xvi) of the two manuscripts comprising a separate translation (the fifteenth-century manuscript of this translation is fragmentary); see M. H. Green 1997a, 87–88 (I thank Monica Green for drawing my attention to this attribution).

[6] "Johannes de Burgundia"; printed in Schöffler 1919, 145–308; see also eVK 723 and Norri 2004, 103.

[7] John of Bordeaux (D. W. Singer 1916, 177); see also eVK, Manuscript Index, under BL, Sloane 989, for a list of individual items.

[8] eVK 504.

the words "bodies that bien cleene and nat necligent ne recheles . . ." (lines 23–26). Presumably the scribe's exemplar was damaged in some way, and material that would have filled approximately one and a half lines of text has been omitted. This first treatise breaks off abruptly in mid-line on fol. 156v with the words "the herte peyned or grevid wherfor . . . ."

This treatise is an incomplete copy of a Middle English translation of the so-called "Long Version," with an astrological prologue, of John of Burgundy's *De epidemia*.[9] The numerous Latin manuscripts of John's original treatise fall into two main types, primarily distinguished by the presence or absence of an astrological introduction explaining the theoretical causes of plague and introducing the author and his other works.[10] Both types are found in manuscripts of English provenance and both were translated into English, in at least six independent translations, several unique, none of which seems to have had any widespread circulation (Matheson 2005).

The incomplete treatise in the Trinity manuscript was reproduced in the sixteenth-century partial copy of the manuscript, TCC O.8.29 (part I, fols. 1r–32v, with the *De epidemia* on fols. 25r–29r), but a full text is found in London, BL, Sloane 3449 (fols. 5v–12v). Sloane 3449 is a fifteenth-century manuscript which also contains a version of an anonymous text (*inc.* "Hit is to vndrestond that euery man lyvyng haþe iiij humours like to the iiij elementis") often found with the Middle English translation of Gilbertus Anglicus's *Compendium medicinae* (fols. 1v–5r); a Latin phlebotomy tract (fols. 12v–14v); and a small group of medicinal recipes added in the sixteenth century (fols. 14v–15v).[11] The English Long Version texts in TCC R.14.52 and Sloane 3449 are not very close and suggest that other intermediary copies must have once existed.

John of Bordeaux, *Medicine Against the Pestilence Evil*

Immediately after the incomplete English Long Version of John of Burgundy's *De epidemia*, the scribe begins a second plague treatise with a decorated initial capital letter and the second letter capitalized: "Here bigynneth a noble treatice made of a goode phisicien John a Burdews for medicyne agenst the pestilence evil and it is departed in iiij parties or chapiters." Apart from materials found only in the preceding Long Version treatise,

---

[9] Edited from the Latin (with many errors) in Sudhoff 1912, 61–69. A good modern English translation, slightly adapted, is in Horrox 1994, 184–93.

[10] Sudhoff 1912, 59–61; Singer and Anderson 1950, 39–42.

[11] Singer and Anderson 1950, 42–43 (where the text in T is not noted); see eVK 1227, 3212, 5700, and Getz 1991, lxxi–lxxii.

considerable overlap between the two treatises develops in their phlebotomy sections. It is possible, then, that the guiding spirit behind the compilation of the Trinity manuscript realized this belatedly and instructed that
the scribe discontinue his copying of the first treatise.

Despite the promise of four chapters in the incipit, the text does not
include an explicit for the third chapter, a heading for the fourth, or a sentence such as "The fourth chapter telleth how that a man shall be kept that
is fallen into this sickness" (cf. Harvard University, Countway Library of Medicine, MS 19 in Harley 1985 for 1982, 184, lines 94–95), and so the text of
the third chapter continues without interruption or marker into that of the
fourth. The oversight is not the scribe's fault, however, for an analogous situation occurs in other English four-chapter texts of similar type (for example,
Lincoln, Cathedral Library, MS 91; both texts in Oxford, Bodleian Library,
Additional MS A.106 [though a paraph and spaces are inserted in the second
text]; London, BL, Sloane MSS 963 and 983).[12] This second plague tract ends
on fol. 158r with the words "And thurgh the grace of God he shal escape and
be delivered from this sikenes. Here endith the treatice of John de Barba and
John of Burdeux made agenst the sikenes pestilencial, whiche is the sikenes
epidymal. *Anno Domini Millesimo CCC^mo nonogesimo* [i.e., 1390]."

This is a copy of a plague tract that is usually attributed to a John of
Bordeaux, alias John de Barba.[13] This work was very popular in fifteenth-
century England and survives in over forty Middle English copies and
at least eight Latin copies written in England; there are also Dutch and
Hebrew translations, most likely made in the Low Countries. The contents
are derived from John of Burgundy's *De epidemia* (probably the type without the astrological introduction) and presented in the form of four short,
practical chapters dealing with: (1) regimen and diet to avoid the pestilence; (2) how the disease enters and attacks the body; (3) detailed blood-
letting instructions to combat the disease in a person who has contracted
it; (4) diet and medication for an infected person.

The English four-chapter texts can be divided into three groups, according to whether they contain a short colophon ascribing the composition of
the treatise to the year 1365, to the year 1390, or, sometimes by simply omit-
ting the colophon, contain no date at all.[14] The three manuscripts that note
the year 1365—Oxford, Bodleian Library, Ashmole MSS 1444 and 1481, and

---

[12] See also Explanatory Note 34 below.

[13] Modern editions are Sudhoff 1912, 73–75 (BL, Sloane 2320, with many errors of
transcription); Ogden [1938] 1969, 51–54 (incorporated in the *Liber de Diversis Medicinis*; Lincoln, Cathedral Library 91); Harley 1985 for 1982, 182–85 (Countway 19).

[14] See Singer and Anderson 1950, 31–33, 34–38; Keiser 1998, 3856; additional
detail is given in Matheson 2005.

London, BL, Sloane MS 965—name the author as "Maister John de Bur-geyne," also known as "La Barbe." However, these texts contain verbal elaborations and idiosyncrasies typical of texts that passed through the revising hand of John Shirley, the well-known anthologist and scribe,[15] and this form of the text cannot directly underlie the 1390 and undated groups. The text in TCC R.14.52 belongs to the large group of texts that usually name the author as John of Bordeaux, alias John de Barba, and contain the date 1390 in a colophon. In fact, the third group of four-chapter texts, that containing no date, should be rolled in with the 1390 group, as the presence of the date is, for various reasons, of limited diagnostic value; thus, for example, in TCC O.8.29 (the sixteenth-century copy of R.14.52) the scribe simply omitted the colophon that contains the date, although it was present in his exemplar.

The 1390 and undated four-chapter texts are usually ascribed to John of Bordeaux, but at least two of the undated texts, in TCC O.2.13 and London, BL, Harley MS 3383, name the author as John of "Burgo(y)n," i.e., Burgundy, and may, therefore, represent an early stage in the text's development. It is just possible that a John of Bordeaux was responsible for the reworking of John of Burgundy's *De epidemia*, but it is more likely that the name arises from a misreading of the Latin "*Johannis de Burgundia*," i.e., Burgundy, as "*Johannis de Burdegalia*," i.e., Bordeaux.

The four-chapter version may well have been made in 1390, for some form of virulent disease broke out in England in that year. The Westminster Chronicle reports: "About the beginning of June intensely hot weather set in and continued until nearly September. This was the cause, owing to the rankness of the air, of a great and deadly pestilence, which was epidemic in various parts of England (though it never raged everywhere) until Michaelmas, its victims being rather the young than the old. Even so, some illustrious knights died in this time of plague."[16]

An Approbate Treatise for the Pestilence

The third plague tractate in the Trinity manuscript occurs on folios 174r to 175v. It is a compilation of several pieces, as detailed below, and does not specify the name of any supposed author, though most of its material is

---

[15] See Connolly 1998, 176–77 and 186–87 n. 32 (citing A. I. Doyle). See also n. 17 below.

[16] Translation in Hector and Harvey 1982, 439 (the Latin text is on the facing page). This was almost certainly not bubonic plague, but one should keep in mind that, as Shrewsbury points out, "John [of Burgundy] had no conception of bubonic plague as a specific disease entity," and what was considered a "plague" "might be any one of a dozen or more communicable or transmissible diseases of man" (1971, 140, 141).

drawn from John of Burgundy/Bordeaux. A second copy appears in London, BL, Additional MS 5467, fols. 85r–87r, a collection of practical, medical, and historical works, several of which are connected with or translated by John Shirley; this manuscript was written in the second half of the fifteenth century and may have belonged to Selby Abbey in the West Riding of Yorkshire.[17]

The component parts of the *Approbate Treatise* in the Trinity manuscripts are as follows:

1) A heading (lines 312–315): "And folowyng here next bigynneth an approbate treatise for the pestilence studied bi the grettest doctours of phisik amonges the vniuersites of Cristendom and amonges al Cristen naciouns in the tyme of Seynt Thomas of Caunterbury."

Dorothea Singer (1916, 174 n. 3) suggests that this St. Thomas "can hardly be Thomas à Becket, who occupied the See from 1162 to 1170. The reference is probably to Thomas Bourchier, Archbishop of Canterbury from 1456 to 1486." This is unlikely for two reasons: first, John Shirley may, again, have been involved in the present text and he died in 1456; second, Bourchier was not canonized. The reference is probably to Becket, a cheerful anachronism designed to give venerable authority to the text.

2) Material (lines 316–384) abstracted without attribution from John of Burgundy/Bordeaux, especially from the section on bloodletting, beginning "For the vniuersal goode of al Cristen people to lierne the most soverayne medicyne of diete, of bloode leetyng, and of herbis and moche other counsails of solempne doctours for the Epedemye cleped the pestilence," and ending "that diete is goode and medicynable for the pestilencial sikenes."

3) A section on, first, the general virtues of phlebotomy and, second, the dangers of over-recourse to it (lines 385–396), beginning "Thiese bien the vertues and the goodenessis that folowyn bicause of bloode leetyng in competent and dewe tyme," and ending "It is the norice also of the gowte; the straitnes of the brest cometh therof also and many another malady and sikenes." TCC R.14.52 includes a very similar passage on the virtues of bloodletting earlier in the manuscript,

---

[17] For descriptions of the contents, see the entry in British Library online catalogue of manuscripts, http://molcat.bl.uk/msscat; Manzalaoui 1977, xxxvii–xxxviii; Matheson 1999, 7–10. On links with Shirley, see Connolly 1998, 121–40, 175–78; Matheson 1999, 11–12. For connections between manuscripts associated with Shirley and manuscripts written by the Hammond scribe, see Connolly 1998, 178–82, and Mooney, chap. 3, 59–60 above.

in the *Liber fleobotomie* (Supplementary Text II, lines 142–149, above). In addition to the two copies of the *Approbate Treatise* in the Trinity and BL Additional manuscripts, closely related texts on the virtues and dangers of bloodletting are found in London, BL, Sloane MS 963, fol. 4r–v (which also includes item 4 below); BL, Sloane MS 1315, fol. 32v (also item 4); Edinburgh, National Library of Scotland, Advocates' MS 18.3.6, fol. 1v (also item 4); San Marino, Huntington Library, MS HM 64, fols. 9r (virtues), 82v (dangers; also item 4); Helmingham Hall, MS LJ.II, fols. [2v–3v]; TCC O.9.10, fols. 73r–74r (virtues).[18]

4) A short preventative recipe against gout (lines 397–399), also found in the four manuscripts indicated in the previous item.[19] The Trinity copy is closer to the other instances of this recipe than that in BL, Additional 5467, though both alter the recommended date for taking it from the first Thursday in May (as in the four other manuscripts) to "the first day."

5) A section on uroscopy (lines 400–413), beginning "And for þe knowyng verily bi the disposiciouns what maner of sikenessis men and wymmen bien in, biholde bi the morow if þe vryne be white al bifore mete," and ending "Bi thiese ensamples ye may have notice of your estatis." The second surviving manuscript of the *Approbate Treatise*, BL, Additional 5467, ends at this point with the word "Explicit." The uroscopic signs given in this section appear to be a subset of those found in some of the Middle English uroscopy tracts that begin with a form of the phrase "Urine white on the morrow and brown after meat." In particular, the signs given here derive from a version of the tract that characterizes certain urines of women as shining like silver and gold,[20] though the normal form of this tract contains more than the six diagnoses given in the extract included in the *Approbate Treatise*.

6) The Trinity copy of the *Approbate Treatise* contains a few concluding lines (lines 414–417) on three ("the" in the manuscript) perilous days of the year for bloodletting "bi writyng and doctryne of Seynt

---

[18] eVK 3121 and 3502; 3121 and 6877; 3122 and 3501; 1297 and 3500; 7285; 1298. On BL, Sloane 1315, see also Brown 1994, 5–6.

[19] eVK 888; 883; 2932; 882.

[20] The "bright as silver/red as gold" version of the text can be found in BL, Sloane 963, fols. 12v–13r and 54r–55r; BL, Royal 17.a.iii, fols. 60v–61v; Bodleian Library, Ashmole 1393, fols. 61v–62r, and Ashmole 1438, part I, p. 117. The Voigts-Kurtz electronic database records twenty-six items with some form of the "white/brown" incipit, but the majority of those texts do not contain the silver/gold signs. My thanks to Tess Tavormina for information on these Middle English uroscopic texts.

Beede"; this segment ends incompletely in mid-line with the words "and thiese creatures of man that letith hym bloode vpon any of thiese iij daies he shal [be dead]." These lines may be an addition to the original compilation. Very similar though not identical materials occur independently of the *Approbate Treatise* in BL, Additional 5467, fol. 69v (*inc.* "By th'ynstrucioun, good counsell, and doctryne of Seynt Beede ther bene certeyne days of the yere that been defendid an ynhibet that no mane lete hym blood vppon hem ne et no flesshe of gees . . . ") and, especially, fols. 71v–72r (under the title "Mede-syns approbate for mortall sekenessesse by Saynte Beede," begin-ning "Mane to let hym blode vppon, by the writyng and waryne of Sante Beede; and by theos, what criaturs of manekynde that leteth hyme blode vpon any of thies iij dayes, he shall be dede withynne six dayes nexte that folowyn . . . ").[21]

Editorial Practice

The principles and conventions listed in the preface to this volume have been followed, but the following points should be noted:

1) Since the English translation of John of Burgundy's *De epidemia* (Long Version with Astrological Prologue) is previously uned-ited, a full collation with the second surviving text in London, BL, Sloane MS 3449, fols. 5v–12v (with the siglum **S**) has been provided. Selected variants in the Latin (**Lat.**) texts are cited from London, BL, Royal MS 12.G.IV, fols. 158r–160r (**R**); Oxford, Bodleian Library, Ashmole MS 1443, pp. 351–75 (**A**); Cambridge, University Library, MS Kk.6.33, fols. 39r–42v (**U**); and Sudhoff's 1912 edition, 61–69 (**Su,** used with caution; includes variants from Erfurt, Amplonian Library, MS Q.192, fols. 146r–148v [**Am**] and the privately-owned Rosenthal manuscript, fols. 58v–62r [**Ros**]). The French translation in Paris, BN, fonds français, nouv. acq. MS 4515 (formerly 4516), fols. 97r–102v (**BN**; ed. D. W. Singer 1916, 201–12) is occasionally cited in the Explanatory Notes. For reasons of length and redundancy of general content with materials in the two subsequent treatises, the remainder of the English Long Version, found only in **S**, has not been printed in the present volume.

---

[21] Edited in Furnivall and Pollard 1904, 188. The word "approbate" occurs in BL, Additional 5467 in this title, in the title of the *Approbate Treatise*, and in the phrase "doctours approbate of the vniuersall scool of Athenes" (fol. 70r). See *MED*, s.vv. *approbat* ppl., *approbaten* v.

2) In light of the many surviving texts of John of Bordeaux's *Medicine Against the Pestilence Evil* and their complex textual relationships, only a very selective collation is provided in the Textual and Explanatory Notes, to elucidate errors in the Trinity copy or to present substantively significant variant readings. The manuscripts used are Cambridge, Jesus College, MS 43 (Q.D.1), fols. 137r–139r (**J**), and three texts from the Sloane Group: Harvard University, Countway Library of Medicine, MS 19, fols. 43r–49r (**C**; ed. Harley 1985 for 1982); Cambridge, Gonville and Caius College, MS 336/725, fols. 148r–150v (**G**); and London, BL, Sloane MS 2320, fols. 16r–17v (**Sl**; ed. Sudhoff 1912, 73–75; used with caution).

3) Since *An Approbate Treatise for the Pestilence* is also previously unedited, a full collation with the second surviving text in London, BL, Additional MS 5467, fols. 85r–87r (**Ad**), has been given.

JOHN OF BURGUNDY:
TREATISES ON PLAGUE

De epidemia (Long Version with Astrological Prologue)

[fol. 153v] Bicause that al thynges here in erth, as wel þe elementis
as thynges spryngen and compowned of the elementis, bien graunted
and ladde bi the bodies tha[t] bien in the spieris or cerclis of the firmament, as Moises Hallac seyn in their bookes of interpretaciouns,
5 *Capitulo accio,*[1] the bodies aboven bien founden to bryngen into al the
bodies that bien vndir their sercles essent or beyng, nature or kyndely
in substaunce, vegetacioun or drivyng, livyng and dieng. As nowght
long [sithen], of influence or impressioun of the hevenly or high bod-
10 ies, both causatiefly and effectually the aire was corrupt and bigan pestilencial in effect. Nought that the aire was corrupt in his substaunce,
for it is a symple or vnmedled body, but it corruptith be encheason of
the evil vapours medled toguyders, wherof *Epedimia* or pestilence in
many costis folowen. And yit now in ful many placis his tracis or his
15 steppis appieryn, as it shewith wele, for many on is infect, and namly
suche as bien replet and stuffed ful of humours that bien mystempered
with evil qualitees.

---

1. *Titles for the three treatises that follow are editorial.*

3. graunted] governed S

4. that] S, than T   bien] *foll. by* above S

5. Moises Hallac . . . bookes] Mosehallac seith in his boke S

6. Capitulo accio] *in display script; marg. in later hand:* Commyng of the pestelens

7–8. kyndely in] kynde S

8. drivyng] thryvyng S   and] or S

9. sithen] S; feedyn T

10. bigan] bicom S

12. or] þing or an S

13. Epedimia] *prec. by paraph and in display script*

14. now] *om.* S   ful] *om.* S   or his] and S

16. ful of] with S

17. qualitees] qualite S

But yit corruptyng of the aire is nat al-only cause of moreyne, but
also habundaunce of humours corruptith in hym þat dien, as **Galien**
20 saith in his *Booke of Fevers*; the body suffrith no corrupcioun but if the
matier of the body be prompt or redy to and in maner subiect or obe-
dient to the corruptible cause.[2] For right as the fuyre may nat brenne
but in matier that be combustible (able to brenne), right so nother
[pestilence ne pestilencial aire noyeth nat but if it fynde matier redy
25 and obeyeng to corupcioun, wherfor] bodies that bien cleene and nat
necligent ne recheles in purgyng and clensyng of hemsilf abiden and
enduren in holsumnes and helth.

Also, thei abiden hole whos complexioun is contrary to þe aire that
is chaungid or corrupt, and ellis al folke shuld corrupte and die in the
30 aire at oones. The aire, therfor, so chaunged and corrupt bredith or
engendrith in dyvers folke dyvers sikenes or soris after the variaunce
or [**fol. 154r**] diuersitees of their humours. For every worcher or every
thyng that worchith parformyth his werk after the habilite and disposicioun of the matier that it werkith ynne.

35 And bicause that many maisters ther han bien, grete and fer lierned
in theoric or in speculacioun and groundly in sight of medicyne, but
thei bien but litel proeved in practic and therto al ful ignoraunt in the
science of astronomyc, the whiche is in phisik wonder nedeful, as wit-

---

18. al-only] alone S

19. corruptith] corupt S   dien] *add. in right marg. by scribe*   Galien] *prec. by
paraph and in display script*

21. to] þerto S   in] *foll. by* a S

22. as] as (*line end*) as S

23. be] is S   combustible] *foll. by* or S

24–25. pestilence . . . wherfor] S; T *leaves a half line and then three lines blank bef.
recommencing with a paraph*

26. ne] nor S

28. abiden hole] *om.* S   is] *om.* S

29. corrupt] *foll. by* abiden hole S

29–30. in the aire] *om.* S

30. chaunged and corrupt] corupte and chaunged S   or] and S

31. or] and S   variaunce] variauncez S

34. it] he S

35. many maisters . . . grete] þer haue ben many grete maistirs S

36. in (2)] *om.* S

37. ful] fully S

38. whiche] *foll. by* science S

nessith Ipocras in *Epedimia sua,* seyeng: what phisicien that ever he be,
40 and he can non astronomye, no wise owith to put hymsilf in his handis,
&c.[3] Forwhi astronomy and phisik rectifien eche other in effect. And
also that oon science shewith furth many hid thynges of that other. For
al thynges in every thyng mown never be declared.

    And I, bi xix yeere and more,[4] often tyme proeved in practisyng
45 that a medicyne yoven contrarie to the constellacioun—although it
were wele compowned or medled and ordynatly wrought after the science of phisike—yit it wroght nother after the purpos of the worcher
ne to the profite of the pacient, as if I have yoven a medicyne laxatief
to purge dounward, the pacient hath cast it out ageyn above, although
50 he lothid it nought.

    Wherfor thei that han nat drunken of that sweete drynke of astron-
omy now put to this pestilencial sores no parfit remedy; for bicause they
knowe nat the cause and the qualite of the sikenes, they may nat hele
it, as saide the prince of medicyne, **Avicen**; how shuldistow, he saide,
55 hele a sore and thow knowest nat þe cause, *quarto canone capitulo, de
curis febrium.*[5] He that knowith nat the cause, it is impossible that he
hele the sikenes. The Comentor, also, *super secundum phisicorum,* saith
thus: a man knowith nat a thyng but if he knowe the cause both fer
and nygh.[6] Sithen, therfor, the hevenly or firmamental bodies bie of
60 the first and prymatief causis, it is bihoueful to have the knowyng of
hem, for if the first and the primytief causis bien vnknowen, men may
nat come to knowe the cause secundarie. Sithen, therfor, the first cause

---

40. non] not S   wise] *foll. by* man S   hymsilf] hym S
41. &c.] *om.* S
42. hid thynges of that] thinges hidde in þe S
43. every] one S   mown never] may not S
44. bi xix] 90 S *(see Explanatory Note)*   often tyme] haue oftyn tymes S   prac-
tisyng] practise S
46. were] *foll. by* both S
48. ne] ner S   as if I have] And when some men haue S
52. now] mowe S   bicause] *foll. by* þat S
54. saide (1)] seith S   medicyne] phisik S   Avicen] *in display script*   saide
(2)] saith S
55. knowest] knowe S   quarto] iij S
56. impossible] vnpossible S
60. knowyng] knowlechyng S
61. the (2)] *om.* S   men] we S
62. cause (1)] causez S

bryngith in more plentevously his effect than the cause secundarie, as
is had *primo de ca[u]sis*,[7] **[fol. 154v]** therfor it shewith wele that with-
65 oute astronomye litel availith phisik, for many a man is perisshed for
defaute of his conseillour.

I sawe, therfor, a certeyne receite made for pestilence that cam from
the maisters of Coloyne[8] that was sent to Lyons,[9] that ther shuld be
made a confeccioun of rue, figges, and walnotis, salt and hony, to pre-
70 seruacioun of pestilence, and yit nevertheles it hadde no maner respect
agenst the pestilence but in preseruacioun agenst venemous matier of
poisounyng. If ther be any man drede venemous drynke, it is goode to
lette the venym til other remedies mown be had. But agenst pestelence
thei han no maner effect, ne no man have ful affiaunce therin.

75 And therfor I, Johannes de Burgundia, *artis medicine professor*,[10] here in the
bigynnyng of thiese pestilencis made a treatice of the causis and kynde
of the aire corrupt after the jugement of astronomy, of the whiche many
hadden the copie and it bigynneth thus: *Deus deorum dominus qui simpli-*
citer & absolute omnium ensium est conditor et prima causa, &c. And also I
80 made another treatice of distincciouns or markes of pestilencial sores,
how thei shuln be knowen from other, and that bigynneth thus: *Cum*

---

63. than] *foll. by* doth S

64. is had] hit shewith S   causis] S, casis T

65. availith] vayleth S   a] *om.* S   is] *foll. by* praised *canc.*   for (2)] in S

67. therfor] forsothe S   receite] nota *sign in marg. in later hand; marg. in an-*
other hand: Henricus v^{tus} H   for] *foll. by* the S   that] and S

68. Lyons] Leons S

69. rue] *foll. by* and S   walnotis] *foll. by* and S

70. nevertheles] nerthelees S   hadde] hath S

72. poisounyng] *marg. in very late hand:* Ag^t venemous drinke   If ther be . . .
it] Iff eny man haue dronkyn eny venemous drynke or be fferde of eny suche
drynke the said receipt S

73. the] suche S   mown] may S   had] ordeyned S

74. ne] þerfore S   man] *foll. by* owith to S

75–76. here in . . . made] for the pestilence haue made S

76. pestilencis] *marg. in later hand:* pro pestilenc *with flourish on* c   treatice]
marg. in same very late hand as above (line 72): Tractatus Johannis de Burgundiâ
de Peste &c. Eiusdem Tractatus

77. the (3)] *om.* S

78. thus] in this wyse S

81. shuln] schulde S

nullum preter instans tempus epidimale, &c.[11] In whiche, so ever hath the
copies, he shal fynde therin many thynges both to preseruacioun and
to cure. But yit nat al tho thynges that perteynen therto, as it askiþ now
85 in this present pestilence, that (as to me) is fallen on al new, and yit eft
and eft bien to fal mo divers bi successioun of tymes, for thei bien nat
yit at an end.

Therfor I, in the moreyne of the people havyng pite and compassioun, busily desiryng with hool herte al mennes helth, and therto
90 with al my busynes to profite bi divyne helpe and counsail, first lowly
biseche (I thynke) in thiese fewe wordis fully to declare both the preseruacioun [and] the cure of thiese wounderful sores. So that vnneth
any man shal have neede of any phisicien and leche, governour, pre-
server, and heler.

95 F[i]rst, therfor, to preseruacioun is nedeful every man to flee or eschewe
overmoche repleccioun of mete and drynke, and lete hym eschewe hote
bathes or stiewes and al thynges that **[fol. 155r]** rarefien wynden of muscles of the body[12] and open the pooris of issues of the skyn and flessh. For
whan the pooris or issues bien open, the venemous aire entrith, thrillyng
100 the body and defoulyng the spirites. And above al thynges coite or lechery is to be eschewed and fledde.

Of fruytes, forsoth, he may ete but litel or non, but if it be sowre
fruytes. And lete hym vse metis that bien of easy and light digestioun or
defieng and drynke aromatike (or wyne of riche odoure) and alaied with

---

82. tempus epidimale] *om.* S   so] who so S

84. to] *foll. by* the S

84–91. as it askiþ now . . . fully] accordyng to this pestilenciall tyme that now
is present ne to the pestilenciall tymes þat ben to done. Therfore I with goddis grace here folowyng in fewe wordis purpose S

92. and] S, of T

92–94. So that vnneth . . . heler] *om.* S

95. First] *dec. cap.* F *over* fi   to (1)] *foll. by* the S   preseruacioun] *foll. by* hit S

96. drynke] *marg. in later hand:* To be diot for þe pestilens   lete hym] also
to S

97. that] *catchword* rarifien

97–98. wynden of muscles] or wyden the mascles S *(see Explanatory Note)*

100. and (1)] *foll. by* coruptyng and S   And (2)] *om.* S

101. eschewed and fledde] left S

102. forsoth] *om.* S

103. fruytes] frute S   lete hym] *om.* S   of easy and light] easy and light of S

104. wyne of . . . and (2)] ryche odoured wynes S

105 water. Late hym eschewe meth and al other metis and drynkes that bien
medled with hony, and lete al their mete be medled with vynegre.

And in cold tyme and rayny wedir lete fuyre be made in þeir chambre and whan the weder is misty and troubled, whan he risith at morn,
or than he passe his chambre, if he be riche, lete hym vse precious
110 and riche confecciouns of noble redolence, as bien diambra, diamusca,
diantos with *muscis, pliris cum musco,* and suche other. And if, forsoth,
he be but poore, lete hym vse zedwale, gilofre, notemuges, macis, and
suche other; and oones or twies in the wike lete hym take of goode triacle and proeved, to the quantite of a beane, and lete theym bere in
115 their handis pomum ambre[13] or sum other aromatikes that bien most
excelent in redolence. And at nyght, or than he go to his bedde, after
the wyndows of the chambre bien shit and the chambre is close, lete
be made a blaase of the tree and of the braunchis of iuniper tree,
that the smulder and the heete may fille and overspreede al the cham-
120 bre. Or ellis lete put iij or iiij quik coles in a crusel of erth and lete

---

105. water] *marg. in later hand:* Metis & drynkis for þe pestilens   Late hym]
and S

105–106. other metis . . . with (2)] drynkes medled with hony and with alle
metys vse S

107. tyme] sesoun S   lete fuyre be made] haue fyre S   þeir] youre S

108. whan he . . . morn] þan in the mornyng S

109. than he] ye S   passe] *foll. by* his passe *del.*   his] youre S

109–110. if he be . . . and riche] a ryche man take S

110. confecciouns] *marg. in later hand:* precius & Riche confeccions   bien]
om. S

111. muscis] muske S   cum musco] with muske S

111–112. And if forsoth . . . hym] A pore man may S

112. notemuges] notemyg S

112–113. and suche other] *om.* S

113. lete hym] *om.* S   of] *om.* S

114. and (1)] *om.* S   to] *om.* S   and (2)] *foll. by* ete yt or drynke it and S
theym] hym S

115. their handis] his hande S   pomum] pome S

116. than] *om.* S   his] *om.* S

117. is] be made all S

118. made] make S; *marg. in later hand:* for þe pestelens T   tree (2)] *om.* S

119. smulder] smoke S   heete] *foll. by* þerof S

120. lete (1)] *om.* S   crusel] *badly formed* cr; *cross in inner marg.* T; litill panne S

120–121. lete do thervpon] cast vppon the coles S

do thervpon a litel of this powder; and lete hym receive the breth bi
his mowth and nose and anon vpon that ley hym doun. Take frank-
ence and white olibanum an vnce, lapdanum *di.* an vnce, storax,
calamynte or timiama[14] vj peny weight, lignum aloes iij peny weight.
125   Lete thiese be made into a wounder smal powder and lete this powder be vsed as often as in the aire is felt other stenche or evil odour.
And if it be the wil of God, that is above al other thynges, in cold tyme
and frosty wedir and corrupt he may be preserved and kept from evil
accidentis and from th'effecte of pestilence.
130   [fol. 155v] Yi[f], forsoth, in tyme of pestilence the weder is outrageous in heete, than vs bihovith to kepe another governaunce and to
vse more cold thynges than hote and to ete lasse than in cold tyme and
to excede more largely in drynkes than in meatis, and lete his wyne be
white wyne wele alaied. In his metis lete hym vse vynegre grete plente
135   and agrista, that is, an egre verious. Ne lete hym nat than vse hote spices,
as is peper, galingale, greyne parice,[15] and suche other.
        Bi the morow, forsoth, ar than he go out of his chambre, yif the
weder be reyny and the aire evil disposed, than lete hym smel rosis, violettis, floures of nemyfore,[16] sandalos, and rubias[17] and muscatelinos and
140   camfre. Triacle, forsoth, mai be take but litel in hote tyme. And yit non
take it but thei that bien fleamatik and suche as bien of cold complexioun. But thei that bien sangwyne or colric shuln take no triacle in hote
weder, but lete theym vse pomegarnettis and pome d'oranges or pomes

---

121. powder] *foll. by* þat folowith aftur S   breth] *foll. by* þerof S
122. anon] *om.* S   ley hym doun] lete hym lye downe &c. T   Take] Recipe S
123. di.] half S
124. timiama] *marg. in later hand (though prob. not referring directly to* timiama*):*
id est spurge or Esula; *cross in inner marg.*   peny (1)] d S
125. into a wounder] in S   lete (2)] vse S
126. as often] ofte tymes S   other] *om.* S
130. Yif] And if S, Yit T   Lat.: Si R   forsoth] *om.* S
130–131. is outrageous] be outrage S
131. vs bihovith . . . to (2)] we must S
132. more cold thynges] thynges more colde S
134. In] And in S   vynegre] *foll. by* in S
135. verious] vergeous S   Ne] but S   vse] *foll. by* to S
137. Bi] And by S; *marg. in later hand:* ffor þe pestelenc T   forsoth] *om.* S
than] *om.* S   yif] yf S, yif and if T   Lat.: si R
140–141. non take it but thei] it is not for to be takyn but of theym S
142. shuln] shulde S   triacle] *marg. in later hand:* Tryacle is not good &c.
143. lete theym] *om.* S   and] or S   d'oranges] orynges S

citrinis condutes or citronade or triasandis or the letuarie *pigra frigida*
145 cophyns,[18] and suche other, and lete hym pur[v]ey cucumbres, gourdes,
fenel, violarie, beetis, borage or lang de boef, and suche other.

And lete hym eschewe garlik, oynons, leekis, and suche other thynges that overmoche heten, as pepir, grayne, &c., but gyngier, canel, and
other that bien attempre mown bien vsed; and if for fervence of the
150 weder he otherwhile thurst strongly, lete hym amonge sovpe[19] cold water
medled with vynegre.

Also, if any man feele any stiryng or mocioun of bloode, fleeyng or
flikeryng, prickyng or punchyng, anon lete menuse hym on the same
side and of the next veyne therto. And the pavyng, strawyng, or floore
155 of the chambre that he lith in be spreynt with cold water and vynegre
medled. Or ellis, if he be riche, with water of rosis and vynegre, and
that twies or thries in the day.

Also, *pillule rosarum*[20] bien woundirly excelent of preseruacioun
in hote tyme if thei bie received oones in the wike, and thei availen
160 in every complexioun and in every tyme, hote and cold, save that thei

---

144. triasandis] trisandali S

145. cophyns] cophonis S   lete hym] *om.* S   purvey] purrey TS   Lat.: utatur

146. or] *om.* S

147. And (1)] *marg. in later hand:* Dyatyng in þe pestelens tyme   suche] all S

148. grayne] greynes S   Lat.: granum paradisi

148–149. and other] and other (*line end*) and other S

149. attempre] temperate S   mown] may S

150. amonge sovpe] among S   Lat.: aliquociens . . . sorbeat

151. medled with vynegre] and vynegre medled togyder or lete hym drynke
ptisans for they profiten myche and namely to them that ben hote bodies and
drye that ben slendre. And in no [*ins. above, with caret in text*] wyse hit is not
gode to suffre myche thurst in suche tyme S

152. Also] And S

152–153. or mocioun . . . punchyng] flikeryng or prychyng S

153. menuse hym] hym blede S

154. of] on S   And (2)] *foll. by* that S   pavyng] pavyment S

155. spreynt] sprynkeled S   cold] the coldest S

156. if he be riche] *om.* S   vynegre] *foll. by* medlet S

156–157. and that twies or thries] ij or iij tymes S

158. rosarum] *marg. in later hand:* pullule Rosarum A good preservatiue for þe
pestelens; *same hand in lighter ink:* ones In þe wek

159. availen] vailen S

160. that] *om.* S

bien nat accordaunt but to theym that bien replete. And other doctours
commenden hem moche, sauf that they bien sum- **[fol. 156r]** what laxatief, but the corrupt humours bi litel and bi litel þei avoiden.

165 And also thiese pillules bien ful profitable. Take aloue cicotryn thre
half peny weight, safron and myrre bi evene porcioun vj peny weight:
lete make therof pillules wiþ surip of fumetory; and of iiij and ob. peny
weight; lete be made vij pillules and oon of hem be yoven at ones.

And he that vsiþ this gouernaunce may be preserved from the marcial
deth, corrupcioun of the aire,[21] if the helply wil of God be with hym.

170 Now, forsoth, if any man for defaute of goode governaunce be fall in
pestilencial infirmyte, it is to be purveied of þe remedy, how it is therin
to procede for this maner pestilencial sores and infirmytes that bien
conformed and fastned[22] withyn a day, þat is, withynne xxiiij houres,
wherfor it is behoveful hensfurth to applie to the remedie.

175 But at the first it is to wite in mannes body bien iij principal membris, that is to wite, the herte, the liver, and the brayn, and everiche of
thiese hath his purgyng halkes (that bien clepid emunctories), whider
he purgith his superfluites, as the arm-holis bien the emunctories of the

---

161. And] Avicenna and S   other] *cross beside line in outer marg.*

162. that] *om.* S

163. bi (2)] *om.* S   avoiden] voiden S

164. pillules] pilles S   profitable] *foll. by* made in this wyse S   Take] Recipe
S; *marg. in later hand:* The Makyng of pillules Rosarum T; *marg.* Medicina pre-
seruatiua S   aloue] aloes S; *cross beside line in inner marg.* T   thre] iij S

165. porcioun] porciouns S

166. pillules] pilles S

166–167. of iiij . . . pillules] make þerof vij pilles of the weight of iiij pens &
an halpeny S

167. hem] *foll. by* to S

168–169. the marcial . . . hym] that mortall corupcion of the aire but yf the
will of god be herto contrary S *(see Explanatory Note)*

170. Now forsoth] And S; nota *sign in marg.* T; *marg. in later hand:* Pestilens T
in] *foll. by* this S

171–172. purveied of þe remedy . . . procede] knowen what provisioun shall be
made þerfor and howe men shall procede theryn S

172. that] *om.* S

173. conformed] confermyd S

174. hensfurth] *long* s *written over sigma-shaped* s T; hens forward S

175. wite] *foll. by* þat S

177. thiese] *foll. by* iij S   clepid] *om.* S

178. purgith] p *over another letter, prob.* h T; puttith S   emunctories] S; *only six
(rather than seven) minims for* mun T

herte; the emunctories, forsoth, of the lyver bien the gryndes; and the
180 emunctories of þe brayn bien vnder the earis and vnder the tunge.

Now mote yee vndirstonde that every venym takith his cours o[f]
distroyeng of the stomac, as it shewith wele in bityng of adders and serpentis and other venemous beestis. And so this venemous aire, whan it
is medled with the bloode, anon cometh to the herte, as to fundament
185 of the kynd and lif, to fordo that and distroie it and sle it.

The hert, forsoth, bi his cleene sensibilite apperceivyng that noyous aduersarie comyng, as in defence of hymsilf he dryvith that empoisouned or venemous bloode to his emunctories; bute if that venemous
matier fynde his weyes stopped, that he may nat have his cours, anon
190 he sekith to that other principal membre, that is, the liver, that bi hym
he myght distroie the kynd. The liver, forsoth, repugnyng and defend-
yng thervpon, lettith and drivith that noyous matier to his emunctories. This same is þe brayn.²³

Wherfor, bi suche maner accidentis, that bien distincciouns and
195 **[fol. 156v]** signes to the phisicien, may be wist in what place that avoided
or fastned matier²⁴ lurkith and bi whiche veyne may be avoided and

---

179. emunctories forsoth . . . gryndes] gryndes ben emunctories of the lyver S
and] *om.* S

180. the (1)] *foll. by* ij S

181. Now mote yee] And now ye must S; *marg. in later hand:* The places wher
pestilences ffixithe T   of] S, os T

182. of (1)] from S

184. cometh] hit coveitith S   to (2)] *foll. by* the S

185. it (2)] *om.* S

186. cleene] alone S   apperceivyng] perceivyng S

187. comyng] *foll. by* than S

187–188. empoisouned] empoysonde S

188. bute] and S

190. sekith] sechith S   membre] membres S

191. forsoth] *om.* S

192. thervpon lettith] hym silf betyth S   drivith] *foll. by* awey S

192–193. emunctories] emunctory S

193. This same is] and in like wyse dothe S   þe brayn] þe *foll. at end of line in
right marg. (in John Fortho's hand) and cont. in left marg. bef. and after* brayn *in next
line thus:* (þe) grindes þere þe [stop *canc.*] passadge stoppte in flyeth to the
(brayn) which sendes to the eares T

195–196. avoided or fastned] the S

196. and (1)] *foll. by* hideth hym self and by suche mene hit may be knowen S
whiche] what S   veyne] *foll. by* hit S   avoided] devoided S

draw oute. Forwhi if that infect and empoisouned bloode be sent or brought to the arm-holis, it is wele wist therby that the herte peyned or grevid, wherfor

200 **John of Bordeaux,** *Medicine Against the Pestilence Evil*

Here[25] bigynneth a noble treatice made of a goode phisicien John a Burdews for medicyne agenst the pestilence evil and it is departed in iiij parties or chapiters.

The first tellith þat how a man shal bere hym in tyme of pestilence,
205 that he fall nat in that evil. The secunde tellith how this sikenes cometh. The thrid tellith medicyne agenst this evil. The iiij, how he shal be kept therin.

This clerk saith in the first chapitre that for defaute of goode rule and dietyng in mete and drynk, men ful often fallen into this sikenes.
210 Therfor whan the pestilence reyneth in the cuntre, a man that wil be kept from this evil hym bihovith to kepe hym from al outrage and excesse in mete and drynke, that he vse no bathes nor swete nat moche, for al this openyth the pooris of the body and makith venym to entre and distressith the lifly spirites in man and enfieblith the body, and in
215 especial lechery, for that enfieblith the kynde and openeth the pooris þat wikked aire may entre and envenyme the spirites of a man.

Also, vse litil that tyme of fruytis but if thei bien sowre fruytes, and ete litel or nought of garlik, oynons, leekis, or other suche metis þat bryngith a man to vnkynde heete. Also, suffre nat gretly thurste that
220 tyme. And if thow thirst gretely, drynke but mesurable, both to slek thi thirst and thyn heete. And the best drynke were cold water menged with vynegre or tisan, for þat maner of drynk is right goode, namly to theym that bien colryke of complexioun, for thei bien hote and dry and comunely leene of body. *Explicit primum capitulum.*

---

197. empoisouned] poysynd S
197–198. sent or brought] flemyd and dryven downe S
198. it is wele wist therby] þerby hit may be knowen S   herte] *foll. by* is S
199. wherfor] *text breaks off in mid line and is immediately foll. by next tract* T; *text continues for 3½ more folios* S
202. medicyne] *marg. in later hand:* Remedy for pestestilens (*sic*)
212. moche] *marg. in later hand:* Swet ne to moch
217. fruytes] *marg. in later hand:* Ete lytill ffrut but hit be Sowre
218. other] r *ins. above*
222. vynegre] *marg. in later hand:* Water & veneger

225   The secunde chapitre tellith how this sikenes cometh and what is
the cause therof. In a man is iij principal parties and membres—the
herte, the liver, and the brayne—and ech hath his clensyng place wher
he may pute out his superfluite and clense hym.

    The herte hath his clensyng place vnder **[fol. 157r]** [the] armes;
230 the lyver hath his clensyng place bitwene the thighes and the body and
in the thigh-hoolis both;²⁶ the clensyng of the brayne or hernys is vnder
the earis and vnder the throte. Than this evil comyth þus: whan the
pores [bien]²⁷ open for sum cause aforsaide, that the venyme entreþ
and also mengith with mannes bloode and so renneth to the herte, þat
235 is ground and lif of mannes kynde, for to distroy it and sle the man.
The herte kyndely fleeth that is ageyne it and contrarious to it and puttith it to his clensyng place. And for that place is stopped, that it may
nat passe oute, than it passith to the principal part next, that is, for to
distroy the liver. And it on the same wise puttith it to his clensyng place,
240 and for that it is spered, that it may nat oute, than it passith to the thrid
principal party, that is, the hernes, and he puttith it out to his clensyng
place. And yit it may nat oute ther. And thus a long tyme it is moeved
or it reste in any place xij houres and more, and than at the last withyn
xij houres, if he²⁸ be nat passed out with bledyng, he fasteneth in sum
245 place and castith a man into agwe and makith a bocche in sum of the
iij clensyng placis or neere theym. ***Explicit secundum capitulum***.

    The third chapitre tellith help agenst this evil and whan it may be
wele helped. Whoso feelith prickyng of bloode or flakeryng, it is token-
yng toward that sikenes. Therfor thei shuld bleede soone, if it myght
250 be withyn the first houre or withyn the vj hour after. And if it be nat
than, drynke nat nor ete nat or it be. And tary nat over xij houres, for

---

225. cometh] *marg. in later hand:* The commyng of pestelenc *with flourish on* c

229. the (2)] CGSl, his T, hese J

231. brayne or] *joined by add. letter, poss.* e *or* c

233. bien] ben CGJSl, earis T *(see Explanatory Note)*

239. clensyng place] *underlined; inner marg. in John Fortho's hand:* videl: þe groyne

241. hernes] *underlined; marg. in John Fortho's hand:* or braine

241–242. clensyng place] *underlined; inner marg. in John Fortho's hand:* vid: vnder
þe eares; Throate

244. with bledyng] *underlined and asterisked above* bledyng; *marg. in John Fortho's
hand: asterisk foll. by* in 12 howers space

249. bleede] *nota sign in marg.; marg. in later hand:* Blode lattyng ffor pestelens

251. tary nat over xij houres] *underlined; marg. in John Fortho's hand:* not in 12
howers

al that tyme the matier is moevyng for cause forsaide. And certainly
bledyng be-tyme on the veynes that I shal telle [shal have it awey], but
ther passe xxiiij houres—the matier than is gadred and harded and wil
255 nat passe oute of the veyne if it be striken. Neuertheles, if a man bleede
than, it shal nat harme, but it is nat siker that it may helpe.

If than ther be matier that be gadred vnder either arme-hoolis, it
cometh of the herte veyne, that is cald the cardiacle,[29] and on the same
side that the evil is in, or ellis ther is two harmes: oon, if thow bleede
260 on that other side, the goode bloode and cleene in thi side nat corrupt
nat venymed shal be drawen out of, and the evil bloode shal dwel stil
ther. And than the body is fiebler for defaute of goode bloode that wold
han holpen the kynde. And the harme is more, **[fol. 157v]** for than the
bloode that is venymed shal passe overthwert the herte and venymeth
265 it and hastith a man to his endyng.

If the sikenes be bitwixt the thighes and the body, it is of the lyver,
and than if the matier appiere in the inner side bi the prevy thynges,
bleede on the foote on the same side and on the veyne bitwixt the thomul-
too and the too next it; for if the bocche be ther and thow bleede on
270 the arme, the matier wil draw vp ageyn to the principal partis of þe
herte or the liver and do harme. Also, if matier be more outward to the
side and further from the prevy thynges, bleede on the vayne betwixt
th'ancle and the heele or on the veyne that is evene vnder the ancle,

---

253. shal (2) . . . awey] CGSl, wylle help J, *om.* T

253–256. but ther passe . . . it may helpe] *underlined; marg. in John Fortho's hand:*
Bleedinge after 24 howers hurts not [*cropped?*] so it secure not

257–259. hoolis; herte veyne; on the same side] *underlined; marg. in John Fortho's
hand:* For swellinge vnder armc hooles bleede one þe harte vaine one þe same
side vid: cardiac: seu <u>Media</u>[<u>na</u>] [*cropped*]

261. nat] ne CGJSl

263. for] nota *sign in marg.*

266. If] *marg. in later hand:* God to Bled for the Pestilenc *with flourish on* c

266–269. bitwixt the thighes and the body; bi the prevy . . . too next it] *underlined; marg. in John Fortho's hand:* For swellinge in þe groyne bleede one þe
vaine one þe foote betweene þe greate toe and þe next. vid: a brainch of þe
saphena which is seated ouer þe inside of þe ancle & is deriued from þe flank
&c. <u>one same side:</u>

271–273. if matier be more outward; further from the prevy thynges; on the
vayne betwixt . . . vnder the ancle] *underlined; marg. in John Fortho's hand:* For
swell: more outewarde from þe flank: bleede one þe vaine betwene þe anckle
& heele scil: ischiadica one þe owte side of þe foote or saphen: on þe inside or
Box þe thigh: &c. <u>one same side</u>

that is cald sophen,[30] or ellis be thow ventused on the thigh with a box
275 beside the bocche.

If the matier appiere in the clensyng place of the hede or on the
[armes], bleede on the hede veyne on the same arme, that is cald cephalica[31] (the hede veyne), that liggith above the body veyne, that is to say,
cordiacle, in the bowght of the arme; or ellis bleede on the veyne that
280 is above the hand, bitwene the thumb and the next fynger; or ellis be
ventused bctwix the shuldres with boxes[32] til the bloode be drawe oute.
And the principal [membre] thus clensid, the herte shal be comforted
bi cold electuaries to temper the grete heete therof. Wherfor, it were
goode to have water stilled of thiese herbis: beteyne,[33] pympernel, tor-
285 mentil, and scabious, and this medicyne is goode in this sikenes and
to be kept from it.

But while[34] a man is in this sikenes, he shuld be dieted the more
mesurably, ffor the fever agwe is euermore with this sikcnesse; and while
a man is in this fever agwe, he shuld nat ete flessh gretely, but it were
290 litel chikens soden with water or fresshwater fissh or other smal fissh
fressh rosted to ete with vynegre.

Also, it is goode to ete potage of almaundis and drynke tisan or
drynke smal ale and thynne. And if the sike man coveite gretely to drynke
wyne, gyf therfor hym vynegre medled with moche water. But white wyne
295 of þe Ryne is bettir than rede, mesurable put therin.

Also, it is goode to vsc a powder that is goode agenst venyms[35] that
is made of thiese herbis (or sum of theym that may best be goten), that
is to say, betayne, pympernel, tormentil, scabious, boole armoniac, &
terra sigillata. The ij last, spicers han to selle. Ilkon of thicse herbis or
300 spicery braied bi theymsilf and drynke with wyne or ale, that castith

---

277. armes] CGSl, hernes T

278–279. the body veyne; cordiacle] *underlined and joined across two lines of text
by lighter line; inner marg. in John Fortho's hand:* Scil: aboue þe Mediane

280–281. above the hand . . . next fynger; ventused betwix the shuldres with
boxes] *underlined; marg. in John Fortho's hand:* For swell: vnder eares. Throate
[*left brace*] Cephalic: Saluatell: a quibusd: dict: consul: vesal: lib: 3. p: 273 linea 6; Cupping &c.

282. membre] CGSl, membris J, *om.* T; *cf. Lat.* De epidemia: membro R

284. water] *marg. in later hand:* Gode Waters to Drynk ffor þe Pestilenc *with
flourish on* c

289. ete] *marg. in later hand:* Dyot In pest

296. powder] *marg. in later hand:* A good powder for þe Seknes; *pointing hand
indicating recipe for powder against venoms at bottom of leaf*

[**fol. 158r**] out venym bi the same place wher it had entre, if a man be venymed.

Therfor, whoso dredith hym of this sikenes, kepe he hym from thynges in the first chapitre named. And whoso is therin, do he bi-tyme as
305 þat other chapitre tellith and rule hym after the techyng of this treatice. And thurgh the grace of God he shal escape and be delivered from this sikenes.

Here endith the treatice of John de Barba and[36] John of Burdeux made agenst the sikenes pestilencial, whiche is þe sikenes epedymal. *Anno*
310 *Domini Millesimo CCC^{mo} nonogesimo.*[37]

[*Followed in the manuscript by text on "Eight Manners of Medicines" (fols. 158r–159r; see Supplementary Text III below) and medical compendium beginning "As Salamon saith" (fols. 159r–173d verso).*]

An Approbate Treatise for the Pestilence

[**fol. 174r**] And folowyng here next bigynneth an approbate treatise for the pestilence, studied bi the grettest doctours of phisik amonges the vniuersites of Cristendom and amonges al Cristen naciouns in the tyme
315 of Seynt Thomas of Caunterbury.[38]

For the vniuersal goode of al Cristen people to lierne the most soverayne medicyne of diete, of bloode leetyng, and of herbis and moche other counsails of solempne doctours for the **Epedemye** cleped the pestilence.[39] Whan the people bien enfect of that sikenes, loke for sure
320 and notable doctryne men to forbere the etyng of leekis, of garlik, of oynons, and al other metis that bien hote of nature. And if a man thurst moche, it is goode otherwhile to drynke cold water of the welle menged with aisel or tysan (if it may bien had), ffor thei bien goode and medi-

---

312. And . . . next] Here Ad   treatise] treite Ad

313–314. the vniuersites] thunyversite Ad

314. Cristendom . . . al] *om.* Ad

315. Caunterbury] *foll. by title set off by blank lines from incipit and text:* An approbate medicyne for the Epidemye Ad; Medecyne approbate | ffor the Epidemye *used as running head, fols. 85v–87r* Ad

318. solempne] loke and rede *marg.* Ad   Epedemye] *in display script*   the (2)] *om.* Ad

320. to] doo Ad

323. tysan] with tisane Ad

cynable, and specialy for the bodies that bien hote and dry, that is to
325 say, to hem that bien of colerik complexioun, for in that tyme a grete
thirst shuld in no wise be suffred.

Also, whan a man feelith moevyng or stiryng or prickyng of his
bloode, lete hym bloode anon vpon the same side of the veyne whiche
is next to the place where the moevyng [i]s, the same houre if it may
330 be and at the lest withyn vj houres next folowyng. And if that may nat
be, looke that the pacient abstene from mete and sleepe and drynke til
he be laten bloode, but looke that the bloode leetyng be taried in no
wise lenger than xij houres, withyn þe whiche the sikenes of the pestilence is confermed evermore, and the evil bloode than is so ronne
335 so thikke that it may nat vse ne go out of the veyne that is smyten with
flewme or with launcet.

Now if a man be infecte with the sikenes of the Epedemy bicause
of the evil dietyng or bi any other forfaiture of gouernaunce, takeþ
heede, for in this wise he shal fynde remedy. Ye shuln vndirstonde that
340 in mannes body is ther iij principal membris, that is to say, the herte,
the liver, and the brayn, and alwey this pestilencial [sikenes] is engendred in oon of thiese iij. And everiche of thiese iij membris han issues
bi hemsilf.

The herte hath his issue vnder þe armpit. The liver at the grynde
345 of the thies. The brayn vnder **[fol. 174v]** the eeris and vnder the tunge
in the throte. And evir the evil approchith til oon of thiese iij placis.

---

324. for the] to Ad

327. or (1)] *om.* Ad   prickyng] pricchyng Ad

328. bloode (2)] *marg. in later hand:* Bloodlettinge

329. moevyng is] mevyng is Ad, moevynges T

330. be] *foll. by* looke that the pacient abstene *canc.*

331. looke] loke and rede *marg.* Ad   abstene] *foll. by* hym Ad

332. bloode (1)] nota *sign in marg.; marg. in later hand:* Blodlatyng; *marg. in different later hand (same as in Textual Note to line 328):* Bloodlettinge B

332–333. leetyng . . . than] lesse yn no wise taried to Ad

333. withyn] *prec. by* wi (*with curl and beg. of ascender of* h?) *canc.* Ad

334. ronne] ronnyne togiddirs Ad

335. vse] isshe Ad; *cf. Textual Note to line 352 below*

338. the] *om.* Ad

340. is ther] ther be Ad

341. alwey] loke and rede *marg.* Ad   sikenes] sekenese Ad, *om.* T

342. thiese (1)] thieese

346. the evil] *om.* Ad

The gadryng and the cause of this evil ye shul thus conceyve: that this
venemous aier whiche that is infect entrith into the man bi the poores
that bien open; and whan the aier is medled with the evil bloode, anon
350 it passith vnto the herte; and whan the herte feelith the greuaunce, it is
busy for to defende itsilf and castith out the bloode that is envenymed
to his owne issues. And whan the venymous matier fyndith th'issue
stopped, it goeth streight to the liver, and the liver in the same wise castith the matier to his issues. [And in the same wise doeth the brayne to
355 his issues.]

Herby may a man knowe bi what veyne shal the evil bloode be so
voided, ffor if the bocche appiere vnder the armpitte, thanne it cometh
from the herte; than shal the bloode be leeten of þ[e] hertes veyne.[40]
In the same wise of the liver and of the brayn. And draw out the bloode
360 ay vpon the same side ther as thow feelist the bocche in, ffor if it be
drawen out on that other side, ther cometh ij harmes therof. The first
harme is that the cleene bloode that is nat infecte [is] so drawen out.
The secunde is [the bloode that is] infect shal passe to the regioun of
the herte, and anon bryngeth in deth with hym. And if ther be nought
365 in thiese issues of the liver, than drawe bloode on the veyne on the right
hand that lith bitwene the litel fynger and the leche fynger.

---

347. this (2)] the Ad

350. vnto] to Ad

351. for to] to Ad

352. issues] *prec. by* vse *canc.*   And] *foll. by* yn the same wise bothe the brayne
canc. Ad   th'issue] isshue Ad

353. stopped] stoppid *(corr. from* stoppithe *with* d *over* t *and* he *canc.)* Ad   and
the liver] *om.* Ad

354. to (1)] *with curl above* o *like ascender of* h T, till Ad

354–355. And . . . issues] and yn the same wise doth the brayne to his isshues
Ad, *om.* T; loke and rede *marg.* Ad

356. bloode] and the blode Ad

358. of] owt of Ad   þe] þ *with* er *abbreviation mark* T, the Ad   hertes] hart
Ad

360. vpon] on Ad

362. is (2)] Ad, shal passe to the regioun of þe herte T *(scribal anticipation)*

363. the bloode that is] the blode that is Ad, *om.* T *(scribal eyeskip)*

364. bryngeth] bryng Ad

365. thiese issues] th isshues Ad   on (2)] vpon Ad; loke and rede *marg.* Ad

And if the liver put the matier towardes the grynde of the thigh,
or if the bocche appiere toward the prevy membris toward the neither
partie, than drawe bloode on the same side in the veyne of the foote
370 bitwene the grete too and the next too. For if the bloode be drawen
oute vpon the arm, the evil shal draw to the liver, and that were a grete
err[our]e. And if the evil appiere vnto the bak or the side, lete draw the
bloode bitwene the ancle and the heele, or ellis to be boxed vpon the
shuldre. And the evil appiere at the side of the brayn, draw bloode at
375 oon of the hed veynes,[41] that is above the myddil veynes,[42] or ellis on
the veyne vpon the hand bitwene the thumbe and the shevyng fynger,
or ellis vse for to boxe the bitwene the shuldres.

And whan the bloode is in this wise **[fol. 175r]** drawen oute from
the herte, than bihovith the herte to be comforted bi cold lectuaries
380 that wiln aswage the heete from the herte: that is goode and a soverayne medicyne. And also for the same cas, another medicyne: water
stilled, of scabious, dipteyne, pympernel, tormentil, ffumytere. Metis
and drynkes in the tyme of the saide sikenes shuld be fieble and litel,
ffor that diete is goode and medicynable for the pestilencial sikenes.

385 Thiese bien the vertues and the goodenessis that folowyn bicause of
bloode leetyng in competent and dewe tyme.[43] First, it clierith the sight
and clensith the brayne; it tempereth the stomac; it clensith the teeth[44]

---

369. partie] parte Ad   bloode] nota *sign in marg.; marg. in later hand:* Blod-
lettyng

371. the evil shal] the evil shal the evil shal

372. erroure] arroure Ad, erre T   vnto] towardes Ad

374–375. at oon . . . veynes (1)] draw b [*partially formed*] at the on the hed
veyne *canc.* Ad

375. veynes (2)] vayne Ad

378. drawen] nota *sign in upper marg.*

380. a] *om.* Ad

381. cas] *om.* Ad

382. dipteyne] deteyne Ad   ffumytere] ffunyter Ad

384. the] that Ad

385. vertues] vertuous Ad; Loke and rede for blodelese *marg.* Ad   goodenes-
sis] godenesesse Ad

386. bloode leetyng] *marg. in later hand:* The vertues of Blodlattyng; blode-
lesse Ad

387. and] a Ad   clensith the teeth] hetith Ad; *curl above first* e *of* teeth *like ascender of* h T

and clensith the heryng and openeth þe eeris; it defieth mete and
drynke. It makith the voice cliere; it sharpiþ the witte; it lighteneþ the
390 wombe; it gaderith the sleepe; it norisshith goode bloode and long
helth in many a body.

And in moche bleedyng thiese sikenesses folowen therof withyn the
body: it makith it cold; it makith the herte feynt; it makith þe hand to
quake and the jaundise is nurisshed therby; it fieblith also the brayn. It
395 is the norice also of the gowte; the straitnes of the brest cometh therof
also and many another malady and sikenes.

Vpon the first day drynke a disshful of the juce of the water of betayne,
al fastyng, and what man that so doeþ, he shal be defended of al maner
gowtes for that yeere.[45]

400 And for þe knowyng verily bi the disposiciouns what maner of sikenessis
men and wymmen bien in, biholde bi the morow if þe vryne be white
al bifore mete—it is a triewe token that thei bien infect with non evil.[46]
And if the vryne be rede as bloode, it is a token that the bladder is hurt
with sum sikenes withyn. And if the vryne of the womman be white,
405 thynne, and bright as silver, that is token that the wommans stomac is
fieble and that she hath non appetite to mete and drynk but for to have

---

388. mete] the mete Ad

390. goode] the gode Ad

391. helth] hele Ad   many a] manes Ad

392. in] ynto Ad   bleedyng] *marg. in later hand:* To Moche Bledyng   sike-
nesses] sekenes Ad

393. it (1)] and Ad   it makith the herte feynt] and hit makithe the hart faynt
hit maketh [the hart *catchword*] the hart faynt Ad

395–396. therof also] also therof Ad

396. sikenes] sekenessis Ad

397. the juce . . . betayne] juysse or of stilled water of ditaygne Ad

398. that] *om.* Ad   maner] *foll. by* of Ad

399. yeere] yere &c. Ad

400. sikenessis] sekenes Ad

402. bifore] tofore Ad   that] *om.* Ad

403. a] *om.* Ad

404. vryne] *marg. in later hand:* Vrens

404–405. And if the vryne of the womman be white thynne] *om.* Ad

a vomyte, and that bitokenyth that she is with chield. And if the wommans vryne be rede as gold and hevy, it bitokeneþ that she desirith the
felawship of man. And if a man or a womman have the agwe and ther
410 be in the vryne a blac compas above,⁴⁷ it is a grete token of deth. If the
vryne of a womman **[fol. 175v]** that never was acompanyed with man
be cliere, it is a token of goode hele.

    Bi thiese ensamples ye may have notice of your estatis.

Ther bien also the daies of the yeere that bien most perilous and sike-
415 liest any man for to leete hym bloode vpon, bi writyng and doctryne of
Seynt Beede, and thiese creatures of man that letith hym bloode vpon
any of thiese iij daies he shal⁴⁸

---

407. that (1)] *om.* Ad   chield] *marg. in later hand:* Tokyns to be with Child

410. the (1)] thare Ad   deth] *marg. in later hand:* Signum mortis; (*different ink*) Nota bene

411. womman] wo *ins. above with caret* Ad   acompanyed] compayned Ad
man] *om.* Ad

413. ye may] may ye Ad   estatis] Ad *ends here and adds* Explicit

417. shal] *Text breaks off in mid line and is immediately foll. by next item in MS; the
next words should read "be dead" (see Headnote, 576)*

Explanatory Notes

[1] **Moises Hallac seyn in their bookes of interpretaciouns,** *Capitulo accio***:** The author's name (Messahalla) has been erroneously taken as a plural; cf. S.

[2] **But yit . . . Galien saith . . . cause:** Cf. Galen, *De febribus* 1.6 (Kühn 7:289–94).

[3] **as witnessith Ipocras . . . handis, &c.:** Cf. Hippocrates, *Epidemics* 3, 15–16 (trans. W. H. S. Jones; Loeb ed. 1:256–57); *Airs Waters Places* 2 (trans. W. H. S. Jones; Loeb ed. 1:73), where epidemic diseases are mentioned in a defense of the use of astronomy and knowledge of the seasons in medicine.

[4] **xix yeere and more: Lat.:** *annos quadraginta & amplius* R, *annos 40 & amplius* A, *XL annos et amplius* Am. The French translation also gives the author's experience as "XL. ans & plus" (BN). S's highly improbable "90" may represent a misreading of "xl" as "xC."

[5] **for bicause . . .** *quarto canone capitulo, de curis febrium***:** Avicenna, *Canon medicinae* 4.1 passim, though the precise reference remains unidentified.

[6] **The Comentor . . . nygh:** Averroës, *Commentary on the Physics* 2.3.1 (Venice 1562 ed., fol. 59va).

[7] *primo de causis***:** A reference to the pseudo-Aristotelian *Liber de causis*; compare **Lat.** *causa primaria plus influat in effectum suum quam causa secundaria* (Ros RA) with *De causis* 1.1: *omnis causa primaria plus est influens super causatum suum quam causa universalis secunda* (Pattin 1967, 46; for discussion, see Lohr 1986). My thanks to an anonymous MRTS reader for this identification.

[8] **the maisters of Coloyne:** The independent English translation in Oxford, Bodleian Ashmole 1443 also refers to plural "masters" (p. 379), though other texts, such as R and A, refer to a singular master of Cologne. As D. W. Singer (1916, 164 n. 4) points out, the University of Cologne was founded in 1388 and thus the master could not have been a graduate of that university.

[9] **Lyons: Lat.:** *Laodicie* RA. The French translator's interpretation of the Latin as "liege" (BN) is an error, though perhaps a natural one.

[10] **Johannes de Burgundia,** *artis medicine professor***:** So also S. A number of the Latin texts (with and without the astrological prologue), the French translation (with the prologue), and the English translation (without the prologue) in CUL Kk.6.33 add to the author's name an alias and his place of residence: "*Johannes de Burgundia aliter vocatus cum barba ciuis Leodoniensis*" (RA), "Jehan de Bourgoigne autrement dit a la Barbe Cytoien de liege" (BN); "John of Burgoyn or John with the berd burges of Ledye" (U).

[11] *Deus deorum . . . prima causa, &c. . . . Cum nullum . . . tempus epidimale, &c.***:** Neither of John's other works on aspects of the plague can be identified from their incipits; see D. W. Singer 1916, 176–77. Both R and A abbreviate the incipit of the first work to "*Deus deorum.*" *Deus deorum dominus* may echo Ps. 49:1 (Vulg.), though the rest of the incipit does not match the subsequent words of the psalm.

[12] **wynden of muscles of the body: Lat.:** *corpus* 'the body' RASu. S's version of this difficult phrase, "or wyden the mascles of the body," suggests that it was

originally intended to explain the verb *rarefien* 'soften (flesh, muscles, pores)'; *wyden the mascles* may mean 'open the meshes (i.e., the pores seen as spaces between connecting tissues).' The scribe (or an earlier copyist) may have had a text that had lost the conjunction *or* and may then have misread the unusual word *mascles* as *muscles*. If so, *wynden* might just possibly be a desperate guess paralleling the use of the gerund *wrappingis* to mean 'muscle fibers,' attested in Lanfranc's *Science of Cirurgie*. See *MED*, s.vv. *rarefien, maskel, wrapping(e*.

[13] **pomum ambre:** 'a ball of ambergris'; see Riddle 1964.

[14] **calamynte or timiama: Lat.:** *calamite vel t(h)imiamatis* RA; *calamentae seu thimiamatis* Ros; see Latham 1980, s.v. *thymiama* 'incense.'

[15] **greyne parice: Lat.:** *granus paradisi* R; *grana paradisi* Su; page missing in A. The sense is 'grain of paradise (i.e., spice).' The association with Paris rather than Paradise is very common in Middle English texts (see *MED*, s.v. *grain* n., sense 5) and is also found in fourteenth-century Latin texts, in forms such as *granum (de) Paris*' and *granum Parisiense*; see Latham 1980, s.v. *grana*.

[16] **of nemyfore: Lat.:** *veniferas* R (an error); page missing in A; *nenufaris* 'of the water-lily' Su. See Latham 1980, s.v. *nenuphar (-far)*.

[17] **sandalos, and rubias: Lat.:** *sandalos & rubeas* R; page missing in A; *sandalos albos et rubeos* 'white and red sandal-wood' Su. There may have been a confusion in the transmission of the Latin text with *rubia* 'madder'; see Latham 1980, s.v. *rubia*.

[18] **the letuarie *pigra frigida* cophyns: Lat.:** *ellecturio* (sic) *frigido cofonis* R; page missing in A; *electuario frigido* (*Cophoni* add. Ros) Su; **French:** *electuarie froit cophonis* BN. The attribution to the Salernitan master Copho has become obscured in both the French and English translations. For the term *pigra* in the English text, see *MED*, s.vv. *jera-pigra* n., *pigre* n. Cf. also Medieval Latin *pigra Galeni, hiera picra, hiera picra Galeni, hiera pigra, gira pigra, hiera pigra Constantini*, names for various purgatives; see Latham 1980, s.vv. *picria, hiera*.

[19] **lete hym amonge sovpe: Lat.:** *aliquociens . . . sorbeant* (*sorbeat* Ros; om. Su)R; page missing in A.

[20] ***pillule rosarum*: Lat.:** *pilule rase* R, *pillule rasis* (with -*is* abbrev.) A, *pilulae Rasis* Su. The attribution of these pills to Rhazes has been lost in the English translation and, perhaps, in some Latin texts too.

[21] **from the marcial deth, corrupcioun of the aire: Lat.:** *a pestiferi* (*pestiferis* A) *aeris corrupcione* RSu.

[22] **conformed and fastned: Lat.:** *confirmati* 'confirmed, firmly established' RASu; cf. "confermyd and fastynde" in S.

[23] **This same is þe brayn: Lat.:** *hocque* (*hoc* Su) *idem de cerebro est asserendum* RA. John Fortho's marginal addition (see Textual Note to line 193) expands the sense of the rather laconic Latin and Middle English texts.

[24] **avoided or fastned matier: Lat.:** *materia mineriata* R; *materia minerata* A; *materia venenata* ('poisonous matter') Su, poss. a misreadng; **French:** *de la matiere la miniere* BN. The Latin of R and A (followed closely by BN) means 'the root or core matter,' i.e., the precise source of the infection. The word *miner(i)ata* is

derived from *minera* '(fig.) source, origin,' itself descended from *mina* 'a mine, ore' (see Latham 1980, s.vv.). The English translator has failed to recognize the Latin word and seems to have made a stab at some plausible meaning based on the surrounding text.

[25] **Here:** The Sloane Group texts (C, G, Sl, etc.) preface the English text with a Latin incipit, here printed from G: "*Et iam incipit tractatus Johannis de Barba al. dictus Johannis de Burdegalia extractus in lingua Anglicana contra morbum pestilencialem* [*n* canc. between *e* and *s*] *siue epidemialem.*"

[26] **and in the thigh-hoolis both:** & these hooles. But C; and in thee3 holes. But G; and in þe thee3 holys. But Sl; A[n]d J. The reading of T has been allowed to stand since it makes good enough sense, while it is clear from the variant readings (and two others cited in Harley 1985 for 1982, 186) that the scribes of the Sloane Group texts were confused between the demonstrative pronoun "these" and forms of "thigh(s)."

[27] **bien:** If *earis*, the unemended reading of T, is not simply an erroneous repetition of the word from the previous line, then it could represent some form of "are," a generally Northern form, in the exemplar of T.

[28] **he:** the referent is "the venyme" that has entered the body.

[29] **the cardiacle:** cardiak C, the cardiak G, þe corrall J, the cardiac Sl. The cardiac vein of the arm (Lat. *cardiaca*), also called "cordiacle" and "the body veyne" below, was associated with the heart; for the use of the terms *cardiaca* and (much rarer in the vein sense) *cardiacle*, see Norri 1998, 324–25. For the approximate positions of this and the other veins referred to in the text, see the illustrations of "vein men" in Gil Sotres 1994, 142–44 and explanation on 145.

[30] **sophen:** the saphena vein, an inner or outer vein of the foot.

[31] **cephalica:** the cephalic vein of the arm, also called "the hede veyne," associated with the head.

[32] **ventused . . . with boxes:** 'bled . . . by means of cups.'

[33] **beteyne:** 'betony'; here, as below in line 298, CGJSl have forms of 'dittany,' which is also the reading in the corresponding recipes in the Latin Long Version of *De epidemia* (Sudhoff 1912, 66, line 128; 67, line 166).

[34] **But while:** Like certain other manuscripts, T runs together chapters 3 and 4 with no indication of a new chapter. The Sloane Group texts, CGSl (with minor variations), indicate chapter 4 thus: "Capitulum quartum. The fourthe chaptre tellith how that a man shall be kepid that is fallyn into this sekenes. Whils . . . " (G). Like T, J omits this linking sentence and continues "But wyle . . . ." Earlier, however, J inserts "Capitulum iiij[m]" after the phlebotomy instructions and before the instruction for cold electuaries to strengthen the heart; this is also the point at which TCC R.14.32 begins the fourth chapter (Sudhoff 1912, 74, line 92 and n. 1).

[35] **a powder that is goode agenst venyms:** This powder corresponds (in much shorter form) to the recipe and enthusiastic endorsement in the Long Version of *De epidemia* for the wonderful "pulvis imperialis," known in Arabic as "Bethzaer, id est, a morte liberans," which protects infallibly against epidemic disease and all

poisons, including snakebites. John remarks that very few apothecaries have the ingredients for it, and few physicians know of it either. But, in at least one Latin manuscript and in the French translation, John notes that he knows of a certain apothecary in Liège who specializes in it (Sudhoff 1912, 66–67, lines 158–177; D. W. Singer 1916, 208–9). A cynic may be reminded of Chaucer's Physician:

> Ful redy hadde he his apothecaries
> To sende hym drogges and his letuaries,
> For ech of hem made oother to wynne –
> Hir frendshipe nas nat newe to bigynne. (*General Prologue*, 425–428)

[36] **and:** possibly an error for "or."

[37] **Here endith . . . *nonogesimo*:** CGJSl (among other texts of their type) have a Latin explicit, here printed from G with variant readings from J: "*Explicit tractatus Johanis de Barba vel Johannis de Burdegalia* [*Joh. de Burgall J*] *editus contra morbum pestilencialem &* [*pestilencie qui J*] *est morbus epidemialis. Anno domini Millesimo tricentesimo Nonagesimo.*" Like J, several manuscripts (but not T) add two Latin paragraphs between the end of the John of Bordeaux text proper and the explicit: the first suggests flight from an infected area but then rejects it on biblical grounds (Ps. 138:7 [Vulg.] and Heb. 4:13); the second is a recipe for distilled waters mixed with various herbs.

[38] **Seynt Thomas of Caunterbury:** See Headnote, 574.

[39] **For the vniuersal goode . . . the pestilence:** As it stands, the text begins with a grammatically fragmentary sentence. Despite the blank line after the incipit and the decorated initial "F" of T, and despite the blank lines, the interpolated title (see Textual Note to line 315), and the space left for a decorated initial "F" in Ad, the original state of the *Approbate Treatise* may have combined the incipit with what is now the opening sentence, thus presenting a grammatically complete sentence.

[40] **þe hertes veyne:** the cardiac vein of the arm (see Explanatory Note 29 above).

[41] **the hed veynes:** the cephalic veins of the arms, associated with the head (see Explanatory Note 31 above).

[42] **the myddil veynes:** the median cubital veins of the arms.

[43] **Thiese bien the vertues . . . dewe tyme:** The redactor of the *Approbate Treatise* now turns to material drawn from a "Virtues and Vices of Bloodletting" text; see Headnote, 574–75.

[44] **clensith the teeth:** This odd reading appears to have resulted from a combination of an anticipation of "clensith" and a misreading of "hetith" (Ad) as "the teeth." Evidence of scribal hesitation may be indicated by the half-made curl recorded in the Textual Note to line 387.

[45] **Vpon the first day . . . gowtes for that yeere:** This recipe for gout is found elsewhere (see Headnote, 575), where it is advised that it be taken on the first Thursday of May.

[46] **And for þe knowyng . . . with non evil:** The redactor now turns to material drawn from a uroscopy text; see Headnote, 575.

[47] **a blac compas above:** a dark-colored layer of urine at the top of the sample (also called the *circulus urine*) signified imminent death when accompanied by fever. The word *compas* is not recorded in a specifically uroscopic sense in *MED*, s.v.

[48] **Ther bien also the daies . . . he shal:** A version of this text, incomplete in T, occurs at an earlier point in Ad (fols. 71v–72r); see Headnote, 576. Given the "Explicit" in Ad (see Textual Note to line 413), the inclusion of these lines in T may be an individual decision by the compiler of the latter manuscript, though he seems to have changed his mind; for further discussion, see Headnote, 575–76. The ME text in Ad, which follows up on the warning against bloodletting on three perilous days by warning against the conception of children or consumption of goose-flesh on three perilous Mondays, is an adaptation of two paragraphs in the phlebotomy text often attributed to Bede, *De minutione sanguinis* (*PL* 90:960–61, with corrections from Lazenby 1993, 64–65):

> Plures sunt dies Ægyptiaci, in quibus nullo modo nec per ullam necessitatem licet homini vel pecori sanguinem minuere, nec potionem impendere, sed ex his tr[e]s maxime observandi, octavo Idus April, illo die lun[ae], intrante Augusto: illo die lun[ae], exeunte Decembri; illo die lun[ae], cum multa diligentia observandum est, quia omnes venæ tunc plenæ sunt.
>
> Qui in istis diebus hominem aut pecus inciderit, aut statim aut in ipso die vel in tertio morietur, aut ad septimum diem non perveniet; et si potionem quis acceperit, quindecimo die morietur; et si masculus, sive mulier, in his diebus nati fuerint, mala morte morientur; et si quis de auca in ipsis diebus manducaverit, quindecimo die morietur.
>
> [There are many Egyptian days on which by no means nor for any reason is it allowed to draw blood from man or beast, nor to give a draught, but of these, three are especially to be observed: 6th April, the first Monday in August, and the last Monday in December; on that particular Monday much diligence is to be observed because all the veins are then full.
>
> Whoever cuts a man or beast on those days [the patient] will die either immediately or [?] on that very day or on the third day, or he will not last until the seventh day. And if anyone has taken a draught he will die on the fifteenth day following; and if either a male or a female child is born on one of those days, he or she will die a bad death; and if anyone eats goose on those days he will die after fifteen days. (Trans. Lazenby 1993, 59)]

For an Anglo-Saxon version of this text, see Cockayne 1866, 76–77, and Lazenby 1993, 64–67. A number of the ME texts indexed in eVK under the subjects "Bloodletting" and "Lucky and unlucky days" have incipits that mention Bede and days that are perilous in one way or another; these incipits may represent additional versions, but one would need to check the full texts to see if they contain the characteristic warnings about conceiving/bearing children or eating goose. On fol. 105v of Trinity R.14.52, the principal annotator added an abbreviated version of the "three perilous Mondays" text, including the dangers of conception/childbirth, eating goose-flesh, or undertaking good works on those days but not the danger in bloodletting (complete text and selected parallels in Mooney 1995, 56). For a different tradition of vernacular bloodletting texts, see Mooney 1994.

Supplementary Text III

Eight Manners
of Medicines

Between the four-chapter version of John of Bordeaux's plague treatise and the prologue to the medical compendium on folios 159r–173v of Trinity College R.14.52 there occurs a brief descriptive list of eight external therapeutic procedures, beginning *Ther bien viij maners of medicynes mynistred to the parties of the body withoutfurth.* The procedures are prescribed for use against a variety of ailments: dysentery; swelling of the legs from dropsy; bruised, numb, or broken limbs; insomnia in acute fevers; fluxes and raw skin around the anus; and so on. A marginal annotation in a later hand also suggests that they may serve as *Medicyns ffor pestlens,* perhaps seeing them as a kind of sequel to the two plague treatises that precede them, although there is no direct mention of pestilence or its characteristic symptoms in the text itself.

The Voigts-Kurtz database of incipits of Middle English scientific and medical writings (2000) reports no other texts with a similar opening, but the list could easily be an excerpt from a longer, general work on medicine, yet to be identified.[1] The descriptions of the procedures are relatively clear and concrete, and would have been useful to non-latinate readers who encountered the Latinate terms, unglossed, in other texts. Since the procedures themselves are not particularly complicated, lay users of the manuscript might even have been able to follow the descriptions to provide medicinal care for themselves or their households.

---

[1] A similar, but much shorter Latin list of eight procedures—with more concise definitions, a different order, and substitution of *Emplastrum* for *Sacellacioun*—occurs in Oxford, Bodleian Library, Rawlinson MS D.251, fol. 41v, between other short Latin texts on phlebotomy and uroscopy. A text in BL, Sloane MS 783b, fol. 18v, shares the same incipit as the Rawlinson D.251 item ("Emplastrum est dura confeccio"; TK 498.

Eight Manners of Medicines*

[fol. 158r] Ther bien viij maners of medicynes mynistred to the parties
of the body withoutfurth, whiche bien cald in this maner, that is to say:
Encatisme, Synapisme, Epithymye, Cathaplasme, Fomentacioun, Sub-
5 fumygacioun, [Embrocacioun], and Sacellacioun.

Encatisme is a litel setil made in a particulier bath so as he makith
or doeth agenst dissentery, that is a divisioun of fleyng and bloody flux.
Forwhi thei taken stiptic herbis, that is to say, cold and drie of complexioun, so as bien *resta bouis*, arnoglossa, argilla, and suche other, and
10 bien boiled with water in a cawdroun and after that cast al that out of
the cawdroun into a bolle of tree and lete the dissenterik discovere the
parties of his ars and sitte in that bolle vpon tho thynges whiche bien
withynfurth.

Cathaplasme is whan cold herbis alteratief bien broken and the
15 juce out of theym expressed and of that juce the pacientis place be
moisted and after a plaster of the same herbis above be bounde, *vnde
versus:*

Si cathaplasma facis succus ponuntur & herba.

Also cathaplasme is whan sambucus and ebulus and suche
20 maner herbis laxatief bien boiled in water and the legges and feete of
i[drop]ike of that be wasshen. Wherof it availith moche agenst swellyng
and bolnyng fallen in legges and feete, only þat bolnyng cometh ageyn
after v or viij daies. And for this al that inflacioun or bolnyng is nat
take awey.

25 Fomentacioun is that in water of decoccioun or seethyng of herbis
the matier of sikenes or sor biholdyng the parties of an hurt body be
holden. In like wise, ffomentacioun is that in the forsaide decoccioun
or in simple hote water with a spunge or with a **[fol. 158v]** lynnen cloth
iij-fold wet and after vpon the hurt place expressed and after with an
30 hand lightly and softly froted.

Cinapisme is whan the saide fomentacioun made, spreng the powder above as to drie, coart, drive, constreyne, consowde, and hele the

---

* Paragraphs in this transcript reflect decorated initials at the start of new lines in
the manuscript. The handful of paraphs in the text are not recorded here.

2. medicynes] *marg. in later hand:* Medicyns ffor pestlens

5. Embrocacioun] *om.*

18. Si cathaplasma . . . herba] *written on new line*

21. idropike] ipodrike

26. biholdyng] yg *in compressed script with nasal susp.*

membre of the pacient broken bi brusyng, stonyeng, and bi other smytyng, as it was don vpon the ars of the dissinterik or of the pacient
35 with the flayn ars, as with that stiptik powder to coart, he reduce in
the ars an inche issued bi relaxacioun of nerves and synewes of theym
bounden.

Epithemy is whan of juce of herbis with the juce to frote the hurt
membre. *Versus: Dicitur epithimia de succis vnccio pura.*
40 Embrocacioun is whan a man may nat sleepe in the nyght, as it fallith sumtyme in sharp fevers, whan that therfor be cast prively vpon his
face sum swete smellyng water. In this maner be rose water or water of
nymphee put in a viole of glas; after be it stopped with a cap wele cered
and after with a grete nedil be ther made many holis in that cap or cov-
45 eryng and bi tho hoolis the rose water beyng withynfurth be cast vpon
the wounde of þe sike man and it shal provoke hym to sleepe.

Svbfumygacioun is whan brent erth whiche fallith from the ovene
and gallis and other stiptik medicynes brenne we vpon the coles and
the fume or smoke of theym bi chaffyng be tourned entre into the ars
50 to streyne every maner of flux of the wombe or to streyne menstrues
whiche in pacientis for flowyng of the matrice or bi their noses and nosethrilles the bloode from theym outwellith.

Sacellacioun or setillyng is whan mile or otis bien dried in a lynnen bagge, wee bynde and to the pacient thenasmon (that is to say,
55 ars out or wrynggyng of the wombe) we vnderput, that is to say, in
sanguyn, fleame, and malencoly. Forwhy in theym of grosse and grete
humydite bien raw and venemous is made thenasmon and wrynggyng
of wombe. In coler wher thei bien convenient particuliers in dric seedis
hoote and bittir, fforwhi thei oughten to be more duratief to be sowed
60 in a lynnen bagge and in simple water to be boiled and after pressed
out and **[fol. 159r]** put vpon. So only sacellacioun agenst cold or heete
is convenient to riche men. Also thei diffirensen among hemsilf cathaplasme, epithimy, and emplasme, fforwhi cathaplasme is whan the medicyne is rightly put and sette vpon the dolorous and sike placis and nat
65 in compas. Epithemy forsoth is whan it is put aboute the place hurt
and nat rightly vpon. Emplasme is whan it extendith vpon eche side.

---

40. Embrocacioun] *marg. in later hand:* To mak on to slepe
50. flux] *marg. in later hand:* Mekyll Blod
53. dried] d (2) *ins. above line*
65. is whan] is whan is whan
66. nat] t *ins. above line*

Medicyne bi the ars bien received or taken in ij maners, forwhi it is entremeted in dure substaunce and so it is suppositorye, or in liquite and so is it clisterie.

---

69. clisterie] *marg. in later hand:* Clysters

-13-

TEXTS CONCERNING SCIENTIFIC INSTRUMENTS

Edgar S. Laird

It is not altogether surprising to find within a collection of writings mostly devoted to medicine a sub-collection mostly devoted to astronomical instruments. From antiquity through the Middle Ages, medicine was supported by astrology,[1] and astrology in turn was supported by the kind of practical astronomy that uses instruments for the easy and efficient locating of celestial bodies. As Hellenistic medicine and astrology passed westward, often by way of Islam, they were attended by Greco-Arabic astronomy, out of which, during the thirteenth and fourteenth centuries, Europe produced for itself a large number of astronomical works in Latin. Some of these gradually constituted themselves into a standard *corpus astronomiae*, with somewhat variable contents but usually including treatises on the astrolabe, quadrants, and the Jacob's staff, often bound together in the same codex.[2] The writings presented in the present chapter are an English-language counterpart to the Latin *corpus*.

Some of the elements in the English collection—for example the first, on the solid sphere—are unified treatments of a single subject, derived from a single source. Others, such as the ones here called *New Quadrant 1* and *New Quadrant 2*, look like genuine efforts to produce unified treatises from various source materials. Still others, such as the ones referring to the astrolabe, are more fragmentary, associated with one another merely by a

---

[1] Neugebauer 1957, 2. By 1300 the University of Bologna had created a chair of astrology for teaching medical students, and just after mid-century a college of astrology and medicine had been founded at Paris.

[2] O. Pedersen [1974] 1993, 223–28.

common subject and juxtaposition in the manuscript.[3] It is not always easy
to see, in fact, how the elements relate to one another or what principle, if
any, organizes them. Sometimes the principle appears to be free association, as when in an astrolabe fragment an incidental reference to solar altitudes prompts (apparently) the inclusion of the next item, tables of solar
altitudes. The last of these tables mentions "hours of the quadrant," and
so the next item is a set of sketchy instructions on that topic, followed by
a slightly more elaborate set on the same topic. There is some measure of
arbitrariness therefore in the way I have grouped some of the elements and
given titles to the groupings. A brief discussion of each treatise or group-
ing of fragments follows.

The Solid Sphere (fols. 215r–222r)

The treatise presented below as *The Solid Sphere* describes the construction of a physical model of the celestial sphere—a model, that is, of the last
heaven, the outermost layer of the physical cosmos. From early antiquity
through the Middle Ages the cosmos was regularly conceived as a sphere
whose outer surface contains or "bears" the fixed stars and the mythologi-
cal constellations formed of them.[4] In representing this surface, the imagi-
nation imposes on it as many as three sets of circles to form systems of coordinates whereby the stars can be located. One set is based on the celestial
equator and the poles thereof, with some circles parallel to the equator and
others, at right angles to it, passing through the poles—an arrangement
analogous to that of circles of latitude and longitude on a terrestrial globe.
Another set of circles, similarly arranged, is based on the ecliptic circle (the
line tracing the sun's apparent annual course through the zodiac) and the
poles thereof. A third set, arranged in the same way, is based on the circle
of the observer's horizon and his meridian circle, which passes through his
zenith. *The Solid Sphere* describes an instrument on which the horizon and
meridian circles are represented by metal rings concentric with a globe
which is mounted so as to fit snugly within them. The other sets of circles
are inscribed on the globe itself.

   The Solid Sphere is a translation of part of a Latin treatise, *De spera solida*,
that begins, "Totius astrologie speculationis radix . . . " (TK 1576). In most
surviving manuscript copies, the work is anonymous and undated, but in

---

[3] The fragments on the astrolabe taken from Geoffrey Chaucer's *Treatise on the
Astrolabe* appear to have been composed in a fragmentary way and never fully integrated into Chaucer's treatise. See Laird 2000, 410 n. 7.
[4] On the modern misconception that the ancients and medievals did *not* conceive
the earth and the cosmos as spherical, see J. B. Russell 1991.

some of the earliest it is dated 1303 and attributed to John of Harlebeke.[5] The work is certainly no later than the early fourteenth century, and John of Harlebeke, who is probably to be identified with the astronomer and monk of that name at the Benedictine monastery of St. Martin at Tours, is a likely author.[6] The Latin treatise consists of a prologue and two parts, one on the construction of the instrument and the other on its uses. The English treatise translates only the part on construction.

Like manuscripts of its Latin source, the *Solid Sphere* was planned as an illustrated text, with several spaces left for "present figures," diagrams of different components of the sphere and stages in its production. These diagrams were never completed in the Middle English manuscript (see plate 6 for an example of the space left blank on folio 216r), but some sense of what they might have looked like may be garnered from the Latin source as found in Oxford, Bodleian Library, Selden Supra MS 78 (see plates 7–9). The *Solid Sphere* is also noteworthy for its inclusion, uniquely among the texts in TCC R.14.58, of the attributive phrase *Quod Multon*, repeated four times, once with the date 1458 added (folios 215r, 217r, 219r, 222r; see plate 5 and the discussions by Pahta, chap. 1, pp. 3–4, 16, and Mooney, chap. 3, pp. 55, 59–60 above).

As to the instrument's uses, its chief function was the didactic one of displaying the rudiments of astronomy, in particular the dispositions and motions of the stars in relation to coordinate circles. It is, no doubt, to such a celestial globe that Geoffrey Chaucer refers in his *Treatise on the Astrolabe* (1.17) when he says to "litel Lowys" that "thys cercle equinoxiall [i.e., the celestial equator] turnith justly from verrey est to verry west as I have shewed the in the speer solide."[7] More generally, Chaucer says (at 2.26), "The excellence of the spere solide, amonges othir noble conclusiouns, shewith manyfest the diverse ascenciouns of signes in diverse places, as wel in the right cercle as in the embelif [oblique] cercle." The risings of stars and constellations as viewed from various places and as measured by right ascension (in the celestial equator) or in oblique ascension (as viewed by an observer not on the equator) are awkward to describe in words but easy to show on a celestial globe equipped with horizon and meridian rings (see Olson and

---

[5] Many manuscript copies, though not all extant ones, are identified in Thorndike-Kibre.

[6] Lorch 1980, 155. A few manuscripts attribute the work to Accursius de Parma, and that attribution is accepted by Dekker and van der Krogt 1993, 16.

[7] As the explanatory notes to this passage in the *Riverside Chaucer* document, some have believed that Chaucer's reference is to a treatise rather than an instrument. However, it is the instrument that is best suited to *showing* celestial motion, as opposed to *explaining* it.

Laird 1996). To display such risings is the chief point of the instrument, so that, in a broad way, Chaucer has accurately described its function.

The construction of the instrument may be sketched by means of an outline of *The Solid Sphere*, chapter by chapter, as follows:

1. Making a wooden globe on a lathe ("an instrument that rounde thynges bien turned in").
2. Making a meridian ring ("armyl or . . . roundel meridian") and support-pieces ("additamentis").
3. Inscribing coordinate circles on the globe.
4. Marking fixed stars on the globe.
5. Making a horizon ring ("orisont armyl"), fitted with a cursor or sliding pointer ("rule rennyng").
6. Making a quarter-ring for taking altitudes, called an altitude quadrant ("iiij altitude" or "quadraunt of the altitude").
7. Making a hemispherical bowl for holding the instrument, with another bowl to rest on it as a cover.
8. Providing a means for suspending the instrument by four cords, one of which is marked geometrically for reading altitudes indicated by a sliding bead ("almury") on it.
9. Making a decorative device (with "lily levis") from which to suspend the globe by the cords.

The making of globes to represent the sky is an ancient practice. Globes bearing some sort of figures of constellations predate Ptolemy, the great astronomer of antiquity, and after his *Almagest* (ca. A.D. 150), with its systematic spherical coordinates and catalogue of forty-eight constellations and over a thousand stars, celestial globes become truly scientific instruments (Tallgren 1928, 208–10). They can also be very beautiful. Fashioned of wood, metal, or papier-mâché, they are often dark-colored to emulate the night sky (as Ptolemy recommends in *Almagest* 8.4); the stars are generally represented as points of silver; and the images of mythologized constellations are in many cases very decoratively inscribed.[8] Most of the surviving globes from the medieval period are Islamic, but they are generally of the same type (a globe mounted in meridian and horizon rings) as the one contemplated in the *Solid Sphere*.[9] The oldest surviving one from medieval Europe was made in the middle of the fourteenth century.[10]

---

[8] Poulle (1991, 267–68) suggests that the instrument's beauty was important as affecting the emotions of beginning astronomy students.

[9] Savage-Smith 1985, 4. This work contains excellent pictures and diagrams.

[10] A black-and-white photograph of it is printed in Dekker and van der Krogt 1993, 17. It is 10½ inches in diameter and, like the one in the *Solid Sphere*, is made of wood.

New Quadrant 1 and *New Quadrant 2* (fols. 222r–226r; 226r–231r)

The two treatises here titled *New Quadrant 1* (NQ1) and *New Quadrant 2* (NQ2) refer to an instrument called in the Middle Ages the *quadrans novus*, to distinguish it from earlier quadrant-instruments such as the one devised by Johannes or Robertus Anglicus (ca. 1276), which later came to be called the old quadrant (*quadrans vetus*).[11] The new quadrant was invented by Profatius Judaeus (Jacob ben Machir ibn Tibbon, of Marseilles) and is the subject of a treatise by him, written in Hebrew in 1288, translated into Latin in 1290, and often copied, re-edited, and modified thereafter, as for example in the late thirteenth-century treatises *Novus quadrans* and *Ars et operatio novi quadrantis*. The new quadrant is an instrument derived directly from the ordinary planispheric astrolabe by the device of imposing most of the markings from the circular face of the astrolabe onto the quarter-circle of the quadrant. It is as if a circle (the astrolabe) had been folded in half twice to make a quarter-circle (the quadrant). The most widely used medieval treatise on the astrolabe was the *Compositio et operatio astrolabii*, a thirteenth-century Latin compilation wrongly attributed in the Middle Ages to the Arabic writer Messahalla (Māshā' Allāh).

The above-mentioned Latin treatises, all more or less directly relevant to NQ1 and NQ2, will be designated here and in the Explanatory Notes by shortened forms as follows:

> QV = *Quadrans vetus*, ed. N. L. Hahn 1982, 1–113 (TK 585)
>
> Prof = Profatius Judaeus, *Il Quadrante d'Israel*, ed. Boffito and Melzi d'Eril 1922.
>
> Q1, Q2 = *Novus quadrans* and *Ars et operatio novi quadrantis*, respectively, ed. F. S. Pedersen 1984, 571–648 and 731–804.
>
> M = Pseudo-Messahalla, *Compositio et operatio astrolabii*, ed. Gunther 1929, 133–231.[12]

---

[11] In addition to modern editions of quadrant treatises mentioned below, see the following substantial studies: Millàs Vallicrosa 1932, on the old quadrant and its relation to treatises on practical geometry; Anthiaume and Sottas 1910, on the new quadrant, with a cardboard model of the instrument in a pocket at the end of the volume; Poulle 1964, on the new quadrant and its relation to the astrolabe. Photographs of medieval quadrants, astrolabes, and other instruments are printed in Poulle [1967] 1983.

[12] For some of the many manuscripts and versions of M and Prof, see TK's index, s.nn. Messahala: Astrolabe and Profatius Judaeus: New quadrant, with more than ten distinct incipits for each.

Also relevant, though less directly, are some treatises on what was called "practical geometry," which derives less from academic mathematics in the tradition of Euclid than from the practices of Roman surveyors or land-measurers (*agrimensores*). Materials from these treatises were incorporated into both astrolabe-treatises and quadrant-treatises. Exemplary practical geometries are as follows:

> Hugh of St. Victor, *Practica geometriae,* ed. Baron 1966, 15–64.
>
> Anon., *Geometria due sunt partes principales,* ed. N. L. Hahn 1982, 115–65.
>
> Anon., *Artis cuiuslibet consummatio,* trans. into French as *Praktike geometrie,* both ed. Victor 1979.

NQ1 consists of a prologue, naming the features of the instrument, and a series of operations taken from part two (the "operatio" part) of M. The basing of a quadrant treatise on an astrolabe treatise is not an unreasonable procedure. Since the quadrant instrument is a modification of an astrolabe, a treatise on the former can in principle be achieved by modifying a treatise on the latter. NQ1 makes some but by no means all of the necessary modifications. NQ2 consists of operations taken from some version or versions of Profatius's treatise[13] and operations taken from QV. This combining of sources concerning two different instruments is possible because the new quadrant shares some features with the old quadrant, even though its most characteristic features derive from the astrolabe.

Two Fragments on the Astrolabe (fols. 231r–231v; 231v–234r)

NQ2 is followed by two fragments concerning the astrolabe. The first, here called *Inscribing Almucantars on an Astrolabe,* is translated from Pseudo-Messahalla, *Compositio et operatio astrolabii* (again designated M) 1.13. This is the treatise from which adaptations were made to produce material on the quadrant for inclusion in NQ1. But in this fragment no such adaptations have been made, nor could they have been, since almucantars (circles of altitude used in connection with the star-map called a rete) are features of the astrolabe that could not usefully be transferred to the quadrant.

The second fragment consists of four chapters (or "conclusions") from Geoffrey Chaucer's *Treatise on the Astrolabe* (Laird 2000). They are 2.37, 40,

---

[13] Sometimes NQ2 appears to be following Prof very closely, and at other times it is demonstrably closer to Q1 or Q2. The author may have had access to more than one treatise on the new quadrant, or he may have been working from some version not identical with versions in modern editions.

39, and 38, in that order. They are not attributed to Chaucer in the Trinity manuscript and are in several ways adapted to their context therein rather than to Chaucer's treatise. In the first of them, Chaucer's 2.37, the rubric is altered to begin, "A maner of equacioun . . . " rather than "Another maner of equacioun . . . " because Trinity has omitted the first "maner," Chaucer's 2.36. At the end of Chaucer's 2.40, where some manuscripts add an *explicit* to the whole treatise and others simply break off in mid-sentence, Trinity supplies an "&c." so that it can pass without a break to the next item in its own plan of compilation (Laird 1999, esp. 145 and 158–59.). None of the chapters from Chaucer in the Trinity manuscript is accompanied by a diagram nor by such a tag as occurs in some manuscripts, for example, "And for the more declaracioun, lo here thi figure." Nevertheless, each is followed by a blank space where a diagram might be entered.[14]

Tables of Solar Heights (fol. 234v)

Latin collections of astronomical texts almost always include sets of planetary tables of various sorts. The little *Tables of Solar Heights* included here are a minimal gesture toward providing the English collection with a counterpart to what the Latin collections offer. The numbers in the tables are approximate. They are calculated for an observer at the latitude of Oxford, reckoned to be 52° north (rather than, say, 51°50', a figure often employed). Solar altitudes are given for the solstices and equinoxes only, rather than for every day in the year. Tables were usable in conjunction with astrolabes and quadrants, as indicated by Geoffrey Chaucer, *Treatise on the Astrolabe* 2.32 (for astrolabes) and John Somer, *Kalendarium* (for quadrants; ed. Mooney 1998, 101).

Two Fragments on Drawing Hour–Lines on a Quadrant (fols. 234v–235v)

Following the table of "houres of the quadraunt," the last of the *Tables of Solar Heights*, there is appended as if by afterthought a brief set of instructions for drawing the hour-lines on a quadrant. This is followed by a slightly longer set of instructions to the same purpose. Hour-lines are six arcs of a circle inscribed from the apex (right-angled corner) of the quadrant toward six points spaced equally along the quarter-circular border of the instrument. They occur on virtually all types of quadrants, including the

---

[14] Gunther reproduces diagrams accompanying the treatise in Cambridge, University Library, MS Dd.3.53 (1929, 101–7).

quadrans vetus, the *quadrans novus*, and the simplified "horary quadrant," used for time-telling alone.

The Latin quadrant-texts (QV, Prof, Q1, Q2) prescribe the drawing of hour-lines by geometrical methods, using a draftsman's compasses (*circinus*), rather than by the mechanical methods here prescribed, using as well the quadrant's plumb-line ("threed," "perpendiculier") and almury ("margarit," "perle"). The hour-lines as described here are somewhat difficult to visualize, and an illustrative diagram would have been helpful, but none, nor a blank space for one, has been provided in the manuscript. Many medieval illustrations of hour-lines are available in printed reproductions. One of the clearest, because of its simplicity, is a diagram of a horary quadrant from a thirteenth-century English manuscript.[15] Also clear is a diagram of a *quadrans vetus* derived from the thirteenth-century *Liber del cuadrante*, wherein the lines are labelled "La hora prima," "La segunda," etc.[16] Hour-lines and the geometry for drawing them are both represented in a diagram included in one copy of Profatius's treatise on the *quadrans novus*.[17]

The Art of Gauging 1 (fols. 235v–236v)

The treatise here called *The Art of Gauging 1* (the first of two treatises on the subject in the Trinity manuscript) is translated from an anonymous Latin work titled *De arte visoria*, beginning "Si quis velit ex arte vbicumque terrarum fuerit virgam visoria conficere . . . " (TK 1462). Its subject is the making of a gauging rod to be used for calculating the volume of a barrel, in particular a wine barrel (for a general account, see Folkerts 1974). The need for such a rod, for practical persons actually gauging volumes of wine, arises from two facts: first, deriving the volume of a cylinder from measurement of its dimensions requires cumbersome computation; and second, a wine barrel is not strictly a cylinder. The use of a gauging rod allows one to treat the barrel as if it were a cylinder and simplifies the mathematics needed to calculate its volume. Imagine a barrel lying on its side. Its diameters at the ends are the same, but it bulges toward the middle so that its diameter there is greater. By taking the mean between the end-depths and the middle-depth, one reduces the barrel to (approximately) a cylinder.

---

[15] Reproduced in Gunther 1923, 160.

[16] Reproduced in Millàs Vallicrosa 1932, fig. 1. See also N. L. Hahn 1982, xlii and xliii, figs. 2 and 3.

[17] Reproduced in Boffito and Melzi d'Eril 1922, immediately following the text in the facsimile presented as an (unpaginated) appendix. A clear photograph of an English quadrant of the *quadrans-novus* type, showing numbered hour-lines, is printed in Chandler 1985, 217, fig. 176.

The length can then be measured directly by equal divisions marked on one side of the rod, and the volume computed on the basis that the volume of a cylinder is proportional to its length and the square of its diameter. The computation is simplified by unequal divisions for depth measurement marked on another side of the rod. These represent geometrically the squares of diameters, so as to avoid having to figure square roots. The volume is expressed in terms of a standard measure, which might vary from region to region. It is the "cofre" (container, Latin *capsula*), a cylinder in terms of whose dimensions the rod is calibrated.

Unlike the astrolabe, the solid sphere, the quadrant, and the Jacob's staff, the gauging rod is an instrument of commerce without direct links to academic learning, even though it is founded on the same kind of practical geometry that was taught in the schools. Treatises on the gauging rod (as distinct from the instrument itself, which had long been in use) appear comparatively late, mostly in the fifteenth and sixteenth centuries, and are almost as likely to be written in a vernacular language as in Latin (Folkerts 1974, 2, 36–37). The gauging rod appears to be an instance of "man's coming to terms with numbers in the interest of his palate" (Meskens et al. 1999, 72). Its treatment along with other instruments discussed in the Trinity manuscript may be justified on the principle that, considering measurement abstractly, it is, like the other instruments, an instrument of measurement. Moreover, the geometry of determining volumes, on which the gauging rod depends, appears to have been derived from the treatment of stereometry at the end of QV (Thorndike 1949). Finally, the commercial functions of the gauging rod link this collection of texts with the reference to calculating annual expenditures and the discussion of the mechanical crafts in the treatise on the liberal arts edited by Mooney below.

The Staff of Jacob (fol. 237r)

The Staff of Jacob is a short and simple treatise on what was, in some of its forms, an important and sophisticated instrument. At its simplest, it consists of a rod ("yerd") perhaps four or five feet long with a cross-piece ("voluel") that slides back and forth upon it, so that when the ends of the cross-piece are made to lie upon the horizon and a star, or upon two stars, or upon two terrestrial objects, the angular distance between them can be read off the graduations on the rod.[18] In its most trigonometrically sophis-

---

[18] An illustration in *Les Premières Euvres de Jacques de Vaulx, pillote en la marine* (Le Havre, 1583) fol. 16r, shows both the Jacob's staff and the method for graduating it. It is reproduced, facing the title page, in Goldstein 1985.

ticated form, it was first described in 1329 by its probable inventor, Levi ben Gerson (also called Gersonides and Leo de Balneolis).[19] It was advertised by him in a poem associating it with the staff of Jacob in Genesis 32:10 ("With my staff I passed over this Jordan") and thus giving the instrument its name.[20]

The Staff of Jacob does not derive directly from Gersonides but is rather a fairly close translation of a short Latin work probably written in the fourteenth century called *De baculo geometrico*, beginning "Ad conficiendum baculum geometricum alias baculum Iacob . . . " (TK 34).[21] The instrument described therein resembles Gersonides' staff but is much simpler and is chiefly intended for terrestrial measurements. The English treatise differs slightly from its original in that the Latin treatise talks in terms of geometrical ratios, whereas the English specifies particular units of measurement—"elnes" (ells), "handful" (hand's breadth or "palm"), and "feete."

Some Uses of the Old Quadrant (fols. 237r–238r)

Some Uses of the Old Quadrant (OQ, for short) is a translation of several sets of instructions from the *Quadrans vetus* (QV). As such, it refers to the old quadrant, and two forms of that instrument are discussed. One is equipped with a cursor, which is a curved, graduated band representing the zodiac and made to slide alongside the fixed scale of degrees in the limb or curved border of the quadrant, thus making the instrument adaptable to various latitudes. The other form, without the cursor, is older but was still widely used in the later Middle Ages. As compared with, for example, *The Art of Gauging 1*, OQ is a very lucid exposition with a good mastery of its source. It will be noted that it covers some of the same ground as NQ1 and NQ2, their sources, and the practical geometry on which they all depend.

---

[19] The description occurs in the astronomical section (in book 5) of Gersonides' *Wars of the Lord*. That entire section was translated into Latin under the title *Astronomia* during Gersonides' lifetime, and the sub-section on the Jacob's staff was Latinized in a different translation in 1342 and dedicated to Pope Clement VI. It is printed by Curtze 1898.

[20] Roche 1981 (esp. p. 9), describes how the name came to be transferred to similar instruments, even ones constructed on different mathematical principles.

[21] Thorndike 1956, 391–92.

The Art of Gauging 2 (fol. 238v)

The Art of Gauging 2 may be regarded as the last item in the sub-collection on instruments. (It is followed by an astrological treatise—*The Seven Planets*, edited by Carrillo Linares below—which, being astrological, belongs to a different category altogether.)[22] *The Art of Gauging 2* begins with an unparsable sentence that implies, both by its content and by its referentless pronouns, something that ought to go before but is missing. At the end it breaks off abruptly at mid-line. In between is a good deal of imperfect syntax, though the intent is easy enough to follow. One can imagine a collector of these instrument-texts, nearing the end of his project, looking back at what has been collected, seeing the inadequacy of *The Art of Gauging 1*, and adding *The Art of Gauging 2* in an attempt to compensate. This last text bears the marks of a hasty ending.

A Note on Technical Terminology

Concerning the instrument-texts in general, perhaps a word should be said about technical vocabulary, although it represents comparatively few problems. The texts are entirely free of astrological terms. Geometric and arithmetic terms in them have for the most part become standard (at least temporarily, as in the case of *abate* meaning "subtract") and are fully documented in the historical dictionaries. Terms associated with the instruments themselves, often derived from Arabic through Latin, became fixed early and remained unchanged as long as the instruments continued in use. Moreover, because Latin instrument-texts were used for educational purposes, terminology from them (e.g., *azimuth*, *zenith*) passed into more general astronomical use. Serious ambiguities occur with only three words: *almury*, *volvel*, and *oilet*.

Almury (Arabic, *al-murī*, "the little hand, indicator") entered Latin and the European vernaculars as the name of a feature of the astrolabe, a projection on the rete (or star-map) that points to degrees on the rim of the instrument. The word is so used in NQ1.8, 9, etc. It was transferred to the movable bead (also called *pearl*, *margarite*) on a quadrant's plumb-line, where it performed an analogous pointing function, as in NQ2.1, 3, 4, etc. Thence it was transferred to the bead on the cord of a suspended solid

---

[22] The standard instrument-treatises are self-consciously on the border between theoretical astronomy, with its mathematical proofs, and practical astrology, with its consequences in human action. See Laird and Fischer 1995, 10–12.

sphere, as in *The Solid Sphere*, 8 and 9. A serious complication is introduced
into the Trinity instrument-texts when, in the prologue to NQ1, *almury*
is given a definition that properly belongs to *almucantar* (from Arabic *al-
muqanṭarāt*, "the arched bridges, arcs"). Almucantars are circles of height
on an astrolabe, but NQ1 says "almuries bien cercles of height." Thereafter,
wherever the term *almucantar* should be used, the Trinity instrument-texts
fairly consistently substitute *almury*. NQ1 does so when rendering *almucantharat* from its Latin source; and even when reproducing the English text
of Chaucer's *Treatise on the Astrolabe* 2.39, Trinity substitutes "almuries" for
Chaucer's "almykanteras." The exception to this consistency is in the fragment on inscribing almucantars on an astrolabe, wherein "almecantrades"
is *not* replaced by *almuries*.

From the various uses to which the term *volvel* is put, it may be inferred
that its general meaning is "a rotating or moving part, especially on an
astronomical instrument." It sometimes, though rarely, refers to the rete on
an astrolabe, as it does in NQ1.5. It is also used to name the cross-piece that
moves along the rod of a Jacob's staff, as in *The Staff of Jacob*. In relation to
quadrants, it refers to a calendrical scale on the back of the instrument, a
system of graduated disks used for finding the approximate places of planets on any given date without having to have recourse to the more accurate
sets of planetary tables calculated for the purpose. A complication attending this usage arises from the fact that a pointer in the form of a rotatable
ruler, used to indicate points on the disks, was sometimes called a *novella*,
a term which, apparently by scribal error, became confused with *volvella*.[23]
Some such confusion appears to have occurred in the prologue to NQ1,
which refers to "the voluel and . . . the reete." In this context "voluel" probably refers to the ruler and "reete" to the disks.

Oilet (= *oillet*, *eyelet*), meaning "a small hole or perforation," is not really
a technical term but a common one used descriptively in the instrument
texts. In *Some Uses of the Old Quadrant* it refers to the holes in the sighting
vanes on the edge of the instrument. In *The Art of Gauging 1* it refers to the
holes pierced in the gauging rod to mark graduations. The most puzzling
use is in the second fragment on drawing hour lines, where *oilet* seems to
refer to some sort of device for drawing circles, suggested as an alternative
to draftsman's compasses.

In a few places the Trinity instrument texts are not as completely translated, so to speak, as they might have been. NQ1.12, for example, translates
the same chapter from Pseudo-Messahalla as does Chaucer's *Treatise on the*

---

[23] F. S. Pedersen 1984, 673; also 24, 418, 740.

Astrolabe 2.16; and where NQ1 has "semycercles," "hiemal," "estyval," "merid-ional," and "septentrional," Chaucer translates "halve cercles," "wynter," "somer," "southward," and "northward." On the whole, however, the Trin-ity texts are not notably Latinate and are generally in the mainstream of development in the growing English technical vocabulary.

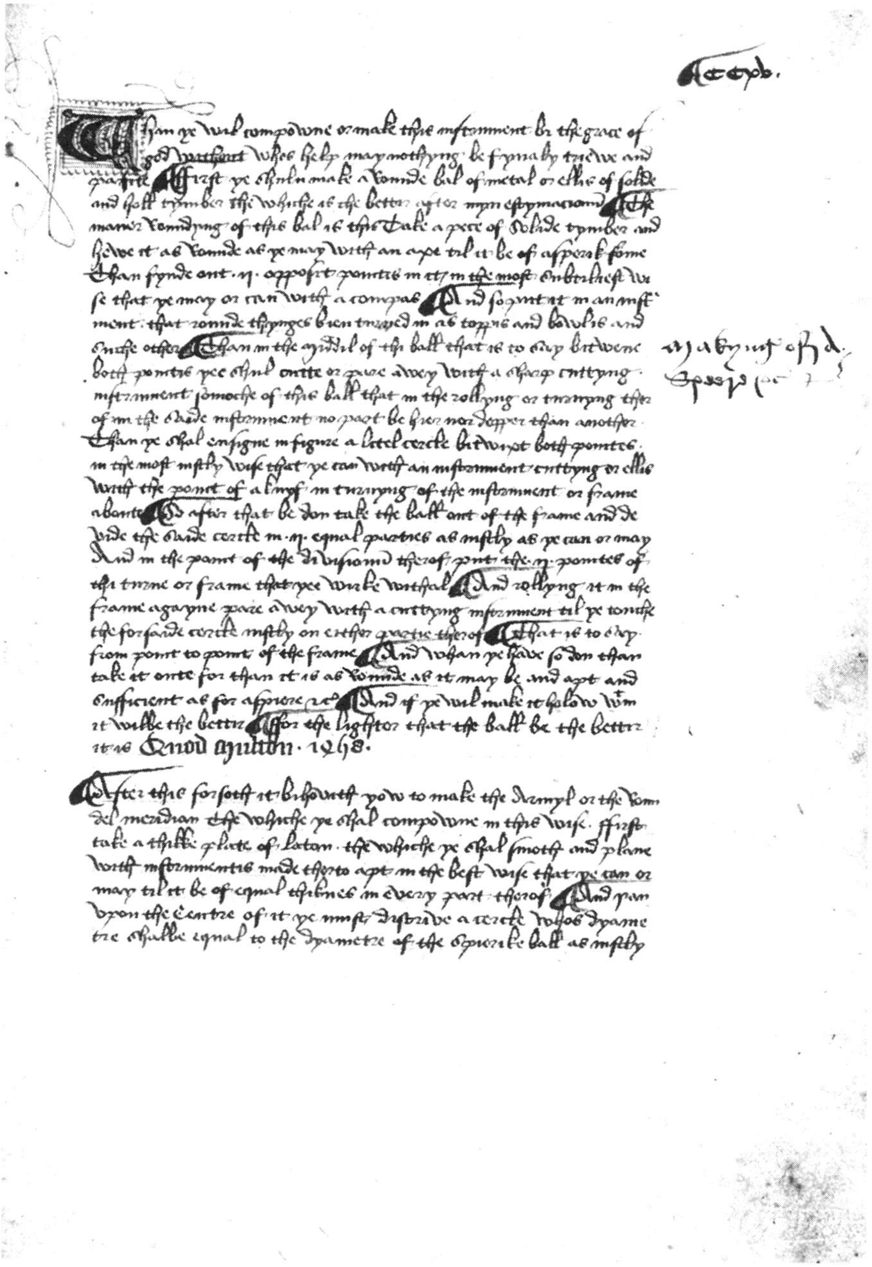

Plate 5. *The Solid Sphere*, chaps. 1-2 and "Quod Multon. 1458" attribution. Cambridge, Trinity College, MS R.14.52, fol. 215r. By permission of the Master and Fellows of Trinity College, Cambridge.

TEXTS CONCERNING
SCIENTIFIC INSTRUMENTS

[The Solid Sphere][1]

[fol. 215r]
[Chapter 1]
Whan ye wil compowne or make this instrument, bi the grace of God,
without whos help may nothyng be fynaly triewe and parfitc, ffirst ye
5 shuln make a rounde bal of metal or ellis of solide and holl tymber, the
whiche is the bettir after myn estymacioun. The maner roundyng of
this bal is this. Take a pece of solide tymber and hewe it as rounde as ye
may with an axe til it be of a sperik fourme. Than fynde out ii opposit
pointis in it in the most subtiliest wise that ye may or can with a com-
10 pas. And so put it in an instrument that rounde thynges bien turned
in, as toppis and bowlis and suche other. Than in the middel of thi ball,
that is to say, bitwene both pointis, yee shul cutte or pare awey with a
sharp cuttyng instrument so moche of this ball that in the rollyng or
turnyng therof in the saide instrument no part be hier nor depper
15 than another. Than ye shal ensigne in figure a litel cercle bitwixt both
pointes in the most iustly wise that ye can with an instrument cuttyng
or ellis with the point of a knyf in turnyng of the instrument or frame
aboute. So aftir that be don, take the ball out of the frame and devide the saide cercle in ii equal parties as iustly as ye can or may. And in
20 the point[es] of the divisioun therof put the ii pointes of thi turne or
frame that yee wirke withal. And rollyng it in the frame, agayne pare
awey with a cuttyng instrument til ye touche the forsaide cercle iustly
on either partie therof, that is to say, from point to point of the frame.
And when ye have so don than take it oute, for than it is as rounde as
25 it may be and apt and sufficient as for a spiere, &c. And if ye wil make
it holow within, it wil be the bettir, ffor the lighter that the ball be the
bettir it is. **Quod Multon. 1458.**[2]

---

11. Than] *marg. in later hand*: Makyng of a Speere &c
20. pointes of the divisioun] point of the divisioun   S puncta divisionis
27. Quod Multon. 1458] *in display script*

[Chapter 2]

After this forsoth it behovith yow to make the armyl or the roundel
30 meridian, the whiche ye shal compowne in this wise. First take a thikke
plate of laton, the whiche ye shal smoth and plane with instrumentis
made therto apt in the best wise that ye can or may til it be of equal
thikness in every part therof. And þan vpon the centre of it ye must
discrive a cercle whos dyametre shal be equal to the dyametre of the
35 spierike ball as iustly **[fol. 215v]** as ye can mesure it, the whiche cercle ye shal divide in iiij equal parties in pointes ABCD. Be A point the
poole se[pten]trioun; and point C poole meridian; and point B poole
equinoxial in the angle of the yrþ;³ and point D the poole equinoxial
in the myddil of hevene. And ye shal draw diametrely ABCD. Afterward
40 ye shal divide every fourth partie in lxxxx partis equaly.

Furthermore ye shal drawe another cercle vpon the same centre
larger than the first and that but litel. And bi the centre bi the pointes⁴
of divisiouns of the first cercle ye convey right lynes vnto the secunde
cercle, and ther shuln be your degrees. Yit vpon the same centre ye
45 shal make another cercle larger than the secunde, and in the space
bitwene ye shal write the nombre of þe degrees, in either of theym
lxxxx and that twies, oones furthright and oones returnyng ageyn contrarie to the first. And than after ye shal write from A toward B from
j til lxxxx and so from B til A in like wise from j til lxxxx. And so do
50 in the remenaunt of the quarters. Than ye shal make the fourth cercle vpon þe same centre gretter than the thridde and, in the space bitwene, the mynute holes⁵ bi gree and gree or ellis bi ij and ij as it pleasith yow best.

Also vpon the same centre ye shal make the fift cercle larger al awey
55 than the fourth cercle. And than cut awey al that is without the circumference of this cercle of your plate, and cut also al that is withyn the first
cercle. And than remayneth your armyl meridian. Enrounde it withyn
and without as wele as ye can.

Furthermore, as touchyng the additamentis⁶ therof, ffirst ye must
60 take ij platis of laton of like thikkenes that thyn armyl meridian is of,
and lete the longitude of either of hem be of x degrees of the grees of
the armyl meridian or ellis more or lesse after that the quantite that
the armyl is of. The latitude forsoth of theym shal be of the latitude
of þe armyl meridian or ellis litil lasse. Than ye shal devide either of
65 theym bi the middil bi a right lyne. And after that ye shal apt⁷ thiese

---

37. septentrioun] semptrioun   S septentrionalis
56. cut also] cut (*end of line*) also cut

additamentis or platis vpon the armyl meridian—oon, that is to say, at
the septentrional poolis parte and that other on þe meridional pooles
part, so that the lyne dividyng the longitude [**fol. 216r**] of either of hem
lith directly to the lyne passyng bi the pooles of þe meredian armyl,
70 the whiche is lyne AC. Than ye shal fastene thiese additamentis surely
vpon the saide armyl that thei moeve nat afterward in no maner ne bi
no meane. After that ye shal boore this armyll in both pooles, the holes
goyng bi the latitude of the armyl iustly bi lyne AC so that half the thikkenes of the holes be in the armyl and half in the additamentis. Than
75 make ij round nailis or pynnes the whiche ye shal put in the holis of
the armyl as oft as it is bihoveful vnto your vse. And this is the figure of
the armyl meridian, &c.

[half page left blank for illustration]

[Chapter 3]
After this forsoth it bihovith yow to discrive your necessarie cercles in
80 this spirek ball. Wherfor it is nedeful that ye fynd out opposed pointes
in the saide ball with a compas as iustly as ye can. And than put it in
the armyll meridian and enfast it surely with ij nailes thurgh the holis
of the armyl into the ij pointis of the spicre and that firmably. Than fix
the armyl surely with nailes vpon a perforate boorde. And take a sharp
85 knyf and set the [**fol. 216v**] longitude therof iustly vpon the lyne DB.
And piche⁸ the knyf softly in the spiere and than turne it aboute, and
so ye shal discrive a cercle the which shal be the cercle of the equatour
of the day.

And this cercle shal ye devide in iiij equal parties iustly bi iiij point-
90 is. Than put the armyl meridian vpon oon of thiese iiij pointis and so,
the spiere standyng vnmoevable, ye shal discrive a cercle after the longitude of the armyl meridian, that is to say, passyng bi the pooles of
the world. And this shal be oon of the colures, and lete it be colure
equinoxial. And this nedely must passe bi the ij opposed pointis in the
95 equatour assigned,⁹ or ellis ye han erred in youre craft and in your werk
is nat iustly triewe.

Than afterward ye shal put armyl vpon another assigned point¹⁰ in
the spiere. And þe spiere standyng alwey vnmoevable, discrive another
cercle with the point of your knyf after the longitude meridional. And
100 þi[s] shal be colur solsticial.

---

71. saide] *foll. by* additamentis *canc.*

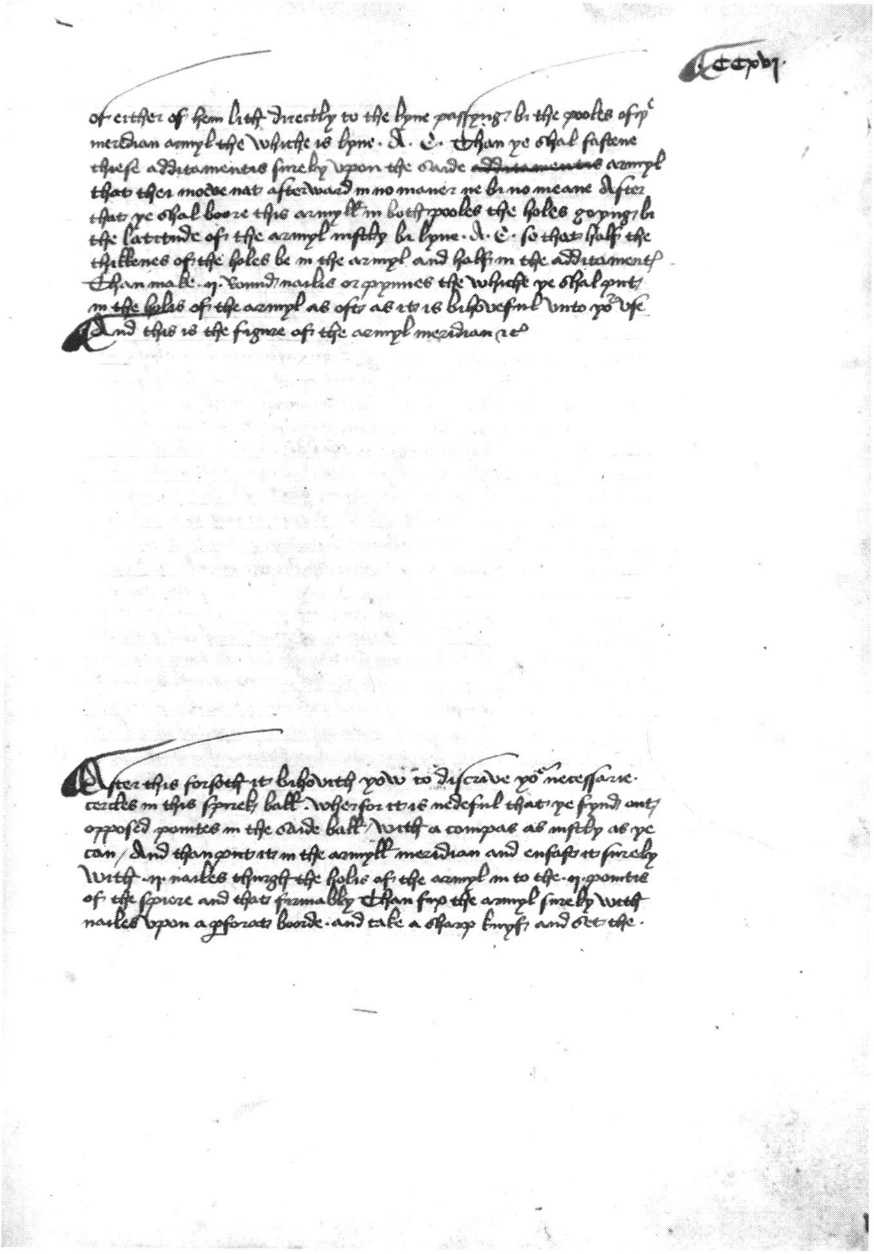

of either of hem lieth directly to the lyne passyng by the pooles of ye
meridian armyll the whiche is lyne .d. c. than ye shal fastene
these adiamentes fixely upon the saide armyll
that they moeve nat afterward in no maner ne be in no maner After
that ye shal boore thise armyll in both pooles the holes goyng by
the latitude of the armyll nyghly by lyne .d. c. so that half the
thiknesse of the holes be in the armyll and half in the adiaments
than make .ij. rownd nailes or pynnes the whiche ye shal put
in the holes of the armyll as ofte as it is behovefull unto yo use
And this is the figure of the armyll meridian &c

After this forsaide it behoveth yow to descrive yo necessarie
cercles in this spherik ball wherfore it is nedefull that ye fynd out ij
opposed pointes in the saide ball with a compace as nyghly as ye
can / And than contrit in the armyll meridian and enfast it fixely
with ij nailes thurgh the holes of the armyll in to the ij pointes
of the spere and thats firmably than fast the armyll fixely with
nailes upon a forsaid boorde. and take a sharp knyft and cut the

Plate 6. *The Solid Sphere*, chaps. 2-3 and space left blank for "the figure of the armyl meridian." Cambridge, Trinity College, MS R.14.52, fol. 216r. By permission of the Master and Fellows of Trinity College, Cambridge.

So after this ye shal divide everiche of thiese iij circulis in ccclx
equal parties. And than take in the armyl meridian from B toward A
xxiij grees and xxxiij mynutis, and therto put the point of the knyf,
enfastnyng it softly in the spiere, and so turne it aboute, discrivyng a
105 ci[r]cle of equal distaunce to the equatour. And that shal be the circule
of Capricorn.[11] And then ageyn take from A toward B xxiij grees and
xxxiij mynutis, and so voluyng the spiere aboute yee shal make another
circule with the point of your knyf. And þat shal be Circule Articus.
Than take from D toward B the same wise xxiij degres and xxxiij
110 mynutis and so ye shal cut the Circule Antartik.
And whan al this is iustly parformed, take out the nailes from þe
pooles and put down the spiere from the armyl in oon of the placis wher
the Circule Artike kervith the colure solsticial, and ther set a marke. For
that shal be the septentrional poole of the zodiac. And in his contrary
115 parte, where the Circule Antartik kervith the colure [solsticial], set
another marke, for that shal be þe meridian poole of the zodiac.
Than put the spiere in the armyl and fast the nailes bi the holis that
bien in the armyl into the pooles of the zodiac surely. And so put the
point of the knyf vpon B point of þe armyl and so fixe it softly in the
120 spiere and turne it aboute and ye shal **[fol. 217r]** make a circule. And shal
be the ecliptike or ellis the zodiac. And this shal be alwey touchyng ij
circulis of equal distaunce to þe equatour, that is to say, of Cancer and
Capricorn, in ij opposed pointis; ellis have ye erred in your werkyng.
And it shal be divided bi the ij colures in iiij equal partis, of the whiche
125 iiij ye shal divide aither in iij equal partes, and thei shuln be the [x]ij
signes.
Than afterward ye shal put the meridian armyl vpon the kervyng
place of the equatour and of zodiac and so, the spiere restyng vnmoevable, ye shal with þe point of your knyf discrive a circule after the lon-
130 gitude of the armyl, that is to say, passyng bi the poolis of the zodiac.
Than put the armyll ageyn vpon the point of the divisioun of the first
quarter of þe zodiac. And the same wise ye shal make another circule
after the longitude of the armyl, the spiere restyng vnmoevable. And
so ye shal do til yee complete vj circulis vpon the vj assigned pointis in
135 the zodiac, þe whiche shal divide the zodiac and also the spiere in xij
equal partes.
Than afterwarde ye shal divide every part of the zodiac in xxx partes equal and so ther shal be in al ccclx. Than take in þe armyll merid-

---

103. xxxiij] *first* x *written over another letter, poss.* p
115. solsticial] equynoxcial   S solstitialem
125. xij] ij   S 12

ian from B toward A vj grees and from B toward C other vj grees and set
140 ther a marke. And vpon every mark ye shal discrive circules wi[th] the
point of a knyf, turnyng the spiere aboute softly, of the whiche everichon is equal distaunt to the zodiac. And bitwene thiese ij circulis shal
be the latitude of the zodiac.

Than yee shal write vpon every signe his propir name and the nom-
145 bre of his grees. And ye shal drawe the zodiac circule and his equal distaunt circulis and also the circulis passyng bi the poolis of the zodiac
with sum notable colours, and the circule of the equatour with his equal
distaunt and the colures with sum other diuerse colures, so that ye may
discerne lightly bi youre dyuers colures your circulis of dyuers spieres,
150 as it representith and shewith plainly in this present figure, &c. **Quod
Multon.**

[fol. 217v]
[Chapter 4]
The iiij chapiter, tellyng the inwrityng of the fix sterris and the shap of
the celestial bodies above, &c.
155   Whan ye have fulfilled iustly al the forsaide thynges so that non
errour be left therin, than it bihovith yow to put the fix sterris and the
celestial images bi writyng in [t]his forsaide spiere, vnto þe which werke
it is nedeful that ye looke wele in the table of the verified fix sterris vnto
what sterre that ye lust and bihold iustly the longitude of it and in what
160 signe that it be and in how many degrees of the signe. And than put the
armyl meridian vpon the same degree in þe spiere. Afterward biholde
how moche is the latitude of the sterre and whether it be septentrional
or meridional and take so ma[n]y degrees meridian in the armyl, from
B toward A if it be the latitude of a sterre septentrional or ellis toward C
165 if it be of a meridian sterre, and set ther a mark. And directly over that
marke make a pointe in the spiere with the point of a knyf, for ther is
the centre of that sterre.

The same wise ye shal enplace al the sterris of al the images of
hevene, whiche bien M[l]xxij sterris.[12] But ye must make sum of hem
170 more and sum lasse after their due quantite. Wherfor ye must have v[j]
siluer wires[13] or ellis tynne wires of the whiche the first shal be gretter
than the secunde and the secunde than the thridde and so after that

---

140. with the] withe
148. distaunt] *foll. by* and also the circulis passyng bi the poolis of the zodiac
150–151. Quod Multon] *in display script*
170. vj] v   S 6

proporcioun of the remenaunt. And than whan ye lust to enplace a
sterre of the first magnitude, take the grettest wire and make a sharp
175 naile therof and fast it in the place of the longitude and the latitude
of the sterre inplanyng [and] infilyng it smothly wiþ the spiere. Than
make a litil hole in the myddil therof, and that shal be the centre of
the sterre. And so must ye werke bi the remenaunt of the fix sterris after
their quantite, writyng their names directely over hem, as many, that is
180 to say, as ye have names for.

Also after this ye must enwrite the ymages of hevene. Wherfor
it bihovith yow to looke surely, in the forsaide table of verificacioun
of the fix sterris, what sterris arn in especial longyng to every image,
and so ye shall draw the images vpon the spiere comprehendyng their
185 owne sterres and non other, shapyng the membris of the images ordynatly with the sterris that bien content therin and parteyneng therto,
&c. Than ye shal enfigure the myddel circulc[14] in this spiere after that
yee **[fol. 218r]** may fynde oute bi tables. Al thiese images ye must drawe
with dyvers colours, enplanyng hem faire with the spiere so that ther
190 be non embosyng nother concavyng but of equal fernes in every partie
of the spiere, every thyng havyng his propir name ordynatly, &c. Whan
al this is iustly don, than is it a parfite spiere, &c., as this present figure
representith yow ensample, &c.

[half page left blank for illustration]

[Chapter 5]
195 The v chapitre tellith the makyng of orisont armyl.

Whan ye have parformed your spiere craftily, than must ye make a
roundel that is cald the orisont armyl, the whiche ye shal contrive and
make in this wise. First take a thynne plate of laton sumwhat more than
the plaate meridian is made of. And vpon the centre þerof drawe a cir-
200 cule equal to the l[e]st circule of the armyl meridian, and than square
it with ij diametours, that is to say, AC and DB. Let A be orient and C
occident, B meridian and D septentrional. Than divide every partie
in lxxxx degrees. And so drawe another circule vpon the same centre sumwhat larger than the first that ye may make your grees bitwixt
205 both formaly.

[fol. 218v] Than make another circule vpon the saide centre gretter than the secunde, and in the space bitwene write the nombre of the

---

176. inplanyng and infilyng] inplanyng infilyng   S liminando
200. lest] last   S minime

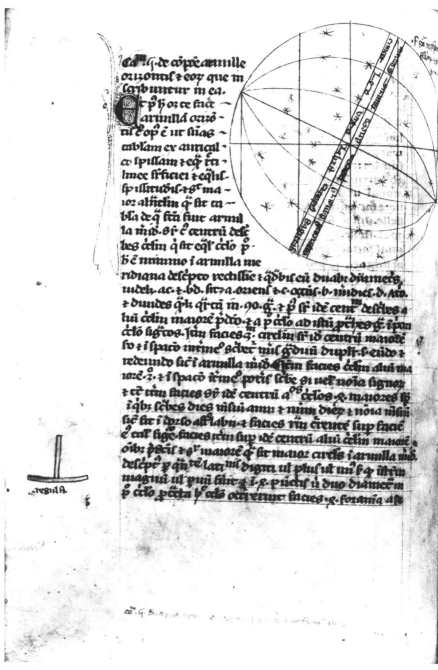

Plate 7. *De spera solida*, chap. 5, with illustrations of a celestial sphere with stars and the Zodiac (cf. chap. 4) and a cursor or *regula* (ME "rule running"; cf. chap. 5, line 219) for the horizon ring. Oxford, Bodleian Library, Selden Supra MS 78, fol. 74v. By permission of The Bodleian Library, University of Oxford.

grees of þe signes double wise [as] it is don in the armyl meridian. Yit
make another circule larger than the last vpon the same centre that
210 ye may write the names of the signes in the space bitwene and ye lust.
Draw yit another circule litil larger than the last, in the whiche ye shal
make holis of equal gretnes directly tofore every signe so perpendiculerly that the pointel that is enfastned to it with the orisont causith right
angles every wey.
215 Than draw other iiij circulis vpon the saide circule proporcionaly,
in the whiche ye shal write the daies of the monethis of the yeere and
the nombre of the daies and the names of the monethis as it is don on
the bakside of the astrolabie.
And þan make a rule rennyng vpon the face of it after this figure, &c.

[half page left blank for illustration]

220 Yit ye shal make another circule larger bi a fynger length þan the
grettest circule of the armyl meredian or ellis more or lesse after that
your instrument is of quantite. And in the iiij pointis **[fol. 219r]** wher
the ij diametours arn concurrent ye shal make iiij holis, kepyng iustly
equal distaunce; atwixt the whiche, ye shal put iiij cordis, as we shuln
225 telle yow herafter. Than cut awey al that is withoute this circule of youre
plate, enroundyng the remenaunt in the best wise that ye can. And
than make another circule vpon the saide centre equal to the grettest
circule of the armyl meridian—that is to say, of the vtter circumference
therof—iustly. And so cut awey al that is withyn the inner circule of
230 youre plaate, and this that remayneth is cleped the orisont armyl, &c.
After this ye shal take from D toward A how moche is the thikkenes of
the armyl meridian iustly, and ther set a marke, and than from B toward
A the same wise and set ther another marke. And bi both markes ye shal
drawe a lyne of equal distaunce to the lyne BD and than file awey the
235 broken space bitwene both lynes til the first declared circule, bigynnyng
at thy ynner part of the armyl from both parties—that is to say, septentrional and meridional—so þat ther be a concavite or holownes in the
whiche the armyl meridian may fal iustly after his thikenes.
The discripcioun of al this saide thynges in this folowyng figure,
240 &c. **Quod Multon.**

208. as] *om.*
222. wher] *folio misnumbered* ccix (*for* ccxix)
240. Quod Multon] *in display script*

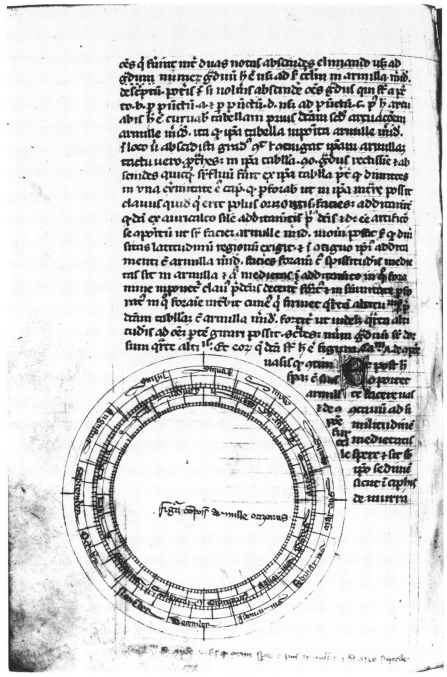

Plate 8. *De spera solida*, chaps. 6-7, with illustrative "figura compositionis armille orizontis," the design of the horizon ring (cf. chap. 5). Oxford, Bodleian Library, Selden Supra MS 78, fol. 75v. By permission of The Bodleian Library, University of Oxford.

[half page left blank for illustration]

[fol. 219v]
[Chapter 6]
The vj chapiter, of composicioun of the iiij altitude.[15]

After that ye make your orizont armyl, than must ye make the quadraunt of the altitude. And that is, first, that ye take a plaate of laton
245 whos latitude shal be as the thikenes of the armyl meridian. And the thikenes therof shal be as the latitude of the grees in þe armyl meridian. The longitude forsoth of it shal be more þan half the diametre of the armyl meridian. Afterward, take in the armyll meridian from B toward A xxiiij grees and put ther a marke, and the same wise from C toward
250 D other xxiiij grees and set ther another marke. And al the grees that bien made bitwene boþ markes ye shal cut awey, filyng til the nombre of the grees, that is to say, vnto the secunde circule declared in the armyl meridian. Ye may also, and ye wil, cut awey al the grees that bien from the point B bi point A and point D til point C. Than enarke or bowe
255 this saide litel table after the enarkyng of the armyl meridian [so that] in the place wher the grees bien cut awey [it] may touche the armyl truly. Than ye shal drawe in this litil table lxxxx grees iustly and than cut awey al that is wastful over of the plaate, except that ye leve in oon of th'extremytees þerof an hed, whiche ye shal bore that a nail may entre
260 in it, the whiche shal be the poole of the orizont.

Than ye shal make an additament of laton like the additamentis afor-saide. And that bihoviþ to do artificialy, that it may be moved vpon the face of þe armyl meridian after that the diuersite of latitudis of regiouns requirith. And in the saide additamentis ye shal make an hole with the
265 armyl meridian, of whos thikenes half shal be in the armyl and that oþer half in the additament; in the whiche hole ye put the saide nail, havyng a litel hole in that oon eend therof wher a litel wegge shal be set to ferme the quadraunte of the altitude—that is to say, the saide litil table—strongly with the armyl meridian þat the altitude quadraunt
270 may be turned to every part. Than write the nombre of grees vpon the [baake] of the quadraunte. And this the figure of al, &c.

---

255. so that] *om.*   S ita quod
256. it] *om.*   S ipsa tabella
271. baake] booke   S dorsum

[fol. 220r]

[half page left blank for illustration]

[Chapter 7]

The vij chapiter tellyng the composicioun of þe vessel that conteyneth the spire with his armyls, &c.

275   Whan ye have made your altitude quadraunt parfitly, yee must make an holow vessel after the symilitude of half the spiere, havyng a litel foote as a masor [is] wont to have.[16] Lete the depnes of the vessel be as moche as half the diametre of the vtter circumference of the armyl meridian and more bi a fynger brede, and ye lust. The mouth of the vessel must

280 be of so grete capacite that it may receive and conteyne the armyl of the orizont withyn hym. Than lete be made beside the mowth of this vessel withynfurth a lymbe or a bordoure after the thikenes of the orisont. [And let be made without the mowth of the vessel another lymbe], of al the hole instrument that the covertour may falle and rest[17] thervpon

285 whan neede **[fol. 220v]** is.

After this ye shul make a litel forke. Wherfor ye must take a plaate of laton whos longitude shal be of ij fyngres brede and latitude of oon fynger brede, the whiche ye shal enforke at that oon ende, craftily filyng awey of both sides so moche þat the armyl meridian after the thikenes

290 may entre and fal iustly into the kerf therof. And than ensharpe that other ende therof and fast it surely in the bottum of this vessel withinfurth, and nat directly in the centre but a litel beside, that is to say, bi half the thikenes of the armyl meridian. Than set the spiere with his forke and armyls in this vessel iustly as we shuln teche yow herafter. And

295 this is the figure of þe vessel, &c.

[half page left blank for illustration]

[Chapter 8]

The viij chapitre tellith the makyng and the divisioun of the iiij cordis and the makyng of the almury, &c.

---

272. *At the top of fol. 220r:* The vij chapiter tellyng the *canc.*

277. is] foote or

282. the (1)] the the

283. And let be . . . lymbe] *om.*   S sit extra labium vasis alius limbus

293. the (1)] the the

As touchyng the makyng of yowre cordis to hang youre instrument
300 by, ffirst ye must take iiij cordis of white colour **[fol. 221r]** and of on
length and of equal thikenes. And lete the length of either of hem be
after the longitude of the iiij diametres of þe armyl meridian or ellis
more, and ye wil. Also looke that thei be wele twyned and iplited toguyder. After that ye must divide ij of the saide iiij cordis—oon, that is to
305 say, to take the altitude of the sonne and the sterris and that other to
take shadewes and other mesures.

First ye shal divide the corde to take the altitudes in this wise. Draw
a right lyne vpon a playne boorde equal to oon of the cordis iustly the
whiche shal be lyne BC. And than ye cut from this lyne also moche as is
310 half þe diametre of the armyl meridian iustly in point A. After that ye
shal enhaunce[18] vpon point A a lyne orto[goni]aliter vpon the lyne BC
and lete that be lyne AD equal to the diametre, the whiche lyne fallith
betwixt the meridian hole and his contrary part in the orizont armyl
iustly. The same wise vpon BC ye shul enhaunce the lyne CE egal and
315 of equal distaunce to the lyne AD. Than drawe the lyne DE. And so the
vttermest of AE shal be the parolel right angle, &c. After, vpon point
D, after the quantite of DA, ye shal discrive quadraunt FA, the whiche
ye must divide in lxxxx degres equal. And than ye shal put arcanlier[19]
vpon point D and vpon everichon of lxxxx grees of quadraunt FA bi
320 and bi.[20] And wher thi ruler so iset bi and bi techith lyne AC, set ther
notis or markis. Than take another corde and dispose it vpon lyne BC
iustly and in his direct point make a notable marke, and þat shal be cald
the point of the orizont. The same wise in the evene directis of everichon of the notis signified in lyne AC ye shal make a signe in the corde
325 with ynk or with sum oþer thynge ellis, as it shewith in the figure[21] of
it in the corde.

So after this ye shal divide that other corde to take shadewes, &c.,
in this wise. First ye must draw a right lyne vpon a playn borde equal to
your corde, the whiche shal be lyne BC, and than cut agayn as moche
330 therof as ye have don of the first figure iustly in point A. Afterwarde of
[fol. 221v] A,[22] lyne AC ye shal [cut ageyn] lyne AG equal to lyne AD of
the first figure iustly. And than devide lyne AG bi xij diuisions equal,
whiche bien the xij pointes of the shadewe. The same wise of point G, if
ye wil, ye may take lyne GH equaly to lyne AG and devide it in xij equall
335 parties. And so ye may do bi the remenaunt, that is to say, AC, if ye lust.

---

311. ortogonialiter] orto*concin*aliter (?)   S ortogonaliter
331. cut ageyn] *om.*   S resecabis

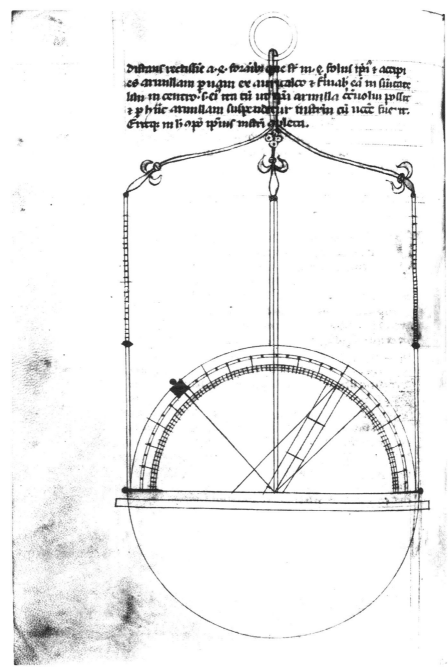

Plate 9. *De spera solida*, chap. 9, with illustration of a celestial sphere in its container, suspended with cords from a ring and the "lily levis." Oxford, Bodleian Library, Selden Supra MS 78, fol. 77v. By permission of The Bodleian Library, University of Oxford.

Than take the same corde, a[t] length disposyng it vpon BC iustly. And
in direc[t] of point A ye shal make a notable marke in the corde, and
that shal be cald the point of the orizont as it is saide in the first corde.
The same wise, in direct of point G and point H ye shal make notable
340   markes in the cordis, and so ye shal in al othe[r] pointis signified [in]
the cord of lyne [A]C. And this is the figure þerof, &c.

[*space of twenty-five lines on left half of page for illustration*]

    After al this ye shal take an almury, that is to say, a perforate mar-
garite or perle or sum other thyng like. Put it and set þat corde <þat ye have
divided to take the altitude in it, and so put this cord> with his almury in
345   the meridian hole of the orizont armyl and ferme it therin surely that he
go nat out ageyn. And this shal be cald þe meridian corde, &c.
    Than shal ye take another almury and put the cord that [ye last]
devided to take þe shadewes into it, and so set þe cord with his almury
in septentrional hole of the orizont armyl and fast it surely therin. And
350   þat shal be cald the septentrional cord. So afterwarde take that othe[r]
ij cordis and put hem in that other ij holis of þe **[fol. 222r]** orizont and
ensure hem fast therin and thei shuln nat out lightly, &c.

[Chapter 9]
The ix chapitre, of the makyng of the lily levis, &c.
355   Whan ye have parformed your almury and disposed your cordis
therin iustly, than ye must make an instrument of laton, iiij levis after
þe shap of iiij lily levis transuertid, in whos endis ye shul make iiij holis
of equal distaunce asunder iustly. Than lete the diametour bitwene
every ij contrary holis be equal to the diameter of the orizont armyl and
360   so sette the iiij saide cordis in thiese iiij contrary holis, fastynge hem
surely therin. And loke wele and diligently that thiese saide cordis be of

---

336. at] a

338. is] is is

340–341. signified in the cord of lyne AC] signified the cord of lyne BC   S
in linea .a.c. signata

343–344. that ye have divided . . . cord] *corr. by orig. scribe in marg.*

346. þe] þe (*end of line*) the

347–348. ye last devided] lest devided   S ultimo divisisti

350. septentrional] septententrional

356. must] *foll. by* ye

357. lily] *marg. in later hand:* lylly

361. cordis] os (*at end of line, poss. for* of) cordis

egal length. Than afterward ye must make a litel hole in the over part
of this lily of equal distaunce to þe iiij holis that bien in the levis therof.
And than take a litel round ryng of laton and put it thurgh the centre
365 therof, that al the instrument may hang thervpon, &c. And this is the
figure therof on that other side of the lef, &c. **Quod Multon**.

Deo gracias

[New Quadrant 1][23]

It is to know that this instrument is the newe quadraunt, fulfillid with
370 al the astrolaby of oone regioun. Forwhy in the breede is the quadraunt
with his point to take heightis, and in his right side is *corda recta* and
corda versa[24]—the *recta* inward ascendaunt to lx, *versa* in descendaunt
bi lx and eft ascendaunt bi as many and so is into cij.[25] And in the lift side
is a lyne of height descendaunt from the equinoccial to the poole bi
375 lxxxx grees and other ascendaunt forn agenst hym bi as many grees
and above the equinoccial toward the est, and þat is the declynacioun
of al the meridie.
    Bitwixt thiese ij sides arn writen iij parilels[26] of Cancer, equinoc-
cial, Capricorn; wiþ the ecliptik as wel to knowe bi the quadraunt as bi
380 þe astrolaby be .a.[li 27] and bi nomber; with the sterris and writyng of þe
names of hem and of the signes in the whiche thei bien; and with cercles of vj houres.
    Over the quadraunt[28] is the scale of height; a- **[fol. 222v]** bove the
whiche is nomber of a ferre cercle replied iiij sithes[29] wiþ divisions, and
385 so the equinoccial cercle is fulfilled bi a semysercle, as it is shewed in
the Alnot,[30] at the last the nombre of the zodiac is writen with his divisions. And thus is the playne of that side fulfilled.
    In that other side[31] is first set the voluel[32] and than the reete,[33] in
whiche lymbe is a cercle of tyme with the monethis, nomber of daies, and
390 his divisiouns. Withynne is a myddel cercle, that is to say, the zodiac with
his signes, nombre, and grees, and their divisiouns; and the sterris, sum
within and sum without, is ficched and sette, but tho that bien writen in
the zodiac bien septentrional and tho without bien meridional.
    But aboute the centre is the label[34] of the mone, to fynde hir myddel
395 place and hir mansioun in the last cercle vndir the reete.[35] First is þe

---

366. Quod Multon] *in display script*
371–372. corda recta, corda versa, recta, versa] *in display script*
378. iij] iiij

cercle equinoccial as the maner is with a waxing nomber, among the whiche bien the houres equals. Ther withyn vnder the reete is þe cercle of the equinoccial, Capricorn, and Cancer. With the almuries bien cerclis of height, and the azimutis[36] bien cerclis shewyng the quarters
400 of the world and their parties. And thus is filled that oþer side.

<i> For to fynde the grees of sonne bi daies of the moneth and agaynwarde.
Sette thi rule vpon thy day[37] that fallith withyn on the stide of the sonne in the zodiac, and note what gree and what is his opposite. And
405 thow shalt fynde of the moneth in settyng thi rule vpon the gree of the sonne þat touches oute with[38] the day of the moneth.

<ij> To fynde the height of the sonne or of a sterre.
Sette the corner of the quadraunt to the sonne or to the sterre, and lift vp the quadraunt or avale it to[39] the sonne beame passe thurgh
410 both holis thereof. And than note what gree of the cercle equinoccial the threede of the perpendicle[40] touchith, for that is the gree sought.

<iij> To fynde houres and grees ascendaunt and also of other principal angles.[41]
Moeve the gree of the sonne or the centre of the sterris on suche
415 an height as thow hast founde, on the orient half of it bifore the lyne meridian or vpon the occident half [i]f it have passed the sonne lyne. And the naydar of the sonne shal shewe the hour inequal of the day passed, or ellis the same gree of þe sonne shal shewe the houre inequal of the nyght if thi worchyng be on **[fol. 223r]** the nyght. The signe for-
420 soth and the gree beyng so in the oriental is clepid the clymyng, and that in the occidental is the goyng doun, and that in the lyne meridian (the whiche is clepid the middil of hevene) is the centre, and the opposite therof is the corner of þe erth.

<iiij> Of the crepuscle and of the morowtide or of the eventide.
425 Looke whan naydar solis hath comen xviij grees[42] in the almuries[43] of th'occident half that is not writen but to the dawyng.[44] And if

---

401. *Section numbers written by the original scribe in the margins of* New Quadrant 1 *and 2 are indicated by angle brackets and bold font.* moneth] *foll. by* fallith within on the stide of the sonne *canc.*
416. if] of
420. is] *foll. by* the *canc.*

this werk be on the orient half than it is th'endyng of the crepuscle at nyght.

<v> To fynde the arcus of the day or of the nyght.

430   Set the gree of the sonne on thi orizont occidental[45] and turne the voluel[46] vp the gree of the sonne, and than the grees that bien bitwene þe lyne meridian and the rule is half the arke of the day. Than double hem and than thow hast the hole day and ark, þe whiche withdrawe [from] ccclx grees and this that levith is the ark of þe nyght. Thus shalt

435   do of the sterres ficched if thow wilt wite how long thei dwellen above erth or vnder erth.

<vj> To fynde the quantite[47] of houres inequal.

Divide þe ark diurne day bi day bi xij and thow shalt have the quantite of an houre inequale, of the whiche if thow subtract it of xxx this

440   þat levith is the quantite of houre inequale of the nyght.[48]

<vij> Of the quantite of the houres equal of the day with half the ark of the day.

Thow shalt fynde the houres equal and their parties answeryng to hem, the whiche thow double and thow shalt have thyn entent. Than

445   withdrawe thilke houres from xx[iv] houres and ther shal leve to the the houres equale of þe nyght.

<viij> To fynde the partie of the houre passed bi the almury[49] with þe nomber of the grees in the lymbe from the bigynnyng of the houre right into the almury of tyme founden.

450   And as þe nomber hath hym to al the houres, right so a partie of the houre passed is to al the houre. Bi this maner the excesse is evened bitwene þe almuries in the astrolaby.[50]

<ix> Of the number of the houres equal in the day passed.

Note the place of almury[51] *in lymbo*[52] to thi tyme founden and turn

455   ageyn the gree of the sonne to the orizont oriental and eft note þe place **[fol. 223v]** of the almury. And afterward accompt the grees bitwene the first note and the secunde, and divide hem bi xv, and the houres equals shal appiere that bien passed. Right so thow shalt do on the nyght bi the sterris and naydar solis.

---

434. from] *om.*   levith] l *written over another letter, poss.* v
445. xxiv] xx (*at end of line*)

460   **<x>** Of reduccioun of houres inequals to houres equals and ageynward.

Take the nomber of the grees of the houres inequals and divide hem bi xv, and thow shalt have the houres equals. And so thow shalt do of houres equals in bryngyng hem into grees ageyn and divide bi
465   a quantite of an houre inequal, the whiche is the xij part of the grees aforsaide, and than shalt thow come out to the houres inequals.

<xi> To have the meridian height.

Set the gree of the sonne vpon þe almuries[53] in the lyne of the middil hevene and the nombre of þe almuries from the place of the ori-
470   zont is the height meridian that thow seekist. And so thou do of sterris that bien ficched.

<xij> A chapiter that goeth bifore to certcyn thynges that folowen further.

Wite thow that the cercle of signes is divided in ij semycercles, of
475   the whiche oon bigynnyth from the hed of Capricorn ther the solsticial hiemal is, ascendaunt bi Aries to the bigynnyng of Cancer ther the solsticial estyval is; another forsoth descendaunt from that stide bi Libra to the bigynnyng of Capricorn. Also wite thow that both the semycerclis bien like fer of grees from either of the solsticial and of oon declyna-
480   cioun meridional or septentrional, and the daies and the nyghtis bien like evyn in length and in shortnes, and their heightes bie evene in the mydday for evermore.

<xiij> To have bi the reete the vnknowen gre of the sonne.

Set a mark vpon the meridian height that thow hast founde and
485   turne thi reetis and ij grees shuln falle vpon their markes. Than whiche of hem thow shalt knowe that bi the gree of the sonne bi the signe of the moneth that is a day, of whiche day and vnto whiche day it is evene, that thow shalt wite bi the grees like fer from þe solsticial, for the daies of it bien evene, as it is saide biforn.

490   **<xiiij>** To fynde the sterre that mydlith the hevene.

Set the sterre vpon the lyne of the myddil hevene and the gree of the zodiac þe whiche **[fol. 224r]** shal fal theron is the gree that thow seekist. And so do thou to the orizont for his risyng and his fallyng.

<xv> For the length[54] of a sterre.
495   The gree forsoth of the length thow shalt have bi the reete[55] set above the poole of the zodiac and the declynacioun of the sterre founden.

\<xvj\> Of the azimutis[56] and the height of the sonne or of the sterre.

Sette the gree of the sonne vpon the almuries[57] to the height yeven and looke what accordith therto of the azimutis, for needely it must be
500 oon of thiese iiij, that is to say, septentrional-oriental or oriental-merid-ional or meridional-occidental or occidental-septentrional. Also in this maner do with the sterris.

\<xvij\> Of the azimutis[58] of the risyng of the sonne and of the sterres.
505   Set the gree of the sonne or the centre of the sterre vpon þe ori-zont oriental and bihold what bifallith hym of the azimutis and above whiche it is risen, and that shal be the azumutis of his risyng. And vpon his likeness shal be his fallyng on that other side.

The iiij partis of the world to knowe, take the height of the sonne
510 or of the sterre and marke the vmbre of sum stable thyng at ij houres afore mydday and than discrive a cercle that passith by ij markes of the whiche the centre bi hevene of that thing vpstreight. And than from the myddil point of the porcioun of þe cercle bitwene the markes draw a diametre, for that shal shew the meridie and the septentrional. And
515 the lyne forsoth of another diametre dividyng that shal declare the ori-ent and the occident.

\<xviij\> To have the declynacioun of eche gree.

Set hym on that lyne of the myddil of the hevene and than wite thow the height of þat from the orizont. Afterward knowe the height
520 of the hed of Aries and Libra in the same lyne meridional. The whiche so knowen, take the difference of hem, the whiche difference is the declynacioun of that gree. [I]f septentrional, the declynacioun is sep-tentrional; if it be meridional it is meridional.

Wite also that the grees of the signes septentrional bien higher than
525 the equinoccial and the meridionals lower, forwhi more declynacioun is in the hede of Cancer than in the hede of Ca- **[fol. 224v]** pricorn.[59] In the same maner thow shalt fynde the declynacioun of ficched sterris.

\<xix\> Of the breede[60] of the regioun that is the reryng[61] of the pole of the world above the orizont.
530   Loke the height of the sonne in the meredie and take that out of lxxxx if it be in the bigynnyng of Aries and Libra, and this that levith

---

500. thiese iiij] *written as one word, with dividing stroke after* thiese
522. If] of

is the breede of the regioun. And if the sonne be in any other gree,
avise wele the height of þat gree, the whiche if it be septentrional, take
it from the height meridional, or ellis adde it if it be meridional, and
535 so shal come oute the height of *capitis Arietis*. And whan thow hast don
that, worche as it is beforesaide.

<xx> Or ellis thus: Take the meridional height and also the height of
what sterre thow wilt and the breede therof and worche as is biforn saide.
Or thus: seeche the overest height and the lowest partie of what sterre
540 þow wilt that fallith[62] nought and joyne hem both toguydre, and than
take the half therof, for that is the height of the poole in that regioun.

<xxj> Of the ascenciouns in signes in a right cercle.
Set the be[gyn]nyng of a signe or of a gree vpon *semidiatrum orientis*,[63] and the grees of þe cercle equinoxial founden vnder the almury
545 shewith thyn entent.

<xxij> Of the ascenciouns in signes in cercle oblique.
Set the bigynnyng of the signe or of the grees vpon the orizont on
the orient half, and the grees of the cercle equinoccial that bien vnder
the almury[64] founden bien the grees that ascenden with the same por-
550 cioun.

<xxiij> For to knowe the vnknowen sterris that bien sette in the
astrolabye.
Take first the height of sum sterre that thow knowest and set it vpon
suche an height like in the almuries.[65] Afterward looke the sterre that
555 than thow wilt wite of, bi how moche [he]ight it lith vpon the almuries.
And in that partie that it be the whiche so seyn, the more[66] sterre that
thow seest thurgh the holis of the pynnels,[67] havyng suche height in þat
partie of hevene that thow sie the sterre in, is the sterre that þou seekist.

<xxiiij> In whiche maner sterris nowght set in the astrolaby shal
560 be knowen.

---

543. begynnyng] benyng
547. vpon] vpont
554. an] and
555. height] light   M altitudinem

Abide til [the] sterre be comen nygh to the lyne meridian and þan
turne aboute thi reete to looke if any sterre set in thyn astrolaby accordith with that height. And if it be so, that is he that thow seekist. And
if ther be non suche, than bihold sum sterre that thow knowest weele
565 the **[fol. 225r]** place of in the astrolabie that is next that height. And
after the height þerof ordeyne the reete and in the directis of[68] that
gree of the signes that be in the lyne of the myddil hevene shal be that
sterre vnknowen. And þe breede is shewed in accomptyng the almuries[69] from the marke of that height vnto the equinoccial.

570   **<xxv>** For to wite in what gree of a signe the moone is.
Looke the height of the mone in the almuries[70] in that side that
she is in knowen; þan ordeyne sum sterre after his height, and the cercle zodiac that fallith in the almuries[71] vpon the marke of the height of
the mone shal be the [gree] of the mone. And if it appiere in the day,
575 do in the same maner with the height therof and of the sonne. In the
same maner thow may fynde the placis of the planetis, if thow wilt on
nyghtis marke þe height of hem.

          <xxvj> To fynde the place of the planetis better.[72]
Take the height of a planete bifore the lyne of the myddil hevene
580 and take the ascendaunt in the same houre bi sum of the sterris ficched
and kepe that with the houre. Than looke the descence like to the ascendyng and eft take the ascendyng and the houre bi sum sterre ficched.
Than take the halfuendele bitwene the first ascendaunt and the secunde
bi the almury *in lymbo*,[73] and the gree þat fallith than vpon the lyne of
585 the myddil hevene, in that is þe planete.

          <xxvij> Of the breede[74] of a planete from the wey of the sonne.[75]
Take heede [i]f þe height of a planete that thow hast taken whan it
was in the lyne of þe myddil hevene be evene to the height of the same
gree or more or lasse. For if it be evene it hath no breede; if it be more

---

561. the] *blotted*   be comen] becomen

570. For to wite . . . moone is] *marg. in later hand:* What gre of a signe þe mone
is in

574. gree] *om. at end of line*

580–581. bi sum . . . houre] *foll. by* by sum of the sterris and kepe that with
the houre

587. if] of   M utrum

590 it is semptentrional; and if it be lasse it is meridional. And as moche is
his breede as is that difference.

<xxviij> Of the retrogradacioun or direccioun of planetis, whiche
thow wilt of hem take in mynde the height and the height of sum other
sterre ficched.

595 Than after the iij or the iiij nyght, in the whiche is sensible moevyng,
with a sterre that bifore had the same height bihold the height of the
planete. The whiche height if it be [lasse], þan his first height it is
streight; if it be more, it is retrograde. And þat if the sterre be on the orient half, but if it be on th'occident side it bifallith th'opposite.

600 [fol. 225v] <xxix> Of the evenyng of the house[s] xij.⁷⁶
Set the gree ascendaunt vpon þe viij houre of the lyne.⁷⁷ Than the
gree that fallith vpon the lyne of mydnyght is the bigynnyng of the
secunde hous. Than leede ageyn the gree ascend[aunt] vpon the lyne
of the x houre, and the gree founden vpon the lyne of mydnyght is bi-
605 gynnyng of the thrid house. Reduce that same gree in the orizont oriental, and the gree of the lyne of mydnyght is bigynnyng of the iiij house.
Set than the naydar gree ascendyng on the lyne of the secunde hous,
and the gree on the lyne of mydnyght shal shewe the bigynnyng of the
v hous. Set yit the forsaide naydar on the lyne of the iiij houre, and the
610 gree on the lyne of mydnyght is the bigynnyng of the vj house. Thiese
other vj houses forsoth bien had bi th'opposites of thiese, for the first
is opposite to the vij house, the ij to the viij, the iij to the ix, the iiij to
the x, the v to the xj, the vj to the xij.

<xxx> Of the aspeccioun⁷⁸ of the planetis.

615 Looke how many grees bien bytwene hem of whom thow wilt wite
the aspect. For if ther be lx degrees, the aspect is the sextile; if lxxxx,
quartile; if [cij], iij;⁷⁹ if cviij,⁸⁰ th'opposite; if nothyng, thei are ioyned; if
v lesse, it is applied to the aspect; if it be more, it is departed.⁸¹ And note
wele that the aspectis are knowen bi the grees equals, after sum men.
620 Nevertheles bi Tholome thei arn knowen bi þe grees of the ascencioun
of a streight cercle. And after sum other thei arn set after the gree of
a cercle oblique.

---

597. lasse] *blotted*   M minor   his] his (*end of line*) his
600. houses] house
603. ascendaunt] ascend
617. cij] M¹ (*see Explanatory Note*)   cviij th'opposite] cviij if thopposite

<xxxj> Of the science worldly or naturally,[82] that is to say, to knowe
þe introite of the sonne into Aries, what signe and what gree ascend-
625 ithe every yeere.
    Set the ascendaunt gre of that yeere past on the orizont oriental.
After that, meve the almury[83] from the place that he was in vnto lxxxvij[84] grees and xix minutis, and than the gree that fallith on the orizont shal be ascendent of the yeere folowyng. And if ther be mo yeres,
630 for eche moeve the almury after the succession of the signes so many
grees and so many minutis and thow shalt have thyn entent.

    <xxxij> To knowe the houres equals bitwene yeeris yisen.[85]
    Diuide the grees of the perambulacioun, that is to say, bi al the
goyng aboute of [fol. 226r] the almury[86] in maner aforesaide bi xv.
635 And the nomber that goeth oute in the divisioun is the nombres of the
houres equals among the yeeris yesen.[87]
    And note wele that as for the worchyng of the quadraunt (wont
to be sette in the astrolabie, þat is),[88] in this next treatice, shewyng
the whiche is appropred thereto, shal be declared openly þe rulis of
640 mesuryng of heightis, and of lengthis of playnes, and of depnes of pittis. Therfor in this treatice I wil sey nothyng thereof.[89]

[New Quadrant 2][90]

    <j> **Vppon this maner** thow shalt fynde the declynacioun of the
sonne and of the sterris from the equinoccial.
645   Set the thridde[91] vpon þe gree of the sonne *in lymbo*, and sette the
almury in the ecliptike. And leede the threede withyn the almury to
the lyne of the height þat is in the lift side, and the grees that bien bitwene þe equinoccial and the almury is the declynacioun of þe sonne,
þe whiche is septentrional if the place be septentrional or ellis meridi-
650 onal if it be meridional. And right so it is of a sterre.

    <ij> If thow wilt wite the meridian height of the sonne and of þe
sterris.
    Looke the nombre of the grees descendaunt from the equinoxial
to the orizont, and that nombre shal declare the height of Aries and
655 Libra. To þat height adde the septentrional declynacioun of þe sonne

---

643. Vppon this maner] *in display script*
655–656. declynacioun . . . sterres] *marg. in later hand*: Declynacioun of þe
son & sterres

or of þe sterres; or ellis take out the meridional declynacioun therfro, and than the meridional height that thow worchest for shal arise out. But of the sterris that gon nat doun, this rule servith of nought.

<iij> If thow wilt knowe the quantite of houres inequal of the day
660 passed.

Looke first the meridian height[92] and set the threede in the equinocciall vpon it, and wher the threde kervith the lyne of the vj houre, ficche the almury. Than turne the corner to the sonne, that þe sonne beame even thurgh both smale holis, and the sight[93] of the almury bi-
665 twene the arke of the houres techith the houres. But þe parte of the houre passed thow shalt fynde bi the viij chapitre of the astrolabie tofore writen.[94]

<iiij> If thow wilt fynde the ark of the day and of the nyght and the quantite of the houre inequal of the day or of the nyght and also the
670 quantite of houres equals of eche day.

Set thyn almury vpon the gree in the ecliptik with the whiche thow worchest [**fol. 226v**] and leede furth the threede til the almury fal vpon the orizont þat thow wilt worche fore. And looke than the grees of þe equinocciall how many bien bitwene the threed [and] the riet ori-
675 zont,[95] the whiche is cald Capricorn,[96] on the right hand. The whiche thow adde to lxxxx grees if the gree proposed be septentrional; or if it be meridionall, take it from lxxxx grees. And double the nombre that comeþ þerof, and so shalt thow have the holl arke of the day. The whiche take it out of ccclx grees, and the residue shal be the ark of the
680 nyght. After that, devide the arke bi xij and thow shalt have the quantite of the houre inequal of the day. Take thow out of xxx grees and thow shalt fynde the quantite of the houre inequal of the nyght. Divide eftsoones the forsaide arke bi xv and so hast thow the houres equals of the day. The whiche houres take hem out of xxiiij houres and thow
685 shalt have the houres of the nyght.

[v.a][97] For to knowe the ascenciouns in the right, that is to say, *in circulo directo.*[98]

Set thi threede in that gree in the zodiac that thow worchest with, and it shal fal in the cercle equinoccial vpon the grees that ascenden

---

672. almury] l *ins. above line*
674. and] of   Prof et

690 with hym. And note weele that, knowen ascenciouns of iij signes, al
thiese other bien knowen as in that table.⁹⁹

[v.b] To fynde ascenciouns and grees of signes in the cercle
oblique.¹⁰⁰
        Wite first the ascencioun of that gree that thow worchest for in the
695 right spiere. Than set the threde vpon that gree in the zodiac and sette
the almury in the ecliptik. And, he so ficched, leede furth the threede
til the almury fal vpon the orisont; and the grees of the cercle equinoccial that fallen bitwene the reetis orizont¹⁰¹ and the threede adde thow
vpon the ascendens in the right spire if the gree be meridional. And if
700 it be septentrional, withdrawe hem. And so the ascenciouns therof shal
appiere in the cercle oblique.

[vj] For to declare the grete ascendaunt and the bigynnyng of oþer
xij houses.¹⁰²
        Wite first how many houres inequals and how many parties of houres
705 in the day bien passed and reduce thiese houres and their parties into
grees and mynutes. And hem thow adde to the ascenciouns of grees of
the sonne in þe cercle [fol. 227r] oblique ifounden. And looke than bi
thyn instrument or ellis lightlier bi thi table of thi regioun, the grees
of the zodiac aunsweryng this ascendyng. For that without doute is the
710 ascendyng and bigynnyng of the first house.
        After, from that ascencioun abate lxxxx grees if thow may; and ellis
adde ccclx and than withdrawe it. And the remenaunt that levith looke bi
thyn instrument in the grees of the zodiac to whom in the reetis spiere¹⁰³
the nombre accordith; forwhi that is the myddel of the centre¹⁰⁴ and shal
715 declare the bigynnyng of the x house. Over that, take out þe nombre
of an houre inequale of thyn arke of the day in the gre ascendyng and
double it. And that doubled, adde thow to that ascencioun of the x hous
tofore had. And the grees of the zodiac accordyng to this ascencioun
in the right spiere tellith þe bigynnyng of the xj house. Efte, the same
720 houre tofore doubled to the ascencioun that thow fonde in the xj house
joyne thow. And the gree of the zodiac accordyng to this ascencioun in
the right spiere shewith the bigynnyng of the xij house. Therto yit eft,
enjoynaunt the houre doubled toforesaide to the ascencioun of the xij
house and the grees of the zodiac joyned to this ascencioun in the rec-

---

707. cercle] *catchword* oblique
714. the (3)] *foll. by* spiere *canc.*

725 tis spiere shewith the gree ascendaunt founden first. Furthermore, the
double houre bifore withdrawe from lx grees and adde the manaunt to
the ascencioun last bifore founden. And the gree of the zodiac that his
ascencioun accordith withyn the right spiere shewith the bigynnyng of
the secunde hous. Than the same remenaunt eft adde thow to the next
730 ascencioun tofore founden, and the gree of the zodiac that it accordith
to in the right spiere shal bigynne the thrid house.

Thiese vj houses thus knowen, thiese other vj shal be knowen bi the
naddair of hem. Forwhy the x is naddair to the iiij, the xj to the v, the xij
to the vj; the first to the vij, the ij to the viij, the iiij to the ix opposite.
735 The houres passed thus thow shalt knowe. The arke bitwene the
gree ascendaunt and the gree with the whiche the sonne ascendid in
thyn orizont bi partis of an houre inequale of the day divide thow for
to have þe houres [fol. 227v] inequals. But for the houres equals, divide
hem bi xv, and þe nombei that cometh therof shewith the houres that
740 thow sechist.

<vij> For to fynde the ark of the day and of the nyght of a sterre
fix and þe gree of the sterre with the whiche he mydlith[105] the hevene
[and its] risyng and fallyng.[106]

F[or] the arke of the day and of the nyght of the sterre, it is to do
745 as it is saide bifore of the sonne in the iiij chapitre therof.[107] But as for
the secunde point, set thi threede vpon the centre of the sterre, and
with the gree of the zodiac founden vnder the threede the same sterre
mydlith heven. For the thrid point, the whiche is risyng and fallyng,
adde to the ascencioun of the gree of the sterre wherwith it mydlith
750 hevene lxxxx grees. And of that toguyder ioyned take oute the half
arke of the day of that sterre and the gree of the zodiac perteyneng to
that ascencioun lefte in the cercle oblique with the sterre shal rise. But
if thow to that ascencioun in the right spiere the grees of þe sterre with
the whiche he mydlith hevene to lxxxx gadred toguyder with half the
755 ark diurne of that sterre do toguyder, than the naddayr of the sonne to
whom this ascencioun in the orizont oblique accordith with the same
sterre fallith doun.

---

743. and its] *om.*
744. For] from
755. of (2)] of (*end of line*) of

<viij> For to knowe the gree ascendaunt and the bigynnyng of other
houses, with the houres of the nyght equals and inequals bi the sterres.

760   Seeche the houres[108] inequals and the partis of the houres of the
sterre þat thow worchest with that bien passed, the whiche arke thow
withdrawe. And if þis sterre be bifore the meridie, kepe this ark found-
en[109] from al the arke diurn of the same sterre and kepe the nombre
that levith. After that, þe half of the arke diurne of that sterre with-
765 drawe, if it be meridie, from half the ark diurne of the gree with the
whiche he mydlith hevene. And the excesse therof adde thow vnto that
grees[110] of the whiche bifore thou reduced into houres. And if it be septentrional, withdraw from thilke grees the excesse founden bi the half
arke of the sterre and of that gree with whiche it medlith the hevene.
770 And that levith of the forsaide grees after the addicioun or subtraccioun adde thow to the ascencioun of that gree with the whiche the
sterre is in the myddil of hevene in the spiere oblonge.[111] And the gree
of the zodiac that accordith to that ascencioun in the spiere oblonge is
the ascent. Withdraw lxxxx grees and than the grees of þe zodiac **[fol.**
775 **228r]** to whom the ascendaunt accordith in the right spiere shewith the
bigynnyng of the x house. The bigynnyng of th'other houses forsoth
thow shalt fynde vnder the forme of the ar[t] seide bifore.
        Than afterwarde withdrawe thyn ascenciouns of *naddair solis* in
the spiere oblonge from the grees ascendaunt, and that levith over shal
780 be the token the ark passed of the houres of that nyght. The whiche
if thow divide bi the parties of the houre inequal of that nyght for to
have the houres inequals or bi xv for the equals, the nombres quociens
shewith the houres that thow seekist and hir parties.

        <ix> The ark of the cordes and the corde[112] of the ark to arken.
785   Sette the threede in the equinoccial vpon as many grees as thow
wilt and leede thyn almury vpon the seccioun of the threede of the
vj houre. The whiche than bere thow to the right orizont, for ther he
shewith his *corda rect*[a] of the grees. Or ellis, the *corda recta* knowen,

---

762. withdrawe] *in marg.*   kepe] *foll. by ins. mark, poss. erroneously placed here instead of after* thow *in prec. line of MS*

773. oblonge] b *written over another letter, poss.* s *or* f

777. art] ark   Prof artis

782. nombres quociens] nombre squociens

786. the (3)] *foll. by* threede *canc.*

788. recta (1)] rect *with final* -e *flourish; no other occurrences of* corda recta *and* corde recte *mix Latin and English endings*

thow shalt fynde þe ark, settyng thyn almury vpon the *corda*. And thanne
790 bere it furth ageyn vpon the vj houre, and the touchyng of the threede
in the equinoccial shewith the ark of the corde founden. And if thow
wilt knowe the *corda versa*, set the threede vpon as many grees as thow
wilt, and in the towchyng of the threede of the cercle opposite set thyn
almury. The whiche than thow bere furth to the right orizont vpon the
795 partie of *corda versa*. There the sight of it shal teche the his corde verse
or, supposed *corda versa* with the ark thcrof, as in *corda recta*. Nowe is
shewed whereof *corda recta* cresceth into lx ascendaunt and *corda versa*
in descendaunt to lx and in ascendaunt to c[xx].

But it is to wite, if the grees of *corda versa* bien sought from i into
800 lxxxx or from clxxx into cclxx, considre the almury in the partie
descendaunt of *corda versa*. And if thei bien from lxxxx into clxxx
or from cclxx into ccclx, it is to considre the almury in the nombre
ascendaunte of *corda versa*.

Note also if thow have ij almuries, settyng that oon vpon the vj houre
805 and that other vpon the cercle opposite, than both the cordes thow
may knowe toguyder and also the ark, if thow wilt.

<x>[113] If thow wilt fynde the *vmbram rectam & versam*[114] bi the
height.[115]

Sette thi threede in the equinoccial vpon the height of the sonne,
810 and set the first almury[116] vpon the cercle opposite and þe secunde [**fol.
228v**] vpon the meridional, and bere furth thi threede to the right
orizont. And the parties of *corda recta* vnder the first almury founden
multiplie thow bi xij and the product therof divide thow bi þe parties
of the same *corda* founden vnder the secunde almury. And the nom-
815 bre quociens[117] shal shewe the signes[118] of *vmbram rectam*. And if thow
multiplie the parties of *corda recta* founden vnder the secunde almury
bi xii, dividaunt the nombre that goth out therof bi the parties found-
en vnder the first almury, than shal the nombre quociens notifie to the
vmbra versa.

820 Neuertheles thow may do this lightlier[119] settyng thi threede vpon
the height of the sonne wherof thou wilt the *vmbra*. Forwhi if this height
be lesse than xlv grees, þe threede [fallith] vpon the point of *vmbra
versa*; and if it be more, vpon *vmbra recta*; and if it fal precisely vpon xlv,

---

798. cxx] c 	Prof 120
814. And] a *written over* q
822. fallith] *om.*

than the *vmbra* is evin to the height of eche thyng that is evene streight
825 and perpendiculerly set vpright.

And *econverso*, settyng the threede vpon *vmbra recta* or *versa*, the
height of the sonne shal be knowen. For wher the threede touchith the
equinoccial, ther the height of the sonne shal be knowe accordyng to
that vmbre.

830   And if thow wilt knowe bi the corde verse the corde recte *econverso*,
divide the corde verse[120] founden bi þe nombre of the scale, the whiche
is cxliiij, and the nombre quociens therof shal shewe the corde recte
and *econverso*.

<xj> To shewe the houres of the day and the ark bi the height of
835 the sonne; and the houres of the nyght and the ark bi the height of the
sterris.

Set the threede vpon the present height of the sonne and the first
almury vpon the cercle meridional, and bere the threede furth vpon
the myddil ark diurne. And sette the secunde almury vpon the cercle
840 cenyth[121] and multiplie [the] corde recte founden vnder the first almury
bi the corde verse vnder the secunde almury, kepyng the nombre of the
secunde almury and þe productis. And the threede set vpon the meridian height therof and þe almury vpon the cercle cenyth, and divide thi
nombre product before founden and kepe the corde recte vnder the
845 almury now founden. And do awey the nombre quociens from *corda versa*
of the secunde almury first kept, and vpon the residue set the almury in
corda versa. And leede hym than to the cercle of cenyth, and **[fol. 229r]**
than the threede shal shere in the equinoccial the ark of the houres bitwene the tyme of the taken height of the meridian; the whiche thow
850 withdrawe from the myddil ark diurne if it be bifore the meridie, or adde
it to the same if it be after the meridie. And than shal come out the ark
from the sonne risyng vnto the houres tyme founden; þe whiche if thow
divide by the parties of the houres inequals of the day or ellis bi xv, the
houres inequals or equals shuln com out and þe parties of hem subtil-
855 ier than thei dide bifore.

---

834. height] *foll. by* and the height
839. secunde] *foll. by* ark *canc.*
840. the (1)] and
841. the (2)] *foll. by* first *canc.*
845. versa] *foll. by* and leede hym thanne *canc.*

<xij> Over that, thus thow shalt know[122] of nyghtis bi the sterris þat thow knowest the gree ascendaunt and the bigynnyng of thiese other houses.

Take the *corda versa* of the myddil ark of that sterre ffirst and sith
860 the cord recte of the present height, and than multiplie the *corda versa* first founden bi the *corda recta* secunde founden, kepyng that product and the cord *prima*. After that, take *corda recta* of the meridian height of that sterre and bi that departe the product that thow keped bifore and do awey the nombre quociens of *corda versa* bifore founden and
865 kept. And of the residue seeke the ark versa and take that out of the ascencioun in the right spiere of the grees with þe whiche it mydlith the hevene of the height taken bifore the meridie; or if it be after the meridie adde it therto. And the gree of the zodiac to whom this ascendent accordith in the right cercle sha[l] shewe the bigynnyng of the mydde
870 hevene. And to this ascendaunt adde lxxxx grees, and the gree of the zodiac to whom this ascendaunt accordith to in the cercle oblique is the ascence. Of this ascence withdrawe the ascencioun of *naddair solis* in the cercle oblique, and than shalt thow leve the ark rerid from the sonne fallyng to the tyme of the taken height; þe whiche divide thow
875 for the houres inequals and equals, as it is set bifore.[123]

<xiij>[124] For to knowe the height of thynges ireised perpendiculerly on an evyn playn.[125]

Go towardes or ellis frowardes the thyng til the threde fal vpon xlv degrees, the height seen thurgh the ij smale holis. Than mesure the dis-
880 taunce bitwene the stacioun and the base of the thyng, to the whiche adde the quantite of hym that mesurith it from his eyen to the erth, and ther shal come out al the height of þe þinge.

Another maner: if the height be lesse than xlv grees, the threede
[fol. 229v] wil fal vpon *scala versa*. Than what proporcioun is xij to
885 thiese pointes the same is of distaunce to the height. But what is the proporcioun of pointes of *scala recta* to xij the same is of distauns to the height.[126]

Or on another maner, if the thynge be inaccessible (þat is to seyn, if a man may nat com therto), take the nombre of pointes of *vmbra versa*,
890 the height wele iseen tofore; the whiche pointes thurgh grace of ensample[127] bien iiij that in xij thries arn conteyned. From thens go bacwardis

---

867. taken] *foll. by* be
874. tyme] *foll. by* .o.[R]   Prof presentis temporis

bi a right lyne til the threede falle on the pointes the whiche iiij sithes
arn conteyned in xij. Take þan oute the lasse habitude of proporcioun
from the more, that is to say, the triple from the quatriple, and ther lev-
895   ith an vnite. Mesure than the distaunce bitwene the secunde stacioun,
for that distaunce is or shal be evyn to the height. And if ij leven it shal
be double the distauns, if iiij triple, and so furth. And alwey adde therto
the stature of hym that mesurith, from his eye vnto the erth.

     <xiiij> To mesure the length of a playne.
900   Biholde thurgh the smale holis the terme of the playne that shal be
mesured. The corner of the quadraunt set to the eye; and whiche com-
parisoun of pointes of *scala versa* is to xij, suche is of the stature of hym
that mesurith from the eye to the erth vnto the length of the playne.

     <xv>[128] To mesure the depnes of a pit.
905   What so is the proporcioun of pointes of *scala recta* to xij (the angle
of the quadraunt turned vp as bifore and the beame visuale passyng bi
the side of the pitte to the terme of depnes of the side opposite whiche)
is the dyametre of the pitte to al his depnesse.

     <xvj>[129] And for to make the quadraunt, make a rounde cercle
910   wherin thow wilt make thi quadraunt. Lyne it in the iiij quarter and than
set A in the myddis of the cercle. And than shal the quadraunt be the
quarter of the cercle. And that nedith to be round, for the astrolabye
shal be on that oon side and the quadraunt of that other side. And thus
thei must both be made in that oon quarter, as it is saide bifore, that
915   oon vpon that on side and that other vpon that other side.

     <xvij> Of geometry ij parties bien:[130] theoric and practik.[131] The-
orike is that one bi speculacioun of thought ensesyng þe quantites and
proporciouns of thinges. Practik is when we mesure þe **[fol. 230r]**
vnknowen quantite of any thyng bi sensible point of artificiall mesuryng
920   that is clepid practic. Thre spechis ther bien: altimetric, pleynmetric,
and steriometric.[132] Altimetric is when we seeche al-holely the height of
any thyng. Pleynmetrik is when we seeche in mesuryng the breede of
any thyng. Steriometric is when we seeche the length, breede, and depnes of any thyng. In the first maner, the streight mesuryng we mesure; in
925   the secunde, the superficial; in the thridde, the sadde bodily mesure.

---

892. right] bright   Prof rectam   the (1)] the the

Therfor the treatice in whiche we shal teche for to knowe the
mesures of al thyng as it parteyneth to the inleedyng of this craft in
ij parties we diuiden. Forwhi in the first partie we shuln treate of the
quadraunt and of the iiij parte of the cercle forseide whiche it con-
930 teyneth; and in the secunde parte, of the worchyng that is don bi hym
and of the profites therof.

<xviij> The quadraunt forsoth is an instrument that conteyneth þe
iiij part of a cercle and certeyne outdrawyng of lynes bi þe whiche we
may gete the grees of the sonne and the declynacioun, and the height
935 of sterris; and the houres of the tyme discryve, and þe height of thynges, the fernes of citees, the length of londis, and the depnes of pittis.
Therfor the quadraunt shal be made in this maner: a plaate of bras
or tree or coper shal be take and founde to[133] the iiij part of a compas.
Than shal a cercle be made in sum pleyne boorde of the whiche cer-
940 cle the iiij part sha[l] be mesured by compas to the quadraunt, and
after the mykelnesse therof shal the quadraunt be made. And withyn
the sides of the quadraunt a space shal be left on eche side to draw in ij
streight lynes markyng alwey a streight corner[134] and withyn the corner
the quadraunt, the whiche cornere shal be cald A, bi this craft.
945 Ther shal be drawen a subtil draught[135] from the corner B of the
quadraunt to the corner C, and þat shal be divided in ij evene partis.
And in the point of the middil divisioun shal the standyng foote of the
compas be ficched, and þat other foote of the compas shal be strecched
to sum partie bisides A,[136] of the whiche partie[137] thow wilt drawe ii right
950 drawghtis bisides the half[138] of the quadraunt, the whiche [fol. 230v]
shal close in with hem the iiij parte of the sercle. The moevyng foote of
the compas vnto that right, aftirwarde bi that settyng it shal be moeved
to the B and C, and so the place shal be marked in a subtile lyne so
drawen whan the moevable foote of þe compas shal touchen that lyne.
955 And fro that point biforsaide bisides A to the point bisides B and C shal
be led ij lynes that shal within hem close a right corner, and vnderneth
drawyng the iiij parte of a cercle circumferencial that shal contene the
iiij parte of a trew cercle. And that nether draught goyng in compas is
cleped *lymbum*, and that other ij parties withoute shal be cald the sides
960 of þe quadraunt.

---

940. shal be] shabbe
946. ij] iij   QV duas
956. ij] iij   QV dua

And on the right half of the quadraunt shal be ij tablettis sette eche even from the ex[tr]emites of the side A and C. And they shuln be perced with ij smale holis evenstandyng from þe lyne A and fallyng to the lyne C.

965   Also, biside the lyne vnderneth that is circumferencial (that is to say, BC) shal be drawe ij lynes in cercle iliche from other; bitwixt the whiche, spaces bien left [below whiche can be inscribed], in the neither space biside *lymbum*, eche gree. And in that binethe, that nomber of the grees may be writen, as it shal be knowen herafter. And the neither lyne, BC, 970 be divided in ij evene parties; and eche partie of CB be divided in iij; and echon of the parties, in oþer iij. And the lynes of divisioun shal be drawen from the lyne circulier bineth vnto the iij lyne circulier aboven, occupyng ij spaces betwixt the occupied [x]viij spaces.[139]

    And the neither partie *in lymbo*[140] echon shal be divided in v equals, 975 and certeyn lynes of the neither cercle shal be drawe into that other lyne circulier folowyng, occupieng the first space. And ther shal be lxxxx grees. So many shal ther be in þe zodiac of eche cercle.[141] And that space so ordeyned bi grees is cleped *lymbum*.

    Afterward shal be divided and left a space of ij fyngres and an half 980 or nere that, and a lyne circulier shal be drawe, departyng the space vnder from that above. And that lyne shal be cald FG; and that lyne divided in vj even parties, and thei shuln be cald pointis of diuisioun, so that thei bien cald and knowen HIKLMN. And þan shal the quadraunt be set in a playn table and so fastned with nayles that it be nat lightly 985 moeved of the stiede.

    And than another table shal be ioyned therto in evene breed in the point of the table toward **[fol. 231r]** C. Than the foote of the compas [shal be put] in the point A, and þat oþer foote shal strecche from the ly[ne] AH.

990   Afterward a point shal be soughte in the lyne AC toward A to that[142] other foote of the compas moevable pas thurgh the point A. Than shal the compas be restrayned, and another point eft sought in the forsaide lyne towarde A to the moevable foote of the compas pas thurgh the

---

966. ij] iij   QV due
967. below whiche can be inscribed] *om.*   QV infra que describi possint
970. ii] iij   QV duas
971. and (1)] *foll. by* nat   QV et quelibet illarum partium in alias tres
973. ij] iij   QV duo   xviij] viij   QV 18
981. FG] *first letter unclear*   QV FG
988. shal be put] *om.*   QV ponetur

lyne AK. And do so ay in sechyng a poynte towardes A in the lynes AC
995 to vj, [vnto] lynes circumferentals bien drawen from the point A to the
vj pointes HIKLMN. And thiese lynes shuln be of houres, bi the whiche
the houres of daies artificials shuln be take.

[Inscribing Almucantars on an Astrolabe] [143]

For to make the almecantrades, thow shalt sette the cercle of Capricorn
1000 ABCD, and the diametres shuln kerve vpon the point E. The cercle of
Aries and Libra shal be the cercle ZHTK, and the point allilakas[144] shal
be the pointe A. Thanne thow shalt divide the cercle ZHTK by ccclx
divisiouns. Afterward thow shalt sette the arc KL as the latitude of the
regioun and the ark HM like hym and the ark ZG. Also afterward þou
1005 shalt joyne G with H, and thow shalt kerve the diametres AC vpon P,
and the point P shal be the point of the cenyth. Afterward ioyne H with
L and thow shalt kerve the diametre AC vpon S.[145] After that thow shalt
ioyne H with M, and thou shalt drawe out HM for-to it joyne vpon N,
and NS shal be the diameter of the cercle of the emyspiere (that is, of
1010 the orizont), þe whiche thou shalt departe bi the half. And thow shalt
make that first part of the cercle kervyng the cercle of Capricorn vpon
the point[is] VF, and if this partie V[S]F go vpon the point[is] H[S]K,
than is thi werk triewe and ellis nat. Afterward þou shalt kerve from
the point M toward Z of iij grees or v or x or as many as thow wilt, and
1015 it is the ark MR and the ark LQ.

Also afterward ioyne H with R and drawe a lyne for-to it kerve the
diametre NS vpon [O]. Than divide O[I] by half and that on part of
the cercle shal kerve the cercle of Capricorn vpon YX, and the ark is Y-
X. And thus thow shalt nat cese to do til thow come to the cenyth[146] P,
1020 and thow shalt write vpon [fol. 231v] the almycantrades the nomber of
hem that thei arisen by and in the azmutis also.[147]

[fourteen lines left blank]

---

995. vnto] *om.* QV donec
1012. VSF] vcf   M vsf *or [MS var.]* arcus sfv   pointis HSK] point hck   M
punctos hsk
1017. O] c   M o   OI] o   M oi

[from Chaucer, *Treatise on the Astrolabe*] [148]

[2.37] *A maner of equacioun of houses bi the Astrolaby.*

Take thyne ascendaunt and than hast thow the iiij angles; for wele thow
1025 wost, the opposite of thyn ascendent, that is to say, the bigynnyng of
the vij house, sit vpon the west orizont, and the bigynnyng of the x
house sitte vpon the lyne meridional, and his opposite vpon the lyne
of mydnyght. Than ley thi label on the gree ascendent and reken from
the point of thi label al the grees in the bordure til thow come to the
1030 meridional lyne; and than departe al thiese grees in iiij evene partis,
and take ther the evene porcioun of iij houses; for ley thy label on everiche of thiese iij parties and þan maist thow see bi thi label in the zodiac
the bigynnyng of everich of the iij houses from the ascendent; that is
to say, the xij house next above thyne ascendent, and than from the
1035 bigynnyng of the xj house, and than the x house vpon the meridional
lyne, as I first saide. The same werke from the ascendaunt downe to the
lyne of middenyght, and thus hast thow iij other houses; that is to sey,
the bigynnyng of the ij the iij and the iiij house. Than is þe naddair of
thiese the bigynnyng of iij houses that folowen thy lyne meridional.[149]

[fol. 232r]

[nineteen lines left blank]

1040 [2.40] *To knowe with whiche gree of the zodiac that any planete ascendith in the*
orizont whether that his latitude be north or south.

Knowe bi thyne almynak the gree of ecliptik of any signe in the whiche
that the planete is rekened for to be and is clepid the gree of this longitude. And knowe also the gree of his latitude f[ro] the ecliptik north
1045 or south. And bi this ensample folowyng maist thow werke in general
in every signe of the zodiac:

The gree of the longitude, peraventure, of Venus or of any other
planete was vj grees of Capricorn, and the latitude of hir was northward ij grees from the ecliptike lyne. Thanne toke I a subtile compas
1050 and clepid that oon point of my compas A and that other point F. Than
toke I the point and set it in ecliptike lyne in my zodiac in the degree of
the longitude of Venus, that is to say, in the vj gree of Capricorn; and
than set I the point of F vpwarde in the same signe bicause that the
latitude was north vpon the latitude of Venus, that is to say, in the vj

---

1042. Knowe] To knowe
1044. fro] for

1055 gree of Capricorn. And thus have I ij grees betwixt my ij prikes. Than
laide I doun softly my compas **[fol. 232v]** and sette the gree of the longitude vpon the orizont. Tho toke I and wexed my label in maner of a
peire tablis to receive distinctly the prikes of my compas. Than toke I
this forsaide label and leide it fix over the gree of my longitude; than
1060 toke I vp my compas and set the point of A in the wex of my label as
even as I coude gesse over the ecliptik lyne in the end of the longitude.
Than toke I vp my compas and sette þe point of F endlong in my label
vpon the space of the latitude inward and over the zodiac, that is to say,
northward from the ecliptic. Than laide I doun my compas and looked
1065 weele in the wey vpon the prikes of A and F. Than torned I my reete til
the prike of F sit vpon the orizont. Than sawe I wele that the body of
Venus in hir latitude of [ij] grees septentrional ascendid in the vj gree
from the hede of Capricorn.

And note that in this maner maist thow wirke with any latitude sep-
1070 tentrional in al signes. But sothly the latitude meridional of a planete
in Capricorn may nat be take bicause of the litel space bitwixt the ecliptik and the bordure of the astrolaby; but in al other signes it may be.

Also the gree, peraventure, of Jupiter or of another planete was in
the first gree of Piscis in longitude and in his latitude was iij grees merid-
1075 ional. Than toke I the point of A and set it in the first gree of Piscis on
the ecliptik and set the point of F dounward in the same signe bicause
the latitude was sowth iij grees, that is to say, from the hede of Piscis, and
thus I have iij grees bitwixt both prikes. Also set I the longitude vpon
the orizont and toke my label and laide it fix vpon the gree of the longi-
1080 tude; than set I þe point of A on my label evene over the ecliptike lyne
in th'ende of the gre of longitude and than set the point of F endlonges
in my label the space of the latitude outward from the zodiac, that is to
say, southward from the ecliptik towarde the bordure. And thoo turned I
the reete to the prike of F sat vpon the orizont, and than I seyng that the
1085 body of Jupiter in his latitude of iij grees meridional ascendid with the
xiiij gree of Piscis *in horoscopo*; and in this maner maist thow wirke with
any latitude meridional, as I first saide, [save] in Capricorn.

And if thow wilt pley this [craft] with þe arisyng of the mone, loke
thow rekene wele the cours houre bi houre, for she dwellith nat in a
1090 gree of his longitude but a litel while, as thow **[fol. 233r]** wele know-

---

1067. ij] *om. (cf. line 1049 above)*
1072. but] *foll. by* it *canc.*
1087. save] *om.*
1088. craft] cast

est. But nevertheles if thow rekene hir moevyng in thi tables houre bi
houre, &c.

[*fifteen lines left blank*]

[2.39] *Discripcioun of the meridional lyne, of longitudis and latitudis of citees*
and townes, as wel as of a clymate.

1095 This lyne meridional is but a maner of discripcioun or a lyne imagyned
that passith vpon the poolis of this world and bi the cenyth of our hede,
and it is clepid the lyne meridional, ffor in what place any man is at
any tyme of [yer, whan that] the sonne, be moevyng of the firmament,
come to his veray meridional place, than is veray mydday, that we clepe
1100 noone as to that man. And therfor it is clepid the lyne of mydday. And
note that evermore of any ij townes or of ij citees of whiche þat oone
towne approchith nerrer the est than doeth that other towne, trust wele
that thiese townes han dyuers meridians. [Nota] also that the ark of the
equinoccial that is conteyned and bounded bitwixt ij meridians is clepid
1105 longitude of the towne. And if ij townes have ilike meridians, than is
the distaunce of hem both iliche from the est, and the contrary; and
in this maner thei chaunge nat hir meridian, but sothly thei chaunge
ther [almykanteras] for enhaunsyng of the poole and the distaunce of
the same.

1110   The longitude of a clymate is a lyne imagyned from the est into þe
west [**fol. 233v**] ilike distaunce from the equinoccial.

         The latitude of a clymate may be cleped the space of the erth from
the bigynnyng of the first clymate into th'ende of the same clymat evene
direct agenst the poole artik. Thus seyn sum auctours, that if men
1115 clepen the latitude of a cuntre the ark meridiane that is conteyned or
intercept bitwixt the cenyth and the equinoccial, than sey they that þe
distaunce is from the equinoccial into the end of a clymat.

[*eleven lines left blank*]

[2.38] *To fynde the lyne meridional to dwel fix in any certeyne place.*
Take a rounde plate of metal; for worchyng, the bradder the bettir, and
1120 make thervpon a just compas a litel withyn the bordure; and lay the

---

1098. yer whan that] *om.*
1103. nota] *om.*
1108. almykanteras] almuries

rounde plate vpon an evene grounde or on an evene stone or on an
evene stok ficched in the ground; and ley it evene bi level. And in the
centre of thi compas stike an evene pyn or a wire vpright, the smaller
the bettir. Set thi pyn bi a plom rules end and even vpright. And lete
1125 this pin be [no] lengger than a quarter of the diameter of thi compas
from the pin. And waite busily aboute x or xj of the clok whan the sonne
shyneth and whan the shadewe of thi pin entrith any thyng withyn the
cercle of thi compas on hir mole[150] and marke ther a prike with a thyng.
Abide than stille waityng on the sonne after oon of the clocke, til the
1130 shadewe [of] the wire [or] the pyn passe amoevyng oute of the cercle
of the compas, be it never so litel, and set ther anothe[r] prike.
    Take than a compas and mesure even the myddil bytwene both the
prikes and set ther a prike. Take than a rule **[fol. 234r]** and drawe a
strike evene a-lyne from the pyn vnto the middill prike, and take ther
1135 thi lyne meridional for evermore as in that same place. And if thow
drawe a crosse lyne overthwert þe compas iustly over the lyne meridional, than hast thow est and west and south. And *per consequens* the opposite of the south lyne is the north.

[Tables of Solar Heights][151]

1140 **[fol. 234v]** To the height of the sonne in the solsticial of wynter[152]

houres bifore mydday	ix	x	xj	xij
houres after mydday	iij	ij	i	o
grees	v	x	xiij	xiiij

The heightis of the sonne at al the houres in the equinoccial[153]

[houres bifore mydday]	vj	vij	viij	ix	x	xj	xij
[houres after mydday]	vj	v	iiij	iij	ij	j	o
[grees]	o	ix	[xviij]	xxvj	xxxij	xxxvj	xxxviij

1125. no] *om.*

1130. of the wire or] or the wire of

1138. north] *foll. in later hand after 8 blank lines by:* this boke of medycynes is
provid & tryede to be true you may be well assuryde that every kynd of medy-
cyne ys wounderfull good for the disease hit speakith of as any be in all the
worelde

1146. o] *foll. by* planetis

The heightis of the sonne at al the houres in the solst[ic]ial of somer

[hrs. bifore mydday]	iii	v	vj	vij	viij	ix	x	xj	xij
1150 [hrs. after mydday]	viij	vij	vj	v	iiij	iij	ij	j	o
[grees]	ij	viij	xviij	xxvij	xxxvj	xlv	liij	lix	lxij

To the height of the sonne in the vpper part at al houres of the quadraunt[154]

iiij	v	vj	vij	viij	ix	x	xj	xij
1155 lix	xlix	xxxviij	xxvij	xvij	v	x	xiij	xiiij

[Drawing Hour-Lines on a Quadrant]

[I.] Sette the threed in thyn instrument vpon the gree xxxv and the margarit or perle[155] vpon the lyne meridional. And than drawe the threde vnto the lvij gree and an half. And ther restith the knot, set ther
1160 thi cercle and ther drawe for the iiij and th[e] v houre of the day. Set doun the knot eftsoones bi oo gree and than drawe the threede to lviij grees, and wher þe knot abidith set ther the cercle and drawe for the vj houre. Yit drawe the threde to lxvj grees, and wher the knot abidith set ther thi cercle and drawe for the vij houre. To the xxxiiij gree and the
1165 knot vpon the lyne meridional and drawe vnto lxxv, and ther set for the viij houre. Also set the threede vpon xxxiij and the knot vpon meridional and drawe vnto lxxxij grees, and that for the ix houre. Also set the threede vpon xxxij gree, and drawe furth to lxxxvij grees for the x houre. Also set the threede vpon xxxj gre and drawe furth to lxxxix
1170 grees and a litel more for the xj houre.

    [fol. 235r] [II]. It is to be noted that if thow wilt make houres equal[156] in the quadraunt, than thow owest to werke in þis maner.[157] Take a rule or a threede perpendiculier from the poole [to] the myddis of lxij grees, and signes of pointis wher that he metith with the lyne
1175 meridional.[158] Take than a compas or oilet[159] of a foote and sette into the poole and another into the pointe remembred, to drawe agenst the lift part of the quadraunt. And cal that lyne A.[160] Evene in like wise do thow to the xxxviij gree, and cal that lyne B; and to the xv gree,

---

1149. xij] *foll. by* planetis
1150. o] *foll. by paraph and* xiij. xxvj. xxxix. xlix. lix
1158. or perle] *interlinear*
1174. wher] r *written over* t
1175. or oilet] *interlinear*

and cal that lyne C. Knowe thow þerfore that al the houres bien deter-
1180 myned at the lyne or cercle of A. But thei ascenden nat all neither to
B neither to C.

To have the foote of houres,[161] do in this maner: drawe the threede
to lix gres, signes[162] and pointe wher he touchith the lyne of A, and ther
is the foote for the xj houre. In like wise do thow to liiij gree for x, and
1185 to xlvj for ix, to xxxvij for viij, to xxviij for vij, to xix for vj, to x for v,
and to ij for iiij houres.

And note that ther bien many holl houres whan the daies bien
long[er] than xvj, though it be exces after sum mynutis.[163] Knowe thow
therfor sum of thiese houres oughten to kerve the lyne of B in ascend-
1190 yng. And to knowe wher this ought to be, drawe the perpendiculier to
xxxvij grees and signes the point wher that he kervith bitwene the B,
forwhi ther he shal passe the xj houre. Evene in like wise do thow to
xxxiij for x, to xxvj for 9, to xviij for viij, and to ix for vij; vj forsoth ter-
myncth and endith in the point termyneng the vj houre.

1195   Forsoth many houres ascenden nat to the lyne of B. To knowe wher
al houres han above furth to be determyned, note that al-only iij ascend-
en vnto the lyne of C—that is to say, ix, x, xj—and ther bien termyned
and ended. Drawe therfor the perpendiculier to v grees and signes the
point wher he kervith the lyne of C, forwhy ther shal be termyned ix;
1200 and to ix, x; and to xiij, xj. Forsoth the viij houre endith in the lift side
of þe quadraunt in the cercle corespondent and evene answeryng xviij
grees; vij after the corespondent xxviij gres; vj after the corespon- [fol.
235v] dent xxxviij grees; v after corespondent xlix gres; iiij after corespondent lix grees.

1205   To knowe therfor wher the foote of the compas or oilet ought to
be set for to make thiese houres, drawe the perpendiculier to ij gres
and mark the point wher he touchith the lyne of C, and cal that point
D. Also drawe the perpendiculier to xxix gres and signes the point
wher he kervith the vj houre cornerd—that is to say, the lyne meridi-
1210 onal—and cal that point E. Set therfor the foote of thi compas or oilet
in D to drawe from E vnto the right partie of the quadraunt softly a lyne
or a cercle, and in that cercle ought to be set the foote of þe compas or
oilet to al the houres to be made. Therfor require and seeke bi pointes
memoratief remembred in ABC lynes. And that compas or oilet shal
1215 alwey passe bi tho pointes, and thow shalt have the houres equals.

1205. or oilet] *interlinear*
1209. houre] *foll. by* kerued *canc.*

Note that the foote of the ladder[164] hath to stonde vpon the lyne
A in point equal vpon xlv grees and be made the lower part of hym in
the right side of the quadrant and in like wise in the lift side after corespondent xxxix grees and in the vpper after corespondent xxxv grees
1220 in either partie or side of the quadraunt; and diuide both and either
vmbre or shadewe as wel direct as oblique equaly in xij; be made half
the part of it after corespondent of xxxvij grees.

[On the Art of Gauging 1][165]

Iff thow wilt of craft to make a yerd visory or gawgyng yerd everywher
1225 of londis, take of þe cofre.[166] And of that latitude take the diametre, and
that, as often as thow maist into oo side of the yerde thow signe marke
or oilet,[167] thow do [so] oft. And if so, at the first front or sight thiese
signes shuln be, forwhy with the same oilet therof the first signe shal
dwel and abide vntouched.[168] But the secunde bi thries ought to be
1230 touched inequal, the thrid bi v inequals, the fourth bi vij equals, the v
bi ix equals, the vj bi [xj] equals, the vij bi xiij, the viij bi xv and so alwey
into ascendyng bi doublyng[169] in nombre as al that space be divided in
xix equal parties, of the whiche take viij for the first signe, **[fol. 236r]**
vj for the secunde, and v for the thrid. Forsoth v signes inequal of the
1235 thrid space so taken as al that space be divided without in tables[170] in xx
parties equals, of the whiche take iiij with an half for the first signe, iiij
with iiij without the half for the v.[171] Forsoth the remenaunt kept to the
forsaide nombre bien equals amonges hemsilf. And this part of þe rod
or yerd [is] now made, that is to say, to mesure the depth of vessels.
1240   After this, in that other side of the rod owen to be set and put
other signes whiche bien saide longitudes or lengthes of a yerd or rod.
In al londis may the first part of the same yerd dwel and abide, that is to
say, the depthis. But the secunde part—that is to say, to the longitude
or lengþ—ought to varie after the variacioun of mesure in al londis.
1245 This maner or as þe cofre first taken, she[w]ith the mesures of water
to what he wil, what or whos rod or yerd to be made. And note the

---

1227. so] *om.*

1228. oilet] *foll. by* oilettis

1231. xj] xij   Vis. vndecime

1234. vj] *upper marg. in later hand:* The lord is only my support and he which
doth me keep

1239. is] *om.*   Vis. est

1245. shewith] shedith

ascence of water whiche [is] in the cofre with a litil stike or straw, and this signe afterwarde shal be the first longitude, whiche owith equaly to be replied bi al the longitude of the rod.[172]

1250   And so than to whom it pleasith he may the nombre after the order of signes to either partie of the rod to inscribe or write.

Or otherwise may the rod be made into more subtile maner and more lightly in this maner: as the first signe of profunde depth of hap or fortune he takith to grete or litel pleasure;[173] and than the sccunde,
1255   first equal and bi iij inequals divided. And the thrid signe eftsones to hym equal and bi v inequals divided; and iiij bi vij, and so to ascende as it is aforsaide.[174]

Afterward, or after the maner of a grete vessel, he ought to take the longitude in this maner:[175] as that he take a grete vessel knowen of
1260   quantite and divide the longitude in as many parties as the mesures conteyneth. And of tho equal partis ought to be taken as many for the first longitude as signes of the same equat vessel in his extremytes conteyneth with the half in his profundite. And than the first longitude founden ought to be replied bi al the rod as it is aforsaide.

1265   [**fol. 236v**] Also as yit in thre maners and more lightly yit may be made the profundite or depth of the rod in maner as above happiþ and fortuneth, also as the longitude happith or fortunyth. And so the yerd or rod made shal be fals, nevertheles bc he corrected in maner and forme as withynfurth: as that he see to the proporcioun of triewe
1270   mesure to the fals signe or markc, with his falshed abiect and outcast and the triewe inscribed.

Forsoth a rod made in maner and forme as abovesaide, who wil gawge ought to vse[176] hem in this maner as with the profundite or depth of the rod, that is, with part of the rod in whiche bien signes inequals.
1275   Note and marke the profundite and depth of the vessels in their extremytes, next the bottums, and also in the myddis, next the mowth. And bien they marked in the rod after that bien thei reduced equaly to the half, th'excesse to cast out and to adde the defaute: that is, to take the meane signe bitwene the more and the lasse therof. Take the
1280   longitude of the vessel bi another part of the rod in whiche bien signes equals mesured. Than after this the signes of length bien they multiplied bi signes of depth, and that thyng sought shal be had.

Bi the same rod or yerd if the body of a quadrate vessell if thow wilt mesure, werke in the same maner as of a rounde vessel, that is for to
1285   say, the mesure of his depth or profundite bi the profundite or depth

---

1247. is] *om.*

of the rod or yerd and his longitude bi the longitude of the yerd. Also
multipl[i]e signes of longitudes bi signes of profundites and depthis
or evene turned. And this that cometh therof multiplie bi xiiij and the
product divide bi xj, and it shal shewe the nomber sought bi as often.

1290 And the reason of this maner is forwhy therfor the rod or yerd of gawgyng in maner as above made is made to mesure rounde vessels and cercles. But forwhi the quadrate without the cercle hath hymsilf as xiiij to
xj,[177] therfor the first founden ought to be multiplied bi xiiij and the
product to divide by xj, and it shal shewe.

1295 ## [The Staff of Jacob][178]

[fol. 237r] Iff thow wilt make the Staff of **Jacob**, take a iiij-square yerd[179]
to the length of j or ij elnes, lengger or shorter. Than take the voluel[180]
to the length of j or ij handful. And the longitude or length of that voluel thow shalt signe or marke in a yerd. As often as thow maist therof,

1300 make the same volubil[181] vp or down. And so if it pleasith, write in the
first signe and in the secunde and so of everiche.

And so than bi the saide staf if thow wilt mesure any altitude, set to
sum playne and sette the voluel vpon sum signe of the yerde after the
competent accompt of the distaunce, and nygh to the altitude or with-

1305 drawe from the altitude til th'extremitees of the thyng mesured appieren
precisely to the eye-sight bi both hoolis of the voluel equal with the voluel. Than sette the signe in the place of thi stacioun.[182] From that, nygh
thow to the þing or withdrawe, and the voluel bifore or bihynde sette,
and nygh eftsones or withdrawe til to thyn eye eftsoones hath appiered

1310 to the altitude of the voluel equal as to his both holis. And eftsoones set
the signe in the erth. Afterward biholde how many feete distaunt that
oo signe set in the erth from that other, and so many feete is the height
of the thing to be mesured.

In the same maner do thow of latitudes mesured, that is to say, as

1315 to termyne of latitudes. Thei shuln appiere equal with the voluels sette
at ij signes bi ij staciouns. And if thow wilt fynde the distaunce or the
breede bitwene the [oon] and that other,[183] than multiplie the space bitwene ij staciouns bi the nombre of the signe of the yerd that to the voluel was set, and the product shewith the purpos. Bi grace of exsample,

---

1289. shewe] *foll. by* soug *canc.*
1296. Jacob] *in display script*
1303. yerde] y *written over* r
1317. oon] *om. (see Explanatory Note)*

1320   as if ther bien xij feete bitwene ij staciouns and the voluel was sette in
the v signe of Jacobs Staf, therfor multiplie v bi xij and thow shalt have
lx, whiche shuln be the distaunces.[184]

[Some Uses of the Old Quadrant] [185]

    [1.] To knowe the latitude of a regioun (that is, þe distaunce of
1325   the cenyth of the equinoxial[186] or the height of the poole)[187] what it is
in al.
    Take the height of the sonne at mid- **[fol. 237v]** day whan it is in
the bigynnyng of Aries or in the bigynnynge of Libra and withdrawe
or abate that height of lxxxx degrees,[188] and that levith[189] wil be the lat-
1330   itude of that regioun.
    Yit maistow knowe it in another maner. Take the height of the sonne
in the mydday and of that height abate þe declynacioun of the sonne
of that day if the sonne be in the northen signes or adde it if it be in
southren signes. And this that levith after adde it to the subtraccioun
1335   in abatyng and than, withdraw it of lxxxx degrees,[190] and this that levith shal be the latitude.

    [2.] And yit thow myghtest knowe in another maner bi nyghtis tyme.
    Take the altitude of sum sterre fix notable from the poole[191] whan
she hath most height that it may have. And after, take the lest height
1340   that she may have in that same nyght and withdrawe the lasse height
from the more. And halfuendel the differaunce that thow wilt fynde
thow must adde to the more height,[192] and this that comyth therof shal
be the latitude of the regioun that thow seekist.

    [3.] And if thow wilt fynde the houres in al regiouns.
1345   Know the latitude as aforsaide—as at Parice is xlviij grees and
at Mountpilers nygh xliiij grees—and tel so many grees in the lymbe
of the quadraunt as that regioun hath of latitude. And bigynne to tel
toward the side of C (that is to wite, toward the side of ther the oilettis[193]
stonde). And than put the bigynnyng of Aries eft to the cursure of the
1350   gree wher the latitude shal want,[194] and that shal be the assise of the
cursour for that regioun.
    And whan thow hast the forsaide thynges in this maner, take the
height of the sonne at mydday and moeve nat the perpendicle from the
place where it wil fal. And after, moeve the cursure of the day so long

---

1329. of] *foll. by* with with

1355 that wherof thow takist the height at midday sonne [be] vndre the perpendicle, and that shal be the disposicioun and the perpetuel assise of
the cursour in that regioun.

And whan thow hast thus assised cursour and thow wilt knowe the
houres, put the perpendicle of the day wherof thow wilt knowe the houre
1360 and drawe the perle so long til it be over **[fol. 238r]** last lyne of the
houres (that is, the sixt). And after, do þe sonne beame goo[195] thurgh
the oiletes of the quadraunt and bihold the place of the perle among
the houres, for the place of the perle ther she wil be shal shewe the
houre that than is present.

1365   [4.] Iff thow wilt fynde the houres bi the quadraunt without cursour.
Take the degre of the taryeng in the oilettis of the quadraunt, and
bi that gree entre into the table of the declynacioun[196] and take the
declynacioun as the sonne, that is, agenst that gree. And abate it of[197]
the latitude of the regioun wher þou art if the sonne be in northern
1370 signes, and if the sonne be in southern signes than thow shalt adde
to the forsaide declynacioun. And kepe that thow shalt have after the
forsaide addissioun or subtraccioun, and tel hem so many grees in þe
lymbe of the quadraunt towarde the corner C,[198] and put the perpendicle ther the nombre wantith. And than renne the perle to the cir-
1375 cumferencial lyne of midday, and that shal be the assise of the perle in
that regioun wher thow art atte þat day. And than do the sonne beame
passe thurgh both oilettis of the quadraunt and waite wher the perle
wil be among the houres, for that shal be the houre that thow seekist.

       [5.] Now herafter we wil speke of mesures and heightes of dyuers
1380 thynges wher we may come nygh.[199]
Bihold þe height of any thyng thurgh the ij oilettis of the quadraunt
with thyn oon eye and go toward the thyng and froward til the perpendicle fall vpon the lyne of xlv degrees, that is to say, in middes of
the quadraunt. Than [take] the height of thyn eye from the erth and
1385 gadre therto[200] as moche as is bitwene thyn eye and the erth, and marke
wel þe place. And how many feete bien bitwene that forsaide place and
the bace of that thyng that thow wilt mesure, and so many feete is the
height.

1355. be] *om.*
1384. take] *om.*   QV accipe

[On the Art of Gauging 2]

1390 [**fol. 238v**] Forsoth, to the maner of makyng the rodde or yerd be made
with whiche he wil gauge, owith to vse thoo thynges in this maner
as with the depth of the rodde—that is, with the parte of þe rodde in
whiche bien signes inequal noted. And knowe þe depth of the vessel in
extremytes next the bottums and also in the myddis next the mowth,[201]
1395 and is signed and marked in þe yerd. After that, bien thei reduced to
the half evenly, th'excesse to outcast and the defaute to adde—that is,
to take the myddil signe bitwene the more depth and the lasse therof.
Take þe length of the vessel bi another part of the yerd, in whiche bien
equal signes mesured. Than after, thiese signes of length bien thei mul-
1400 tiplied bi the signes of depth, and he shal have the thyng sought.

Bi the same yerd if the body of the vessel be quadrate, mesure wil
thow to werke in the same maner as thow canst of a rounde vessel—that
is to say, the deepe mesure of it by the depth of the yerd and the length
of it bi the length of the yerd. Also multiplie the signes of the length
1405 bi þe signes of the depth or in contrary wise. And that comeþ therof
mu[l]tiplie bi xiiij, and the product or broughtfurþ divide by xj;[202] and
he shal shewe bi the nombre as often sought.

And of this maner of reason is forwhi vessel roddis, or of gawgyng
yerdis, to what maner it is made to mesure boþ rounde vessels and in
1410 compas. But forwhi the quadrate or iiij-square without compas bihavith
hymsilf as is xiiij to xj, therfor to the first invencioun owght to be multiplied bi xiiij, and the product therof divide by x[j], and it shal shewe.

1405. wise] *foll. by* E *(?), canc.*
1412. xj] x

Explanatory Notes

[1] **The Solid Sphere:** In these notes, comparisons with the Latin original of the treatise on making a celestial sphere are based on a copy in the early fourteenth-century manuscript, Oxford, Bodleian Library, Selden Supra MS 78 (S). The title is supplied from the Latin, *De spera solida*.

[2] **Quod Multon. 1458:** See Pahta, chap. 1, 3–4, 16 above, and Mooney, chap. 3, 55, 59–60 above. Here and in lines 150–151, 240, and 366, the Multon attributions are in display script, represented by bold text in this edition.

[3] **angle of the yrþ:** Opposite of the mid-sky point above the earth (S: *in angulo terre*).

[4] **bi the centre bi the pointes:** *From* the center *through* the points (S: *a centro per puncta*).

[5] **make . . . mynute holes:** Make small holes (S: *foramina minuta*).

[6] **additamentis:** Attachments, as support-pieces (S: *addamentis*).

[7] **apt:** Apply, put in place (S: *aptabis*).

[8] **piche:** Press into (S: *impinges*).

[9] **in the equatour assigned:** Represented (S: *figurata*) in the equator.

[10] **assigned point:** S: *punctum signatum*.

[11] **from B toward A . . . circule of Capricorn:** The English treatise omits the name of the circle at 23° 33' North (the Tropic of Cancer) and then omits the instruction for inscribing the circle or Tropic of Capricorn at 23° 33' South, between B and C, which follows at this point in S, probably because of some kind of eyeskip by a scribe at some point in the textual tradition.

[12] **M^{l}xxij sterris:** Ptolemy's catalogue of 1022 stars in his *Almagest* remained standard at least until Ulūgh Beg's fifteenth-century catalogue.

[13] **vj siluer wires:** Silver wires of differing thicknesses represent the six magnitudes of stars in Ptolemy's catalogue.

[14] **the myddel circule:** The Milky Way (S: *circulum lacteum*).

[15] **of the iiij altitude:** The altitude quadrant (S: *quarte altitudinis*), a movable quarter-ring attached to the horizon-pole for measuring distance from the horizon or attached to the ecliptic pole for measuring distance from the ecliptic (= *quadraunt of the altitude*, S: *quartam altitudinis*, in line 268).

[16] **havyng a litel foote as a masor is wont to have:** Having a base as does a drinking vessel (S: *& sit sub ipso sedimen sicut in ciphis de murra*). A *ciphus de murra* is a mazer, a large drinking bowl.

[17] **And let be made . . . falle and rest:** The sense of the Latin original is, "Let there be outside the mouth of the vessel another rim (*limbus*) on which the cover of the whole instrument falls and rests" (*super quod cadat & requiescat coopercullum instrumenti tocius*). A list of instruments belonging to Merton College,

Oxford, in 1410, printed in North 1976, 3:132–33, includes a solid sphere with container (*speram solidam cum capsulam*).

[18] **enhaunce:** Erect (S: *eriges*).

[19] **arcanlier:** Apparently a ruler or straight-edge (S: *regulam*).

[20] **bi and bi:** One at a time (S: *singulos*).

[21] **as it shewith in the figure:** No figure or space for one is in the manuscript, although S provides a figure at the corresponding point.

[22] **Afterwarde of A:** Afterward *from* A (S: *ex .a.*).

[23] In the notes on *The New Quadrant 1* (NQ1), comparisons are suggested with its Latin source, the *Compositio et operatio astrolabii*, designated M. Comparisons are also suggested with an English treatise that also uses M as a source, the *Treatise on the Astrolabe* by Geoffrey Chaucer, designated Ch. These designations are followed in the Explanatory Notes by the part and chapter numbers of the treatise so designated (e.g., M 2.1, Ch 2.1).

Correspondences between these texts are summarized in the following table:

NQ1, Prologue: I have found no direct source for this prologue.

NQ1.1: Cf. M 2.1; Ch 2.1.	**NQ1.17:** Cf. M 2.18, 19; Ch 2.31, 29, 38.
NQ1.2: Cf. M 2.2; Ch 2.2.	**NQ1.18:** Cf. M 2.20; Ch 2.20.
NQ1.3: Cf. M 2.3; Ch 2.3.	**NQ1.19:** Cf. M 2.21; Ch 2.25; also QV 41–42.
NQ1.4: Cf. M 2.4; Ch 2.6.	**NQ1.20:** Cf. M 2.22; Ch 2.24.
NQ1.5: Cf. M 2.5; Ch 2.7.	**NQ1.21:** Cf. M 2.28; Ch 2.27.
NQ1.6: Cf. M 2.6; Ch 2.10.	**NQ1.22:** Cf. M 2.29; Ch 2.28.
NQ1.7: Not in M.	**NQ1.23:** Cf. M 2.30.
NQ1.8: Cf. M 2.8.	**NQ1.24:** Cf. M 2.31; Ch 2.17.
NQ1.9: Cf. M 2.8.	**NQ1.25:** Cf. M 2.32; Ch 2.34.
NQ1.10: Cf. M 2.9; Ch 2.8.	**NQ1.26:** Cf. M 2.34; Ch 2.17.
NQ1.11: Cf. M 2.10.	**NQ1.27:** Cf. M 2.35; Ch 2.30.
NQ1.12: Cf. M 2.13; Ch 2.16.	**NQ1.28:** Cf. M 2.36; Ch 2.35.
NQ1.13: Cf. M 2.14; Ch 2.14.	**NQ1.29:** Cf. M 2.37; Ch 2.36.
NQ1.14: Cf. M 2.16; Ch 2.18.	**NQ1.30:** Cf. M 2.39.
NQ1.15: Cf. M 2.16.	**NQ1.31:** Cf. M 2.41.
NQ1.16: Cf. M 2.17; Ch 2.33.	**NQ1.32:** Cf. M 2.42.

[24] *corda recta* **and** *corda versa***:** Graduations along one side of the quadrant's face for sine and versine trigonometric functions, sometimes called "sinus rectus" and "sinus versa," as in Q1: "divisiones chordarum vel sinuum versorum et rectum" (F. S. Pedersen 1984, 600).

[25] **into cij:** An error for *into cxx,* 'up to 120.' Cf. Q1: "unus procedit ab uno ad 60 . . . et alius . . . ad 120" (F. S. Pedersen 1984, 600). There appears to be some

kind of confusion or conflation of Arabic positional notation for numbers with the letters used for Roman numerals; similar errors occur on fol. 225v (see line 617 and nn. below).

[26] **parilels:** The parallel circles are those of Cancer, the equinoctial, and Capricorn. The ecliptic is not parallel to the others.

[27] **.a.ˡⁱ :** The meaning of this abbreviation is unclear. Perhaps it represents *alibi*; the general sense of the passage would then be "to know by the quadrant as, otherwise, by the astrolabe, and by number."

[28] **Over the quadraunt:** Around the limb (rim) of the curved side of the instrument.

[29] **replied iiij sithes:** The numbered quarter-circle must be repeated four times to represent the full circle of the equinoctial for measuring right ascension.

[30] **Alnot:** Although this word is similar to the astronomical name 'Alnath' (*MED*, s.v. *Alnath*, and *FrankT* 1280n, 1285n [Benson 1987]: 'a star in Aries; the first mansion of the moon'), the word must pertain specifically to the equinoctial, in particular as it is inscribed on a quadrant. Although Thorndike and Kibre list some texts whose incipits start with "Alnach/Alnath" (TK 84), none of them appears to be a likely source for the information discussed here.

[31] **that other side:** What has just been described is the front side or *face* (*facies*) of the quadrant. Now follows a description of the back side or *dorsum*.

[32] **voluel:** Circular calendrical scales for finding the place of the sun or moon at given dates.

[33] **reete:** This is a badly chosen term for the present context. *Rete* normally refers to a rotatable star-map on the face of an astrolabe, showing the ecliptic, the signs of the zodiac, and certain fixed stars. Traces of these features survive on the *quadrans novus*, engraved directly on the quadrant's face. What is here referred to however, on the back side of the quadrant, is a set of graduated circles that evolved from the zodiacal calendar on the back side of the astrolabe. These are the outer circle, of months and days, and within it the zodiacal circle of signs and degrees. Within these, according to Profatius, are other circles, including one locating the astrological "mansions of the moon"; but instead of describing these latter, inner circles, NQ1 begins to describe the rete of an astrolabe with its fixed stars.

[34] **label:** The pointer, a swivelling ruler used for indicating which lunar mansion the moon is in. See the preceding Explanatory Note.

[35] **reete:** The author now reverts to description of the face of an astrolabe.

[36] **almuries . . . azimutis:** *Almury*, meaning literally "pointer, indicator," is apparently misused here. The "circles of height" are properly called *almucantars*, and the *azimuths* are circles of direction (compass bearings). Almucantars and azimuths are features on an astrolabe that could not be usefully transferred to a quadrant.

[37] **thy day:** The present day (M: *diem presentis*).

[38] **touches oute with:** Points to (M: *ostendit*).

[39] **to:** Until (M: *donec*).

[40] **threede of the perpendicle:** Whereas the astrolabe performs this function with a rule (M: *regula*), the quadrant employs a plumb-line, called in Latin a *perpendiculum*, as in *Artis cuiuslibet consummatio* 2.37, where "a perpendiculo" means "by the plumb-line."

[41] **ascendaunt . . . angles:** The ascendant is the astrologically significant portion of sky on the eastern horizon. Together with the portions on the western horizon, at mid-sky above the earth (at the "lyne meridian") and at mid-sky beneath the earth (the nadir or opposite of the line meridional), it is one of the "principal angles" for horoscopes. On astrological significance, see Chaucer, *Astrolabe* 2.4, "A special declaracioun of the ascendent."

[42] **xviij grees:** The limit of the crepuscular periods is achieved when the sun is 18° below the horizon rising or setting, though some authorities say 20° or some other number.

[43] **almuries:** Mistake for *almucantars* (M: *almucantharat*).

[44] **that is not writen but to the dawyng:** Altitudes are not measured below the crepuscular line, which is inscribed below the horizon line (the lowest almucantar) to mark, on the eastern side, the beginning of morning twilight, which Chaucer calls "the sprynge of the dawenyng" (*Astrolabe* 2.6).

[45] **orizont occidental:** The first almucantar (M: *primum almucantharat*) on an astrolabe.

[46] **voluel:** Not the volvel (calendrical scale) mentioned in the prologue to NQ1. *Volvel* is used here to refer to an astrolabe's rete. It is sometimes so used elsewhere, as well; e.g., in the labelled figure of a rete in Oxford, Bodleian Library, Selden Supra MS 78, fol. 57r.

[47] **quantite:** The number of degrees (M: *numerum graduum*) of rotation corresponding to an unequal hour.

[48] **subtract it of xxx . . . houre inequale of the nyght:** Unequal hours vary in duration according to season (with daylight hours longer in summer and shorter in winter), but at all seasons one unequal hour of the day plus one of the night yields a total corresponding to 30° rotation of the equinoctial (Laird 1997, 55–56).

[49] **almury:** The account here is not of a quadrant's almury (sliding bead on the plumb-line) but of an astrolabe's almury (pointer on the rim of the rete).

[50] **Bi this maner . . . astrolaby:** Not in M.

[51] **almury:** Again, the pointer on an astrolabe's rete.

[52] *in lymbo:* On the limb (rim or outer border, Lat. *limbus*) of the circular face of the astrolabe.

[53] **almuries:** Mistake for *almucantars.*

[54] **length:** ecliptic longitude (M: *graduum . . . longitudinis*).

[55] **reete:** *Rete* cannot be correct. M has "filium," but his procedure too is faulty.

[56] **azimutis:** Azimuths, circles on an astrolabe that indicate compass-bearings (M: *cenith*).

[57] **almuries:** Mistake for *almucantars* (M: *almucantharat*).

[58] **azimutis:** See above NQ1.16 and Explanatory Note 56.

[59] **Wite also . . . Capricorn:** The greatest declination northward is the head (beginning) of Cancer, the greatest southward that of Capricorn.

[60] **breede:** Latitude.

[61] **reryng:** Altitude.

[62] **fallith:** Sets. Stars near the poles (circumpolar stars) do not appear to set but are seen to circle the poles.

[63] *semidiatrum orientis*: Presumably the east horizon-line on an astrolabe. M (and Chaucer following him) says to place the beginning of the sign over the meridional line, but in any case, NQ1 has omitted several steps from the procedure.

[64] **almury:** The pointer on an astrolabe's rete, but again as in NQ1.21, several steps have been omitted, so that what remains is incoherent.

[65] **almuries:** Mistake for *almucantars* (M: *almucantharat*).

[66] **more:** Larger (M: *maior*).

[67] **pynnels:** Pinnules, vanes or small plates pierced with pin-holes to serve as sights on an astrolabe's sighting-rule or a quadrant's sighting-edge.

[68] **in the directis of:** In line with (M: *directo*).

[69] **almuries:** Mistake for *almucantars.*

[70] **almuries:** Almucantars.

[71] **almuries:** Almucantars.

[72] **better:** M has already given, in M 2.32, one way of locating planets. Now he offers another and better way (*in alio modo . . . et verius*).

[73] **bi the almury** *in lymbo*: This is the almury (pointer) on an astrolabe, not the almury (bead) on a quadrant. It points to a degree in the limb (border) of the astrolabe's face.

[74] **breede:** Angular distance.

[75] **wey of the sonne:** The sun's apparent diurnal path.

[76] **evenyng of the houses xij:** The equal dividing ("evenyng") of the sky into astrologically significant segments ("houses"); usually termed *equation of houses* (M: *equatione 12 domorum*; Ch: *equaciounes of houses*).

[77] **þe viij houre of the lyne:** The eighth hour-line (M: *super lineam 8*).

[78] **aspeccioun:** Establishing the astrologically significant *aspects* (degrees of separation) between planets. The important aspects are *sextile* (60°), *quartile* (90°), *trine* (120°), *opposition* (180°), and *conjunction* (0°).

[79] **if cij, iij:** Context makes it clear that this compact expression should mean "If 120°, [the aspect is] trine." However, the manuscript here actually reads "if M^l iij." Based on the earlier erroneous reading of *cij* for 120 (see Explanatory Note 25 above), the immediately-following mistake of *cviij* for 180, and the similarity of a capital M to a hastily written *cij* with lower-case *c*, it seems possible that the scribe's exemplar actually read (albeit erroneously) *cij*.

[80] **cviij:** An error for 180°. See Explanatory Note 25 above.

[81] **applied . . . departed:** These words refer to technical astrological concepts called *applicatio* and *separatio*. See Lemay 1962, App. III.

[82] **worldly or naturally:** Reference is to the astrological "year of the world" or "natural year" (M: *anni mundani vel naturalis*).

[83] **almury:** The almury or pointer on an astrolabe.

[84] **lxxxvij:** Various manuscripts of M give figures varying between 87 and 93.

[85] **yisen:** I.e., passed (M: *preteritum*; cf. *MED*, s.v. *isen* v(1), in an extended sense of "experienced, seen as they went by").

[86] **almury:** The almury on an astrolabe.

[87] **yesen:** I.c., passed (M: *exientium*).

[88] **(wont to be . . . þat is):** The sense of this somewhat awkward parenthetical comment is "When I say 'quadrant,' I don't mean the instrument of that name but rather that part of an astrolabe that can also be called a 'quadrant.'"

[89] **I wil sey nothyng thereof:** The matters here postponed (until NQ2.13–17) are the ones treated in the succeeding chapters of M (2.42–47). The "quadraunt" referred to in this paragraph is not the instrument that is the subject of the treatise but the "shadow square" that is inscribed on both astrolabes and instrument-quadrants. See NQ2.10 and notes below.

[90] Being based on quadrant-treatises rather than an astrolabe-treatise, NQ2 contains fewer confusions in terminology than does NQ1. *Almury*, for example, consistently refers to the bead on the plumb-line, and there are no references to the *rete* or *almucantars* or *azimuths*, which are features of the astrolabe. In these notes, Prof is cited by chapter number and Q1, Q2, and QV by paragraph number.

Correspondences between these texts are summarized in the following table:

NQ2.1: Cf. Prof 3, Q1.47, Q2.45.   **NQ2.5b:** Cf. Prof 9, Q1.50, Q2.48.

NQ2.2: Cf. Prof 4, Q1.47, Q2.45.   **NQ2.6:** Cf. Prof 10, Q1.52, Q2.50.

NQ2.3: Cf. Prof 6.   **NQ2.7:** Cf. Prof 11.

NQ2.4: Cf. Prof 7, Q1.48.   **NQ2.8:** Cf. Prof 12.

NQ2.5a: Cf. Prof 8, Q1.49, Q2.47.   **NQ2.9:** Cf. Prof 14, Q1.61, Q2.59.

NQ2.10: Cf. Prof 15, Q1.63, Q2.61.

NQ2.11: Cf. Prof 16, Q1.66, Q2.63.

NQ2.12: Cf. Prof 16, Q1.67, Q2.64.

NQ2.13: Cf. Prof 18, Q1.68, Q2.66, QV49.

NQ2.14: Cf. Prof 19, Q1.76, Q2.71.

NQ2.15: Cf. Prof 2, Q1.87, Q2.73.

NQ2.16

NQ2.17: Cf. QV.1.

NQ2.18: Cf. QV.3–7.

[91] **thridde:** Thread, i.e., the plumb-line.

[92] **meridian height:** The sun's meridional altitude.

[93] **sight:** Site.

[94] **viij chapitre of the astrolabie tofore writen:** Reference is to NQ1.8.

[95] **riet orizont:** Right horizon; i.e., the horizon of an equatorial observer.

[96] **cald Capricorn:** Evidently a mistake, and not grounded in sources.

[97] NQ2.5a, 5b, and 6 are not numbered in the manuscript, which resumes numbering with NQ2.7.

[98] **the right, that is to say, *in circulo directo*:** The celestial equator, called the equinoctial circle or the right circle.

[99] **that table:** Prof refers to the "Toledan tables" (*tabulis toletanes*) derived from Azarquiel (ca. 1029–1087). By the fifteenth century these had been superseded by the Alfonsine tables.

[100] **cercle oblique:** Oblique circle or oblique horizon (Prof: *orizonte obliquo*; Q1: *circulo obliquo*), i.e., the horizon of an observer not on the equator.

[101] **reetis orizont:** Right horizon (Q1 and Q2: *horizontis rectis*); see also Explanatory Note 103 below.

[102] **ascendaunt . . . oþer xij houses:** Strictly, the ascendant, on the eastern horizon, is itself one of the twelve astrological "houses." It is the first, and the others are numbered counter-clockwise to a total of twelve.

[103] **reetis spiere:** Right sphere (Prof: *spera recta*), the celestial sphere as seen by an equatorial observer, for whom the north and south celestial poles lie on the horizon (the "right horizon") and all stars rise at right angles to that horizon.

[104] **myddel of the centre:** Mid-sky (Prof: *gradum medij celi*).

[105] **mydlith:** Transits, crosses the line of mid-sky.

[106] **risyng and fallyng:** Rising and setting. NQ2 omits Profatius's discussion of circumpolar stars (which do not rise and set).

[107] **iiij chapitre therof:** Fourth chapter of the present work (NQ2.4). Instead of cross-referencing, Prof repeats the instructions in brief.

[108] **Seeche the houres:** NQ2 omits Profatius's detailed instructions on how to do so.

[109] NQ2 has garbled Profatius's instructions by omission. Between "founden" and "from" should be some such words as "and if the star be west of the meridian, subtract the degrees and minutes . . . " (Prof: *et si stella sit versus occidentem substrahe gradus et minuta*).

[110] **vnto that grees:** To the degrees of that star (Q1, Q2: *ipsius stellae gradibus*).

[111] **spiere oblonge:** Oblique sphere, i.e., oblique horizon (Q2: *in horizonte obliquo*).

[112] **ark . . . corde:** Discussing the conversion of arcs to chords and the reverse, Prof prefers the term *sinus* for "chord," whereas Q1 and Q2 prefer *chorda*.

[113] This chapter employs the "shadow square" or "shadow scales," consisting of a square of which two adjacent sides, called "umbra recta" and "umbra versa," are graduated into twelve parts or "digits" each. Angular altitudes of objects are taken by sighting; and the shadow scales, by use of tangents and cotangents, allow heights and distances to be calculated. The shadow square was a feature of the old quadrant borrowed for use on the astrolabe and (hence) on the new quadrant. Cf. QV.30 and M1.3.

[114] *vmbram rectam & versam:* The numbers (*digitos*) on the scale of *umbra recta* or *versa*.

[115] **bi the height:** By the sun's altitude (Prof: *per solis altitudinem*).

[116] **first almury:** The first of two beads now assumed to be on the plumb-line.

[117] **nombre quociens:** The outcome of dividing (Prof: *egrediens*); the quotient (Q1, Q2: *numerus quotiens*).

[118] **signes:** Number of digits (Prof, Q1, Q2: *digitos*).

[119] **thow may do this lightlier:** From here to the end of the chapter, NQ2 ceases to correspond to Prof but follows Q1 and Q2 closely (Q2: *Facilius tamen hoc scire poteris,* etc.).

[120] **divide the corde verse:** NQ2 says here to divide the number of digits in corde verse by 144, whereas the corresponding Latin texts say to divide 144 by the number of digits (Q1: *divide 144 per numerum digitorum umbrae versae*).

[121] **cercle cenyth:** This is a semicircle constructed on one straight side of the quadrant, opposite the semicircle that is the sixth hour-line (Prof: *cercle cenit*). Q1 and Q2 call it "circulum zenith vel circulum oppositi."

[122] **Over that, thus thow shalt know:** You shall also know by the method sketched in the preceding chapter. NQ2 is here translating Prof (*sic etiam scies*), but cf. Q1 and Q2: *Hoc autem modo poteris etiam scies . . . .* Throughout the chapter Prof specifies the sightings and manipulations of plumb-line and almury that yield numbers for use in calculation. NQ2 omits these and deals only with the calculations, perhaps because the method has already been sketched. As a result, NQ2.12 is scarcely intelligible.

[123] **as it is set before:** As has already been explained (in NQ2.8).

[124] **NQ2.13–17:** These are the chapters that were promised at the end of NQ1. They concern terrestrial measurements (Q1: *De mensuratione rerum inferiarum*) and preserve a tradition shared by treatises on practical geometry and on geometrical instruments such as the astrolabe and the quadrants.

[125] The operation is illustrated in a good drawing that accompanies the corresponding section of QV in a fourteenth-century English manuscript, reproduced in Murdoch 1984, 168. For related instructions on practical geometric

calculations, see the treatise on the seven liberal arts edited by Mooney, chap. 15 below, lines 371–562.

[126] ***scala recta . . . distauns to the height:*** This ratio, for *scala recta*, should be of height to distance, the reverse of the ratio for *scala versa* (Prof: *argumentum erit econverso*).

[127] **thurgh grace of ensample:** This phrase would appear to be a translation of *exempli gratia,* but no such phrase (and no worked example) appears in Prof, Q1, or Q2.

[128] NQ2.15 corresponds to the last chapter of Prof, as the title of the corresponding chapter of Q2 acknowledges ("capitulum ultimam novi quadrantis Prefatii Iudaei"), although Q2 continues with nine more chapters.

[129] The editors of Prof print, from a single manuscript, a tractate called "compositio istius quadrante." It is brief, though longer than NQ2.16, and is about inscribing a quadrant rather than construction. Q1 and Q2 begin with instructions for making a quadrant, but they are much more elaborate than those in the present chapter.

[130] **Of geometrie ij parties bien:** A standard beginning for treatises on practical geometry, incorporated into the first chapter of QV.

[131] **theoric and practik:** In their basic senses, going back to Aristotle and Boethius, *theorica* signified cognitive knowledge and *practica* signified moral action. But in the Middle Ages a habit developed of identifying practical (meaning "applied") aspects of all arts and sciences, even theoretical ones such as astronomy and geometry. Hugh of St. Victor, in his *Practica geometria,* first so divided geometry and was followed by others. A key factor in the division is that the practical employs instruments, whereas the theoretical is "only mind works," as Robert Recorde says at the beginning of his *Pathway to Knowledge* (London, 1551).

[132] **altimetric, pleynmetric, and steriometric:** The terminology is standard, although instead of *stereometric* some writers use *cosmimetric* or, occasionally, *crassimetric.* The liberal arts treatise edited by Mooney below refers to "Altimetrie, Planymetrie, and Profundymetrie" (chap. 15, lines 372–373).

[133] **take and founde to:** Shaped in the form of, reduced to (QV.4: *reducatur ad*).

[134] **streight corner:** Right angle (QV.4: *angulum . . . rectum*).

[135] **subtil draught:** Fine line (QV.5: *linea subtili*).

[136] **bisides A:** beside A (QV.5: *iuxta A*).

[137] **of the whiche partie:** From which point (QV.5: *a quo puncto*).

[138] **bisides the half:** Near the side (QV.5: *iuxta latere*).

[139] **xviij spaces:** The manuscript reads "viij spaces," but see the preceding sentence: $2 \times 3 \times 3 = 18.$

[140] **the neither partie *in lymbo*:** In the lower (nether) part, in the border (limb), i.e., near the rim of the curved side of the quadrant.

[141] **in þe zodiac of eche cercle:** This is an ill-advised interpolation (not in QV), commenting that like the curve of the limb, the curves representing segments of the zodiac also contain 90°.

[142] **to that:** Until the.

[143] The designation M in the following notes again refers to Pseudo-Messahalla, as cited above. The present fragment is taken from M1 (the part on "composition" or construction of astrolabes), chap. 13.

[144] **allilakas:** The point, at the top of the astrolabe, where the suspending ring (Arabic, *halka*) is attached. Here (M1.13) the Latin reads "allidadath," but in M1.12 the same point is called "alilacat."

[145] **vpon S:** M reads "super h," but the English text is correct and agrees with the attendant diagram in the manuscript of M.

[146] **cenyth:** Zenith (M: *cenith capitum*).

[147] **and in the azmutis also:** Not in M, which ends, "and inscribe the numbers over each almucanthar, as you see in the figure." In the English manuscript a space has been left blank but no figure has been supplied. In the Latin manuscript there is a figure but the numbers have not been added.

[148] For the text of these chapters as established in the context of Chaucer's whole *Treatise on the Astrolabe*, see the edition in *The Riverside Chaucer* (Benson 1987).

[149] **thy lyne meridional:** This phrase does not appear in the modern editions of Chaucer.

[150] **on hir mole:** Several manuscripts of Chaucer's *Astrolabe* 2.38 here use the phrase *an heer mele* (meaning, apparently, "a hair's breadth") and one reads "one heer brede."

[151] In these tables the meridional (midday) altitudes of the sun are 62° at the summer solstice, 38° at the equinoxes, and 14° at the winter solstice. These figures imply that the tables are made for a location approximately 52° north latitude, the approximate figure usually given for Oxford, as in Chaucer's *Astrolabe* 2.23.

[152] **To the height . . . solsticial of wynter:** The first line gives the times before midday (9 A.M., 10 A.M., etc.), the second gives times after midday, and the third gives the sun's altitude above the horizon, in degrees, for each of those hours.

[153] **The heightis . . . in the equinoccial:** Again, the first two lines give the hours A.M. and P.M., and the third gives the sun's altitude in degrees. The degrees for 8 A.M. and 4 P.M. are missing in the manuscript and have been supplied from Nicholas of Lynn's fourteenth-century *Kalendarium* (ed. Eisner 1980, 80). Nicholas gives 18°13', which I have rounded off to 18°, in keeping with the tables' use of whole degrees.

[154] **To the height . . . of the quadraunt:** This table is puzzling. The "houres of the quadraunt" are presumably the "unequal hours" employed by quadrant instruments, and if these are designated in the first line, then the first five numbers in

the second line look like solar altitudes at unequal hours of the summer solstice (when one equal hour = one hour and 20 minutes in unequal hours). The
last four numbers, however, simply repeat solar altitudes at equal hours at the
winter solstice.

[155] **margarit or perle:** The almury (sliding bead) on the quadrant's plumb-line.

[156] **houres equal:** The procedure here described produces lines used in reckoning equal hours (hours in the modern sense) in relation to *un*equal hours
(obtained by dividing periods of daylight and darkness each into 12 equal
parts). Equal hours (obtained by dividing the whole period of one diurnal rev-
olution into 24 equal parts) would be reckoned from curved lines intersecting
the lines of unequal hours at the equinoctial circle (indicating that when the
sun is at the equinoxes, equal and unequal hours are the same). Poulle notes
that neither extant medieval new quadrants nor medieval treatises thereon include lines of equal hours (1964, 154). They are, however, present on some Islamic astrolabes, as described by Hartner 1968, 297–99. They are also present
on some horary quadrants, described by Poulle 1981, 40.

[157] **werke in þis maner:** The first step results in drawing quarter-circles for
Cancer, the equinoctial, and Capricorn—the figures 62°, 38°, and 15° repre-
senting the sun's meridional altitudes in those three places for an observer in
Oxford (52° north latitude: see *Tables of Solar Heights*, above).

[158] **lyne meridional:** The scale of meridional declination marked on the side
of the quadrant opposite the sighting vanes.

[159] **oilet:** Possibly a form of *oilet* 'eyelet'; in any case, obviously a device for drawing an arc, mentioned as an alternative to compasses.

[160] **lyne A:** Lines A, B, and C are segments of circles. See below, "lyne or cercle of A."

[161] **foote of houres:** One end of each hour-line is the apex of the quadrant; the
other is "foot" of the hour, also so called ("pes dicitur horarum") by Ascelin of
Augsburg, *Compositio astrolabii* (ed. Burnett 1998, 348).

[162] **signes:** Set a mark. *Signes* is an imperative verb in a form common in northern dialects. Cf. Latin *signa* ("set a mark") and Old French *signez de point*
("mark with a dot").

[163] At Oxford, the day at summer solstice was reckoned to be 16½ (equal) hours
long.

[164] **ladder:** Apparently the shadow square or shadow scale (*scala*, "ladder").
Chaucer, *Astrolabe* 2.12, uses both terms, "skale" and "laddres."

[165] Comparisons with the Latin source *De arte visoria* (Vis.) are, unless otherwise noted, based on the early (mid-fifteenth-century) copy in Munich, Bayerische Staatsbibliothek, Clm 11067, fols. 207rb–208ra.

[166] **cofre:** A cylindrical container (Vis.: *capsulam figure columpnare*) used as a
standard measure of volume.

[167] **oilet:** A small hole (eyelet). A wood-cut from an early printed book (1485), reproduced in Folkerts (1974, 22), shows a gauging rod with holes punched in it to mark the graduations.

[168] **vntouched:** Undivided (Vis.: *intacta*).

[169] **ascendyng bi doublyng:** Rather, increasing by twos (Vis.: *ascendendo per dualitatem*).

[170] **without in tables:** These measures are to be marked outside the rod (*extra virgam*) on a table or board (*in mensa uel assere*).

[171] The main divisions, each called a "signe" (Vis.: *signatura*), are being subdivided into unequal parts. The order of subdivision here given omits some "signes," as does Vis., though not the same ones. Another, later copy of the Latin (Munich, Bayerische Staatsbibliothek, Clm 27001, fol. 167r) fills the omission. It is clear that in the English text "iiij with iiij" means 4¼ (*quattuor et quartam vnius*) and "without the half" means "even" (*precise*).

[172] Using the same container ("cofre"), which is the standard of measure for the region for which the rod is being marked ("in al londis," i.e., in each region; Vis.: *terre in qua velit virgam visoriam conficere*), pour in a measure of water and mark, with a stick or straw, how far it rises.

[173] **of hap or fortune . . . pleasure:** Vis. simply suggests that perhaps the first unit will be measured off with compass (*a fortuna signabit cum circino*) by large units or small, as one pleases (*ad placitum*).

[174] **aforsaide:** I.e., the previously-mentioned method of increasing by twos (Vis. repeats the formula: *ascendendo per dualitatem*).

[175] **this maner:** The English text abridges the Latin account of this manner by more than half, leaving it not quite understandable.

[176] **Forsoth . . . ought to vse:** Vis. treats the material from here on as a separate section, giving it the heading, "De usu seu practica virge." Again, the English treatise's abridgment is severe, becoming progressively more so until finally it breaks off before the end of its source.

[177] **But forwhi . . . as xiiij to xj:** The proportion of 14/11 was employed at least as early as Archimedes to approximate the ratio of the area of a square to the area of a circle inscribed within it, without having to employ calculations involving π. Q1, in a section (86) preparatory to calculating volumes, gives the same ratio.

[178] Comparisons of this treatise with its source, *De baculo geometrico* (Bac.), refer to the copy in Munich, Bayerische Staatsbibliothek, Clm 11067, fol. 207rb.

[179] **iiij-square yerd:** A square rod (Bac.: *baculum . . . quadratum*).

[180] **voluel:** The wooden cross-piece on the rod (Bac.: *accipe paruum lignum . . . et erit volvella*).

[181] **make the same volubil:** The voluel is to be an integral fraction of the rod.

[182] **sette the signe . . . stacioun:** Mark on the ground the spot where the first sighting was taken (Bac.: *tunc signatur stacio prima*).

[183] **bitwene the oon and that other:** Between the two places where sightings were taken (Bac.: *inter duas staciones*).

[184] **distaunces:** In stopping at this point, the English treatise omits its source's treatment of longitude of a field.

[185] Comparisons of *Some Uses of the Old Quadrant* (OQ) with its source, the *Quadrans vetus* (QV), refer to the modern edition of the latter in N. L. Hahn 1982, 6–113. OQ corresponds to QV 41–49 and is in the same order.

[186] **of the cenyth of the equinoxial:** Of the zenith *from* the equinoctial (QV: *ab equinoctiali*).

[187] **or the height of the poole:** The angular distance from the zenith to the equinoctial is equal to the height (angular elevation) of the pole.

[188] **withdrawe . . . of lxxxx degrees:** Subtract from 90°.

[189] **that levith:** What remains, the remainder.

[190] **And this that levith . . . withdraw it of lxxxx degrees:** Subtract from 90° what remains after the addition or subtraction.

[191] **from the poole:** Near the pole (QV: *iuxta polum*); i.e., take a circumpolar star—one that does not set but rather is seen to circle the pole.

[192] **more height:** This should be "lasse height" (QV: *altitudini minori*).

[193] **oilettis:** The pinnules or pierced sighting vanes (QV: *tabule perforata*) fixed to one of the straight sides of the quadrant.

[194] **put the bigynnyng . . . shal want:** Move the cursor until the first degree of Aries is aligned with the degree in the limb corresponding to the observer's latitude.

[195] **do þe sonne beame goo:** Let the sun's ray pass (QV: *demitte radium Solis transire*).

[196] **table of the declynacioun:** A table showing the sun's declination from the equinoctial at every degree of the zodiac. According to N. L. Hahn 1982, xlvii, such tables frequently follow QV in the manuscripts.

[197] **abate it of:** Subtract it from (QV: *eam substrahe de*).

[198] **corner C:** On the side of the quadrant where the sighting vanes are (QV: *a latere quadrantis super quod infixe sunt tabule perforate*).

[199] **wher we may come nygh:** I.e., on the same plane as the observer.

[200] **gadre therto:** Add to the distance, i.e., back up a distance equal to that between the eye and the ground.

[201] **mowth:** Orifice in the bilge of a barrel.

[202] **multiplie bi xiiij . . . divide by xj:** See Explanatory Note 177 above.

–14–

THE SEVEN PLANETS

María José Carrillo Linares

The human need to explain the order of things within the universe and the desire to find a rational answer to all the questions that trouble our lives have always found expression in beliefs about the influence of the stars upon earthly matters. These beliefs are probably as old as the human capacity for wondering and reasoning about the causes of natural processes. Nor are beliefs in astral influence on mundane affairs entirely irrational, since the connections drawn between the stars and the earth from ancient times onward were rooted in empirical knowledge. Simple observations show that the lunar cycle is related to the tides and that the movements of the sun allow us to establish divisions among different parts of the day or different seasons of the year. We can also observe that nature is governed by the seasons, and that humankind is governed by nature. Following this line of thought, it would not have been difficult to conclude that not only the sun and the moon, but also the rest of the known planets might influence people's lives.

This inference resulted, long before the Middle Ages, in the discipline of astrology, which medieval society inherited in several different forms. Theoretical astrology was based on observations and computations; the works of Ptolemy (A.D. 85?–a. 161) served as the ultimate model for most theoretical astrological tracts in the Middle Ages. Nevertheless, theoretical astrology was a discipline of interest to only a small part of the medieval population. It was a descriptive science with little relevance to the ordinary matters which worried medieval men and women. Beside this theoretical astrology, and based only on its simplest assumptions, one finds in the Middle Ages a practical application of this theoretical knowledge: since the human being is just a microcosm in which the order of things within the macrocosm is reflected, the position of the stars at certain moments determines the nature and quality of the human constitution. Many works with such an orientation circulated during the late Middle Ages. They offered medieval people a way of understanding the nature of things, while at the same time helping them accept their misfortunes with the resignation granted by a rational explanation.

The Middle English text we present here as *The Seven Planets* (SP) is just one further example of the popularity of this kind of writing.[1] It occupies folios 239r to 244v of the Trinity codex and appears under the heading *Of the vij planetis*. Its contents are divided into three main sections. From folio 239r to 240v there is an account of the seven planets arranged according to their position with respect to the earth, from the most distant planet, Saturn, to the closest, the moon. In this first section, each planet is described according to the influence it may have on diverse aspects of earthly conditions. The different realms in which one can see a reflection of the stars are mainly man, the animals, and the events associated with the natural elements earth, water, and air. Each planet also represents different groups of people, according to the deity to whom each of them owes its name. Thus Venus, the goddess of love, is the planet associated with women; Mars, the god of war, with warriors; Saturn, the god of agriculture and the divine representation of the passing of time, is associated with plowmen and old men; Mercury, the god of eloquence, with people involved with culture or with a profession in which eloquence is required; and Jupiter, king of the gods, with people in positions of power, such as judges, consuls, or bishops. The sun and the moon, whose names do not derive directly from Roman gods, are associated with other more generic groups: rich and honorable men for the sun, the common people for the moon.

The second section extends from folio 240v to 242v, and in this part we learn about the disposition of those born under the influence of each of the zodiacal signs, listed in the order of the months of the year from February to December. The sign of Aquarius, which should occupy the first position, is missing in this copy. After the last zodiacal sign there is a paragraph in which we read about the constitution of women born in July and August. The main aspects of human life which are related to the zodiacal

---

[1] For more information about texts of this nature dealing with the seven planets, see Brown 1994. Direct Latin sources have yet to be identified for the first two sections of *The Seven Planets*. The third section, however, is a close translation of a Latin planets text, *inc.* "Sciendum (est) quod si (ali)quis nascatur/nascetur/nascitur" (TK 1395, 1399). Manuscripts containing the text include Oxford, Bodleian Library, Bodley MS 648, fols. 10v–12v; Bodleian Library, Digby MS 29, fols. 194v–196r; Bodleian Library, Digby MS 75, fol. 125r; Bodleian Library, Digby MS 104, fols. 75v–77r; BL, Sloane MS 513, fols. 75v–77v. I am grateful to Tess Tavormina for having called my attention to the Latin manuscripts corresponding to this third section.

signs in this text have to do with five of the seven deadly sins and their corresponding virtues, friendship, the degree of trust that one may offer to friends, and with affections toward one's fellow humans. Thus we find that the signs have to do with the sexual dispositions of human beings (toward lechery or chastity), their disposition towards the acquisition and keeping of material goods (avarice or generosity), their attitudes towards others (envy or charity), their temperament (anger or meekness), and their appreciation of their position among other people (pride or humility). The vices of gluttony and sloth and their opposing virtues do not seem to be related in this text to the effect of the zodiacal signs. There is no apparent reason to exclude these two vices from the discussion here, although both are sins that could be considered more common among the rich and powerful than among people of lower status, who may have been the more usual audience for of this kind of information. In any case, human behavior and human attitudes are clearly connected in this section to the Christian system of values.

The third section runs from folio 242v to 244v; it returns to the seven planets and their properties and influence over people according to their position at the moment of birth. They are arranged in this section in a different order from that found in the first section. Here the sun heads the description of the planets, described as the fairest of them all as well as the originator of life. It is followed by the moon, Mars, Mercury, Jupiter, Venus, and Saturn: an order that matches the days of the week named for these planets (Sunday, Monday, Tuesday, and so on through Saturday). The planets are classified in this section as good or evil; as in the section on the signs, we also find an account of the personality traits of those born under the different planets. The planets are again identified with their corresponding gods and goddesses, although in addition to the psychological features given earlier, we also find reference to the physiognomy, or physical features, of those born under each planet. The physical appearance derived from the influence of good or evil planets represents the materialization of good or evil in the body. In each case, these features agree with the nature of the planet and the personality features of those born under its influence. Thus, one born under the influence of a malevolent planet such as Mars will have a black face, a big mouth, and a long and aquiline nose. These features are described in the pseudo-Aristotelian *Secretum Secretorum* as having the following implications:

> Whose noose is brode and in the myddell declynyng to the height, he hath many wordes and is a lyer. . . . And whan the mouthe to moche is, and to grete, it shewith a gloton, an impacient man, and a wyked, for such mouthes have whales of the see. (Manzalaoui 1977, 105–6)

On the other hand, if one is born under the influence of a benevolent or neutral planet such as Mercury, he will have opposite features, namely a clear and beautiful face, big and rounded lips, equal black eyes, and a straight nose.

At the beginning of the third section there is an obscure passage dealing with the main Christian concern about astrology, namely, the influence of the planets upon human behavior and the contradiction that this influence represents to one of the basic assumptions of the Christian moral code, the idea of free will:

> Therfor it is to be wist that whosumever be born in any tyme or houre of the day in whiche domynacioun of coniunccioun of the vij planetis, more proone and redy shal be to goode or to evil, the secunde influence of that planete in whiche he is born. But only non of hem vij inducith or bryngith in sum necessite. Forsoth bi free arbiterment and the grace of God bifore that comyng and evene werkyng a man may do wele. And in contrarie wise bi free arbitrement and bi concupiscence of herte and of eyen having the fomyte of synne in hemsilf may do moche and many evils. (SP 226–234)

A similar passage occurs in *The Wise Book of Philosophy and Astronomy*, which reads:

> ... it is to undirstande þat whatte man is borne in any oure of þe day in þe wiche regneth any of þe 7 planetis, he shalle be apte and disposid to good or to evell after þe enffluence and þe constellacion of þe planete in þe whiche he is borne in, but never þe latter it is to knowe þat non of hem constreyneth a man to good or to evyll, ffor why be a manys owen good wille, and þe grace of God comynge beffor; and by his owen good levynge may do good, thow he were disposide to do evyll after þe nature and inffluence of his planete.
>
> On þe same maner evere contrarie by a manys owen ffre wyll and by þe coveytinge of a manys herte and his eyn, he may do evell all thowh he were disposid by his planete to do good. (Krochalis and Peters 1975, 8)

Thus, human beings have the power to decide the course of their actions since God has granted them free will; God's power is superior to the power of the stars, which are also under his dominion.

Although the first and the third sections both deal with the seven planets and their influence on human nature, the orientation in the two sections, as we have seen, is different. The first section emphasizes the relation between man and the physical environment, with nature and with other non-human living creatures. The third section complements the first, emphasizing the relation of man with himself and with his fellow men. The second section, dealing with the zodiacal signs, rounds out what one should know about the influence of the stars upon human behavior. The text as a whole constitutes general information for laypersons, based in a general way on classical works of astrology, such as the works of Ptolemy, but with the incorporation of a Christian element, both as support and as the hinge on which human relationships turn. In spite of the medical nature of many of the texts in TCC R.14.52, the approach in *The Seven Planets* is not that of astrological medicine. The planets and the zodiacal signs are not used to prognosticate illnesses or to recommend remedies or the timing of remedies for those illnesses. That kind of information is provided elsewhere in the Trinity codex, for example, in *The Book of Ypocras* (fols. 143r–145v), a text that complements the non-medical material we find in this treatise.

The third section of the *Seven Planets* text in TCC R.14.52 circulated in other Middle English versions, often in conjunction with other astrological texts, much as it accompanies the first two sections of the Trinity *Seven Planets*. We find different versions of section three in *The Wise Book of Philosophy and Astronomy* (Krochalis and Peters 1975, 3–17), as noted above, and in the seven planets text found in BL, Sloane MS 1315 (Brown 1994).[2] The contents of treatises like these must have been very well known, and they probably served medieval authors such as John Gower as sources or models for their own works. In book 7 of *Confessio Amantis*, in Genius's poetic dissertation on astrology, Gower lists a number of astronomical authorities, including Ptolemy's *Almagest* (7.739, 983, 1460) and Abū Ma'shar (as "Albumazar," 7.1239).[3] The similarities between several passages in *Confessio Amantis* and some of the seven planets texts, including the version edited in

---

[2] According to the information provided in *The Index of Middle English Prose* a similar text is also found in Bodleian Library, Ashmole MS 393 (Eldredge 1992, 19, item 12; Mooney 1995, 61–62, item 52). This text nevertheless shares with the Trinity text only the widely-used theme of the seven planets. It is a much shorter text and the planets are defined by their gender status in the first place (Saturn, Jupiter, Mars, Sol, and Mercury are manly planets, while Venus and the Moon are womanly planets). We also get information in the Ashmole text of the things that every planet is good or bad for. The similarities between the Trinity text, some sections of *The Wise Book of Philosophy and Astronomy*, and the Sloane 1315 seven planets text are, as mentioned above, much stronger than those between the Trinity text and that in Ashmole 393.

[3] Glossed by Sarton ([1927–1948] 1975, 1:568–69) as Abu Ma'shar, astrologer born in Balkh, Khurasan, who died ca. 886. He was frequently quoted in the Middle Ages and many works of astrological nature have been attributed to him.

this volume, show the diffusion and modification of all this material. Thus, the expositions of the sun in *Confessio Amantis* and *The Seven Planets* begin with the following passages:

> Next unto this Planete of love
> The brighte Sonne stant above
> Which is the hindrere of the nyht
> And forthrere of the daies lyht,
> As he which is the worldes ye.
>
> (*CA* 7.801–805)

The sonne is the eye of the world, the beaute of the firmament, the lighter of the mone and of al other planetis. Of whom also the day takith to be his, fforwhi the day is non other than to the spredyng of the sonne vpon the erth. (SP 254–257)[4]

Editorial Practice

The spelling of the manuscript has been reproduced with as few emendations as possible. Editorial practice generally follows that of other texts in this volume, but paragraph divisions of the manuscript have been mostly retained, with a few alterations made in order to follow what seems to be the arrangement intended by the compiler.

---

[4] The SP version seems to be missing something in this passage. In *The Wise Book of Philosophy and Astronomy*, the passage reads: "þe sonne is þe eye of þe world, þe ffayreste of þe ffirmament, the lyghter of þe mone, and of alle oþer planetis, of whom þe day takiþ his leynge. Ffor þe day is no þinge but þe spredinge of þe sonne uppon erthe." (Krochalis and Peters 1975, 14). The Latin text in Bodley 648 has "Sol est mundi oculus firmamenti pulcritudo luna & aliarum planetarum illuminator. A quo & dies accipit esse suum. Nam nichil aliud est dies quam latio solis super terram" (fol. 11r).

OF THE VII PLANETIS

[fol. 239r] As ther bien vij planetis, **Saturnus** of al is hier in his cercle, and he is the signifior[1] and tokener of auncient riche men, and riches, and religious, and erth tiliers or ploughmen, and of auncient and old men, whiche as he is impedyment or letter in houre and tyme of reuo-
5 lucioun, a distroier of whatsumever is in his domynacioun of thynges. If he be in signes of a man,[2] signifieth that ther shuln fal infirmites long tyme and fer of, and to be facciouns or weikenes of body to drynes and leenes and fevers quarteyn; also fugaciouns and involuciouns or wrappynges of aungwisshis, dreede, and deth; and to interfeccioun or
10 slaughter of riche men, and to distruccioun of lifly thynges and vitailes, and riche men bien made poore. Poore forsoth shuln die and be of evene grete sorowe. And if he be in an erthly signe, it signifieth the dist[ru]ccioun of hem whiche bien of his seedis, that is to say, penurie of trees and of their detrymentis or hurtis of wormes and locustes or
15 dogflies. And if he be in airely signe, signifieth grete cold and moche ise and frost, and with clowdis and the corrupcioun of complexioun of the aire, thundres and lightnynges with shynynges and impedymentis of multitude of reynes. And if he be in a watery signe, ther shuln falle many impedimentis in floodis and sees, ship-brechis and of many other
20 watres that shippes shuln suffre. If he be apt and of vtilite or profitable, that is to say, without impedyment in houres and tymes of reuolucioun, and if he be fortunate without any other impedyment, signifieth to the contrary of thiese thynges whiche I have saide, and the conuersioun of evil into goode—and this openly shewith in the booke of natures[3]—
25 and to more a[c]tioun in al his beames. And biholde the evil that lettith hym, whiche is Mars and the tail of the dragon,[4] that is to say, bi con-iunccioun and Mars bi aspect coniunccioun. And propirte of Saturne is as I have saide. In like wise it shal be to the variacioun in other signes so as of a partie is saide of Saturne. So forsoth, as he biholdith hym in
30 the houre and tyme of the conuersioun and turnyng of the yeere, for-tunes or evil shewynges after the strengger in his place and he whiche

---

1. As] *marg. in later hand:* here begyn   Saturnus] *in display script*
6. signifieth] *in marg., marked for ins.*
13. distruccioun] distinccioun
25. actioun] aptioun
26. Mars] *corr. from* Mart?

is the more testimonial shal nat be **[fol. 239v]** in vayne but if the werk
be fieble, forwhi he doeth his werke to al but if he be fieble.

Ivpiter is of signes and of juges and of bisshoppes and consules
35 and of religious and of sectes of citezenis, the whiche if he be letted he
suffrith detryment and hurt of al his. Whiche if he be in [signes] of
mankynde, signifieth deieccioun of riche men and scarste of tho thynges, and after the name of hem þe order and busynes is agenst neighburghs. If he be in an erthly signe, it signifieth distruccioun of londis
40 and scarste of fruytes, distruccioun of trees and of whete and barly, and
a grete fall of vitails and of lifly thynges. If he be in a signe airly, it signifieth scarste of raynes with corrupcioun of wyndes and with corrupcioun of the aire. If he be in a watery signe, it signifieth perdicioun and
losse of shippes in the see by consumpcioun of water and litel fissh. If
45 he be in a bestiall signe, it shal be of impedymentis in bestis of thiese
thynges whiche parteynen vnto men, that is to say, of propir whiche
parteynen to that signe. If he be in an evil place or fortunat, turne the
mone and sey into the place of evil, goode. And say thow in the place of
iniurie or wrong, iustice, and in the place of deieccioun, subtilite, &c.
50 And biholde the planete impedient or lettyng hym in what signe so he
be and evene medle hym and to speke after that I have expowned to
the in thyng of Saturne. And in like wise in the aspect of Jupiter with
fortune or evil shal be the narracioun as abovesaide.

Mars signifieth counseillours and actours or doers of batailes and
55 of werre and of hym whiche sekith vnrightwisnes and falshed and abscisours or cutters of wey[n]es. Whiche if he be in mannes signe, it signifieth multitude of bataile and werre agenst the kynges deth, also sodeyne
and multitude of infirmyte and grete fevers and tercians and abscisours
of wey[n]es and of high fallis. If he be in a erthely signe, it signifieth
60 distruccioun of trees bi the brennyng of heete in hem and with grete
wyndes and noyful, and the combu[s]t or brennyng of new fruytes in
place **[fol. 240r]** in whiche they renne. If he be in a signe airly, signifieth the fewnes of planetis and gretnes of heete and floodis and noyful
heetis. If he be in a watery signe, it signifieth brekyng of shippes with
65 wyndes and strong blastis. If he be in signe quadrupet or iiij-footed,
it signifieth detriment and hurt in al iiij-footed beestis, and of thiese
thynges the whiche parteynen to that signe. After this bihold the planete impedient or lettyng hym in whiche signe he be and medle hym
and to speke as above in Saturne.

70   Sol signifieth the grete riche and honurable men. Whiche if he be in the
houre and tyme of reuolucioun the impedyment, detryment, or hurt

---

36. signes] thynges

he suffrith what it is of hym, that if he be in kyndely signes of mankynd
it shal be in impediment in thiese signes whiche parteynen in hym of
men. If he be in an erthly signe, it shal be impedient of hym in this that
75 is of the substaunce of the erth and of metals. If he be in a signe airly,
it shal be, &c. If he be in a watery signe, it shal be impedient, that is, of
hym of beestis. If he be in place of evil forme or shap, turne the sentence: say into the place of evil, goode, and in contrarie. And biholde
the planete impedient of hym in what signe he be and medle hym and
80 say of hym as above. Knowe thow that thou oughtest to biholde the necessarie nature, forwhi in so moche thow knowist that signifieth of every
planete in their essence and beyng and what shal be to everiche.

Uenus is the marker and bitokener of wymmen and of spadouns
or geldynges of maydenes. Whiche if she be impedient in houre and
85 tyme of reuolucioun, he lettith and al that is of hym. If he be in kyndly
signes of man impedient, signifieth what that is of hym in men and of
men. Also if he be in signes erthly, he distroieth what that is of hym of
the substaunce of the erth and so of the remenaunt.

Mercurius is marker, signator, and bitokener of writers, arsmetricers
90 and other negocioners or busyers, and of chieldren scole-maisters I have
opened. Whiche if he be **[fol. 240v]** lettid of his reuolucioun, he suffrith
detryment what it is of this. And shal be to the variacioun vpon tho thynges whiche parteynen to hym and vpon his descencioun, if he be in signis of mankynde, erthly, airly, watery, bestial, and with aspect or sight of
95 evils and fortunes to hym, as it is abovesaide of Saturne.

Luna is signeres of legaciouns, ambassiatis, and of al the vniuersite
of the comune people and of their liflode and continence and of their
quiete rest every day. Whiche if he be letted in tyme and houre of hir
revolucioun, distroieth al that parteyneth to hir of this. And to the var-
100 iacioun vpon that whiche bien of hir and the presence of hir in signes
erthly, airly, watery, and bestial with the aspect of evil fortunes vpon
that, so as it is abovesaide of Saturne.

[The Months and Their Signs]

Who that is born in Februarie in the signe of Piscis is disposed as to
105 be a grete lechour and of light beryng and a grete purchasour. And bi
many contrariousites shuln come vnto hym but he shal wele escape.
Many folk wold noye hym and thei shul nat prevaile. Bi envie he shal
suffre many blames. His counsail is goode and glad of felawship. With

---

93. whiche] *foll. by* and vp *canc.*
102. Saturne] *marg. in later hand:* here ende

whom he lovith thow maist trustily treate and thi secretis to hym shewe.
110 He can nat be curious for his friendis damage. He hath suche a passioun whiche is saide "Amor Ereos."⁵

Who that is born in the signe of Aries in Marche is disposed as that
he be habundaunt and plentivous of richesse, forwhi he is coveitous
and busy agenst tho thynges as that he gadre money and juels. Whom
115 he lovith, he lovith nat parfitly nor his love shal nat longe endure, and
whan he is wroth, vnneþ he may be peased. He is curious and sumtyme
liberal but only it is nat to trust in hym nor shewe hym nat thi secretis,
forwhi if he be to the offended, he saith al the evil that he may. He is
disposed as that he be gret in honour and worship. But as I have saide
120 he is nat constant or abidyng in love but for a tyme.

Who that is born in Aprille in the signe of Tauri he is excelent in
goodenes and wounder feithful, holl, and triewe. He lovith non adula-
tours, flaterers, nor swete wordis but the **[fol. 241r]** holl trowth. Many
vnkynde shal he fynde whiche yielden hym evil for goode. He kepith
125 pees nor soone wil be troublid but if it be of grete cause. He is high of
herte and therfor he wil nat be gladly in any mannes daungier nor he
chargith nat if any hym haate without cause. If he fynde any feithful
and triewe, he shal be right kynde and free vnto hym. With hym thow
maist surely treate. If thow may have his benevolence and goode wil
130 shewe to hym thi secretis. If forsoth thow gretely offende hym, of light
thyng he shal receive the into his love and friendship.

Who that is born in May in the signe of Geminis he shal be prevy
and sapient and wounder ware. Never shal he shew his veray secrete. But
sumwhat he shal say to the with guyle as that thow trust in hym to have
135 his confidence and so warely profreth and bryngith furth his wordis
as they mown be turned to either partie. Sielden or never shal he be
treatid with any famulier felauship. But for lucre and yiftes gladly he
shal yeve yiftis, but nat of veray kyndenes but that as he bynde the taker
vnto hym. Ne be thow nat overfamulier with hym nor shewe thow hym
140 thi secretis, fforwhi whan he knowith al, he shal lightly dispise the and
as sodainly haate the.

Who that is born in Jun in the signe of Cancri comune he is paale
as that he be envious and malicious in his seyenges, and suspecious and
proone and redy to al filthede and vices, and to man haateful, and as to
145 craft a nygramansier, leche, or cirurgien. In like wise with suche thow
treate nat but as charite requirith. Sumtyme he shal have faire wordis
agenst the, as that he aspie thi secretis to thi confusioun and nat to
goode. And he is wounder malencolik and hard and double in wordis.
Beware the of suche for sielden shal thow fynde hem goode or felawly.

150   Who that is born in Jull in the signe of Leonis shal have grete eyen.
Disposid he is to be a grete lechour and that he lovith moche. Alwey
he shal be biloved and worshipped, so as he growith in honure; and
men whiche treaten with hym shuln trust to his feithfulnes, forwhi he
is veray feithful and kynde. And vnneth or never shal he have chield.
155 And if [**fol. 241v**] he have many wymmen, he shal be gracious at grete
men. But a wounder it is he livith nat above xlix yeere; wele he may die
at his half⁶ but biyonde that shal he nat passe bi disposicioun of nature.
With hym thow maist wele treate and thi secretis shewe. And thow shalt
fynde that his right side in herte is synister or left; or body or knees or
160 the right partie of his hede he shal have his signes.

    Who that is born in August in the signe of Virginis he appierith
meke and innocently bifore men and if he be agreved he is malencolious and malicious. And if any suche is, he is of rede colour, vnpacient,
colerik, and malicious, sapient and wise to bie and to selle, and coveit-
165 ous as that he habounde in juels and other worldly thynges. And he
shal have grete and gracious felawship of wymmen for the famuliarite
that he pretendith in his wordis and beryng. Sielden shal he aught yeve
and if he yeve a litel he shal repute i[t] moche and grete; and if he be
wroth he shal shewe and tel whatsumever he knowith. Whan he is wroth,
170 vnneth may he be peased. While he is poore or simple, he bihavith hym
simply and mekely and fallith in amonges men simply. But whan he hath
power or domynioun, he put furth his hornes of pride and shewith his
malice.

    Who that is born in September in the signe of Libre is disposed as
175 that he be holl, jocunde, and myrry, and a grete lechour, and that he
set al his love in sum womman. And she shal be a litel womman and
shal have grete eyen of suche, that is to say, to hym evene pleasith, and
alwey shal have sufficiente of money; gladly shal yeve and moche shal
spende and in many thynges shal be founde vnkynde. And therfor sum-
180 tyme he shal cease to be liberal and disposed as he have grace of many
men; and wele knowith to treate with hem and namly with matrones
and old wifes and to have goodis of hem he can wele praie and beg.
Whan he is gretely agreved he is feithful and free.

    Who that is born in October in the signe of Scorpionis he is dis-
185 posed as that he be strong. And wher he lovith [**fol. 242r**] moche, he
shal have an high herte and therfor he wil nat be overcome. He is wordy

---

168. it] is
177. is] is is

in wordis and wrothful; and whan hym grevith, he wrothith highly no
difference from a woode man. Ne shewe nat thy secretis to hym, &c.

190 Who that is born in Nouember in the signe of Sagittarij he is wrathful, but no while it endurith; soone he suffrith. Prone and redy is to
the concupiscence of wymmen and soone ravisshed with love and taken
with sum delectable sight, in whiche to hym wele pleasith. To man and
womman he is feithful and triewe and moche lovith and gladly yevith.
195 He is free and triewly lovith, he is woundirly vnwitty, and comunely if he
be a clerk, he writith and redith wele, forwhi forsoth of his deedis he is
necligent, that is to say, he chargith nat. Often he shal have grevaunces
and damages. If he love any he shal shewe al his secretis in so moche þat
parfitely he trustith of hym. Whan he lovith, thow maist feithfully and
triewly shewe thi secretis, forwhi than the more he lovith the. To magik
200 craft he is disposed, otherwise named "gemancie." And of this maner
and to that experience wher to whom any newe thynges bien aduersarie,
ful dul is he in malice or vengeaunce but nat only the more persecucioun
be don vnto hym. No man he hatith but for malice or vnkyndenes.

Who that is born in December in the signe of Capricornij is dis-
205 posed as that he be sapient and with wymmen a grete avoutrer. Sielden
wroth in this that he conceivith, &c., so he conceivith that non trowith ne bileevith th'opposite and if he swere. Of al biloved and that is to
say he shal be worshipped and namly in straunge cuntreys he is felawly
and free. Shewe nat hym thi secretis for he can nat covore ne concele.
210 He shal have grete tribulaciouns and sum membre of hym shal be broken and shal have infirmyte. And gladly shal yeve and exspende, but
nat of kyndenes but of sum magnificence as that he purchace the name
of laude and praisyng.

A womman whiche is born in the moneth of **[fol. 242v]** Junij is
215 moche felawly and curious and namly straungiors, and hir felawship shal
be perceived in hir wordis of no moche lawghter. But prively or lightly she
lovith, and lovith more straungiers than neighburghs. And what womman be born in August moche amiable and felawly and curious and free,
but it bihovith þat she kepe hir wele, forwhi vnneth she shal be virgyne
220 vnto xx yeere. And often suche whiche in their yowth knowen of men
han litel teatis and chielden with grete labour. Vnneth I remembre me
to have seen a womman in this tyme born, but if she be wounderly yong
spoused, forwhi she hath be take and lad from hir husbond.

---

195. be] *foll. by* and *canc.*

Rede yee what folowith of the planetis and of their
225 **vertues.**

Therfor it is to be wist that whosumever be born in any tyme or houre of the day in whiche domynacioun of coniunccioun of the vij planetis, more proone and redy shal be to goode or to evil, the secunde influ-ence[7] of that planete in whiche he is born. But only non of hem vij
230 inducith or bryngith in sum necessite. Forsoth bi free arbiterment and the grace of God bifore that comyng and evene werkyng a man may do wele. And in contrarie wise bi free arbitrement and bi concupiscence of herte and of eyen having the fomyte of synne[8] in hemsilf may do moche and many evils. Therfor whosumever knowith in what day and tyme that
235 he was bore, rede he thiese wordis folowyng, and in his deedis goode or badde of the wordis folowyng he may reherse the trowth.

Of setting of the planetis in the firmament.
It is to be noted that among al planetis the mone is the lowest. Forsoth after the mone is sette Mercury; after Mercury, Venus; after Venus, Sol;
240 after Sol, Mars; after Mars, Jupiter; after Jupiter, Saturnus alwey ascend-yng. Wherof Sinty,[9] that is to say, the mone, Mercury, Venus, and Sol, Mars, Jupiter, Saturne; therof goode influence. The verse of planetis: "Sum planetis bien holsum and wounde[r] beneuolent and wele willed ass Jupiter and Venus. Forsoth, sum bien **[fol. 243r]** malivelous and evil
245 willed after their influencis, as to be trowed Mars and Saturne. For-soth sum bien meanes, so as Mercury and Luna. Sol also among hem lie accomptith." *Vnde versus: "Jupiter atque Venus bona sunt; Sat[urnus] Marsque maligni; Sol et Mercurius cum Luna sunt mediocres."* And biholde so as the sonne is sette in the firmament in the myddis of planetis,
250 and in microcosme—that is to say, in the lasse world (the whiche is man)—holdith the herte in the mydde place.

Of the sonne and a chield whiche is born vnder his
constellacioun.
The sonne is the eye of the world, the beaute of the firmament, the
255 lighter of the mone and of al other planetis. Of whom also the day takith to be his, fforwhi the day is non other than to the spredyng of the sonne

---

224–225. Rede . . . vertues] *marg. in later hand:* here begyne

228–229. secunde influence] *marg. in seventeenth-century hand:* secundum influ-entiam (according to influence &c). *See Explanatory Note.*

230. sum] *corr. from* any

239. Mercury (1)] M *written over* l (*perhaps orig. for* luna)

vpon the erth, and of whos heete meanely humours spryngen and al
corruptible thynges vpon erth. Forwhi as the Philosopher[10] saith, men
without vertu of the sonne men[11] spryngen nat, fforwhi man gendrith

260 man. And the sonne vnder whos constellacioun a man is born benyngne,
facunde, swete, soft, to disciplyne capax, excelent of wit, most duryng
bi ornat and manerly spekyng, many goodis purchasyng; tho thynges
purchaced, with glad chiere theym expendyng; without bost, moche
amiable and sapient, but only with wymmen overmoche lovyng, al the

265 remenaunt with discrecioun doyng. The signes of the sonne in mannes
body bien, that is to say, faire cliere face & ruddy, a meane mowth, the
lippes sumwhat tumous and rede, and al the body ornatly garnysshed
bi birth.

Of the mone and of a chield that is born vndir his
270 **constellacioun.**
The mone is folower of the sonne, and of the sonne beames lightned,
solace of mansiouns, sheweres of sorcery and wichecraft. Vnder whos
constellacioun a man is born shal be vagabunde, moche wakyng, in
hymsilf moche thynkyng, vnwarely spekyng, with cold lightly sike, light

275 cause in hevy drawyng;[12] but and lightly injury foryevyng, nat lightly his
owne thynges departyng, moche **[fol. 243v]** gold and silver gaderyng
and nat expendyng, bi his goode will nat sittyng or restyng, and with
an inconstaunt soule al aboute biholdyng. The signes of the nativite of
the mone in man be thiese: with pale face and sumwhat declyneng to

280 whitnes, a litel mowth, his nose soone holowyng, and to erthly thynges
hastyng above maner.

Of Mars and of the chield that is born vndir his
constellacioun.
Mars is bitter, contrarious, and a malivelous planete. Vnder whos con-

285 stellacioun bien born kynges of batail, cursers, shrewd seyers; sedicious,
hote, and ware people, fforwhi they bien nat lightly disceived; but and
of lande to be coveitous and bostyng, praisyng their owne werkis, other
mennes dispisyng or ellis also blamyng. And this for a constaunt abidyng witholde, that whosumever be born vnder Mars, be he kyng or

290 pore man, he shal be fiers and ful of fightyng, fforwhi his hand is agenst
al men and al men agenst hym. The signe[s] of Mars his[13] natiuite in
mannes body bien thiese: blac face and leene, a grete mowth, often
apt to strives and detracciouns, wiþ a long nose and a gibbous. And this

---

258. erth] *marg. in later hand:* Mone

holde for a certeyn that hosumever have a long nose lift vp in the myddis
295 as an egle or a kyte, naturaly he shuld be fals.[14]

Of Mercurie and the chield that is born vnder his constellacioun.

Forsoth Mercurie is a goode planete and with al goode planetis accordith. Vnder whos constellacioun bien born philosophers coveitous of al
300 liberal sciences and craftes; also laise[15] men of mecanic craftes wounder
wise and wele itaught. Forwhi Mercurius makith men vnder hym born
proude, facunde, of goode wit, and of goode memorie, moevable and
light, goyng into dyvers regiouns, as alwey they mown noveltes and
straunge thynges vnknowen. And also Mercurius makith his men
305 trustyng their owne counsails and refusyng the counsail of other men;
makith men also many thynges purchacyng and gladly expendyng. The
signes of Mercurye in the nativite of mannes body bien thiese: cliere
face and beautevous and of light rede, grete lippis and rounde, equal
[fol. 244r] blac eyen, streight nose nat gibbous, and of wymmens love
310 gretely he shal be loved.

Of Jupiter and the chield that is born vnder his constellacioun

Jvpiter is a goode planete and a cliere, to al thynges holsum temperat
and myrry. Vnder whos constellacioun a man is bore religious and holy,
315 of whatsumever condiciuon that he be. Jupiter makith men large, glad,
and hardy; moche biloved and gracious, annexed to Venus of natural appetite, but voluntarily spiritualy drawyng to chastite; and vnneth
com they to old age. The signes of natiuite of Jupiter in mannes body
bien thiese: cliere face vnder-rede, eyen citryne, teth vneven and divers,
320 streight nose nat gibbous, in goyng of his with temperat maner.

Of Venus and of the chield that is born vndir his constellacioun.

Uenus is a passyng light sterre and to lower thynges sparyng, goodely
and temperat, cold and moist. Vnder whos constellacioun a man be bore
325 shaply and faire, but lecherous, jocunde, and joyful, appetyng of divers instrumentis as organ, harp, cymphon, sawtry, and trumpes blow-

---

309. blac] *upper marg. in later hand:* per me Edward Furtho sonn to William
Furtho grocer in the old chaindge in Londoun at the roase and crowne in the
old chaindge
322. constellacioun] *marg. in later hand:* Moone

yng. He shal be delicious, noble in beryng and lovyng, and he shal be appetyng vayne praisyng; he shal be moche wroth and lightly foryevyng and his owne counsails more than other mennes trustyng or bilevyng.

330 Furthermore if he be riche, moche of his facultes to pore men he shal yeve. If he be poore, the mercy that he may nat parforme in deede, with goode wil and compassioun myghtily he shal fulfille. Also he shal be woundirly large, more only to poore men þan to riche. And he shal be of goode wit; of that only that he hath lierned, lightly he shal yeve to

335 the foryeteful. Whatsumever only he may lierne to al men freely and wilfully he shall departe.

Of Saturne and the chield that is born vnder his constellacioun.

Saturne is a planete derk and maliuolous or evil willed, cold and drie.

340 Vnder whos constellacioun he shal be tymerous, dredful, and coveitous, havyng oo thyng in þe herte, another in the mowth. He shal be a man envious and sorowful, a traitour and solitarie alone, litel spekyng and maliciously; **[fol. 244v]** but and whan he saith wele he symulith, evil hotith. He fortreatith and (that worst is) lightly he offendith and of hard

345 pleased. Also of hard he pleasith. Also of hard science he conceivith. But whan he hath science of light he leesith it nat.

Therfor al men knowyng vnder what con[s]tellacioun that he was bore rest he to my counseils. If forsoth he were born vnder a beniuolent constellacioun, joie he and do wele vnwerily without ceassyng. Forsoth

350 if he be bore vnder a maliuolous constellacioun, from that evil that it is of kynde, declyne he everlastyng and drawe he into a goode chaunge, that if he so do worthy, rewardes of goode God he shal take, that is to say, everlastyng lif.

---

353. lif] *marg. in later hand:* here ende

Explanatory Notes

[1] **signifior:** The planet that symbolizes or represents a person, group, or event. Cf. the quotation given in the *OED*, s.v. *significator*, from Lilly's *Christian Astrology* (1647): "When we name the Lord of the Ascendant, or Significator of the Querent, or thing quesited; we meane no other thing then that Planet who is Lord of that Signe which ascends, or Lord of that Signe from which house the thing demanded is required"; and the related definition of the word *signifier* as "One who or that which signifies; a significator" (both words recorded in *OED* from the sixteenth century).

[2] **signes of a man:** The medieval classification of astrological signs could be made according to a variety of parameters. In this text we find several classes of signs: human, bestial, four-footed or quadruped, watery, earthly, and airy (fiery signs are not mentioned, but are implied by the other elemental classes). These classifications can be found in most astrological tracts of the time, where one finds among the human signs Gemini, Virgo, Aquarius, and the first half of Sagittarius (those whose representation is human or half human); the four-footed signs are Aries, Taurus, Leo, Capricorn, and the second half of Sagittarius (all quadruped animals); the bestial signs are Aries, Taurus, Leo, the second half of Sagittarius, Capricorn, Scorpio, Cancer, and Pisces (any animal sign); among the watery signs one finds Cancer, Scorpio, and Pisces; the earthly signs include Taurus, Virgo, and Capricorn; the airy signs are Gemini, Libra, and Aquarius.

[3] **the booke of natures:** No authorities are cited by name in this text, and consequently the reference to *the booke of natures* is difficult to trace. It could be a reference to Pliny's *Historia naturalis*, or to any other similar encyclopaedic work circulating at that time.

[4] **tail of the dragon:** One of the two points, or "nodes," where the orbit of the moon intersects the ecliptic. The node at which the moon passes to the south of the ecliptic—the "descending node"—is known as the "tail of the dragon" (*cauda draconis*), that at which the moon passes to the north of the ecliptic—the "ascending node"—as the "head of the dragon" (*caput draconis*).

[5] **Amor Ereos:** The disease of love, a concept inherited from classical medicine; according to Aristotle it was a disease of the heart, while Galen localized it in the brain. In both the classical and the medieval period, there is general agreement as to the symptoms of the malady, some of which are shared with other mental illnesses, such as melancholy or mania. The main symptoms described are loss of appetite, insomnia, inability to concentrate, sunken eyes, and jaundice. Amor Ereos was attributed to a variety of causes, ranging from a malfunctioning of the estimative faculty to an excess of humours in need of expulsion. As a cure for the illness, most medieval authors recommended intercourse, wine, baths, conversation, music, and poetry. For more information about lovesickness, see Wack 1990.

[6] **nat above xlix . . . at his half:** This passage seems to suggest that those born in July under the sign of Leo are predisposed to die no later than age forty-nine (often earlier), an age that in the later Middle Ages was considered to be in the period of maturity for men, quite close to elderly. The passage seems to imply also that these people are more likely to die at about twenty-four or twenty-five (half of forty-nine). This may be related to the idea expressed earlier in the paragraph that they do not have many children, despite their proclivity to lechery and apparent personal charisma.

[7] **secunde influence:** As the marginal note points out, this phrase appears to be an error in translation; the ME rendering should have read something like "[a person is more prone to good or evil] according to the influence of the planet under which he is born." The hand of the correction appears to be that of John Fortho, who also commented and expanded on the geometrical exercises on fols 254r–255r.

[8] **fomyte of synne:** lit. 'kindling of sin' (= Lat. *fomes peccati*), i.e., the tendency toward sin inherent in human beings as the result of original sin, even after the baptismal removal of original sin from the soul. On the use of the Latin word *fomes, -itis* in medical contexts of infection (*fomes morbi*) and the theological discourse behind it, see Nutton 1983, 34 (Addendum to p. 25, n. 107).

[9] **Sinty:** I.e., Cynthia, the moon. Cf. the reading *Scincia* in Bodley 648, fol. 10v.

[10] **the Philosopher:** Probably a reference to Aristotle.

[11] **men . . . men:** The second *men* may be a pleonastic repetition of the first use of the word (as subject of the clause) or a direct object of *spryngen* used as a transitive verb with the sense "generate," though the *MED* does not record transitive uses of *springen* 'to arise, originate, begin.' Alternatively, the second *men* could be a misspelling or misreading of *mei*, a form of the verb *may*.

[12] **light cause in hevy drawyng:** Perhaps equivalent to 'tending to convert simple matters into serious ones,' or making a mountain out of a molehill. Cf. "And he dothe make a lytyll cause a grete cavse" in the version of this text edited by Brown (1994, 17) and the reading "lenem (*or* leuem) causam in grauem trahens" in Bodley 648, fol. 11r.

[13] **Mars his:** Mars's (possessive, construed as 'Mars his').

[14] **nose lift vp . . . be fals:** Aquiline or hooked noses were associated with Jewish physiognomy in the later Middle Ages as well as in the modern era, so this comment may be implicitly anti-Semitic. The illuminated codex containing Alfonso X's *Las Cántigas de Santa María* copied ca. 1280, and preserved today in El Escorial as MS T.1.1, includes several illuminations in which the Jews are portrayed with this physiognomic characteristic. See also the dozen images listed in the Index Iconographique, s.v. *nez busqué, courbe, crochu etc.* in Blumenkranz 1966, 150; according to Lipton (1999, 162 n. 38), citing Zafran 1973 and Mellinkoff 1993, "the topos of the crooked nose does not seem to have become a commonplace until the fifteenth century," although instances can be found from the thirteenth century on.

[15] **laise:** Possibly a rare spelling of *less,* meaning 'of lower rank or position.' Or perhaps a miscopying of *laie* 'lay': the sentence appears to be contrasting men who incline toward study of the liberal arts and those who pursue the "mecanic craftes." Cf. the version of this passage in the seven planets text edited by Brown: "Also lewyd men and vnleyttryde, þey that ar bore vnder Marcury, ar wyse and ware and sly and argus in all maner of harde craftys, as in goulde-smythe crafte, wrytyng, sewyng, schapyn, and all other crafte of honde" (1994, 19) and the reading *laici* in Bodley 648, fol. 11v.

– 15 –

THE SEVEN LIBERAL ARTS

Linne R. Mooney

A unique Middle English text on the seven liberal arts survives in Trinity College, Cambridge, MS R.14.52.[1] Latin texts on the seven liberal arts were certainly in circulation in medieval England, but this text is, to my knowledge, the earliest one written in English.[2] It thereby offers evidence of the vernacular English reader's knowledge of (or access to the knowledge of) the arts that were the foundation of medieval university education. This text is also unique in that it includes in its chapter on grammar an attempt to describe the phonetic production of the letters of the alphabet, providing the only surviving contemporary approximation of the pronunciation of medieval English, and in that it adds a chapter on the mechanical sciences, relating them as does no other medieval author to the English craft guilds.[3]

---

[1] This article is reprinted (with authorial deletions and revision) by permission from Mooney 1993b.

[2] The seven liberal arts were also described in Middle English in longer works, such as *The Court of Sapience*, lines 1807–2205 (ed. R. Harvey 1984), Stephen Hawes's *Pastime of Pleasure*, lines 519–2933, passim (ed. Mead 1928); and William Caxton's *Mirrour of the World*, chaps. 5, 7–13, pp. 27–29, 33–43 (ed. Prior 1913). The earliest recorded copy of *The Court of Sapience* is, interestingly, also written by the Hammond scribe (Harley 2251), and the second earliest copy in Cambridge, Trinity College, MS R.3.21, which was partly written by the Hammond scribe (see Mooney, chap. 3 above). Caxton's *Mirrour* would have been translated soon thereafter (ca. 1480) and Hawes's *Pastime* somewhat later (1505–6). For Latin texts available in English manuscripts, see for instance Pseudo-Seneca, *De septem liberalibus artibus*, in Glasgow, University Library, Hunter MS 231 (U.3.4), pp. 123–29, of the fourteenth century. (My thanks to Professor Laurel Means for drawing my attention to this manuscript.)

[3] For general background on the liberal arts, see Abelson 1906; Masi 1981; Wagner 1983; Machielsen 2003, 1–24.

The text on the seven liberal arts is preserved on folios 244v–254r, copied by the main scribe of the manuscript, the Hammond scribe. It is not a holograph—it contains errors of the kind one would associate with the copying, not the composing, of a work[4]—so we must assume a date of composition previous to or contemporary with the writing of the manuscript, that is, before 1485. The author of this Middle English text (or of the Latin source or sources from which he was translating) makes frequent references to his authorities, including St. Paul; Robert Grosseteste, especially his *De artibus liberalibus*; Priscian, *Ars major* and *Institutiones grammaticae*; Remigius of Auxerre, *Expositio super Donatum*; Porphyry, *Isagoge*; Aristotle, *Topics* and *Elenchi*; Pseudo-Aristotle, *Secretum secretorum*; Boethius, *De divisione*, *De institutione arithmetica*, *De musica*, and commentaries on Cicero's *Topics* and Porphyry's *Isagoge*; Isaac Judaeus, *De diaetis universalibus*; Ptolemy, *Tetrabiblos*; Euclid, *Elements*; and Quintilian, *Institutio oratoria*. Many of these texts were required reading at Oxford for the degree of bachelor of arts.[5] This writer's knowledge of some of them (e.g., Porphyry's *Isagoge*, Priscian's *Institutiones grammaticae*, Euclid's *Elements*) seems thorough enough to suggest that he had studied them. His knowledge of others, however, seems so superficial that he may have known them only through summaries or encyclopedias of the arts that cited these authorities.

The Middle English text as we have it is organized after and drawn from earlier writers on the seven liberal arts, including Boethius, Hugh of St. Victor, Martianus Capella, Remigius of Auxerre, John Scottus Eriugena, and especially Robert Grosseteste, but it is clearly a compilation of texts, abridged or altered to suit its audience or compiler. The process of abridgment and alteration seems to have taken place in more than one stage (whether in Latin or English) before producing the text that survives.

Apparently the base to which other materials were added in the course of compilation was Grosseteste's *De artibus liberalibus* (ed. Baur 1912, 1–7). In the text edited here, the defense of the seven liberal arts in the introduction, in the review preceding the chapter on geometry, and in the conclusion[6] is drawn from Grosseteste's defense of the arts in *De artibus liberalibus*. Grosseteste is specifically named in the introduction and in the review

---

[4] See, for example, the loss of text at the turning of a page, discussed below.

[5] See Fletcher 1992, esp. 323–24. The required texts in the second half of the fifteenth century included, for instance, Porphyry's *Isagoge*; Aristotle's *Elenchi*; Priscian's *Institutiones grammaticae*; Boethius's *Topics*, *Arithmetica*, and *De musica*; and Euclid's *Elements*.

[6] Lines 1–57, 256–341, and 585–593, respectively.

preceding the chapter on geometry;[7] and his defense of the arts is trans-lated almost word for word in two passages of the introduction.[8] Further, portions of the expositions of the arts of rhetoric and especially of music are drawn from Grosseteste's work.[9] The compiler of the first recension of this work, then, seems to have begun with Grosseteste's *De artibus liberalibus*, drawing on his defense of the arts and on his exposition of two of the arts. He then apparently added material from other sources for his exposition of the other five arts: from Priscian on grammar, from Boethius and Porphyry on logic, from Quintilian and Grosseteste on rhetoric, from Boethius on arithmetic, from Boethius and Grosseteste on music, from Pseudo-Aristo-tle on astronomy, and probably from Euclid on geometry.[10] At this stage the work would have ended around the present line 341; it may be seen that the compiler sums up his defense of the arts at lines 334–341, echoing his intro-ductory defense[11] and writing as if he had treated all seven arts already,[12] before the chapter on geometry.

The author/compiler of the next recension must have discarded the chapter on geometry (which had probably come between arithmetic and music, as in other descriptions of the arts) and added to the end a much

---

[7] At line 30, "as Lincoln saith," and at line 340, "as Lyncolniens saith."

[8] Lines 39–42 translate Grosseteste, p. 1, lines 19–21, and lines 44–49 translate Grosseteste, p. 4, lines 10–14. I quote the first pair of passages here:

Aspectum grammatica recte informat. Recte informatum quale sit logica sine errore dijudicat. Ut judicatum quale sit moderate fugiat affectus vel appetat, rhetorica persuadet.

As for our vndirstandyng Gramer enformyth hym with congruyte in spekyng, in writyng, and due pronunciacioun; Logik shewith without errour whe[r]with he is enformed; and than folowith Rethorik persuadyng what thynge mannes wil shuld mesurably flee or desire.

[9] Lines 160–167 on rhetoric are drawn from Grosseteste's *De artibus liberalibus*, p. 2, lines 2–9; lines 250–268 on music are drawn from Grosseteste's *De generatione sono-rum* (which was often treated as a continuation of *De artibus liberalibus*), p. 7, lines 5–24; and lines 290–299 on music are drawn, again, from *De artibus liberalibus*, p. 4, line 35, to p. 5, line 20.

[10] See the Explanatory Notes to the edition below.

[11] For instance, "thiese vij special sciences . . . bien partis and pilers of philosophie" at lines 336–337, echoing "other vij pilers as the vij special sciences to helpe man to directe hym in his werkis and to purge al errours" at lines 28–29.

[12] He writes, "thiese vij special sciences bifore rehersed bien partis . . . " (lines 336–337) and "therfor thiese vij afore other mown wele be cald sciences and konnyng-es" (line 340–341).

longer summary of that science, devoting almost as many lines to his explanation of geometry as to the other six arts combined: 221 lines on geometry as compared with 294 on the other six arts.[13] This chapter on geometry
is excerpted from a version of Euclid's *Elements*, which was independently
translated from Latin to Middle English in at least one other version, as preserved in London, BL, Sloane MS 213, at folios 121r–124r.[14] In the text as it
survives here there are no fewer than four specific references to Euclid in
the exposition of the science of geometry, at lines 433, 476, 504, and 507;
and in this chapter no other writer is referred to, other than "Pictagoras
with his folowers, [who] commendid gretely geometry" (line 347), and "the
Philosopher," who commended sight among the five wits as that through
which we gain the greatest knowledge of things (lines 365–367)—both

---

[13] This special focus on geometry may be connected to material in other texts in
Trinity R.14.52: on the one hand, to Bacon's theoretical claims for geometry and
perspective as means to achieving long life ("In Due Rule of Body," ed. Tavormina,
chap. 9, lines 8, 98–99, 183, 272, above); and, on the other, to the practical scientific, commercial, and architectural applications of geometry described in the
treatises on scientific instruments edited by Laird above (chap. 13, lines 916–926,
1295–1322, 1379–1412, etc.).

[14] Lines 342–343 and 371–428 correspond to portions of the Middle English text in
the Sloane manuscript. This latter text was edited by Halliwell (1839, 56–71). The
text in the Sloane manuscript begins, "Geometri es saide of þis greke worde geos
þat es erthe on englisch and of þis greke word metros þat es mesure on englisch,"
obviously drawn from the same source as lines 342–343 for the title to the chapter
on geometry: "Geometrie is saide of geo in Greeke that is lond and metron that
is mesure." The ultimate source is Euclid, but both writers could also have taken
this etymology from Balbus, which might have been available to them in the copy
recently printed by Gutenberg (Mainz, 1460). Thereafter the Sloane text (cited by
page and line references to Halliwell's edition) corresponds to the text here edited
as follows: lines 371–382 here to 57.4–58.16 in Halliwell; lines 382–386 to 59.28–30
and 61.10–14; lines 386–393 to 62.29–63.6; lines 394–404 to 66.4–17; lines 406–
416 to 68.1–15; and lines 417–428 to 70.14–25. To illustrate its being an independent translation of the same text, I give here the Sloane version for comparison
with lines 394–404 of the text edited below:

> If you wilt mesure þe heght of any thyng by a myrure. lay þe myrure in þe
> playne grounde, and go toward and froward til you se þe toppe of þat thing in
> þe mydel of þat myrure. þan multiply þe playne bitwene þe foundement of þat
> thyng to be mesured and þe myrure by þe space fro þethen to þe erthe. and
> þat comes þereof departe by þe space bytwene þi fote and þe myroure and þe
> noumbre howe ofte it be es þe heght of þat thyng. Also als fro þethen to þe
> erthe has it to þe space bytwene þi fote and þe myrure so þe heght of þat thyng
> has it to þe playne. Whilk es bitwene þe rote of þat thyng to be mesured and
> þe myrure and so ageyne (ed. Halliwell, 66.4–17).

The *Elements* was translated from Arabic to Latin by Adelard of Bath.

named in the introductory defense of geometry, not in the exposition of it. Finally, either at the same time or in another recension, there was added a brief exposition of the seven common or mechanical crafts and, to conclude, a brief explanation of their utility in relation to the arts. At some point in this process of alteration the text was translated into English.

Whatever its specific sources and however it came to be compiled or translated, this text on the seven liberal arts is a significant witness to English vernacular knowledge of (and attitude toward) the arts in the second half of the fifteenth century. The chapter on grammar includes, unique to Middle English writings, an attempt to describe the phonetic production of twenty letters of the alphabet: the five vowels, six semivowels (*l, r, n, x, s,* and *m*), and nine mutes (*f, b, p, d, t, k, q, c,* and *g*). The pronunciation of the semivowels is particularly revealing of the vernacular character of this phonology:

> The semy-vowels bien vj, and thei bien gendred thurgh touchyng of the tung to on of the palatis of the mowth. And if it touche the over palate with streyneng out of the tunge so that the pointe of the tunge towchith the palat so is *l* causid, but if þe tunge be more bowed and in maner with a tremelyng folowyng afterward than is *r* gendred. And if the tung be in party streyned right and in part bowid so that the sowne goth nat oute completely bi the mowth but bi the nosethrillis so is *n* caused. And if the tunge touche the lower palate twics so is *x*. And if it touche but oones with an hissyng sowne than is *s* gendred, for the sides of the tunge bien joyned to the sides of the palate. And if it touche the outward part with coniunccioun of the inward part of the lippis so is *m* caused. (87–98)

Compare Martianus Capella's description of the pronunciation of Latin letters, drawn from classical texts:

> L is a soft sound made with the tongue and the palate. . . .
>
> R is a rough exhalation with the tongue curled against the roof of the mouth. . . .
>
> N is formed by contact of the tongue on the teeth. . . .
>
> X is the sibilant combination of C and S. . . .
>
> S is a hissing sound with the teeth in contact. . . .
>
> M is a pressing together of the lips.[15]

---

[15] Martianus Capella, *The Marriage of Philology and Mercury,* in vol. 2 of *Martianus Capella and the Seven Liberal Arts* (trans. Stahl and Johnson 1977, 75; for the Latin text, see Martianus Capella, ed. Dick [1925] 1978, 95–96).

The "tremelyng folowyng afterward" in pronunciation of the letter *r* in the Middle English text is unique to this text and clearly indicates its vernacular character.

The chapter on grammar follows Priscian's *Institutiones grammaticae*, or rather a medieval recension of it that dealt with orthography, etymology, syntax, and prosody, in that order.[16] The author describes each of these studies in order, referencing Priscian; but he spends most of the chapter on his description of the phonetic production of the letters. Such a description is not to be found in the classical Priscian, nor, as suggested by this author at line 67, was it provided by Remigius of Auxerre in either his *Expositio super Donatum* (or *In artem Donati minorem commentum*) or his *Commentum in Martianum Capellam*; but it is to be found, as noted above, in Martianus Capella's *De nuptiis Philologiae et Mercurii*, in the third book, on grammar.[17]

The author begins by listing the parts of the body involved in the generation of speech, and then more fully describes the shape of the cavity inside the mouth as it changes for generation of the five vowels, explaining the shape of the letters in relation to the shape of the mouth when each is produced.[18] Unfortunately, the description only compares the pronunciation of vowels with one another, so we learn nothing from it of how far to the front or back the whole range was pronounced. The author then distinguishes semivowels from mute consonants. This is immediately followed by descriptions of the generation of each of those letters, beginning with the semivowels, as quoted above. His semivowels are *l, r, n, x, s,* and *m*; his mute consonants are *f, b, p, d, t, k, q, c,* and *g*.[19] His descriptions of the letters *l, r,* and *n* are easy to comprehend, and by following them one produces the expected result.[20] The explanation for this author's description of letter *x* may come

---

[16] See Explanatory Notes 5, 8, and 9.

[17] Ed. Dick [1925] 1978, 95–96. For Remigius's commentaries on Martianus and Donatus, see the editions of Lutz (1962–1965) and Fox (1902). However, there might well have been a medieval text on pronunciation of the letters attributed to Remigius. See the postscript to Pinborg 1982, on the attribution to Remigius of a "huge family of treatises dealing with Latin morphology or accidence" (65).

[18] See Explanatory Note 7.

[19] Priscian's semivowels are *f, l, m, n, r, s,* and *x*, but he adds, "sed f multis modis ostenditur muta magis." See Priscian, ed. Hertz, in H. Keil [1855–1880] 1961, 2:9. Priscian's mutes are *b, c, d, g, h, k, p, q,* and *t* (ibid.). The two lists are the same, except that this author moves *f* to the list of mutes and for some reason omits *h* altogether.

[20] By comparison, Martianus's descriptions for these three are "L is a soft sound made with the tongue and the palate"; "R is a rough exhalation with the tongue curled against the roof of the mouth"; and the confusing "N is formed by the contact of the tongue on the teeth" (trans. Stahl and Johnson 1977, 2:75). The Latin reads, "L lingua palatoque dulcescit"; "R spiritum lingua crispante corraditur"; and "N lingua dentibus appulsa collidit" (ed. Dick [1925] 1978, 96).

from classical texts, where, for example, Martianus describes *x* as "the sibilant combination of C and S."[21] Here the author seems to be suggesting a sequential combination of *c* and *s* as he describes each of them: "And if the tunge touche the lower palate twies so is *x* [caused]."[22] The touching of the lower palate with the tongue to produce the letter *s* is unusual, since both modern dental /s/ and lisped *s* involve contact of the tongue with the teeth.[23] Perhaps some form of an alveolar /s/ is intended. The description of *f* is also unusual, involving as it does the contact of the lower teeth with the upper lip (exactly the opposite of what we would expect).[24] The descriptions of the other letters and their groupings—*b* and *p*; *d* and *t*; *k*, *q*, and *c*; and *g* by itself—are all comprehensible and produce the expected sounds. The author's apparent difficulty in accurately describing some letters, and his divergence from classical descriptions, suggests that he was trying to work out the pronunciation on his own, and therefore in most (or perhaps all?) cases giving us a description of at least one fifteenth-century Englishman's pronunciation of the letters.

Also unique to this text is the association of the seven common crafts with the craft guilds of medieval England. The idea for including the seven common crafts in a treatise on the liberal arts may ultimately derive from Varro through Martianus Capella's *Marriage of Philology and Mercury*, but the specific crafts named as the seven and the brief descriptions of them more closely follow the description of the seven mechanical sciences in book 2 of Hugh of St. Victor's *Didascalicon*, chapters 20–27.[25] Hugh's seven mechanical sciences are fabric making, armament, commerce, agriculture, hunting, medicine, and theatrics, in that order. Hugh wrote of them:

> These sciences are called mechanical, that is, adulterate, because their concern is with the artificer's product, which borrows its form from nature. Similarly, the other seven are called liberal either because they require minds which are liberal, that is, liberated and practiced (for

[21] Trans. Stahl and Johnson 1977, 2:75. The Latin, "X quicquid C atque S formauit exsibilat" (ed. Dick [1925] 1978, 96).

[22] Lines 94–95. Both *c* and *s* are produced by touching the tongue to the lower palate, so the instructions given for *x* could be a shortened form of instructions for sequential productions of *c* and *s*: "if the tung touche the lower egge of the teeth" halfway between a "grete openyng of þe mowth" and a "litel openyng . . . so is c [gendred]" (lines 104–107) and "if [the tunge] touche [the lower palate] but oones with an hissyng sowne than is s gendred" (lines 95–96).

[23] So also the classical authors. Martianus describes it as "a hissing sound with the teeth in contact" (trans. Stahl and Johnson 1977, 2:75); the Latin, "S sibilum facit dentibus uerberatis" (ed. Dick [1925] 1978, 96).

[24] Martianus describes it as we would expect: "F is made by the teeth pressing on the lower lip" (trans. Stahl and Johnson 1977, 2:75); in the Latin, "F dentes labrum inferius deprimentes" (ed. Dick [1925] 1978, 95).

[25] See Explanatory Note 48.

these sciences pursue subtle inquiries into the causes of things), or because in antiquity only free and noble men were accustomed to study
them, while the populace and the sons of men not free sought opera-
tive skill in things mechanical.[26]

Three centuries later, this Middle English author (or his source), perhaps
aware of the greater social breadth of his readership or perhaps himself
related to the artisan class, wrote:

> Bvt beside thiese vij sciences ther bien other vij that bien nat cald spe-
> cial sciences, but rather vsual or comune craftis and hand werkis the
> whiche bien daily vsed and exercised of comune artificers and werk-
> men, as tilieng, venery, phisik, theatrik, lanyfice, armery, navigacioun.[27]

In adapting Hugh's text, the fifteenth-century writer has made a number of significant changes to suit the list to his audience or his purpose.
First, he has modified the traditional understanding of social stratification
which had been accepted by Hugh. Second, he has changed the order of
the crafts—with agriculture, hunting, and medicine, which serve primary
bodily needs, now corresponding to the trivium, and theater, weaving,
armament, and navigation corresponding to the quadrivium. The seven
crafts are described as "beside thiese vij sciences," as if the writer intends
them to be seen as comparable to the seven liberal arts; and they are further described as the "vsual or comune craftis and hand werkis the whiche
bien daily vsed and exercised of comune artificers and werkmen," in contrast to Hugh's more disparaging description of the craft of artisans and
laborers. In the Middle English text the seven common crafts or mechanical sciences represent the lowest of the three orders of sevens given to man
by God after the Fall: the first "pilers" cut out of God's passion were the
seven sacraments (lines 25–26), the second order of "pilers" the seven liberal arts (lines 28–29). The crafts are never referred to as "pilers," but are
called the "other vij" that are "beside thiese vij sciences" (line 563). As such,
the crafts are seen as serving a practical (and mundane, in the best sense
of the word) purpose, as compared with the arts, which, as the author takes
pains elsewhere to make clear, serve to broaden the knowledge of man and
thus bring him closer to God.[28]

---

[26] Hugh of St. Victor, *Didascalicon* 2.20 (ed. and trans. J. Taylor 1961, 75).

[27] Lines 563–567.

[28] Lines 1–57 of the edition below, which, as noted above, draw heavily upon Grosseteste's defense of the arts. The author's failure to distinctly trace the relationship
among the three sevens may come from his compilation of different source materials, the first two being described and compared clearly in the introduction drawn
from Grosseteste, the second and third being compared only in the added chapter
on the seven common crafts.

Finally, and apparently uniquely among treatises of this sort, the author has attempted to relate the crafts to the guilds of medieval England. "Venery," he says, "conteyneth al occupacioun in huntyng, fowlyng, ffisshyng, with al dightyng of metis and drynkes and generaly al craftis of fisshmongers, bochiers, tauerners, and brewers." "Lanefice [or wool-working] conteyneth al maner of wevyng and werkyng in wulle threde, cloth, skynnes, baskettis, or mattis and so furth, as tailours, hosiers or drapiers, fullers, shermen, and skynners." Apparently a portion of the text is missing at a page break, where the author is comparing the kind of skill necessary to perform these crafts with that required for study of the liberal arts. What we have is this:

> And þiese vij be not cald sciences or veray konnynges propirly and |[29]
> mercers, grocers, and suche other comunely, that is to say, a maner
> of knowlache in a thyng, and therfor thei bien cald but instrumen-
> tis and mynistres to philosophie and to the vij liberal and special sci-
> ences, namely to the iiij mathamatical. But specialy to Geometry and
> his partis, for ther is more certitude and evidence in demonstracioun
> in deduccioun of his conclusioun, bi the whiche demonstracioun ve-
> ray kunnyng is caused and brought into mannes [soule] . . . , than in
> many other sciencis. (580–589)

Here, to the extent that we can reconstruct his argument, the writer appears to be defending the common crafts and the skill required to perform them as "instrumentis and mynistres to philosophie and to the vij liberal . . . sciences."

As a whole, the comparison of the liberal arts with the worldly crafts that serve them and the association of those crafts with guilds are just what we would expect in a manuscript prepared for use by a member of London's merchant class, like Sir Thomas Cook. It seems plausible, then, that the final revision of this text, that is, the addition of the longer description on geometry which complements other texts in the volume (see n. 13 above) and the comparison with the crafts drawn from Hugh of St. Victor and then adapted to compare with the work of craft guilds, was done for its inclusion in this volume.

---

[29] Here the page break occurs, apparently (from the grammar and sense) with some loss of text.

THE SEVEN LIBERAL ARTS

[**fol. 244v**] Glorious and mervailaus God, in al his werkis the verray craft
of wisdam of the fader of hevene, whiche in the bigynnyng beyng bifore
al creatures, as witnessith scripture [cf. Colossians 1:15], made al creatures of nought, and man after the image and symilitude of the holi
5 Trynite, puttyng hym in so high and grete dignite indowed hym with so
grete giftes both in body and in soule, and in so myrry and pleasaunt
place of paradice that he myght nat wele have be put in a more jocunde
place but if he shuld atteyne to the veray sight of the godhed, so that the
body was hole and nat corrupt and greved nat the soule, for the lawe of
10 the flessh was nat contrarye to the lawe of the soule [cf. Romans 7:25] but
his outward and inward wittis obeied to reason, reason to his wil, and his
wil to God alone. This was cald the state of our rightwisnes: and in figure to kene therof, man is made of right stature in body that he shuld
be also in his soule. But oure first fader, thus put in so grete grace, whan
15 he was in honour and worship vndirstode it nat, and disobeyeng the
comaundement of his maker, had a grevous falle both in werkis of his
soule and of his body, so that the light of his vnderstandyng was made
derke bi ignoraunce, and his desire in wil and affeccioun cam nat to
a due terme or ellis passed without mesure his due terme and ende,
20 and also the moevyng power of his body was made fieble and vnparfite
thurgh the corrupcioun of the clog of his flessh. Wherfor the Lord of
all [**fol. 245r**] vertu and God of al connyng, *the veray wisdom of þe fader*
[cf. 1 Corinthians 1:30, Colossians 2:3], consideryng the fowl fall both
in origynal and actual synne ordeyned remedie whan plener and ful
25 tyme cam, as Seynt Paul seith,[1] and cut out of his passioun vij pilers [cf.
Proverbs 9:1], that is to say, vij sacramentis wasshyng awey bi theym both
origynal, venyal, and actual vnclennes. And bifore this tyme he cut out
of the grete tresour of his wisdam other vij pilers as the vij special sciences to helpe man to directe hym in his werkis and to purge al errours,
30 ffor that is th'office of the vij liberal sciences, as Lincoln saith,[2] to rectifie a mannes operaciouns and to deduce hem from errour to perfecci-

---

1. Glorious] *marg. in modern hand:* Incipit 7 Sciences

10. nat] *foll. by the* canc.

22. the veray wisdom of þe fader] *underlined in text*

26. vij sacramentis] x *above* vij, *with line leading to marg. note in later hand:* s. la
ma m (*canc.*) sacra

oun; the werkis that bien in mannes power, they bien in the knowlache
of his reason and vndirstondyng or in affeccioun and desire of his wil
or in bodily moevynges or in bodily desires. Mannes soule considrith ij
thynges: ffirst þe thynges that he considerith bi his reason he knyttith
toguyder or dividith and sundrith after their propirte and offrith hem
to the wil that he may cheese and pursue suche thynges as bien convenient, or flee and eschewe theym that bien noyous and disconuenyent.
As for our vndirstandyng Gramer enformyth hym with congruyte in
spekyng, in writyng, and due pronunciacioun; Logik shewith without
errour whe[r]with he is enformed; and than folowith Rethorik persuadyng what thynge mannes wil shuld mesurably flee or desire;[3] and so
thiese iij sciences rectifie the vndirstandyng of mannes soule and bryng
it to perfeccioun as it shal be saide afterward. Furthermore if we bi our
moevyng intende any other thyng beside our moevyng than we divide
þinges joyned toguyder or ellis conteigne thynges divide or assigne to
gyve order and situacioun or ellis we make figures and discripciouns
or take mesuris of height playne and deepe thynges with suche other
many, in the whiche Arsmetrike and Geometry maken direccioun.[4] And
if we attende to rectificacioun of our moevyng and nat to thynges that
bien made bi bodily moevyng, therfor is Musike specialy orday- **[fol.
245v]** ned. But yit in thiese thynges we may soone erre, if wee knowe
not the situacioun and order of the parties of þe world. Also nat al our
werkis be ordured but if thei bien mesured bi certeyne space and tyme,
for Astronomy is necessarie þat techith to discerne and knowe the situacioun of the worde with distynccioun of tymes, bi the moevyng of hevene
and cours of sterres.

Gramer

First the office of Gramer is to enforme our soule with vndirstondyng
and with due writyng and thynges vndirstondyng duely to pronounce
with congruyte as it is declared in the iiij parties of Gramer. For the
first part that is cald Ortographie informyth in rect and congrue writ-
ynge, and it is taught of Prescian in his more volume[5] from the bigynnyng vnto that part wher he saith a letter is þe last part of mannes voice.
But for more cliere knowlache of þis part we shuln vndirstonde the
nature of our lettris, and firste of the v vowels the whiche han divers
placis and dyvers maners of their generacioun. The placis, as Remygius

---

35. his] *foll. by* power *canc.*

58. *Centered headnotes are also centered in the MS.*

61. Gramer] *marg. in later hand:* Grammer

saith,[6] bien v: the lunges, the throte, the palate, the teeth, and the lippis; the maner of generacioun is in this forme, for generaly whan any
70 substancial voice is caused sumtyme of openyng is more in the mowth
outward than withyn toward the lunges and than it is like a triangle[7]
whos foote is in the mowth, and the poynt in the throte, and this is þe
generacioun of the first letter *a*, and therfor it is in figure like a triangle; or ellis it is contrarie-wise and than is *v* caused, and his figure is
75 turned and hath contrarie situacioun. Somtyme the throte is opened
equaly on every part, and so is *i* caused and therfor it hath a rect and
egal figure. The generacioun of *o* is in rounde openyng of the mowth,
so that the tunge and the lippis bowe theymsilf in their myddis; but *e*
is gendrid in the inward of the throte and the mowth so that the mowth
80 drawith to roundenesse more than the throte, and therfor his figure is
half cercle like a bowe with a part of a strynge in t[h]e over ende. And
for bicause that the place of the **[fol. 246r]** complete generacioun of
the letter *a* is bifore the place of *e*, the place of *e* bifore *i*, and *i* bifore *o*,
and the generacion of *o* is bifore the generacioun of *v*, therfor thiese
85 vowels be so ordeyned *a e i o v*. Furthermore the consonauntis bien
divided, for sum be semyvowels and sum mutis; a semyvowell hath the
sowne of a vowel bifore, but a mvte afterward. The semyvowels bien vj,
and thei bien gendred thurgh touchyng of the tung to on of the palatis
of the mowth. And if it touche the over palate with streyneng out of the
90 tunge so that the pointe of the tunge towchith the palat so is *l* causid,
but if þe tunge be more bowed and in maner with a tremelyng folowyng afterward than is *r* gendred. And if the tung be in party streyned
right and in part bowid so that the sowne goth nat oute completely bi
the mowth but bi the nosethrillis so is *n* caused. And if the tunge tou-
95 che the lower palate twies so is *x*. And if it touche but oones with an hissyng sowne than is *s* gendred, for the sides of the tunge bien joyned to
the sides of the palate. And if it touche the outward part with coniunccioun of the inward part of the lippis so is *m* caused. But the mvtis han
iij placis of their generacioun: the lippis with both rowes of the teeth.
100 If it be thurgh touchyng of the lippis, so that the nether smyte vpon the
over lippe so is *ff*, and if this touchyng be more outward so is *b*, or ellis al
without the mowth and so is *p*. And if the tunge touche the over egge of
the teeth moche with so is *d* caused, or ellis it touchith the same place
more withoute neere the teeth and than is *t* gendred. But if the tung
105 touche the lower egge of the teeth with grete openyng of þe mowth so

95. the] *foll. by* palate *canc.*
103. moche with] *prob. scribal error, poss. caused by confusion with* "mowth" *in the
line above or with* "touchith" *in the following line*

is *k*, or with litel openyng and than is *q*, or ellis it is in a meane bitwixt both and so is *c*. And if the mydpoynt of the tunge touche the nether teeth with a maner liftyng vp of the after part and depressioun of the part bifore of the tung so is *g*. And for bicause that a smoth place and
110 holl, moist and hote, is a goode place for sowne, therfor the consonauntis that bien gendred in suche placis bien cald semyvowels, for they sowne wele, but the place of teeth ne is nat playne ne hote [**fol. 246v**] but cold, for thei bien made of erthly grosse matier. Also þe place of the outward part of the lippis is cold for it is withoute the mowth in the aire,
115 therfor the consonauntis that bien gendred in thiese placis bien cald mvtis, for their fieble sown, &c. Gramer also enformeth mannes soule with triewe vndirstandyng of euery part of reasoun bi hymsilf bi the secunde part that is cald Ethymologye, gyven and taught of Precian in th'end of the grete volume.[8] We bien also informed bi gramer in congru-
120 ite and construccioun of partis of reason toguyder bi the third part that is cald Diasintastik, gevyn of Prescian in the lasse booke.[9] Also gramer enformyth mannes soule with a grete and a due pronunciacioun bi the fourth part cald Prosodie.

Logik

125 The office of Logik is to discerne and discusse that is formed and vndirstanden bi Gramer bi wey of argument and reason techyng the forme of resownyng in every faculte. And so, as Boice saith,[10] an argument is cald a reason of a thyng that is doutful make it certitude and feith of thyng that is douted, but many thynges maken feith, as our
130 sight of thynges that we see, but it is no reason and son argument. And it hath iiij kyndes vnder hym, Induccioun, Exsample, Emtymene, and a Silogisme. Induccioun is whan an vniversal proposicioun is proeved bi al his singuliers. Exsample is whan a thyng is proevid bi another like to hym. Emtyme is a short Silogisme includyng only on premisse and
135 oon conclusioun. But a Silogisme is an argument þe whiche hath ij premysses and proposicions bifore the conclusioun, the whiche premisses grauntid muste nedely folowe the conclusioun bi the saide premysses. Logik is divided into iij partis, Diffynicioun, Particioun, and Colleccioun. Of Diffynicioun and his partis is treatid in old logik, as in Porphi-
140 ries predicamentis,[11] &c. Of Particioun treatith Boes in his divisiouns.[12]

---

107. mydpoynt] myd *ins. above line*

128. make it] *prob. scribal error; poss. the infinitive "to make it" is intended*

130. son argument] *poss. for* sond argument

But Colleccioun is treatid in dyvers wises in the newe logik, for a disputacioun sumtyme procedith in triewe and necessarie argument, the
whiche is cald a de- [fol. 247r] monstracioun. And that may nat be but
in a Silogisme wher boþ premisses and the conclusioun bien necessa-
145 rie proposiciouns. Sumtyme the argument is made in probable proposiciouns the whiche have non evidens, and seme to be triewe to the more
partie of wise men, and it is cald a topical reason, as Aristotil shewith in
his topikes.[13] Sumtyme the proposiciouns be fals in the argument, and
semyth to have a diewe forme of a Silogisme, and it hath nat in deede.
150 And this argument longeþ to the Sophister,[14] whos spices and braunchis bien declared in þe *Elynkes*.[15]

Retorik

And in as moche as th'office of every craft and konnyng is that the artificer owith to do after his craft, th'office of an oratour that he owith to
155 do be Rethorik is to say wele, as Quyntilian saith,[16] that is, to say suche
thynges þe whiche bien convenient and sufficient to persuade; wheither
he persuade or nat, so as he do as longith to the craft, for as the Philosopher saith, an oratour shal nat alwey persuade ne a phisician shal
[n]at al tymes make a man [wel] though he do as his craft wil,[17] for the
160 whiche he is cald an oratour. And so he intendith principaly to excite and
awake theym that bien slugges and sleepers, to gyve audacite to fereful
and tymerous, and to m[e]ke theym that bien cruel and boistous, and
therfor Rethorik is cald Mercuries rod, with whos end he makith slep-
ers to awake, and with that other end, wakyng men to sleepe. This is
165 the harpe of Orphe, with whos melodie stones and trees bien divided,
and a love day is made bitwixt the wulf and the lamb, the dogge and the
hare, the calf and the lioun, whan thei here the sweete of this harp.[18]
This harp and instrument of the oratour hath vj strynges, that is to
say, vj partis of the oracioun, as the begynnyng or Introduccioun, Nar-
170 racioun, Particioun, Confirmacioun, Reprehensioun, and Conclusioun.
The Introduccioun is cald þe bigynnyng, wher the juge or the soule of
the auditour is inclyned to take or gyve attendans to swiche thynges as
shal be saide afterward. Narracioun is a cliere exposicioun of þinges don
and in like forme as thei bien don bi divisioun or Particioun [fol. 247v]
175 we open and shewe that is accordyng to the processe and wherfor is a
contrauersie and striff. And also we declare and expowne of what thyng-

---

159. nat] at   wel] *om.*

162. meke] make (*cf. Lat.* truces mitigare)

175. and (1)] *in marg. marked for ins.*

es we take our accioun. Confirmacioun is exposicioun of our argument
with auctorite. Reprehensioun is a dissolvyng and a ful avoidaunce of
contrary reasons. Conclusioun is a crafti end of the oracioun and of the
180 holl processe bifore.

Arsmetrik

The mathematical sciencis bien iiij: Arethmetrik, Geometry, Musike,
and Astronomy, the whiche bien cald doctrynall sciences for the surenes
of their demonstracioun. But among theym Arethmetrik and Geome-
185 try bien more noble for in makyng of the word God disposed al thynges in mesure, nombre, and weight [cf. Wisdom 11:21]. Of nombris and of
craft of nombryng treatith Arethmetrik, the whiche directith vs both in
Musik and Astronomy for the consonauns or melodie of musik standith in proporcioun of nombris. Also we knowe bi nombres the risyng
190 and goyng doun of sterris, the slownes and swiftnes of planetis, with
many other calculaciouns and variaciouns of the mone.[19] This craft vsith
x figures that wern founde of Algo in Inde, and so it is cald Algorisme,
for *rismon* is no more to say in Greke but a nomber in Inglissh. A nomber
is a multitude made of many vnitees. The vnyte is bigynnyng of every
195 nomber and every nombre is evyn or odde. The evyn number may be
divide into tweyne equal partis, but the odde nomber may nat. The x
figures bien made in this forme: 0 1 2 3 4 5 6 7 8 9. The firste is cald
a cifre, and thei gon so furþ in a natural order til ix. And eche figure
in the first place, þat is, on the right hand, bitokenyth hymsilf; and in
200 the secunde place it bitokenyth x tymes hymsilf; in the thrid place C
tymes hymsilf; in the iiij place a M^l tymes hymsilf, and so furth; but the
cifre bitokenyth nothyng hymsilf but occupieth a place and so makith
another figure that folowith to signifie as his place is. This craft hath ix
partis, the whiche bien cald Numeracioun, Addiscioun, Subtraccioun,
205 Duplacioun, Mediacioun, Multiplicacioun, Divi- **[fol. 248r]** sioun,
Extraxioun of the Roote, and Progressioun. Nvmeracioun is a crafty
representacioun of every nombre by competent figures. Addicioun is
a gaderyng toguydre of oon nombre to another to knowe what sum
growith of both the nombres so that ther shal be twey ordres, oon of þe
210 more nombre, the whiche shal be discryved above, another of the lasse
nombre that shal put to the more nombre. Subtraccioun is a drawyng
away of on nombre from another to knowe what levith, and shal have
ij orders of nombres as in Addiscioun so that the nomber that shal be

---

186. of (2)] of of
209. twey] *foll. by* nombres *canc.*

withdrawen shal be writen in þe lower order, and it must be eqwal or
215 lasse than the nombre fro whom it shal be withdrawen. Duplacioun is
a dublyng of a nombre in hymsilf, and it hath but oon order of figures
wherin we shal begynne at the lift hand and also in Divisioun and Multiplicacioun, and in al other we shuln bigynne at the right hand. Mediacioun is invencioun of the prescice half of a nomber to knowe whiche
220 it is. Multiplicacioun of a nomber bi hymsilf or bi another is whan ij
nombres bien purposed to fynde þe thridde nombre the whiche shal
conteyne as many tymes the nomber þat is multiplied as be vnitees
in the multiplier. Divisioun is whan they be purposed ij nombres to
divide the more nombre into as many partis as bien vnitees in the lasse
225 number. Extraccioun of the Roote of a nombre is for to fynde a nombre
the whiche multiplied hymsilf makith þe purposed nomber; as twies ij
makith iiij, and therfor ij that is multiplied in hymsilf is the roote of iiij.
Progressioun is a gaderyng toguyder of nombres bi equal excesse from
on vnyte or fro ij; than the som of al may be had compendiously, and
230 this progres sumtyme is natural and contynued as j ij iiij iiij v vj, &c.;
sumtyme it is discontynued bi puttyng awey alwey on figure as 2 4 6 8
10. And if the natural progresse end in an evene nomber take his half of
that last nomber and multiplie the next nomber folowyng bi the same
half, and so we may knowe how many strokis the hamour touchith the
235 clocke in the day and nyght.[20] And if the end be in an odde **[fol. 248v]**
nomber, take half of the next nomber that folowith and multiplie bi hym
the forsaide end. And if the progresse from the vnyte be vnyformaly
discontynued, endyng in an evene nomber, take the half of the last
nomber and multiplie in hymsilf and put to hym half of the next evene
240 nombre that folowith and that shal be the holl somme as i ij iiij vj viij:
half viij is iiij and iiij tymes iiij is xvj, next viij even nomber is x, whos
half is v, put to xvj makith xxj, the whiche is the somme. But if th'end in
his progresse be odde nomber, tak the prescice half of the next nomber
that folowith and multiplie in hymsilf, and that shal be the somme, as j
245 [i]ij v vij: half viij is iiij, and iiij tymes iiij is xvj, the whiche is the somme,
&c. But and if the progresse be al in double nombres, the last number
conteyneth the hole somme of theym bifore hym and the vnyte more,
as j ij iiij viij xvj.

---

225. nombre (2)] *foll. by* as twies ij makith iiij *canc.*
241. iiij tymes iiij] *foll. by* tymes *canc.*
245. iij] ij (*error for second odd number in sequence*)

Musik

250 Mvsik informeth in which proporciouns of our moevynges is concorde
of melody. And if this mevyng be sumtyme in part with violence yit it
is nat vttirly agenst nature, ffor whan a stryng of a musical instrument
be violently touchid, the partis so touched be constreyned to go oute
of their situacioun and place, the whiche partis han a natural power
255 inclyneng ageyn too their natural place makith theym to passe their
diewe boundis. And so thei gon out agcyne from their natural situacioun, and after this thurgh natural inclynacioun thei turne ageyne
passyng their diewe situacioun, so that in this maner is caused a contynual tremelyng in the smale partis of a stryng so touched til at the last
260 that this inclynacioun compellith nat the partis to passe their place; and
this maner of tremelyng or shakyng is open to touchyng or sight. This
moevyng of a stryng so streyned in an instrument thurgh the tremelyng
of the smale partis, the whiche partis folowe the local moevynge of the
saide shakynges, is cald a sowne or a natural swiftnes to sowne. And
265 whan the partis of a sownyng thyng thus tremelith, thei moeve the heire
next hem, in like as thei bien [fol. 249r] moeved, and that parte of the
heire the next part, and so furth til it come to the heire in our earis,
and so is heryng caused.[21] Thus be like proporccioun the melodie of
mannes voice, with the rest and moevyng of mannes body is rectified
270 and tempred. And in as mochc as it is biforesaide, Musik standith in
proporciouns of mannes moevyng, the whiche proporciouns mown nat
be without noinbres, thcrfor Musik is vnder Arsmetrik, ffor the modulaciouns or melodies of Musik—as diatesseron that conteyneth ij tunys
and an half, or diapent that conteyneth iij tunes and an half, or dia-
275 pason that conteyneth both diatesseron and diapent[22]—mown nat be
knowe without nombris and proporciouns. For a tvne standith in proporcioun bitwix ix and viij, diatesseron bitwixt viij and vj, and diapason bitwix xij and vj, the whiche nombre is double to vj; and so it is
proeved in experience if a stryng streyned vpon a lute stopped in the
280 myddis eche half shal sowne viij notis above the sowne of the same
stryng nat stopped, the whiche dowble to eche part. This science **Pictagoras** fonde in a smythes shoppe:[23] as he passid furth by, he vndirstode how the sowne of certeyne hamers vpon a stith made a mervel-
ous melody, whan on was put awey, but he was in doubte of whom this
285 melody shuld be caused. And therfor he made the hamers to chaunge
their place, and thei gave like melody whan on was put away as thei
dide bifore, so that he perceived that it was nat caused bi the strength

---

281–282. Pictagoras] *in display script*

of man but thurgh the condiciouns of the hamours, and that he knew bi
proporcioun of nomber, mesure, and weight [cf. Wisdom 11:21], for on
290 hamer weyed double another, and so furth after dyuers proporciouns of
Musik. Than sith it is so that a mannes soule folowith the body in his werkis, as the philosopher saith,[24] and the body also folowith the soule, he
that knowith the natural disposicioun of man, and the proporcioun of
hvmours in mannes body, and how mannes bodily spirites bien dilated
295 with joye, and dried with hevynes, may with melodious proporciouns
of sownes in mvsical instrumentis esily chaunge the desires of mannes
soule from the hevynes of ire to joye and myrth, as Boice declarith in
the bigynnyng of his **[fol. 249v]** *Musik*,[25] and so Musik is necessary for
nature and moral science.[26]

300   *Astronomy*
Astronomye also is ful necessarie for nature in eleccioun of conuenyent
tyme to gyve medicynes, to sette plantis, with other transmutaciouns
that longen to natures vse, ffor nature in the erth may nat werke but it
be moevid bi the vertu of the vij planetis and other sterris, among whom
305 the moone hath special power to joyne the saide vertues with the bodies in the erth. For þat whan the moone growith in light with fortunat
planetis shal make the plaunte to growe and to be fruy[t]ful, but the
coldenesse of Saturne sumtyme distroieth, and the brennyng heete of
Mars may lette the plaunte to growe, and dryenes to welke and be bar-
310 eyne, or at the leste to bere but litel fruyte. But specialy for the goode
rule and policie of the comune wele, Astronomye is most necessarie,
for it is nat sufficient for the comune goode to knowe al thynges, but
also it is expedient to promote þinges knowen that bien profitable and
to remoeve that bien noyous. And if it so be that Arsmetrik, Geometry,
315 and Musik helpe moche in this part, yit Astronomy rulith all, ffor the
werkis of al sciencis and every grete werke requirith tyme convenyent
the whiche is knowen and chosen bi consideracioun of Astronomye;
and therfor Aristotil in the *Booke of Secretis*[27] techith Alexander that he
ne shuld ete ne drynke ne do nothyng without counsail of astronomers,
320 for al thynges han convenyent tyme, as Salamon saide [Ecclesiastes 3:1–
8] that was wiser than Aristotil. But peraduenture ye wil say that an
astronomer may nat lette ne chaunge thoo thynges that God hath provided withouten end. Aristotil and other clerkis aunswern to this[28] and
seyn that the deedis of thynges the whiche God hath put in power of
325 man bien nat necessary, but that man may cheese bi his fre wil, whiche
part he wil have, though it so be that God knowith whiche part he wil
take. And so a goode astronomer may remoeve many impedymentis, as

Aristotil gyvith ensample:[29] If a grete cold be comyng, an astronomer
may purvey remedy, ordeyneng hoote placis, hoote clothis, and hoote
330 metis, so that the cold shal nat hurt hym, wheras other that knowen nat
Astronomy shuln **[fol. 250r]** be gretely greved therwith; and in like wise
of deth in the see or in batail, as Isaac seith and Ptholome also saith,[30]
that a wise man is lord of sterris and the reasoun of his soule shal helpe
the werkyng of theym, as a goode tilier helpith the natural strength of
335 the erth if [God] wil. Than sith it is so that ther bien sum werkis only of
nature, and sum that longith both to vse and nature, thiese vij special
sciences bifore rehersed bien partis and pilers of philosophie, and rectifie makyng parfite both our werkis and of nature; and for as moche as
the disposicioun of konnyng is to be a rule and guydyng of our opera-
340 cioun, as Lyncolniens saith,[31] therfor thiese vij afore other mown wele
be cald sciences and konnynges.

Geometrie is saide of geo in Greeke that is lond
and metron that is mesure.

Geometrie that treatith of stable and vnmoevable þinges is a special and
345 a noble sciens amonge th'other that treaten of moevable thynges, like
as rest and stablenes is bifore every moevyng. Also saged enserchers
of konnyng, namly Pictagoras with his folowers,[32] commendid gretely
geometry, for it sharpith moche and orderith mannes wit, and causith
in man grete redynes to vndirstonde many thynges. And it is the comune
350 oppynion and expcriens that it profiteth nat only whan it is lierned as
other sciences, but also it is right profitable and delectable in liernyng.
And nat withoute grete cause right famows men gaf grete attendaunce
and diligence to this science, for the sikernes of geometrical demonstracioun certifieth a man more clierly both in Astronomy, also in per-
355 spectif and in science of ponders and weightis, causith men to be gretely
magnified. For in Astronomy is necessarie both cercle and centre, with
cercles of equal distaunce, as it is shewid in the Spiere.[33] Also the north
poole and the sowth, with the axiltre and many suche other in perspectif is necessarie to knowe the proces and the goyng furth of beames
360 from a mannes eye; and from other thynges bi a right lyne, thurgh whos
touchyng is made a triangle, and the brekyng of the saide beames whan
they come to a more subtil body, with refleccioun of theym in myr-
rours and in other **[fol. 250v]** polite and smoth bodies; and this perspectif is also notable, delectable, profitable, and necessarie sciens.[34]
365 For as the Philosopher saith, bifore al other outward wittis we cheese

---

335. God] goode

and commende the sight, the cause is, for it shewith to vs and makith vs
to knowe many diversitees of thynges more than any other wit, for the
figure, gretnes, and multitude of hevenly bodies we knowe in seeyng
theym with the astrolabie and with other instrumentis,[35] and of thynges
370 in the erth we have experience bi our sight; ffor a blynd man shal nat
gyve no iugement of colours. And namly, in craft of mensuracioun, of
whiche craft is divided in iiij partis: in Altimetrie, Planymetrie, and Profundymetrie.[36] Altimetrie techith to mesure a thyng bi his height, and
we may mesure the height of a thyng in divers wises. As if ye wil knowe
375 the height of a thyng bi his quadraunt or triangle, behold and considre
the hiest part of the thyng thurgh both holis of the quadraunt, and go
toward or froward the thyng til the perpendicule plom fal vpon the
mydlyne of the quadraunt, that is to say, vpon xlv degrees. After this
ye shal take the length fro youre eye to the erth and marke the place
380 of your standyng to the grounde of the thynge that ye mesure, and put
therto þe length from your eye to your foote, and al that toguyder shal be
the mesure of the altitude that ye wil have, as is shewed in picture.[37] Also
whan the sonne is xlv grees high above the orisont, the whiche may be
knowe if the sonne shyne thurgh both hooles of the quadraunt, than
385 ye shal mesure the shadewe, and that is iustly the altitude of the same
thyng. Also if ye wil mesure the height of a thyng bi his shadowe, every
houre of þe day whan it hath shadewe, take a right and a playne wande of
ij foote long or iij, and set vp in a playne and mesure þe wandis shadewe.
After that ye shal mesure the shadewe of the thynge that ye wil mesure,
390 and this shadewe ye shall multiplie bi the length of the wande, and that
growith by multiplicacioun shal be divided bi the shadewe of the wand,
and than the nombre quocient shal shewe the altitude and the mesure
therof, &c.
       [fol. 251r] Also if ye wil knowe the altitude bi a glas vpon the playne
395 grounde and go toward the glas and froward til ye see the hiest poynt
in the myddes of the glas, than yee shul multiplie the space from the
foote of the high thyng to the glas bi the distaunce from your eye to
the erth, and that growith bi multiplicacioun yee shal divide bi the distaunce bitwene your foote and the glas, and than the quocient shal shewe
400 the altitude of the thynge. For as the distaunce from your eye to the erth
hath hym in certeyne proporcioun to the distaunce bitwene your foote
and the glas, in like proporcioun hath hymsilf the altitude of the thyng
to the space the whiche is bitwene the grounde of the thyng and the
glas, as it may be shewid in this picture.

---

393. therof &c] *catchword* Also

405   Planymetrie techith the mesure, the breede, or the length of a
certeyne grounde. And this may be without the quadraunt or triangle:
yee shul take twey evene roddis of a certeyne quantite, and on shal be
cald a b, and that other rodde c d, and the space that ye wil mesure
shal be named B E ; than yee shal ta[ke] a b and reise hym recte vpon
410   the erth, than ye shul joyne c d with a b makyng with a b a rect angule
so that it be in like distaunce in every part from the space; afterward
yee shal put your eye bi the over end of a b, consideryng th'end of the
space that yee wil mesure, than marke the place where the sight goeth
bi the rodde c d. Than yee shal multiplie a b bi the quantite of c d, and
415   that growith bi multiplicacioun ye shal divide bi the quantite of a c and
so shal ye have the mesure of the length, &c.
       Profundemetrie to mesure the depnes of a welle or of a rounde pitte.
And if ye wil knowe the mesure of depnes of a welle bi the quadraunt, ye
shal hold the corner of the quadraunt wher the marke is fixed toward
420   your eye and the circumferens toward the pit or the welle, and shal yee
look thurgh both hoolis from that on side of the welle to that further
side from yow as far as yee may see dounward. Than ye shal considre
the nombre of the poyntes in the quadraunt discribed withyn the triangule, wher the perpendicle **[fol. 251v]** lyne fallith. Than ye shal mesure
425   the diametre of the welle, the whiche yee shal multiplie bi xij, and bi
nomber of the poyntes wher the perpendicle lyne fallith. And the
nomber quocient shal shewe the depnes of the welle, as it appierith in
picture.
       In science also of ponders is necessarie to knowe porciouns and par-
430   tis of cerclis with the strynge and the bowe discrived by rotacioun and
goyng aboute of the beame with proporcioun in longitude and thiknes of
the beame and angulis with triangulis and suche other many, the whiche
al be shewed bi Geometrie. And Euclide techeþ in his booke[38] wher he
treatith of perpendicler lynes with angules, tryangulis, quadraungulis,
435   cerculis, and proporciouns of the same, withoute the whiche edificacioun in stone and tymber, for saluacioun or defence of mannes nature
for grete cold and heete, can nat be hadde, beside the grete craft in
trussyng and ereccioun of high thynges as stepils, the whiche requireth
nat only of konnyng and strength of rect and perpendiculier lyne, the
440   whiche is most strong of al lynes, as the Philosopher saith, but also grete
pollicie in chesyng of convenient matier for the saide trussyng or ereccioun. And this konnyng of the perpendiculier is most shewed in tymber, ffor in trussyng above the erth is proevid the strength of the perpendiculier in this matier.
445   But here we shal vnderstonde that in Geometrie bien iij maner of
quantitees: on that hath but on dymencioun, that is cald length, as a

lyne; the secunde that hath ij dymenciouns, boþ length and breede, as a floore; the thridde that hath iij dymenciouns, length, breede, and depnesse, as a busshel, a galoun, or a house, &c. And generaly to knowe

450 any quantite is no more but to knowe how many tymes a lesse quantite is conteyned in the same. As if ye wil knowe how many greynes of whete in length bien conteyned in a mile, ye shal vndirstande that a myle hath many partis, a furlong, a perche or a rod, a cubite, a foote, an inche, and a grayne: iij graynes in length maken an inche, xij inches maken

455 a foote, a foote and an half makith a cubite, ij cubites makith a degre, ij degres and an half maken a passe, C passis maken a furlong and xxx foote, viij furlonges maken a myle. Also xviij **[fol. 252r]** foote maken a rod, xl roddis maken a furlong, and so bi multiplicacioun and divisioun ye may knowe how many graynes in length maken a myle, and

460 how many ferthynges bien in C li., and how moche he may expende in the yeere that may expende every day iij d.[39] Furthermore the secunde quantite, that hath ij dymensiouns as a floore, sumtyme is made of recte lynes, sumtyme of circulis or partis therof. A floore of rect lynes is sumtyme triangule, or quadrat, or quadraungule, or multi-angule havyng

465 many angulis.

Than if ye wil mesure a quadrate floore, take þe mesure of on rib of the quadrate, as if the rib conteyne ij foote the holl quadrate conteyneth iiij tymes so moche, and so it shal be viij foote.[40] And if ye wil knowe a quadrangule floore, multiplie on rib bi another rib that

470 makith an angule with hym, as if a rib conteyne viij foote and another xx foote,[41] the holl floore shal conteyne lxxx foote. But if it be a floore that haþ ij ribbes equal and other ij of another equal mesure withoute any rect angule, than drawe a lyne perpendiculier from oon side to another, and bi this lyne multiplie the side that he dividith, as if the

475 saide perpendiculier lyne conteyne iiij foote and his rib vj foote, the floore shal conteyne xl,[42] as it is proeved in the speculacioun of Euclide. As for triangule flooris, if the triangule have al sides equal, than ye shal divide on of theym in ij equal partis, and from the poynt of division, drawe a lyne to the angule agenst hym and this lyne yee shul

480 multiply bi an half of the lyne bifore divided; as if this lyne so drawen conteyne iiij foote and the half side ij foote, the holl floore shal conteyne viij foote. And if the triangule have but ij equal sides, drawe a lyne from the myd point of therde inequal side to the angule agenste hym and than multiplie the lyne so drawen bi the half of the inequal lyne

485 as ye dide bifore. And if al the sides of the triangule floore be inequall, drawe a perpendiculier lyne from the lengest side to the angule agenste hym, the whiche lyne yee shal divide in the myddis and bi oon half therof ye shal multiplie the lengest side; as if oon half conteyne ij foote

and the lengest side iiij foote, the hole triangle [**fol. 252v**] conteyneth
490 viij foote. And if it be a floore of many angulis made with rect lynes, ye
shal reduce al the floore in quadraungulis or triangulis, and afterward
mesure eche of theym bi hymsilf after the craft of triangule floores and
that is gadered shal be conteyned in the holl floore and no more.

But for to know reduccioun of a figure into his quadrate yee shal
495 vnderstande that if yee knowe how many cubites or how many foote the
floore conteyneth, than yee shal take the length of al þe floore and
therto yee shal put the latitude contynued with the length, than yee shal
make a perpendiculier lyne at th'ende of the firste length, and put the
foote of the compas inmoevable in the myddis of the hole lyne, dis-
500 crivyng a semycercle. Than marke wher the circumference dividith the
perpendiculier and from that point to the poynt of addicioun of the
latitude of the floore shal be of a quadrate conteyneng the forsaide
floore, as it is shewid in figure and is proevid bi the last conclusioun
of the secunde booke of Euclide.[43] Also if ye wil have a quadrate dou-
505 ble to a quadrate assigned, discrive a lyne from that on angule to that
other angule agenst hym and that shal be a rib of a double quadrate, as
it is proved bi the last conclusioun of the firste booke of Euclide.[44] Also
if yee wil knowe a quadrate conteyneng ij quadratis assigned, discrive
ij lynes dividyng theymsilf perpendiculerly conteyneng the length of
510 oon quadrate in on side of the cros and of that oþer quadrate in that
other side, than drawe a lyne from end to end and that lyne is a rib of
a quadrate conteyneng both, and thus ye may reduce C quadratis into
on quadrate. First make a grete angule and a rect and cut as moche
awey of on lyne as aunswerith[45] to on quadrate, and as moche of that
515 other lyne as aunswerith to that other quadrate. Than drawe a lyne
from poynt to poynt and that lyne is a rib of a quadrate conteyneng ij
quadratis assigned. Afterward make anoþer rect angule and divide on
lyne after the quantite of the forsaide grete rib and in that other lyne
take the quantite of the thrid quadrate and drawe a lyne from poynt
520 to poynt and that lyne shal conteyne al iij quadratis, and so shal yee do
if [**fol. 253r**] yee have C quadratis begynnyng alwey to take mesure at
the rect angule.

And if ye wil mesure a flore havyng the forme of an holl cercle, ye
shal take his diametre, that is to say, a lyne that dividith the circule in ij
525 equal partis, yee shal make iij tymes and put therto the vij part of a dyametir,[46] and than is the circumferens had. Afterward, take half of the
diametir and multiplie bi that half the circumferens and ye shal have

---

494. a] *foll. by* floore *canc.*
520. al] *ins. above line*

the floore of the holl circule;[47] as if the dyametir of a rounde floore be
xiiij foote, treble xiiij and it is xlij, than put to hym the vij part, that is
530 ij, and ye shal have xliiij, the whiche is circumferens of the floore; and
bi vij, that is half the diametre, multiplie half the circumferens, the
whiche is xxij, and ye shal have C [l]iiij foote and that is the floore. And
if ye wil have mesure of a floore rounde as a bal yee shal multiplie the
circumferens bi the dyametir; as if the diametre have xiiij foote, the
535 circumference xliiij, xiiij tymes xliiij makith vj C xvj, the whiche is the
hole floore of the bal or of the spiere. And ye shal vndrestande that if
the diametir of a spiere be double to the diameter of another spiere,
the floore shal be quadruple to the lasse floore, and in like wise in a
playne rounde floore but if the diametir be double the circumferens
540 shal be double. Also if yee mesure a floore havyng part of a circule and
a rect lyne yee shal multiplie half the bowe bi half the rect lyne; as if on
half be iiij foote and that other half vj foote, vj tymes iiij is xxiiij, the
whiche is the holl floore. And if it be a floore made of many divers porciouns of circulis, withoute any rect lyne, yee shal divide the holl floore
545 in dyuers floores, havyng in eche of hem both a part of a circule and
a rect lyne. And than ye shal mesure eche of theym bi the craft bifore,
mesuryng eche floore bi hymsilf, and than put hem al toguyder and
that shal be the holl floore. And I suppose ther is no floore but it may
be mesured in this same craft.
550   Furthermore to mesure a body that hath iij dymensiouns, length,
breede, and profundite or thikenes, we shuln considre if the body be
vnyforme [fol. 253v] in his dymensiouns or no; it is cald vnyforme in
his dymensiouns, whan the body hath equal thikkenes in every part of
his floore. Than if ye wil mesure a body havyng vnyforme thikkenes,
555 first ye shal knowe the floore, the whiche ye shal multiplie bi the thikkenes; as if it be a body havyng ij foote in length, iiij in brede and xx
in thiknes, multiplie ij bi iiij and that is viij, than multiplie viij bi the
thiknes, the whiche is xx, and ye shal have C lx foote, and that is the
veray quantite of the body. And ye shal vnderstonde that whan it is
560 saide, that a thyng conteyneth so many foote or so many inchis, it is
comunely take for a foote square iche wey, and for an inche iche wey,
and so of al other mesures.
      Bvt beside thiese vij sciences ther bien other vij[48] that bien nat
cald special sciences, but rather vsual or comune craftis and hand werk-
565 is the whiche bien daily vsed and exercised of comune artificers and

---

532. C liiij foote] ciiij foote; *marg. corr. in later hand (John Fortho's?):* 154 foote
550. Furthermore] *marg. ann., same hand as* 154 foote *(poss. Fortho's?), symbol for
section* (§)

werkmen, as tilieng, venery, phisik, theatrik, lanyfice, armery, navigacioun. The first is agriculture or tilieng, standith in iiij thynges: In tilieng of fieldis, pastures, woodis, and gardynes. Venery conteyneth al
occupacioun in huntyng, fowlyng, ffisshyng, with al dightyng of metis
570 and drynkes and generaly al craftis of fisshmongers, bochiers, tauerners, and brewers. Phisike considerith the qualitees of mannes body
and techith in werkyng bi medicynes to bryng helth into the partis of
mannes body and to bryng sikcnes [out]. The[at]rik techith craft in
al maner of pleyes ffor the[at]rik is cald the place of pleyeng and of
575 sportis. Lanefice conteyneth al maner of wevyng and werkyng in wulle
threde, cloth, skynnes, baskettis or mattis, and so furth, as tailours,
hosiers or drapiers, fullers, shermen, and skynners. Armery nat only
vsith instrumentis for shippes and bataile but also makith instrumentis
for the same. Navigacioun conteyneth al marchaundise and aventures
580 bi the water and al thynges to bc bought and sold. And þiese vij bc not
cald sciences or vcray konnynges propirly and [fol. 254r] mercers, gro-
cers, and suche other comunely, that is to say, a maner of knowlache in
a thyng, and therfor thei bien cald but instrumentis and mynistres to
philosophie and to the vij liberal and special sciences, namely to the iiij
585 mathamatical. But specialy to Geometry and his partis, for ther is more
certitude and evidence in demonstracioun in deduccioun of his conclusioun, bi the whichc demonstracioun veray kunnyng is caused and
brought into mannes [soule] (as the Philosopher declarith in many placis),[49] than in many other sciencis, and so folowith the contrarie, that
590 is errour and ignoraunce, is expelled and put oute of mannes soule.
For the whiche the vij special sciences bien necessarie and principaly
ordeyned, as it was saide in the bigynnyng of this writyng thurgh the
wisdam of the fader of hevene, who be blessid withouten end. Amen.

A rewle to make a square of a rounde cercle as thus: ffirst make youre
595 cercle and drawe a square from side to side of the cercle; than drawe a
crosse from corner to corner and divide the space from the brymme of
the cercle to the corner of the square in x partis equal and vj partis of
the x partis from the cercle, and in like wise at the corners. And drawe
from vj to vj and take there a parfite square of a cercle, as thus an exam-
600 ple. *The example wantinge: I thoughte good to adde it Joh: Fortho*

---

573. out] *om.*

573–574. Theatrik . . . theatrik] Theorik . . . theorik

588. mannes soule] mannes (*cf.* put oute of mannes soule *below*)

594. *In the three geometrical exercises that follow, roman type represents the hand of the main scribe and italic the additions by John Fortho; underlining by Fortho. I am grateful to Tess Tavormina for her adaptations of Fortho's diagrams in figures 2a–2c below.*

[*diagram drawn in right margin by Fortho; see figure 2a, p. 728 below*]

Also a rewle to turne a square in a cercle as thus: first multiple the proporcioun of the square with xiiij and divide it bi xj. And werke the contrarie to turne a cercle in a square, as thus an example. *The exeample
heere also wantinge vide infra.*

[*diagram pasted in right margin by Fortho; see figure 2b, p. 729 below*]

605 **[fol. 254r, lower margin]** *I haue heere in þe margente sett þe example at þe
ende of þe descriptione, þe first parte of it seruinge to make a circle in a giuen
square, where þe sides of þe square are 2 foote, which 2 multeplied by 14 produce
28 & þat deuided by 11 þe quotiente is 2 foote & 3/14 of a foote, which is þe
diameter of þe circle, þe one halfe whereof describes þe circle within þe quadrate
610 giuen, markt with b b b b.*
  *The 2ᵈ parte serues to describe a quadrate within a giuen circle where þe
worke is contrarye, 2 beinge to be multeplied by 11, þe fact or product is 22 &
þat deuided by 14 þe quotient is 1 foote 8/14 in þe poincted line from c to c,
which makes þe seueral sides of the inmoste quadrate described within þe circle,
615 & markt with d d d d—so I haue ioygned boath in one scheame. John Fortho.
[And] þe like may be donne by any other quadrate or [circle?] whatsoeuer* [illeg-
ible due to cropping]

 [right margin under pasted-in diagram] *That þis is þe true meaninge of
þe authore I doubte not & I haue a litle strainde my compasse to make good his*
620 *conclusion, especially in þe later parte where 1 7/14 came nigher þe truthe þen 1
8/14; but I had rather impute it to my owne error in settinge þe compasse soone
committed then to þe rule þe rather because þe former parte* [illegible due to
cropping].
 A tree of l foote of height felle every day oo foote: whan shall the hede
625 of the tree rest on the grounde? At lxxx daies. To prove that triewe do
thus: take a compas and make a cercle and divide the cercle from the
centre into iiij partis equal; than with the compas divide oon of the iiij
partis that strecchith from the cercle to the centre bi v partis. And that
don, name [fol. 254v] every oon part of tho v partis x, than divide the
630 iiij part of þe cercle aboute bi the same x and the quocient wil shewe
viij, the whiche is x tymes viij, and that makith lxxx, and on that day
shal the hed of the tree rest on the grounde, as thus an example:

---

632. on the] on the on the

[fol. 254v, on pasted-in diagram by Fortho *(see figure 2c, p. 730 below)*]
The tree of 50 foote high
The plaine or grounde þe toppe falls to
635 *The arche þe tree toppe makes in his fall*
So þe headde of þe tree beinge 50 foote highe makes 80 foote circumference in his
fall, and by consequence is 80 dayes eare it towche þe grownde. John Fortho.

So <u>Friar</u> <u>Bacon</u> explained

<Addition of mine}> A tree of 50 f. high makes 80 f. fall in arche, 70 in
640   *hypotenusa.—vt sup.—A.*
    A tree of 30 f. high makes 48 f. fall in arch, 42 in
    hypotenusa.—vt sup.—B

Hence

The same tree of 50 foote highe shall fall to þe grownde
645 *in 80 dayes by fallinge a foote a daye in arche & in 70*
dayes by fallinge a foote a daye in Hypoten.
<Obiect> And þe same tree of 30 f. highe shall touche þe grownde
with his tope in 48 d. by fallinge euery d. a foote in arche
— and in 42 dayes by fallinge euery d. a foote in hypot-
650 *enusa or chorde.*

Againe þe 30 foote high tree tyed to 50 f. highe & fallinge
[fol. 255r, at bottom of page] *boath with one equall*
motion lett downe together, the 50 foote high toppe shall
touche þe grownde þe same daye þat þe 30 foote high shall
655 *— and þe 30 f. high þat þe 50 — whether respectinge*
theire seuerall arches or hypotenusas or mixt.

---

633. The tree of 50 foote high] *along inner side of vertical axis, marked off at origin (labeled 1), 10, 20, 30, 40, and 50 units, with the letters "A" and "B" at 50 and 30 respectively*

634. The plaine or grounde þe toppe falls to] *along inner side of horizontal axis*

635. The arche þe tree toppe makes in his fall] *along an arc from point A on vertical axis to horizontal axis*

636–637. So þe headde . . . grownde. John Fortho] *below diagram*

651. fallinge] *catchword by Fortho:* boath

Figures 2a–2c

Geometrical diagrams after John Fortho's drawings in Cambridge, Trinity College, MS R.14.52, fol. 254r–v.

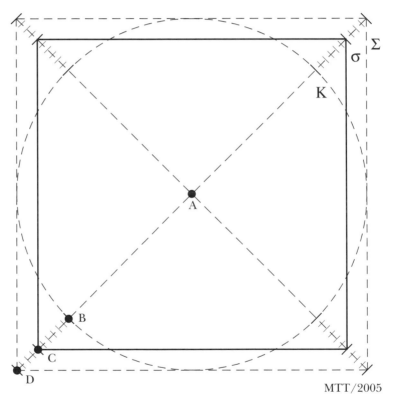

MTT/2005

Figure 2a. Geometrical diagram for squaring the circle, after John Fortho's drawing in Cambridge, Trinity College MS R.14.52, fol. 254r (cf. lines 594–600 above).

K, the circle of radius **AB**, has an area of $\pi(\mathbf{AB})^2$; Σ, the square inscribed around **K**, has an area of $(2[\mathbf{AB}])^2 = 4(\mathbf{AB})^2$.

AD, the half-diagonal of Σ, has a length of $\sqrt{2}\,(\mathbf{AB})$, so **BD** = **AD** − **AB** = $(\sqrt{2}-1)(\mathbf{AB}) \approx (.4142)(\mathbf{AB})$; by construction, **BC** = .6(**BD**) $\approx$ .6(.4142)(**AB**) = (.2485)(**AB**); **AC** = **AB** + **BC** = 1.2485(**AB**).

Thus, the area of σ, the square whose area approximates the area of the circle **K**, is $(\sqrt{2}[\mathbf{AC}])^2 \approx 2[1.2485(\mathbf{AB})]^2 \approx 3.12(\mathbf{AB})^2$, a reasonable approximation of $\pi(\mathbf{AB})^2$. [− *Ed.*]

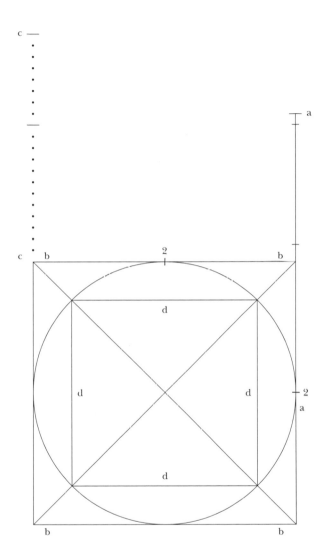

MTT/2005

Figure 2b. Geometrical diagram for calculating the relative areas of a square and a circle inscribed within the square, after John Fortho's drawing in Cambridge, Trinity College MS R.14.52, fol. 254v (cf. lines 601–623 above).

Let **S** = the area of a square with side 2b; let **C** = area of circle of diameter 2b, radius b

$$\mathbf{S} = (2b)^2 = 4b^2; \quad \mathbf{C} = \pi b^2 \approx \left(\tfrac{22}{7}\right)b^2.$$

Then $\dfrac{\mathbf{S}}{\mathbf{C}} \approx \dfrac{4b^2}{\frac{22b^2}{7}} = \left(\tfrac{14}{11}\right)$, $\mathbf{S} = \mathbf{C}\left(\tfrac{14}{11}\right)$, and $\mathbf{C} = \mathbf{S}\left(\tfrac{11}{14}\right)$.

Note that Fortho has misunderstood the proportions to refer to the linear dimensions of the square and circle (sides and diameter), rather than their areas, as well as adding a superfluous "inmoste quadrate" and misdividing 28 by 11 to yield $2\tfrac{3}{14}$ instead of the correct $2\tfrac{6}{11}$. [– *Ed.*]

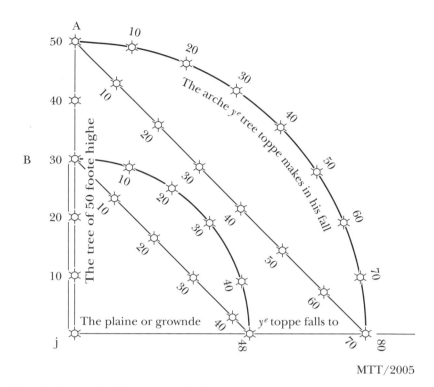

MTT/2005

Figure 2c. Geometrical diagram for calculating the distance traveled along an arc or the chord subtending an arc, after John Fortho's drawing in Cambridge, Trinity College MS R.14.52, fol. 254r (cf. lines 624–656 above).

For a circle of radius 50 and circumference **C**, **C** = $2\pi r \approx 314.16$; ¼ **C** ≈ 78.5.

The chord that subtends the quarter-circle arc is the hypotenuse of a right triangle with equal legs of length 50; its length is thus $\sqrt{2}$ (50), or approximately 70.7.

Similarly, for a circle of radius 30, ¼ **C** = 47.1, and the length of the subtending chord = $\sqrt{2}$ (30), or approximately 42.4.

Fortho's figures of 80 (also given in the original text), 70, 48, and 42 feet are thus reasonably close to the lengths of the arcs and chords drawn in the diagram. [– *Ed.*]

Explanatory Notes

[1] **as seynt Paul seith:** Probably a conflation of texts, including Ephesians 3:9–11, Romans 5, and Gal. 4:4, "ubi venit plenitudo temporis . . . ," quoted notably by Langland in the Tree of Charity scene in *Piers Plowman* B.16.

[2] **as Lincoln saith:** Robert Grosseteste, bishop of Lincoln, *De artibus liberalibus*, ed. Baur 1912, 1–7. See also Baur 1917, 12–25; Callus 1955, 16–22.

[3] **As for our . . . desire:** Grosseteste, *De artibus liberalibus*, ed. Baur 1912, p. 1, lines 19–21.

[4] **Furthermore if we . . . maken direccioun:** Grosseteste, *De artibus liberalibus*, ed. Baur 1912, p. 4, lines 10–14.

[5] **is taught of Prescian in his more volume:** Priscian, *Ars major*; or perhaps the first sixteen books of his *Ars minor* or *Institutiones grammaticae*, called *Priscianus major*. The latter includes a subchapter "De voce" at the beginning of book 1, followed by "De litera," which begins, "Litera est pars minima vocis," which could be translated as here, "a letter is þe last [scribal error for 'least'?] part of mannes voice." Since the short subchapter "De voce" does not deal with orthography, it is difficult to conceive what the author intends here. Perhaps a medieval compilation of texts on grammar, ascribed to Priscian, included a chapter on orthography that preceded the classical Priscian's book 1. No such text is found among the Middle English grammars edited by D. Thomson (1984). For the proliferation of Latin Priscian grammars, see Gibson 1972; for the classical text, see *Grammatici Latini,* ed. H. Keil [1855–1880] 1961, 2:5–6.

[6] **as Remygius saith:** Remigius of Auxerre, *Expositio super Donatum* or *In artem Donati minorem commentum* (commentary on Aelius Donatus's *Ars grammatica minor*): ed. Fox 1902; see also Lutz 1956.

[7] The cavity of the mouth, viewed from the side, is an isosceles triangle whose pointed angle is in the throat for production of the letter *A*, so the letter is shaped like an isosceles triangle. At the opposite extreme, the angle is reversed, with its pointed angle at the opening of the mouth, for production of the letter *U*, so the shape of that letter is like an upside-down *A*. In the middle between these two, the letter *I* is generated when neither end of the mouth is wider, so the shape of the letter is a straight line. The other two vowels are also described in relation to this schema.

[8] **bi the secunde part that is cald Ethymologye, gyven and taught of Precian in th'end of the grete volume:** The "grete volume" might be Priscian's *Ars major*, or perhaps the first sixteen books of his *Ars minor*, as above, Explanatory Note 5. He deals with derivations, similar to etymologies, toward the end of book 2 of the latter (ed. H. Keil [1855–1880] 1961, 2:56–68), but not in books 15 or 16, as suggested by the author here ("th'end of the grete volume").

[9] **bi the third part that is cald Diasintastik, gevyn of Prescian in the lasse book:** The "lasse book" might be Priscian's *Institutiones grammaticae* or *Ars minor*, or only the last two books thereof, called *Priscianus minor*. He does deal

with "gramer in congruite and construccioun of partis of reason" in the last two books (17 and 18). See H. Keil [1855–1880] 1961, 3:106–377.

[10] **as Boice saith:** Boethius, *De topicis differentiis*, commentary on Cicero's *Topics*. See Chadwick 1981, 117–18; Stump 1978. Or perhaps Boethius's commentary on Porphyry's *Isagoge* is intended. See *Boethii In Isagogen Porphyrii commenta* 1.9 (*PL* 64:74).

[11] **as in Porphiries predicamentis:** Probably a reference to Porphyry's discussion of five predicables in his *Isagoge* (to which Boethius wrote a translation and commentary). "Old logic" or *logica vetus* refers to the school of logic based on the first two books of Aristotle's *Organon*, Porphyry's *Isagoge*, and Boethius's commentaries on them, as distinct from the "new logic" which grew up in the second half of the twelfth century. See Crombie 1953, 24–25 and n. 1; Courtenay 1987, 221–40.

[12] **Of Particioun treatith Boes in his divisiouns:** Boethius, *Liber de divisione* (*PL* 64:875–92).

[13] **as Aristotil shewith in his topikes:** Aristotle's *Topics* 1.1 (Barnes 1984, 1:167–277). The *Topics* was translated and commented upon by Boethius (*PL* 64:909–1008).

[14] **Sophister:** Aristotle.

[15] **þe *Elynkes*:** Aristotle's *Elenchi*, or *Sophistical Refutations* (Barnes 1984, 1:278–314); translated by Boethius (*PL* 64:1007–40).

[16] **as Quyntilian saith:** Quintilian, whose *Institutio oratoria* was not available as a complete text in the Middle Ages, though its contents were summarized in medieval encyclopedias.

[17] **as the Philosopher saith, an oratour . . . as his craft wil:** In medieval texts, *philosophus* usually refers to Aristotle; e.g., John Gower repeatedly calls Aristotle by the general title "the philosopher" in his *Confessio Amantis*, book 7.

[18] **And so he . . . the harpe of Orphe . . . sweete of this harp:** Grosseteste, *De artibus liberalibus* (ed. Baur 1912, p. 2, lines 3–9); for other sources, see Baur, p. 2, n. 1. The details about the powers of Orpheus's harp are also found in Martianus Capella, *De nuptiis Philologiae et Mercurii* 9.907 (ed. Dick [1925] 1978, 480–81; trans. Stahl and Johnson 1977, 2:351–52).

[19] **The mathematical sciences bien iiij . . . variaciouns of the mone:** This whole passage is taken from Boethius, *De institutione arithmetica* 1.1.

[20] **how many strokis . . . day and nyght:** The chiming of a clock is taken as an example of a sequence ending in an even number, 12; the arithmetic exercise is that by halving 12 to get 6 and then multiplying that 6 by the next number in the sequence, 13, one arrives at 78, the same figure as one gets by adding the numbers in the sequence 1 through 12, the number of times a clock chimes in a twelve-hour period. For emergence of clock time as the standard in late fourteenth- and fifteenth-century England, see Mooney 1993a.

[21] **And if this mevyng . . . parte of the heire . . . is heryng caused:** Grosseteste, *De generatione sonorum* (ed. Baur 1912, 7–10; for this passage, see p. 7, lines 5–24). The unusual spelling "heire" for "air" may be intended to suggest an etymological relationship to hearing.

[22] **diatesseron . . . diapent . . . diapason that conteyneth both diatesseron and diapent:** Medieval musical theory used these ancient Greek terms for the intervals of a fourth (diatessaron) and a fifth (diapente) and for the interval that includes all tones, that is, the octave (diapason). See Randel 1978, s.vv. *diapason*, *diapent*, and *diatesseron*.

[23] **Pictagoras fonde in a smythes shoppe:** The story of Pythagoras discovering the ratios of consonances in a smithy is told many times, e.g., Boethius, *De musica libri V*, 1.10.

[24] **as the philosopher saith:** Probably also a reference to Boethius, since he discusses the influence of music on both body and soul in *De musica* 1.1.

[25] **as Boice declarith in the bigynnyng of his *Musik*:** Boethius, *De musica* 1.1. See Boethius, *Fundamentals of Music*, trans. Bower, ed. Palisca 1989, 1–8.

[26] **Than sith . . . moral science:** Grosseteste, *De artibus liberalibus* (ed. Baur, p. 4, line 35–p. 5, line 20).

[27] **Aristotil in the *Booke of Secretis*:** Pseudo-Aristotle, *Secretum secretorum*. In the Middle English Ashmole version, written soon after 1445, from Bodleian Library MSS Ashmole 396 and Lyell 36, book 1: "O Kyng most meke, yf it may be, rise not neyther sitte not, ete not, neyther drynke not, neyther in maner no thyng do, with-out the counseill of a perfite astronomyer" (ed. Manzalaoui 1977, 46). Besides its appearance here, the *Secreta secretorum* plays an important role in the Baconian and pseudo-Baconian treatises in the first section of Trinity R.14.52, both in connection with astronomy and as a general source of behavioral advice. See the translations of the pseudonymous *De retardatione accidentium senectutis* (ed. Everest and Tavormina) and the authentic longevity treatises *In debito regimine* and *Corpora Adae et Evae* (ed. Tavormina) in chaps. 6 and 9 above passim, and the Index of Persons, Places, and Works, s.n. *Aristotil*.

[28] **Aristotil and other clerkis aunswern to this:** Pseudo-Aristotle, *Secretum secretorum* 1 (cf. Manzalaoui 1977, 46).

[29] **as Aristotil gyvith ensample:** Pseudo-Aristotle, *Secretum secretorum* 1, immediately following the passages cited in Explanatory Notes 27 and 28 (cf. Manzalaoui 1977, 47).

[30] **as Isaac seith and Ptholome also saith:** Perhaps Isaac Judaeus or Israeli (d. ca. 932), *De diaetis universalibus et particularibus libri II* (Basel, 1570), esp. 1.2; and Ptolemy, *Tetrabiblos* 1.3, ed. and trans. F. E. Robbins 1940, 21–35.

[31] **as Lyncolniens saith:** Grosseteste, *De artibus liberalibus*; see Explanatory Note 2 above.

[32] **namly Pictagoras with his folowers:** See Burkert 1972, 447–48, 465–66.

[33] **shewid in the Spiere:** Probably a reference to the treatise earlier in the manuscript on the making of a celestial globe, or to a similar treatise; alternately, this may be a reference to the instrument itself, as Laird suggests is the case in Chaucer's *Treatise on the Astrolabe* 1.17, "as I have shewed the in the speer solide" (see chap. 13, Headnote n. 7 above).

[34] **Also the north poole ... and necessarie sciens:** The use of congruent triangles based on line of sight measurements is an essential element of many of the practical geometrical calculations described later in this section; they are also often found in treatises on the use of a quadrant, since the quadrant was commonly used to make such measurements. See Laird's edition of *The New Quadrant* 2.13–15, chap. 13 above. The "brekyng" or refraction of beams of light and their reflection in mirrors is part of Bacon's prescription for extending life by concentrating the virtues of starlight upon people and their food and drink; see the translation of his *In debito regimine*, ed. Tavormina, chap. 9 above, lines 94–108, 217–252.

[35] **instrumentis:** Such as the solid sphere, quadrant, and other instruments whose construction and use is described in treatises elsewhere in the manuscript (ed. Laird, chap. 13).

[36] **Altimetrie, Planymetrie, and Profundymetrie:** *New Quadrant* 2.17 refers to "altimetric, pleynmetric, and steriometric" types of measurement (ed. Laird, chap. 13, lines 920–921 and n.).

[37] **as is shewed in picture:** Although the text seems to promise an illustration at this point (and similarly in lines 404 and 427–428 and in the three miscellaneous geometry exercises at the end of the treatise), no space has been left in the manuscript, in contrast to the blank spaces left for illustrations in the *The Sickness of Women* and the treatises on scientific instruments earlier in the volume (plates 2, 4, 6). The last private owner of the manuscript, John Fortho, sought to compensate for the omissions in the geometrical exercises by adding annotated diagrams on folio 254r–v, copied and transcribed below.

[38] **Euclide techeþ in his booke:** Probably cited from a compilation of extracts or a commentary on Euclid's *Elements*. For discussion of these medieval digests, see Heath 1956, introduction. The most popular versions circulating in England in the fourteenth and fifteenth centuries were the translations of Adelard of Bath (particularly the second recension, labeled "Adelard II" by Clagett) and that of Campanus of Novara, based on Adelard. See Clagett 1953; Murdoch 1968. Note that Euclid is mentioned again at line 476 and in lines 504 and 507, discussed in Explanatory Notes 43 and 44 below.

[39] **how many graynes in length maken a myle ... ferthynges bien in C li. ... how moche he may expende in the yeere ...iij d :** Based on the ratios between measurements given here, there would be 207,360 grains in a mile; 96,000 farthings in £100; and an annual expenditure of £4 11s. 3d. While these figures may not all be useful pieces of information in themselves, they do provide examples (perhaps made more interesting by their extremity) of the use of multi-

plication to calculate length or sums of money in different units. Note that the number of feet in the mile as defined here (5760 feet) differs from the modern English statute mile (5280 feet) and that the length of the rod (18 feet) is not that of the usual modern rod (16.5 feet). For a history of English measurement, see Hall and Nicholas 1929, 14, on linear measures (edited from BL, Cotton MS Vespasian E.IX, fols. 86–110, of about the same date as the Trinity MS). Its basis of measurement, as here, is three grains (of barley rather than wheat) to an inch. A daily expenditure of 3*d.* would have been approximately equivalent to the daily wage of an unskilled laborer in England at this time; see Hatcher 1977, 49 (Table II, "Wage-rates, 1301–1540"). The author's attention to practical calculations—or at least to practicing the calculation of measurement and expenditures—is consonant with the interest he shows in the seven common crafts and their associations with English craft guilds at the end of the treatise, and may also reflect the concerns of his intended audience.

[40] **it shal be viij foote:** This calculation for the area of a square is incorrect; it actually gives the formula and solution for finding the perimeter of a square.

[41] **xx foote:** Clearly a scribal error, since the multiplication doesn't come out right; it probably should be "x foote."

[42] **iiij foote and his rib vj foote . . . xl:** This calculation for the area of a parallelogram is incorrect; perhaps the second measure is meant to be "x," ten, instead of "vj," six, to arrive at an area of 40 square feet.

[43] **is proevid bi the last conclusioun of the secunde booke of Euclide:** Euclid, *Elements* 2, proposition 14, explaining how to construct a square equal to a given rectilinear figure (Heath 1956, 1:409–10).

[44] **is proved bi the last conclusioun of the firste booke of Euclide:** Euclid, *Elements* 1, proposition 47, explaining the Pythagorean theorem, not proposition 48, the brief last proposition of book 1, which depends upon 47 (Heath 1956, 1:349–68).

[45] **aunswerith:** The spelling *aun-* here and in the following line is indistinguishable from *ann-*. Although the *aun-* spelling seems the more likely form, at least one unambiguous instance of the less common initial *ann-* spelling for a similar word (*auncient/anncient*) occurs in the translation of the *De coitu* (ed. Matheson, chap. 8 above), where the word is written with a decorated initial A followed by a capital N, with the rest of the word in lower case (line 134n).

[46] **iij tymes and . . . the vij part of a dyametir:** Note that this approximates π times the diameter, the circumference of a circle.

[47] **Afterward . . . holl circule:** Note that this equation for finding the area of a circle arrives at the right answer through a longer equation than would be necessary: to avoid having to find the circumference first, the equation should be half the diameter (i.e., the radius) squared and multiplied by π, though half the diameter by half the circumference gives the same answer, $7 \times 7 \times \pi \approx 154$.

[48] **other vij:** These other seven were treated in Hugh of St. Victor, *Didascalicon* 2.20–27. There they are called the "mechanical sciences" and are given in this order: fabric making, armament, commerce, agriculture, hunting, medicine, and theatrics. See the Headnote above. The seven mechanical sciences or arts were also mentioned in Martianus Capella, *De nuptiis Philologiae et Mercurii* (ed. Dick [1925] 1978, 9.890–91, pp. 471–72), and commentaries on it by Remigius of Auxerre (ed. Lutz 1962–1965, 2:17–18, esp. 4.153.18: " . . . quibusdam divis id est quibusdam deabus, artibus videlicet quales sunt Architectonica, Medicina, et ceterae quae magis in experientia quam in ratione constant" (by certain female deities, that is, by certain goddesses, with arts like Architecture, Medicine, etc. that are based more in experimental knowledge than in reason [my trans.]) and John the Scot (ed. Lutz 1939, 83). See also William of Conches, *De philosophia mundi*, the sections edited by Carmelo Ottaviano (1935); and Hugh of St. Victor, *Didascalicon* (ed. and trans. J. Taylor 1961, 74–79 and 205, nn. 68, 69, and 72).

[49] **as the Philosopher declarith in many placis:** Plato, *Republic*, and philosophers after him, including Aristotle, Euclid, and Proclus in his commentary on the first book of Euclid's *Elements*. Possibly also a reference to Boethius's lost book on geometry (see Chadwick 1981, 102–5; also *Boetii Liber de geometria, PL* 63:1352–64, esp. 1352–53).

APPENDICES
AND
GLOSSARIES

ACCIDENCE[*]

Nouns

The regular plural is normally formed with -s, -es, -is (rarely -ys). A few nouns have endings in -(e)n: eye, eyen (rarely eyn); asshen (alongside asshis, both pl. of *assh); cow/kow, kiene; or in -ren: chield(e), chieldren (rarely children); ey, eyren (alongside eg[ge], egges). (On chieldren/children and ey/eyren/eg(ge)/egges, see Matheson, chap. 4, 80.) Nouns forming their plurals by a change of vowel are man, men; wom(m)an, wym(m)en; kiene (pl. of cow); gees (pl. of *goos); and lise (pl. of *louse). The genitive case is normally marked by an -s, -es, or -is ending, but the relationship noun moder is unchanged in the genitive (always in the phrase his moder wombe Age/582, SW2/39, etc.)[1] and in two instances the pronoun his is used as a genitive marker (God his grace Age/1683; Mars his natiuite 7Pla/291).

Pronouns

The personal pronouns are as follows:

		Sg.	Pl.
1	Nom.	I	we (rarely wee)
	Gen.	myn	our (rarely oure)
	Obj.	me	vs
2	Nom.	thow (rarely thou, þou, thou, thov, þow)	ye, yee
	Gen.	thyn, thy (rarely thyne)	your, youre (rarely yourr, yowre, yovr)
	Obj.	the	yow

---

[*] In the following tables, an em-dash signifies that the form does not occur in the texts edited in the present volume; the symbol φ represents a zero-ending. An asterisk preceding a word indicates a postulated form not found in the texts. Abbreviations for texts are those given in the Headnote to the General Glossary.

[1] The single possible instance of moders as a genitive (moders goynges DHN/291) probably translates matricis exitus 'issues of the womb' (ed. G), though it may reflect maternos exitus 'motherly issues' (ed. A).

3		M	F	N	
	Nom.	*he* (rarely *hee*)	*she*	*it*	*thei, they* (rarely *þei, the*)
	Gen.	*his* (rarely *is*)	*hir* (rarely *her, hire*)	*his*	*their* (rarely *þeir, theire, her*)
	Obj.	*hym*	*hir* (rarely *her*)	*it*	*hem, theym* (rarely *them, theim, þem*)
	Refl.	*hymsilf*	*hirsilf*	*itsilf*	*hemsilf* (rarely *hemself, theymsilf*)

The second-person genitive singular forms *thyn* and *thyne* occur before words beginning with vowels or *h*; *thy* occurs before words beginning with consonants or *h*. The reflexive forms are usually written as two words (*hym silf*, etc.) in the manuscript, but have been combined in this volume to match Modern English word division.

Verbs

The following endings are typically found in regular (weak) verbs:

Infinitive:	*-e, -en, -φ*	
Imperative:	*-e, -φ, -es* (rare; only in Inst)	
Present Participle:	*-yng, -eng* (after *-i-, -y-, -n-,* or *-u-* [rare]), *-ing* (rare)	
Past Participle:	*-ed, -de, -d* (the prefix *i-* occurs on some past participles as well)	
Present Indicative	Sg.	Pl.
1	*-e, -φ*	*-e, -en, -n* (rare), *-φ* (rare)
2	*-est, -ist, -st*	*-e, -φ,*
3	*-ith, -eth, -yth, -eþ, -it* (rare)	*-en, -e, -n, -φ, -es* (rare; only in Inst)
Present Subjunctive	Sg.	Pl.
1	—	*-e*
2	*-e, -φ*	*-e, -φ*
3	*-e, -φ*	*-e, -en, -n, -φ*
Past Indicative	Sg.	Pl.
1	*-de, -ed*	*-de*
2	*-ed*	—
3	*-ed, -id, -t*	*-eden, -iden, -den, -ten, -id* (rare), *-ed* (rare)
Past Subjunctive:	distinctive forms are found only for the verb *to be* (see below)	

Irregular Verbs

The infinitive, imperative, and present tense forms of strong verbs conform to the same patterns as the weak verbs. In the past tense and past participle, strong verbs normally display the following accidence, along with the characteristic changes of root vowels:

Past Participle	*-en, -e, -n*	
Past Indicative	Sg.	Pl.
1	*-e, -φ*	—
2	*-e*	—
3	*-e, -φ*	*-en, -e, -φ*

The forms of the verb *to be* are as follows:

Infinitive:	*be, bien* (rare)	
Imperative:	*be*	
Present Participle:	*beyng*	
Past Participle:	*bien, be* (rare)	
Present Indicative	Sg.	Pl.
1	*am*	*bien*
2	*art*	—
3	*is*	*bien, arn* (rare; only in Inst), *are* (rare; only in Inst), *bie* (rare), *bion* (rare)
Past Indicative	Sg.	Pl.
1	—	—
2	—	—
3	*was*	*wern, were* (rare), *weren* (rare), *wore* (rare)
Present Subjunctive	Sg.	Pl.
1	—	—
2	—	—
3	*be, bi* (rare)	*bien, be* (rare), *bie* (rare)
Past Subjunctive		
1	—	—
2	—	—
3	*were, wer* (rare)	*wern, were, weren* (rare)

Verbs that are irregular in various other ways (e.g., *bryng/broughte, thynk(e)/ thoughte, telle(n)/told(e), calle/cald, meete/met(te), sette/set, go/went, do/dide, have/ had, make/made, wil/wold, may/might, shal/shuld(e), mow(n), dar*) display no striking differences from their usual Middle English forms, which are themselves often close to or identical with their extant Modern English reflexes.

A few past participles and participial adjectives are based on Latin past participial forms (e.g., *abiect, afflict, coct, introduct, intercept, transumpt,* etc.).

Adjectives and Adverbs

Comparative and superlative forms of adjectives and adverbs are normally derived by the addition of *-er* and *-est,* respectively (or by the use of *more* and *most*). In addition to these suffixes, change of the root vowel occurs in the adjectives *old, elder; strong, streng(g)er, strengest;* and *long, leng(g)er* (with *longer* once), *lengest.* In some adjectives and adverbs having etymologically long vowels in the root (*brode, deepe, diere, grete, neere, soone, sweete*), the comparative and superlative forms are spelled with a doubled medial consonant, possibly indicating a shortening of the vowel.

WORD-FREQUENCY LISTS
OF TEXTS IN TCC R.14.52

The frequency lists given on the following pages may serve the needs of scholars interested in a different approach to late Middle English scientific language than those provided by glossaries or by the analysis of scribal dialect. As the lists below demonstrate, the texts edited in this volume differ not merely in regard to subject-specific vocabulary, but also in interesting respect to a number of function words. The latter differences may reflect different modes of discourse (lengthy commentary, instructions for making or using objects or recipes, brief overviews of anatomy or physiology, etc.), different translators (the probable single translator of early texts in the manuscript vs. the several different translators likely to be responsible for the later texts),[1] or different original target audiences. While the lists themselves do not immediately unravel the multiple strands in the lexical fabric of our several texts, we hope that they will offer interested readers suggestive starting points for undertaking such analyses.

We give the fifty most frequent words in each text edited above, with the exception of the supplementary texts and the collection of texts on astronomical and other measuring instruments. For the instrument texts, which were probably translated or composed by several hands (including Chaucer's, in the *Astrolabe* excerpts), we have generated four frequency lists, for the four longest units within this subcollection of texts: *The Solid Sphere*, *New Quadrant 1*, *New Quadrant 2*, and the *Astrolabe* chapters. Although the chapters from the *Astrolabe* are a shorter sample than any of the other texts analyzed for word frequencies, their known authorship and the accessibility

---

[1] Note, for example, the regular occurrences of FORWHI, FORSOTH, and MOCHE in the first five 'top fifty' word-lists (each occurring in four of the five lists) and their relative infrequency in texts from the second part of the manuscript (FORWHI only appearing in the top fifty words of *The Seven Planets*, FORSOTH in the top fifty only in *De epidemia* and *The Seven Planets*, and MOCHE in the top fifty only in *Sickness of Women* and *The Seven Planets*). Given that Matheson's dialect analysis shows that the language of *The Seven Planets* is essentially the same as that of texts in the first part of the manuscript, the hypothesis that *The Seven Planets* might have been translated by the "bad translator" of part 1 seems worthy of investigation. Although it is somewhat more fluent than the texts in part 1, this might be explained by the relatively formulaic nature of its content, and it should be noted that there are still a number of convoluted constructions whose sense might be clarified with the identification of a direct Latin source (e.g., lines 6–9, 50–52, and 78–82, *inter alia*; and compare lines 224–353 with the Latin text in Bodleian Library, Bodley MS 648, fols. 10v–12v).

of the rest of the Chaucerian corpus, scientific and otherwise, seems to warrant their inclusion (with the appropriate caveats about the sample's brevity). The three plague treatises edited by Matheson are also analyzed separately, as they are probably from different sources; again one should note their relative brevity, especially that of the four-chapter treatise *Against the Pestilence* and the *Approbate Treatise*. The frequency lists have been generated with the very helpful Concordance software created by R. J. C. Watt (version 3.2).

Aside from distinguishing the word-forms BE and BI as representing *to be* (v.) and *by* (prep./adv.) respectively, following the scribe's almost universal practice,[2] the lists below leave grammatical distinctions and relationships unmarked. Thus, MAY can represent both the verb *may* and its occasional homograph, the proper noun *May*; similarly, although THE almost always stands for the article *the*, the form also includes a sprinkling of second-person singular objective pronouns (a form of *thee*) and even a very rare alternative spelling of *thei*. Conversely, allographs like the word-forms THE and ÞE or YE and YEE appear separately in the lists (longer lists would have included THEIRE beside THEIR), even if they are or can be variants of the same "word," in the semantic rather than the orthographic or the purely enumerative sense.

In the lists below, "Word(s)" refers to word-forms read by the Concordance program as orthographically distinct, also known as "Types"; these forms include numbers (1, 2, IJ, IIIJ), the ampersand, and the symbols for dram (℈) and ounce (℥). "Tokens" refers to the total number of words in the text, in the sense of an overall word-count of a document (as in "a short story of approximately 3,000 words"). We have not lemmatized the frequency lists to count the number of semantic headwords (i.e., words viewed as dictionary entries) in the texts.

---

[2] Of more than 1300 instances of the spelling BE tallied by the Concordance program from the texts edited in this volume, we have identified only seven used or possibly used as the preposition 'by': *Accidents of Age* 879 (see chap. 6, line 879n above) and 630–631 (*be evene complexioun*); *De coitu* 183 (*be evene temperat*); Bacon's "In Due Rule of Body" 273 (*be light of whos ouersight*); John of Burgundy, *De epidemia* 12 (*be encheason*); *Seven Liberal Arts* 155 (*be Rethorik*) and 268 (*be like proporccioun*). Another occurs in the *Book of Ipocras* (not edited in this volume), on fol. 143v.

We have found the spelling BI for the verb 'to be' only twice in the nearly 650 instances of *bi* in the texts edited above, both representing the subjunctive singular (normally *be*): *De humana natura* 293 (*if any bi goten*); *De coitu* 201–202 (*bifore that mete bi digested*).

ACCIDENTS OF AGE

TOTAL WORDS: 3534   TOKENS: 24737

WORD	INSTANCES (%)	WORD	INSTANCES (%)
AND	1814 (7.333%)	HUMYDITE	118 (0.477%)
OF	1667 (6.739%)	RULE	118 (0.477%)
THE	1269 (5.130%)	SUM	115 (0.465%)
IN	818 (3.307%)	THEI	113 (0.457%)
TO	650 (2.628%)	OLD	112 (0.453%)
THAT	467 (1.888%)	FROM	110 (0.445%)
IS	416 (1.682%)	THIESE	109 (0.441%)
WHICHE	384 (1.552%)	TYME	109 (0.441%)
IT	292 (1.180%)	AL	99 (0.400%)
BIEN	256 (1.035%)	MEDICYNES	90 (0.364%)
MEN	253 (1.023%)	SO	89 (0.360%)
BUT	240 (0.970%)	AFTER	85 (0.344%)
BE (v.)	227 (0.918%)	MADE	85 (0.344%)
AS	193 (0.780%)	ACCIDENTIS	84 (0.340%)
THYNGES	180 (0.728%)	OTHER	84 (0.340%)
WITH	165 (0.667%)	WHAN	81 (0.327%)
AGE	158 (0.639%)	SAITH	77 (0.311%)
NAT	158 (0.639%)	BI (prep./adv.)	75 (0.303%)
THIS	156 (0.631%)	HEETE	72 (0.291%)
OR	152 (0.614%)	CHAPITRE	71 (0.287%)
HE	151 (0.610%)	SAPIENT	70 (0.283%)
A	143 (0.578%)	DE	69 (0.279%)
FORWHI	134 (0.542%)	MAN	65 (0.263%)
NATURAL	134 (0.542%)	ALSO	64 (0.259%)
HIS	129 (0.521%)	BODY	63 (0.255%)

DE HUMANA NATURA

TOTAL WORDS: 981   TOKENS: 3504

WORD	INSTANCES (%)	WORD	INSTANCES (%)
THE	273 (7.791%)	MOIST	16 (0.457%)
AND	190 (5.422%)	SAY	16 (0.457%)
TO	180 (5.137%)	WHOM	16 (0.457%)
OF	140 (3.995%)	IF	15 (0.428%)
IS	71 (2.026%)	OTHER	15 (0.428%)
THAT	64 (1.826%)	DRIE	14 (0.400%)
IN	60 (1.712%)	THER	14 (0.400%)
WHICHE	59 (1.684%)	HERTE	13 (0.371%)
FORSOTH	57 (1.627%)	NATURE	13 (0.371%)
OR	57 (1.627%)	ANY	12 (0.342%)
BI (prep./adv.)	45 (1.284%)	SAIDE	12 (0.342%)
AS	32 (0.913%)	SAME	12 (0.342%)
BIEN	31 (0.885%)	THEI	12 (0.342%)
IT	28 (0.799%)	THYNNE	12 (0.342%)
A	27 (0.771%)	INTO	11 (0.314%)
FROM	27 (0.771%)	NAT	11 (0.314%)
WITH	22 (0.628%)	WHAN	11 (0.314%)
BE (v.)	21 (0.599%)	MADE	10 (0.285%)
COLD	21 (0.599%)	MOCHE	10 (0.285%)
HE	20 (0.571%)	SPIRITE	10 (0.285%)
HYM	20 (0.571%)	SUM	10 (0.285%)
SO	20 (0.571%)	ÞE	10 (0.285%)
AL	17 (0.485%)	VERTU	10 (0.285%)
IJ	16 (0.457%)	WHOS	10 (0.285%)
LITEL	16 (0.457%)	ANOTHER	9 (0.257%)

DE COITU

TOTAL WORDS: 780   TOKENS: 3298

WORD	INSTANCES (%)	WORD	INSTANCES (%)
AND	210 (6.367%)	SHAL	18 (0.546%)
THE	170 (5.155%)	A	17 (0.515%)
OF	138 (4.184%)	HIS	17 (0.515%)
TO	122 (3.699%)	MOCHE	17 (0.515%)
BE (v.)	70 (2.122%)	THIESE	17 (0.515%)
IS	65 (1.971%)	THIS	17 (0.515%)
IT	59 (1.789%)	APPETITE	16 (0.485%)
IN	58 (1.759%)	MOIST	16 (0.485%)
THAT	54 (1.637%)	AL	15 (0.455%)
FORSOTH	53 (1.607%)	BUT	15 (0.455%)
HE	51 (1.546%)	FROM	15 (0.455%)
WHICHE	45 (1.364%)	HOTE	15 (0.455%)
SEEDE	44 (1.334%)	OR	15 (0.455%)
FORWHI	40 (1.213%)	HEM	14 (0.424%)
IF	37 (1.122%)	HYM	14 (0.424%)
AS	32 (0.970%)	THERFOR	14 (0.424%)
BIEN	31 (0.940%)	VERTU	14 (0.424%)
DRIFT	31 (0.940%)	WHOM	14 (0.424%)
NAT	26 (0.788%)	WITH	14 (0.424%)
BI (prep./adv.)	25 (0.758%)	HEETE	13 (0.394%)
WE	23 (0.697%)	SEYN	13 (0.394%)
AFTER	22 (0.667%)	MEMBRIS	12 (0.364%)
BODY	20 (0.606%)	OTHER	12 (0.364%)
WHAN	20 (0.606%)	THEI	12 (0.364%)
COLD	19 (0.576%)	THER	12 (0.364%)

BACON, LONGEVITY TREATISES
TOTAL WORDS: 1529   TOKENS: 7664

WORD	INSTANCES (%)	WORD	INSTANCES (%)
OF	516 (6.733%)	AL	36 (0.470%)
AND	498 (6.498%)	THYNGES	36 (0.470%)
THE	376 (4.906%)	AFTER	34 (0.444%)
IN	231 (3.014%)	FORSOTH	34 (0.444%)
TO	185 (2.414%)	HIS	34 (0.444%)
THAT	158 (2.062%)	MANY	34 (0.444%)
IS	131 (1.709%)	MAY	33 (0.431%)
AS	124 (1.618%)	OR	33 (0.431%)
THIS	92 (1.200%)	NATURE	32 (0.418%)
WHICHE	92 (1.200%)	AGE	31 (0.404%)
BI (prep./adv.)	76 (0.992%)	FORWHI	31 (0.404%)
IT	75 (0.979%)	MANER	31 (0.404%)
THEI	74 (0.966%)	WITH	30 (0.391%)
HE	72 (0.939%)	ONLY	29 (0.378%)
A	69 (0.900%)	OTHER	28 (0.365%)
BIEN	68 (0.887%)	WAS	28 (0.365%)
BE (v.)	65 (0.848%)	BODY	27 (0.352%)
NAT	65 (0.848%)	HEM	27 (0.352%)
BUT	59 (0.770%)	HAN	25 (0.326%)
SO	52 (0.678%)	MOCHE	25 (0.326%)
THERFOR	50 (0.652%)	CRAFT	24 (0.313%)
LIF	48 (0.626%)	HATH	24 (0.313%)
MAN	47 (0.613%)	THIESE	24 (0.313%)
MEN	45 (0.587%)	WHAN	22 (0.287%)
RULE	44 (0.574%)	BOOKE	21 (0.274%)

PROGNOSTICS COMMENTARY

TOTAL WORDS: 2431   TOKENS: 18472

WORD	INSTANCES (%)	WORD	INSTANCES (%)
THE	1244 (6.735%)	THEI	94 (0.509%)
OF	1022 (5.533%)	THIESE	91 (0.493%)
AND	903 (4.888%)	BI (prep./adv.)	90 (0.487%)
IS	581 (3.145%)	WHAN	90 (0.487%)
IN	579 (3.134%)	SIKENES	89 (0.482%)
TO	531 (2.875%)	SIGNIFIETH	83 (0.449%)
THAT	466 (2.523%)	A	79 (0.428%)
OR	334 (1.808%)	VPON	79 (0.428%)
IT	324 (1.754%)	BUT	75 (0.406%)
BE (v.)	203 (1.099%)	THAN	70 (0.379%)
AS	190 (1.029%)	SAITH	66 (0.357%)
HE	183 (0.991%)	AL	65 (0.352%)
NAT	175 (0.947%)	HEM	65 (0.352%)
BIEN	171 (0.926%)	MOCHE	63 (0.341%)
THIS	169 (0.915%)	SAY	63 (0.341%)
IF	165 (0.893%)	DETH	62 (0.336%)
WHICHE	165 (0.893%)	EVIL	59 (0.319%)
FORSOTH	140 (0.758%)	HYM	59 (0.319%)
FORWHI	133 (0.720%)	GALIEN	58 (0.314%)
HIS	120 (0.650%)	SHARP	58 (0.314%)
AFTER	118 (0.639%)	SIGNES	57 (0.309%)
SO	118 (0.639%)	THYNGES	57 (0.309%)
FOR	107 (0.579%)	ALSO	56 (0.303%)
SIKE	106 (0.574%)	EYEN	56 (0.303%)
WITH	104 (0.563%)	ONLY	55 (0.298%)

SICKNESS OF WOMEN 2
TOTAL WORDS: 3620   TOKENS: 23251

WORD	INSTANCES (%)	WORD	INSTANCES (%)
AND	1557 (6.696%)	TAKE	127 (0.546%)
OF	1215 (5.226%)	THEI	121 (0.520%)
THE	1098 (4.722%)	ANA	119 (0.512%)
IN	489 (2.103%)	HEM	117 (0.503%)
THAT	449 (1.931%)	THAN	108 (0.464%)
A	435 (1.871%)	AL	107 (0.460%)
HIR	406 (1.746%)	BUT	103 (0.443%)
IT	400 (1.720%)	OR	102 (0.439%)
IS	336 (1.445%)	1	100 (0.430%)
TO	305 (1.312%)	2	99 (0.426%)
WITH	295 (1.269%)	WOMMAN	91 (0.391%)
ʒ [dram symbol]	205 (0.882%)	ÞE	91 (0.391%)
BE (v.)	179 (0.770%)	PUT	90 (0.387%)
OTHER	168 (0.723%)	CHIELD	89 (0.383%)
MATRICE	162 (0.697%)	POWDER	87 (0.374%)
BIEN	161 (0.692%)	WHAN	83 (0.357%)
FOR	150 (0.645%)	MOCHE	82 (0.353%)
AS	149 (0.641%)	THEIR	82 (0.353%)
IF	149 (0.641%)	ʒ [ounce symbol]	80 (0.344%)
MAKE	145 (0.624%)	SO	78 (0.335%)
&	135 (0.581%)	BLOODE	71 (0.305%)
ALSO	135 (0.581%)	OILE	71 (0.305%)
SHE	135 (0.581%)	WATER	68 (0.292%)
LETE	134 (0.576%)	HIS	66 (0.284%)
THIS	129 (0.555%)	ON	65 (0.280%)

DE EPIDEMIA

TOTAL WORDS: 806   TOKENS: 2328

WORD	INSTANCES (%)	WORD	INSTANCES (%)
AND	145 (6.229%)	WITH	12 (0.515%)
THE	122 (5.241%)	THEI	11 (0.473%)
OF	87 (3.737%)	THYNGES	11 (0.473%)
IN	61 (2.620%)	CAUSE	10 (0.430%)
THAT	61 (2.620%)	MAY	10 (0.430%)
OR	51 (2.191%)	THAN	10 (0.430%)
TO	46 (1.976%)	FORSOTH	9 (0.387%)
BIEN	35 (1.503%)	SUCHE	9 (0.387%)
BE (v.)	34 (1.460%)	ALSO	8 (0.344%)
IS	31 (1.332%)	COLD	8 (0.344%)
IT	29 (1.246%)	MADE	8 (0.344%)
HE	25 (1.074%)	MAN	8 (0.344%)
LETE	25 (1.074%)	MANY	8 (0.344%)
AS	24 (1.031%)	MATIER	8 (0.344%)
BUT	23 (0.988%)	THERFOR	8 (0.344%)
HIS	22 (0.945%)	THIS	8 (0.344%)
HYM	18 (0.773%)	TYME	8 (0.344%)
IF	18 (0.773%)	YIT	8 (0.344%)
OTHER	18 (0.773%)	CHAMBRE	7 (0.301%)
A	16 (0.687%)	CORRUPT	7 (0.301%)
AL	15 (0.644%)	EVERY	7 (0.301%)
FOR	15 (0.644%)	HOTE	7 (0.301%)
NAT	15 (0.644%)	I	7 (0.301%)
BI (prep./adv.)	14 (0.601%)	LITEL	7 (0.301%)
AIRE	13 (0.558%)	MEDLED	7 (0.301%)

AGAINST THE PESTILENCE

TOTAL WORDS: 429   TOKENS: 1365

WORD	INSTANCES (%)	WORD	INSTANCES (%)
THE	114 (8.352%)	BLEEDE	8 (0.586%)
AND	77 (5.641%)	DRYNKE	8 (0.586%)
IS	40 (2.930%)	EVIL	8 (0.586%)
THAT	38 (2.784%)	HERTE	8 (0.586%)
IT	36 (2.637%)	HIS	8 (0.586%)
OF	33 (2.418%)	HYM	8 (0.586%)
TO	27 (1.978%)	MAY	8 (0.586%)
BE (v.)	23 (1.685%)	VEYNE	8 (0.586%)
IN	23 (1.685%)	BLOODE	7 (0.513%)
OR	23 (1.685%)	BODY	7 (0.513%)
A	18 (1.319%)	BUT	7 (0.513%)
NAT	17 (1.245%)	MATIER	7 (0.513%)
THIS	17 (1.245%)	ALSO	6 (0.440%)
FOR	16 (1.172%)	FROM	6 (0.440%)
IF	16 (1.172%)	SIDE	6 (0.440%)
ON	15 (1.099%)	TELLITH	6 (0.440%)
MAN	14 (1.026%)	THER	6 (0.440%)
HE	12 (0.879%)	ÞAT	6 (0.440%)
THAN	12 (0.879%)	AGENST	5 (0.366%)
PLACE	11 (0.806%)	CHAPITRE	5 (0.366%)
SIKENES	11 (0.806%)	ETE	5 (0.366%)
GOODE	10 (0.733%)	OUT	5 (0.366%)
WITH	10 (0.733%)	OUTE	5 (0.366%)
CLENSYNG	9 (0.659%)	PRINCIPAL	5 (0.366%)
SHAL	9 (0.659%)	SAME	5 (0.366%)

AN APPROBATE TREATISE
TOTAL WORDS: 422   TOKENS: 1312

WORD	INSTANCES (%)	WORD	INSTANCES (%)
THE	156 (11.890%)	SHAL	7 (0.534%)
AND	71 (5.412%)	SIKENES	7 (0.534%)
OF	57 (4.345%)	VEYNE	7 (0.534%)
THAT	41 (3.125%)	WISE	7 (0.534%)
IS	30 (2.287%)	AL	6 (0.457%)
IT	29 (2.210%)	ALSO	6 (0.457%)
BLOODE	24 (1.829%)	MAY	6 (0.457%)
IN	22 (1.677%)	SIDE	6 (0.457%)
BE (v.)	21 (1.601%)	THAN	6 (0.457%)
TO	21 (1.601%)	THER	6 (0.457%)
A	18 (1.372%)	VRYNE	6 (0.457%)
IF	18 (1.372%)	WHAN	6 (0.457%)
FOR	16 (1.220%)	ÞE	6 (0.457%)
BIEN	12 (0.915%)	BITWENE	5 (0.381%)
MAN	11 (0.838%)	BRAYN	5 (0.381%)
OR	11 (0.838%)	HIS	5 (0.381%)
BI (prep./adv.)	10 (0.762%)	IIJ	5 (0.381%)
EVIL	10 (0.762%)	ISSUES	5 (0.381%)
HERTE	10 (0.762%)	ON	5 (0.381%)
WITH	10 (0.762%)	OUT	5 (0.381%)
THIESE	9 (0.686%)	SO	5 (0.381%)
LIVER	8 (0.610%)	THIS	5 (0.381%)
SAME	8 (0.610%)	TOKEN	5 (0.381%)
VPON	8 (0.610%)	APPIERE	4 (0.305%)
GOODE	7 (0.534%)	AS	4 (0.305%)

THE SOLID SPHERE
TOTAL WORDS: 725   TOKENS: 4543

WORD	INSTANCES (%)	WORD	INSTANCES (%)
THE	454 (9.993%)	TAKE	32 (0.704%)
OF	224 (4.931%)	LYNE	30 (0.660%)
AND	216 (4.755%)	WITH	30 (0.660%)
YE	125 (2.751%)	ÞE	29 (0.638%)
IN	124 (2.729%)	IUSTLY	28 (0.616%)
THAT	95 (2.091%)	CIRCULE	27 (0.594%)
SHAL	93 (2.047%)	SPIERE	27 (0.594%)
A	81 (1.783%)	WHICHE	25 (0.550%)
THAN	73 (1.607%)	&C	23 (0.506%)
BE (v.)	63 (1.387%)	PUT	23 (0.506%)
IT	63 (1.387%)	IIIJ	22 (0.484%)
ARMYL	59 (1.299%)	MAY	22 (0.484%)
IS	54 (1.189%)	AL	21 (0.462%)
TO	52 (1.145%)	FROM	20 (0.440%)
THIS	46 (1.013%)	ANOTHER	19 (0.418%)
MERIDIAN	40 (0.880%)	CERCLE	19 (0.418%)
SO	40 (0.880%)	MUST	19 (0.418%)
MAKE	38 (0.836%)	WISE	19 (0.418%)
VPON	38 (0.836%)	YOUR	19 (0.418%)
AFTER	36 (0.792%)	GREES	18 (0.396%)
AS	36 (0.792%)	IJ	18 (0.396%)
BI (prep./adv.)	33 (0.726%)	FIRST	17 (0.374%)
POINT	33 (0.726%)	SAME	17 (0.374%)
EQUAL	32 (0.704%)	SAIDE	16 (0.352%)
OR	32 (0.704%)	SAY	16 (0.352%)

NEW QUADRANT 1
TOTAL WORDS: 591   TOKENS: 3218

WORD	INSTANCES (%)	WORD	INSTANCES (%)
THE	473 (14.699%)	BIEN	19 (0.590%)
OF	232 (7.209%)	ON	19 (0.590%)
AND	147 (4.568%)	CERCLE	18 (0.559%)
IS	84 (2.610%)	SET	18 (0.559%)
THAT	83 (2.579%)	WITH	18 (0.559%)
IN	72 (2.237%)	FOR	16 (0.497%)
TO	55 (1.709%)	SHAL	16 (0.497%)
HEIGHT	42 (1.305%)	DAY	15 (0.466%)
IT	41 (1.274%)	TAKE	15 (0.466%)
GREE	38 (1.181%)	AS	14 (0.435%)
THOW	37 (1.150%)	FROM	14 (0.435%)
BI (prep./adv.)	35 (1.088%)	HIS	14 (0.435%)
BE (v.)	33 (1.025%)	HOURE	14 (0.435%)
ÞE	31 (0.963%)	SHALT	14 (0.435%)
IF	29 (0.901%)	SO	14 (0.435%)
GREES	27 (0.839%)	FYNDE	13 (0.404%)
A	26 (0.808%)	HEM	12 (0.373%)
OR	26 (0.808%)	ALMURIES	11 (0.342%)
SONNE	26 (0.808%)	HEVENE	11 (0.342%)
STERRE	25 (0.777%)	ORIZONT	11 (0.342%)
THAN	25 (0.777%)	SUM	11 (0.342%)
WHICHE	25 (0.777%)	ALMURY	10 (0.311%)
LYNE	24 (0.746%)	BIGYNNYNG	10 (0.311%)
HOURES	21 (0.653%)	EQUINOCCIAL	10 (0.311%)
VPON	20 (0.622%)	SAME	10 (0.311%)

NEW QUADRANT 2

TOTAL WORDS: 679   TOKENS: 4263

WORD	INSTANCES (%)	WORD	INSTANCES (%)
THE	629 (14.755%)	THREEDE	25 (0.586%)
OF	259 (6.076%)	OR	23 (0.540%)
AND	203 (4.762%)	ARK	22 (0.516%)
THAT	101 (2.369%)	CORDA	22 (0.516%)
TO	93 (2.182%)	FOR	21 (0.493%)
IN	91 (2.135%)	RIGHT	21 (0.493%)
BE (v.)	68 (1.595%)	SONNE	20 (0.469%)
SHAL	59 (1.384%)	STERRE	20 (0.469%)
THOW	59 (1.384%)	WITH	20 (0.469%)
IS	46 (1.079%)	ASCENCIOUN	19 (0.446%)
ÞE	40 (0.938%)	FOUNDEN	19 (0.446%)
IT	39 (0.915%)	LYNE	19 (0.446%)
GREES	38 (0.891%)	VERSA	19 (0.446%)
BI (prep./adv.)	37 (0.868%)	QUADRAUNT	18 (0.422%)
WHICHE	37 (0.868%)	NOMBRE	17 (0.399%)
VPON	36 (0.844%)	SET	17 (0.399%)
A	35 (0.821%)	THIS	17 (0.399%)
IF	35 (0.821%)	ADDE	16 (0.375%)
HEIGHT	33 (0.774%)	FIRST	16 (0.375%)
HOURES	32 (0.751%)	IJ	16 (0.375%)
THAN	32 (0.751%)	PARTIES	16 (0.375%)
FROM	31 (0.727%)	ZODIAC	16 (0.375%)
ALMURY	28 (0.657%)	DAY	15 (0.352%)
CERCLE	28 (0.657%)	BIFORE	14 (0.328%)
GREE	26 (0.610%)	HOURE	14 (0.328%)

CHAUCER, ASTROLABE 2.37, 40, 39, 38

TOTAL WORDS: 364   TOKENS: 1517

WORD	INSTANCES (%)	WORD	INSTANCES (%)
THE	172 (11.338%)	ANY	10 (0.659%)
OF	106 (6.987%)	EVENE	10 (0.659%)
AND	71 (4.680%)	GREES	10 (0.659%)
IN	43 (2.835%)	THI	10 (0.659%)
A	33 (2.175%)	THIS	10 (0.659%)
THAT	30 (1.978%)	AS	9 (0.593%)
THAN	28 (1.846%)	BI (prep./adv.)	9 (0.593%)
IS	23 (1.516%)	IT	9 (0.593%)
LYNE	22 (1.450%)	BE (v.)	8 (0.527%)
I	21 (1.384%)	F	8 (0.527%)
TO	18 (1.187%)	IJ	8 (0.527%)
FROM	17 (1.121%)	ON	8 (0.527%)
GREE	17 (1.121%)	TOKE	8 (0.527%)
LATITUDE	16 (1.055%)	BIGYNNYNG	7 (0.461%)
MY	16 (1.055%)	FOR	7 (0.461%)
MERIDIONAL	15 (0.989%)	HIS	7 (0.461%)
COMPAS	14 (0.923%)	SAY	7 (0.461%)
THOW	14 (0.923%)	TAKE	7 (0.461%)
VPON	14 (0.923%)	ÞE	7 (0.461%)
LONGITUDE	13 (0.857%)	BUT	6 (0.396%)
IIJ	11 (0.725%)	CAPRICORN	6 (0.396%)
LABEL	11 (0.725%)	ECLIPTIK	6 (0.396%)
OR	11 (0.725%)	HOUSE	6 (0.396%)
POINT	11 (0.725%)	MANER	6 (0.396%)
SET	11 (0.725%)	ORIZONT	6 (0.396%)

THE SEVEN PLANETS
TOTAL WORDS: 1020   TOKENS: 4272

WORD	INSTANCES (%)	WORD	INSTANCES (%)
AND	336 (7.865%)	HAVE	23 (0.538%)
OF	235 (5.501%)	GOODE	21 (0.492%)
HE	200 (4.682%)	GRETE	21 (0.492%)
THE	148 (3.464%)	THYNGES	20 (0.468%)
IN	138 (3.230%)	MOCHE	19 (0.445%)
IS	112 (2.622%)	MAN	17 (0.398%)
BE (v.)	110 (2.575%)	SIGNIFIETH	17 (0.398%)
TO	83 (1.943%)	CONSTELLACIOUN	16 (0.375%)
THAT	82 (1.919%)	EVIL	16 (0.375%)
SHAL	66 (1.545%)	VNDER	16 (0.375%)
A	55 (1.287%)	BIEN	15 (0.351%)
IF	52 (1.217%)	SAY	15 (0.351%)
HIS	47 (1.100%)	THOW	15 (0.351%)
HYM	47 (1.100%)	SIGNES	13 (0.304%)
OR	47 (1.100%)	SO	13 (0.304%)
AS	37 (0.866%)	WELE	13 (0.304%)
BUT	32 (0.749%)	ALSO	12 (0.281%)
NAT	32 (0.749%)	BI (prep./adv.)	12 (0.281%)
WITH	32 (0.749%)	LOVITH	12 (0.281%)
SIGNE	31 (0.726%)	MANY	12 (0.281%)
WHICHE	31 (0.726%)	PLANETIS	12 (0.281%)
BORN	30 (0.702%)	AFTER	11 (0.257%)
MEN	30 (0.702%)	FORSOTH	11 (0.257%)
AL	27 (0.632%)	FORWHI	11 (0.257%)
IT	27 (0.632%)	MARS	11 (0.257%)

THE SEVEN LIBERAL ARTS

TOTAL WORDS: 1396   TOKENS: 7640

WORD	INSTANCES (%)	WORD	INSTANCES (%)
THE	585 (7.657%)	THIS	36 (0.471%)
AND	440 (5.759%)	FLOORE	35 (0.458%)
OF	356 (4.660%)	LYNE	35 (0.458%)
IN	203 (2.657%)	AL	34 (0.445%)
A	202 (2.644%)	NAT	34 (0.445%)
IS	198 (2.592%)	FROM	32 (0.419%)
THAT	145 (1.898%)	MESURE	32 (0.419%)
TO	143 (1.872%)	IJ	31 (0.406%)
AS	96 (1.257%)	OTHER	31 (0.406%)
BE (v.)	79 (1.034%)	PART	31 (0.406%)
SHAL	78 (1.021%)	ALSO	30 (0.393%)
BI	76 (0.995%)	HE	30 (0.393%)
IT	66 (0.864%)	PARTIS	30 (0.393%)
SO	65 (0.851%)	HALF	29 (0.380%)
IF	60 (0.785%)	WIL	29 (0.380%)
OR	60 (0.785%)	IIIJ	28 (0.366%)
BUT	51 (0.668%)	ON	27 (0.353%)
FOR	51 (0.668%)	AN	26 (0.340%)
WITH	50 (0.654%)	CALD	26 (0.340%)
HIS	48 (0.628%)	MANY	26 (0.340%)
BIEN	46 (0.602%)	THYNGES	26 (0.340%)
WHICHE	46 (0.602%)	KNOWE	25 (0.327%)
THAN	45 (0.589%)	NOMBER	25 (0.327%)
YE	44 (0.576%)	YEE	25 (0.327%)
FOOTE	37 (0.484%)	MAY	24 (0.314%)

INDEX OF MANUSCRIPTS CITED

This index records all citations of manuscripts in the preface, chapters, and supplementary texts, with the exception of references to Cambridge, Trinity College MS R.14.52, citations of manuscripts collated in the Textual Notes, and references to manuscripts solely by their LP number in the *Linguistic Atlas of Late Mediaeval English*.

New York, New York Academy of Medicine
MS (ca. 1250):[1] 97, 278, 278n, 280
New York, Pierpont Morgan Library
Morgan Buehler 17: 38
Orléans, Bibliothèque municipale
286: 98, 250n
Oxford, Balliol College
231: 97
Oxford, Bodleian Library
Additional A.106: 572
Arch. Selden. B.35: 149, 343
Ashmole 59: 60
Ashmole 337: 15n, 29
Ashmole 340: 570
Ashmole 342: 564n
Ashmole 393: 685n
Ashmole 396: 328n, 733n
Ashmole 399: 280, 290n, 291, 292, 463n
Ashmole 1285: 323
Ashmole 1393: 575n
Ashmole 1438: 575n
Ashmole 1443: 576, 598n
Ashmole 1444: 572
Ashmole 1471: 280, 290n, 291, 292
Ashmole 1481: 572
Auct. F.5.30: 325
Bodley 178: 457n
Bodley 211: xxii, 147–49
Bodley 438: 147–49, 343
Bodley 483: 461n
Bodley 505: 89
Bodley 591: 462n
Bodley 648: 682n, 686n, 698nn, 699n
Can. Misc. 334: 147–49, 343
Digby 29: 238n, 682n
Digby 67: 15n, 29
Digby 75: 682n
Digby 104: 682n
Digby 218: 343
Digby 235: 343
Douce 37: 465n
Douce 157: 89
Douce 322: 62, 89
e Musaeo 155: 147–49
e Musaeo 219: 291, 292, 296, 297, 306n, 314nn
Laud lat. 65: 324
Laud Misc. 471: 90
Laud Misc. 622: 89
Laud Misc. 724: 463n
Lyell 36: 477, 477n, 480, 733n
Rawlinson C.506: xv n, 6n
Rawlinson D.251: 80n, 570, 603n
Rawlinson D.913: 57, 63n
Rawlinson Poetry 32: 11
Selden Supra 78: xxii, 609, 628, 630, 634, 668n, 671n
Oxford, Corpus Christi College
68: 319–20
201: 89
244: 335n, 337
275: 323
Oxford, Merton College
219 (N.3.2): 97, 100n, 108–14 passim, 280, 291, 292, 297
221 (N.3.4): 325
222 (N.3.5): 325
231 (H.3.5): 321
232 (H.2.6): 322
255 (C.2.6): 325
263 (C.2.14): 320
278 (O.1.6): 98, 250n, 280, 280n, 290, 291, 291n, 292
324 (O.1.2): 291, 292, 296, 297, 306nn, 314nn

---

[1] The NYAM MS is sometimes referred to as NYAM MS Safe or SAFE, referring to its location in the Academy's Malloch Rare Book Room; the manuscript has no formal shelfmark. I am grateful to Ms. Arlene Shaner, Reference Librarian and Assistant Curator for Historical Collections, for clarifying this point.

GENERAL GLOSSARY

This glossary has been compiled by the general editor with the expert assistance of Lister M. Matheson. Though extensive, it remains selective, containing words whose meanings have changed significantly or become obsolete, important or obsolete technical terms (except for the *materia medica* found in the subsequent specialized glossary), and unusual spellings and forms of lexical or dialectal interest (often because otherwise unattested or rare). For the words included in the glossary, the full range of senses found in the edited texts is provided in order to contextualize less common meanings. Predictable plurals of nouns (*-s*, *-es*, and *-is/-ys* endings) are usually not distinguished in the entries, but the more complex accidence of verbs is included in full for clarity. Definitions are intended to explain words and forms in their immediate context or to clarify points of potential difficulty.[1] Isolated Latin words whose meaning is not clear from their immediate context or explained in a note are also included in the glossary (usually under their nominative form), indicated by italics and the abbreviation "(L.)"; the vocabulary of passages of running Latin text, however, is generally omitted. Uncertain or conjectured senses, uncertain instances of a particular sense, and ambiguous grammatical functions are preceded by a question mark.

Headwords, variant spellings, forms of the headwords, and cross-references to headwords are printed in bold type. Phrases using the headword (or a form thereof) follow single-word senses and forms and are printed in italics. A tilde represents recurrences of the headword a) within phrases; b) after variant spellings; or c) after intervening grammatical forms whose spelling differs from that of the headword. The occasional variant spellings of headwords that occur only in phrases are given in bold italics.

References are by text and line number; for hyphenated words or phrases extending over more than one line, the reference is to the starting line. References usually include the first (or an early) occurrence in one or more texts, with additional representative references to illustrate forms or senses; further instances of specific forms or senses are indicated by "etc." Words or forms that result from emendation, or text/line references to them, are indicated by an asterisk. Where appropriate, relevant language, explanatory, or textual notes are indicated by an "n" appended to the text/line reference.

---

[1] Important sources for determining senses of technical terms, in addition to the *MED*, include Latham 1980; Hunt 1989; Getz 1991; Norri 1992; Norri 1998; and Green 2001. Comparisons to Latin vocabulary in the entries are normally based on the known or probable Latin source of the text from which a given citation is taken. Special thanks are owed to Monica Green, Linne Mooney, and Edgar Laird for assistance with individual words from their chapters, and to Juhani Norri for suggestions on particular items; errors that remain are the responsibility of the general editor.

Persons, places, and works mentioned in the texts are listed separately, after the General Glossary and the glossary of *materia medica* named in the texts. For ease of reference, a few words with general as well as pharmaceutical senses appear in both the General Glossary and the *materia medica*.

The order of entries is alphabetical, with the following exceptions: consonantal *i* is treated as *j*, consonantal *u* as *v*, vocalic *y* and *j* as *i*, vocalic *v* and *w* as *u*, palatal *ʒ* as *y*, velar *ʒ* as *gh*, *þ* as *th*, and initial *ff* as *f*.

The following grammatical and lexicographic abbreviations are used in the glossary:

acc.	accusative	*p.ppl.*	past participle
adj.	adjective	*pr.*	present tense
adv.	adverb	*prep.*	preposition
coll.	collective	*pret.*	preterite
comp.	comparative	*pron.*	pronoun
conj.	conjunction	*pr.ppl.*	present participle
fig.	figurative (ly)	*refl.*	reflexive
gen.	genitive	*rel.*	relative
impers.	impersonal	*sb.*	somebody
impv.	imperative	*sg.*	singular
inf.	infinitive	*sth.*	something
interj.	interjection	*subj.*	subjunctive
lit.	literal (ly)	*sup.*	superlative
n.	noun	*vbl.n.*	verbal noun,
phr.	phrase		gerund
pl.	plural	*1 (2, 3)*	first (second,
ppl.adj.	participial adjective		third) person

The following abbreviations are used in references to the individual texts:

Age	*On Tarrying the Accidents of Age*
DHN	*De humana natura*
Fle	*Liber fleobotomie*
Coi	*De coitu*
Bac	Roger Bacon, Extracts on the Prolongation of Life
CHP	Commentary on the Hippocratic *Prognostics*
SW2	*The Sickness of Women*
Plag	John of Burgundy, Treatises on the Plague
8Med	*Eight Manners of Medicines*
Inst	Scientific Instrument Treatises
7Pla	*The Seven Planets*
7LA	*The Seven Liberal Arts*

abasshement *n.* amazement Bac/492

abate *inf.* reduce SW2/355; *impv.* subtract Inst/711, Inst/1329, etc.

abhomynable *adj.* nauseating Age/1072

abide *inf.* remain, stay, etc. Age/881, Age/1736, etc., *impv.* Inst/561, Inst/1129, **abidith** *pr.3sg.* Age/272, Age/430, etc., **abiden** *pr.3pl.* Age/220, Age/859, Plag/26, etc., **abidyng** *pr.ppl.* Age/1782, DHN/79, etc.; ~ *pr.3sg.subj.* survive Coi/4

abidyng *vbl.n.* staying SW2/702; expectation 7Pla/288 [cf. *MED,* s.v. *abiding* vbl.n., 3]

abiect *ppl.adj.* rejected Inst/1270

aborcif *adj.* born prematurely or stillborn Age/1407n

abovtfurth *adv.* on all sides CHP/1485

abovefurth *adv.* above, from above Age/1076, DHN/48, etc., **aboveforþ** CHP/1342

abreviat(e) *adj.* abbreviated, shortened Bac/16, Bac/323, Bac/365, CHP/119, **abreuiate** Bac/33

abscisours *n.pl.* cutters (of veins), bloodletters 7Pla/55, 7Pla/58

absolute *adj.* of words or phrases: in the strict sense CHP/1092, CHP/1101, etc.

absterciouns *n.pl.* acts of cleansing or wiping the skin Age/1540

acces(se) *n.* an attack of illness, a seizure SW2/522, SW2/564, etc.

accidens *n.* a physiological change resulting from disease, aging, or similar processes Age/102, Age/406, Age/479, etc., **accidence** CHP/134, **accidencis, -es** *pl.* Age/140, Age/299, CHP/664, etc., CHP/561, CHP/640, etc.; *accidencis of the soule* mental or emotional disturbances Age/286

accident *n.* a physiological change resulting from disease, aging, or similar processes Age/2, Age/31, Age/384, CHP/194, CHP/351, etc.; a non-essential or temporary property of a thing Bac/582; *accidentis of (the) soule* mental or emotional disturbances Age/186, Age/1626, etc.

accident *adj.* incidental, outside the natural course of things, pathological Age/117, CHP/643

accidental *adj.* incidental, not essential to or inherent in a thing Age/1711, DHN/84, Bac/34, etc.; (as *n.pl.*) **accidentals** DHN/85

accidentaly *adv.* not in the natural course of things Age/1132

accompt *impv.* calculate, measure Inst/456, **accomptyng** *pr.ppl.* Inst/568; **accomptith** *pr.3sg.* includes in a count 7Pla/247, **accompted** *p.ppl.* Age/1738; regarded, considered Bac/44, Bac/52

accompt *n.* a computation or reckoning Inst/1304

accordaunt *adj.* appropriate, suitable Plag/161

accordith *pr.3sg.* agrees Age/370, Age/1018, **accorden** *pr.3pl.* Age/260, Age/1041, etc.; **accordyng** *pr.ppl.* corresponding Inst/718, Inst/721; *accordyng to* suitable for SW2/78; as indicated by Inst/828; harmonious with 7LA/175

actual *adj.* committed by one's own act 7LA/24, 7LA/27

ac(c)ustom *adj.* accustomed Age/88; *han* ~ are accustomed Age/492

acustomd *p.ppl.* in the habit, accustomed (to do sth.) CHP/945; **acustumed** familiar, usual Age/26

adder *n.* a venomous snake Age/1366, Plag/182, **addir** Age/1368, **edder** Age/372

addicioun *n.* addition Inst/770, 7LA/207, 7LA/501, **addissioun** Inst/1372, **addiscioun** 7LA/204, 7LA/213

additament *n.* projection, supportpiece (for the meridian ring of a celestial globe) Inst/59, Inst/261, etc.

adicial *adj.* *part* ~ a vessel from the kidneys carrying choler to the gall

bladder or melancholy to the spleen
DHN/188

admytted *ppl.adj.* granted [error for L.
amittentes 'losing'] Age/541

admyxtioun *n.* the act of mixing together Age/1840

adust *adj.* of a humour: morbidly altered by the body's heat SW2/1527

adustioun *n.* the corruption of bodily humours by heat CHP/410,
CHP/413

aduersarie *n.* adversary, enemy
Plag/187, **aduersary** [error for L.
thesaurus 'treasure'] Age/1166n

aduersarie *adj.* opposing, hostile
Age/16, 7Pla/201

aferde *ppl.adj.* afraid, frightened
SW2/1425

affeccioun *n.* desire, pleasure
Age/804; the soul's capacity for desiring or willing 7LA/18, 7LA/33

afflict *ppl.adj.* afflicted Age/987,
DHN/297, Fle/36

affluxed *ppl.adj.* taken away, lost
DHN/303n

affraieth *pr.3sg.* SW2/86

affrike *adj.* of breath: rough and slow
CHP/1062

afore-past *adv.* beforehand, previously CHP/529

after throwes see **throwes**

age *n.* a stage of life Age/255, Bac/376,
SW2/29, etc.; the number of
years a person has lived Bac/75,
CHP/1352; old age Age/2, Age/31,
etc.; ~ *accident* happening as a result of age Age/117; a period in
history Bac/82; ~ *of decrepite, decrepite* ~ advanced old age Age/165,
Age/168, Age/1691, etc.; ~ *(of) evene
(with)standyng* the prime of life
Age/1698, Age/1727, etc.

ageyn-goten *p.ppl.* regenerated
Age/877

ageyn-lightneth *pr.3sg.* re-illuminates
Bac/7n

ageynseith *pr.3sg.* contradicts, gainsays
Age/707, Age/1452

ageyn-sette *ppl. adj.* placed, set
Age/233, DHN/147

ageynward(e) *adv.* in the opposite direction, away from a place SW2/757,
SW2/1023, etc.; vice versa Inst/461

aggregacioun *n.* ~ *of helth* error for L.
aggregatio saniei 'accumulation of
pus' CHP/1427n, CHP/1432

agitacioun *n.* mental or emotional disturbance Age/717, CHP/1227, etc.

agwe *n.* an acute fever (such as malari-
al fever) Plag/245, Plag/409; *fever* ~
an acute fever Plag/288, Plag/289

ay *adv.* always Plag/360; in each case
Inst/994

air(e)ly *adj.* having characteristics of
the element of air 7Pla/15, 7Pla/41,
etc.

aither *pron.* either Inst/125

ake *inf.* ache, pain SW2/834, **akith**
pr.3sg. CHP/1198, SW2/1070, etc.,
aken *pr.3pl.* CHP/1078, **akyng** *pr.ppl.*
CHP/1183, CHP/1203, etc.

akyng *vbl.n.* ache, pain SW2/308,
SW2/1064

akth *n.* ache, pain CHP/866,
CHP/896, etc., **akthis** *pl.* CHP/1374

alaied *p.ppl.* tempered, diluted
Plag/104, Plag/134

alarged *ppl.adj.* stretched CHP/432

alchitees *n.* dropsy of the abdomen, as-
cites SW2/1365

alday *adv.* frequently, again and again
SW2/1242

algorisme *n.* the art of calculating with
arabic numerals 7LA/192

al-holely *adv.* completely Inst/921

alienacioun *n.* derangement, insan-
ity Age/644, Fle/10, CHP/832,
CHP/839, etc.

alightith *pr.3sg.* becomes limber
Coi/179; **alighten** *pr.3pl.* lighten,
cause to become easy Age/146,
alighted *p.ppl.* CHP/1153

a-lyne *adv. evene* ~ in a precisely
straight line Inst/1134

alkamye *n.* alchemy Bac/7, Bac/89,
etc.

alkamyster *n.* an alchemist Bac/121
allevien *pr.3pl.* lighten, cause to become easy Age/1964
allilakas *n.* the point at the top of an astrolabe where a suspending ring is attached Inst/1001n
almecantrades *n.pl.* circles of altitude marked on an astrolabe Inst/999, **almycantrades** Inst/1020, *almykanteras** Inst/1108 [see Headnote to chap. 13, 618]
almynak *n.* a set of astronomical tables Inst/1042
almury *n.* a projection on the rete of an astrolabe pointing to degrees on the rim of the instrument Inst/447, Inst/449, etc.; a movable bead on a quadrant's plumb-line Inst/786, Inst/810n, etc.; a bead on the cord of a suspended celestial sphere Inst/298, Inst/342, etc.; **almuries** *pl.* error for **almecantrades**, circles of height on an astrolabe Inst/398n, Inst/425, etc. [see Headnote to chap. 13, 617–18]
al-only *adv.* only, solely CHP/1150, SW2/21, Plag/18, Inst/1196
alterat *p.ppl.* changed, altered Age/1664
alteratief *adj.* causing alteration 8Med/14
altimetric *adj.* pertaining to altimetry, the measurement of height Inst/920, Inst/921
altimetrie *n.* the science of measuring height 7LA/372, 7LA/373
altitude *n.* the elevation of a celestial object above the horizon Inst/305, Inst/344, Inst/1338, etc.; height Inst/1302, Inst/1304, etc.; *iiij ~, ~ quadraunt, quadraunt(e) of the ~* a quarter-ring on a celestial sphere, used for taking altitudes Inst/242, Inst/244, Inst/269, etc.
ambassiatis *n.pl.* diplomatic missions or messages 7Pla/96
amyssioun *n. ~ of seede* emission [L. *emissione*] of semen Coi/276

among(e) *adv.* periodically, from time to time Plag/150; *~ thei difference* they differ among themselves Age/751
Amor Ereos (L.) *n.* lovesickness as a medical condition 7Pla/111
anacasym *n.* a method of blood-letting (?on the side of the body opposite the illness) [L. *anakarsin, anacarsim*] Fle/47, **anacaxim** Fle/42, **amacaris** Fle/28
anangred *ppl.adj.* angered, wrathful SW2/1424
ancle *n.* the ankle SW2/610, SW2/718, Plag/273, etc.
angule *n.* a geometrical figure formed by two converging lines 7LA/432, 7LA/434, 7LA/470, 7LA/479, etc; *angle of the yrþ* the point opposite the mid-sky point above the earth [L. *angulo terre*; see also **corner(e)**] Inst/38; *principal (iiij) angles* the four positions in the zodiac located at the cardinal points of the compass Inst/412, Inst/1024; *angle of the quadraunt* the corner or apex of a quadrant Inst/905; *right angle, rect ~* a right angle Inst/316, Inst/213, 7LA/410, etc.
animal *adj.* pertaining to the animating principle of a living creature Fle/79, CHP/1137
anostoma *n.* ?blood-letting by an incision from above [L. *anotoma*] Fle/32 [see also **anotomye**]
anotomye *n.* ?blood-letting by means of an incision from above [L. *anostomo*] Fle/47 [see also **anostoma**]
Antartik *adj. Circule ~* the Antarctic Circle on a globe, at latitude 66° 27' S Inst/110, Inst/115
antrax *n.* a boil or growth CHP/960, CHP/967, CHP/975
aperitief *adj.* of medicines: opening, causing dissolution of an obstruction Fle/161
apertly *adv.* without hesitation Age/1382; clearly, openly Bac/623, CHP/1282

aposory *n.* a form of phlebotomy involving intermittent interruption of the blood-flow [L. *apoforesim* 'a draining'; see Gil Sotres 1994, 152] Fle/55

apostemacioun *n.* swelling CHP/1207, CHP/1215, etc.

apostem(e) *n.* an inflammation or a pathological swelling on or in the body CHP/164, CHP/300, SW2/998, etc., **empostem** SW2/1004, **empostym** SW2/1042, **postem(e)** CHP/806, CHP/975; *cold* ~ an aposteme caused by a cold humour CHP/1362; *hote* ~ *(apostume)* an aposteme caused by a hot humour CHP/619, CHP/1077, CHP/1214, etc., *hote* **apostomes** *pl.* CHP/1385; *light* ~ soft apostemes CHP/1366; *stony* ~ the hardened part of an aposteme CHP/1321

apostemeth *pr.3sg.* becomes swollen or inflamed CHP/1319; **apostemed** *p.ppl.* swollen, infected, inflamed CHP/682, CHP/767, etc.; (as *n.*) infected substance [error for L. gen. sg. *apostematis*] CHP/1431

apparence *n.* appearance Age/989, Age/1460, **apparens** CHP/489

appetief *adj.* *vertu* ~ the faculty of appetite or desiring food Age/546

appetit(e) *n.* desire or drive 7Pla/317; sexual desire Coi/17, Coi/18, etc.; desire for food, hunger Age/2093; *harde* ~ ?limited desire for food CHP/287 [cf. *MED*, s.v. *hard* adj., 3(b)]; ~ *of matier* in medieval philosophy, the tendency of matter to seek its natural goal Bac/136, Bac/140, etc.; *vnskilful* ~ an abnormal hunger SW2/77

appetited *p.ppl.* *light* ~ having a good appetite CHP/283

appetith *pr.3sg.* desires, yearns for, feels desire Bac/136, **appeten** *pr.3pl.* Coi/33, **appetyng** *pr.ppl.* 7Pla/325, 7Pla/328

applie *inf.* devote oneself (to sth.) Plag/174; **applied** *p.ppl.* brought DHN/54, DHN/94, DHN/219; *applied before* of limbs: twisted, malformed DHN/303

applieng *vbl.n.* devotion, application CHP/146

appolexie *n.* apoplexy CHP/1121

appopletik *n.* apoplexy CHP/235

approbate *adj.* proven Plag/312

appropred *p.ppl.* *is* ~ *(ther)to* is characteristic of, is proper to CHP/827, Inst/639

apt *inf.* apply, put in place Inst/65n

apt *adj.* fitting Coi/6, Inst/25, etc.; prone, inclined Bac/594, 7Pla/293

aquosite *n.* of blood: wateriness, thinness Age/1033

ar see **or**

arbiterment *n.* *free* ~ free will 7Pla/230, *free* **arbitrement** 7Pla/232

arc, arcus see **ark(e)**

arcanlier *n.* a ruler or straight-edge Inst/318n

arefaccioun *n.* physiological drying, dehydration CHP/1108

areisen *pr.3pl.* raise, cause to rise Coi/33; **areised** *p.ppl.* incited DHN/206

Aries *n.* the constellation and zodiacal sign Aries, the Ram Inst/476, Inst/520, 7Pla/112, etc.; *Arietis* see *caput Arietis*

ark(e) *n.* an arc of a circle Inst/433, Inst/1004, etc., **arc** Inst/1003; ~ *of the corde(s)* the segment of a circle subtending any chord Inst/784, Inst/791; ~ *of the day (nyght)*, ~ *diurn(e)* the apparent course of a heavenly body above (below) the horizon Inst/432, Inst/434, Inst/755, Inst/764, etc., **arcus** *of the day (nyght)* Inst/429; ~ *of the equinoccial* an arc of the celestial equator Inst/1103; ~ *of the houres* hours expressed as an arc of rotation in the equinoctial circle (i.e., in the celestial equator) Inst/665; ~ *meridiane* an arc along the celestial meridian marking the sun's position at midday Inst/1115; ~ *versa* an arc subtending the cord versa on a quadrant [see **cord(e)**] Inst/865

arken *inf.* convert arcs of a circle to chords and vice versa Inst/784

armery *n.* the trade of making and using military and naval equipment 7LA/566, 7LA/577

arm-holis *n.pl.* armpits Plag/178, Plag/198, **arme-hoolis** Plag/257

armyl(l) *n.* a metal ring attached to a celestial globe Inst/63, Inst/72, Inst/274, etc.; ~ *meridian (meredian), meridian (meredean)* ~ a ring representing the great circle passing through the equatorial poles and the observer's zenith Inst/57, Inst/69, Inst/127, Inst/221, etc.; *orisont (orizont)* ~ a ring representing the observer's horizon Inst/195, Inst/243, etc.

aromatikes *n.pl.* aromatic substances Age/1450, Age/2048, Plag/115, etc.

ars *n.* the anus CHP/547, 8Med/12, 8Med/67, etc; ~ *hole* the anus SW2/1767

arsmetricers *n.pl.* calculators, those who use the art of arithmetic 7Pla/89

arsmetrik(e) *n.* the art of calculating, arithmetic 7LA/49, 7LA/181, etc.

arsnyk *n.* arsenic Age/1020

artetic *n.* pain in the joints, arthritis Fle/15; (as *adj.*) ~ *passioun* pain in the joints, arthritis Fle/114

artificer *n.* a craftsman 7LA/153, 7LA/565

artificialy *adv.* skillfully Inst/262

artificiall *adj.* done by means of an art or craft Inst/919; *daies artificials* the periods of time when the sun is above the horizon Inst/997

artik(e) *adj. Circule* ~ *(Articus)* the Arctic Circle on a globe, at latitude 66°

27' N Inst/108, Inst/113; *poole* ~ the north terrestrial pole Inst/1114

artis medicine professor (L.) *n.* a teacher of or writer on medicine Plag/75

as *conj.* as, such as, like, for example, in the same way Age/49, Age/66, etc., **ass** 7Pla/244; ~ as if Coi/121; ~ *(that, pat), so* ~ so that [translating L. *ut*] Age/15n, Age/26, DHN/4, Coi/8, etc.

ascence *n.* celestial position, expressed in degrees of right ascension (rather than in degrees of the ecliptic) Inst/872; depth (of water) Inst/1247; an ascent Fle/80

ascencioun *n.* rising (of a point or object in the celestial sphere) Inst/542, Inst/694, Inst/711, etc.; *ascenciouns in the cercle oblique (in the right)* the risings of celestial objects from the oblique (right) horizon [see **orizont**] Inst/686, Inst/692; ~ *of naddair solis* the rising of the point on the celestial sphere opposite the sun Inst/778, Inst/872; ~ *of the x hous* the rising of the tenth house [see **hous(e)**] Inst/717

ascendaunt *n.* the degree of the zodiac rising in the east at a given time Inst/580, Inst/775, etc., **ascendent** Inst/868, Inst/1025, etc.; *grete* ~ the first and most significant of the twelve astrological houses, or divisions of the sky, which rises at dawn Inst/702; *ascendent of the yeere* the ascendant at the beginning of the year (i.e., at the sun's entrance into Aries), used for casting the year's horoscope Inst/629

ascendaunt *adj.* ascending, increasing in quantity Inst/372, Inst/375, Inst/476, etc.; *gree* ~ , ~ *gre, gree ascendent* the degree of the zodiac rising in the east at a given time Inst/412, Inst/626, Inst/1028, etc.

ascendens *n.* rising (measured in the equinoctial) Inst/699

asm. *n*. abbreviation for asthma Fle/55

aspeccioun *n*. ~ *of the planetis* the angular distance between two planets (measured along the zodiac), aspect Inst/614n

aspect *n*. the angular distance between two planets (measured along the zodiac) Bac/330n, Inst/616, 7Pla/27, etc.; the influence of a heavenly body (based on its zodiacal position relative to other heavenly bodies) 7Pla/52, 7Pla/94, 7Pla/101

aspiryng *vbl.n.* breathing CHP/291

aspis *n.pl.* asps, venomous snakes Age/1376

ass see **as**

assautis *n.pl.* assaults, ambushes Bac/447n

assellaciouns *n.pl.* sittings at stool, sessions of relieving the bowels Age/1904

assellith *pr.3sg.* moves the bowels, goes to stool Age/1936, **asselle** *pr.3sg. subj.* Age/1935

asshis *n.pl.* ashes SW2/730, **asshen** SW2/110, SW2/1015, etc.

assimuled *p.ppl.* assimilated CHP/634; *be* **assymuled** error for L. *assellare* 'to move the bowels' Age/1934n

assise *n*. ~ *of the cursour (perle)* the correct arrangement or setting of the cursor of a quadrant (or of the almury of a quadrant without a cursor) for a given latitude Inst/1350, Inst/1356, Inst/1375

assised *p.ppl.* positioned Inst/1358

as(s)triccioun *n*. retention Age/1673; constriction Fle/58

assurith *pr.3sg.* assures, confirms [translating forms of L. *asserere* 'to assert'] DHN/107, Coi/225, **assuryng** *pr.ppl.* Age/1227, **assurid** *pret.3sg.* Bac/239, **assured** DHN/129

astate *n*. the third of four stages of an illness, when the climax is reached CHP/53 [see also **state**]

astonyed *ppl.adj.* numb SW2/134

astrolabie *n*. an astronomical instrument, either an astrolabe or a quadrant Inst/218, Inst/565, etc., **astrolaby** Inst/370, Inst/380, etc., **astrolabye** Inst/552, Inst/912 [see Headnote to chap. 13, 611–12]

astromye *n*. astronomy Bac/180, Bac/247

aswage *inf.* relieve, assuage Plag/380, *pr.3sg.subj.* Age/1935, Age/1936

attempre *adj.* temperate, balanced Plag/149

attraccioun *n*. a drawing of a morbid substance out of the body Age/1062; inhalation CHP/811, CHP/882

attractif *adj.* pertaining to the power of inhaling DHN/58, DHN/59

attribute *p.ppl.* attributed DHN/99; delivered, conveyed DHN/138

***attumpne** see **autumpne**

atwixt *prep.* between Inst/224

auctor *n*. an author Age/123, Bac/508, etc., **auctours** *pl.* Bac/88, CHP/201, Inst/1114, etc.; ~ an agent CHP/125 [L. *actor*, var. *auctor*], CHP/190; ~ *of phisik (sikenessis)* a medical writer CHP/895, CHP/904, *auctours of medicyne(s)* Bac/82, Bac/437

audible *adj.* pertaining to hearing DHN/23

augment *inf.* increase, improve Age/805, **augmenten** CHP/907, **augmentith** *pr.3sg.* Age/222, Age/827, Age/1116, **augmenten** *pr.3pl.* Age/1632, **augmented** *p.ppl.* Age/296, Age/2094; in the second of four stages of an illness CHP/58, CHP/62; (as *n*.) the augmented stage of an illness CHP/68

augment *n*. an increase Age/114; the second of four stages of an illness, when symptoms become visible CHP/52

augmentyng *vbl.n.* an increase, augmentation Age/99, Age/108, etc.; the second of four stages of an illness, when symptoms become visible CHP/40, CHP/94, etc.; *straunge* ~ an increase of extraneous substances Age/143, Age/175, etc.

autumpne *n.* autumn Fle/127, ***attumpne** Age/1482, Fle/77

availe *inf.* be effective, avail Age/1443, Age/2049, Bac/350, **availith** *pr.3sg.* Age/513, Age/515, etc., **availeþ** Fle/15, CHP/188, **availen** *pr.3pl.* Age/1408, Age/1450, Plag/159, etc.

avale *impv.* lower Inst/409

avise *impv.* consider Inst/533

avoide *inf.* purge, evacuate Age/1605, **avoidith** *pr.3sg.* Age/1041, **avoiden** *pr.3pl.* Plag/163, **avoided** *p.ppl.* CHP/1345, Plag/195, Plag/196; ~ *inf.* escape, evade Age/1413, Age/1416; ~ *impv.* let blood Fle/128

avoutrer *n.* an adulterer 7Pla/205

awey *adv.* away, out Age/78, Age/101, etc.; *al* ~ by far Inst/54

ax *n.* the axis of a concave mirror Bac/276

axe *n.* an adze Inst/8

axiltre *n.* the axis of the earth 7LA/358

axith *pr.3sg.* asks, requires Age/1779, SW2/7

azimutis *n.pl.* circles on an astrolabe indicating compass-bearings, azimuths Inst/399n, Inst/497, etc., **azmutis** Inst/1021; ~ *(azumutis) of the risyng* azimuths marking the compass-bearing of any point on the horizon where a celestial body is rising Inst/503, Inst/507

bace *n.* base Inst/1387

bal(l) *n.* a ball, spherical object Inst/5, Inst/11, 7LA/533, etc.; a medicinal bolus (to be ingested or used in a pessary or suppository) SW2/1410, **balle** SW2/755, SW2/980, etc.; **ballis** *pl.* ?(bald) heads Age/408

ballidnes(se) *n.* baldness Age/198, Age/401, Age/1005, etc., **baldnes(se)** Age/1000, Age/1002

ballith *pr.3sg.* ?becomes bald Age/1200n

bareyn(e) *adj.* infertile, barren SW2/1332, SW2/1493, 7LA/309, **barayne** SW2/985

bareynesse *n.* infertility Age/827

basilic see **veyne**

be *inf.* be Age/30, Age/46, etc., **bien** Age/910, CHP/204, SW2/168, etc., **am** *pr.1sg.* Age/648, Age/1217, **art** *pr.2sg.* Inst/1369, Inst/1376, **is** *pr.3sg.* Age/19, Age/22, etc., **bien** *pr.1pl.* Age/1716, 7LA/119, **bien** *pr.3pl.* Age/16, Age/52, etc., **arn** Inst/183, Inst/223, etc., **are** Inst/617, Inst/619, **bie** Plag/59, Inst/481, **bion** CHP/22, ~ *pr.3sg. subj.* Age/78, DHN/26, etc., **bie** *pr.3pl.subj.* SW2/473, SW2/1493, Plag/159, **beyng** *pr.ppl.* Age/172, Age/471, etc., **was** *pret.3sg.* Age/24, Age/115, etc., **wern** *pret.3pl.* Age/789, Age/821, Bac/220, etc., **were** Age/318, SW2/1488, **weren** SW2/1063, **wore** SW2/1536, **were** *pret.3sg.subj.* Age/301, Age/1688, Bac/269, etc., **wer** Coi/10, **wern** *pret.3pl.subj.* Age/1663, Coi/121, etc., **were** SW2/1340, **weren** Age/1746, **bien** *p.ppl.* Age/21, Age/83, etc., **be** Age/602, SW2/918, 7Pla/223, etc.; *to* ~ *inf.* (as *n.*) essence, being Age/1678, Age/1683, 7Pla/256

beame *n.* a ray of light from the sun or a star Age/1389, Bac/96, Inst/409, etc.; the fixed leg of a string compass (i.e., a tool for drawing circles by rotating a writing instrument around a stationary axis by means of a taut string) 7LA/431, 7LA/432; ~ *of the aire,* ~ *withoutfurþ* a ray of light from outside the eye CHP/574, CHP/576; ~, ~ *of the visible spirite,* ~ *visuale* a ray believed to pass from the eye to an object seen CHP/575, CHP/1033, Inst/906, 7LA/359, etc.

beautith *pr.3sg.* makes beautiful
Age/1767
bedwardis *adv. to* ~ toward bedtime
SW2/1815
be(e)st(e) *n.* an animal Age/320,
Age/921, Age/2080, Coi/6, etc.,
beastis *pl.* Age/837, Age/1408,
CHP/1020; ~ a pathological growth
in the uterus, the *arpa* or *frater Lumbardorum* SW2/284n; **be(a)stis** error for L. *animalis* 'pertaining to the
soul' Age/183, Age/186, **beastes**
DHN/201
behalve *n. in this* ~ in this matter
Bac/375
beyng see **be**
bely *n.* the abdomen CHP/894,
SW2/849
benethfurth *adv.* below, beneath
SW2/108, SW2/740, etc., **beneþfurth** SW2/1287, **binethfurth**
SW2/584, SW2/590, **bynethfurth**
SW2/59, SW2/1076
benyngne *adj.* gracious, benign
7Pla/260
beperisshed *ppl.adj.* trampled, crushed
SW2/859
berer *n.* a cupbearer Bac/64, Bac/500
beryng *vbl.n.* behavior, bearing
7Pla/105, 7Pla/167, 7Pla/327; producing Bac/305; ~ *of* giving birth to
SW2/706, SW2/765, etc.; *chielde* ~
childbirth SW2/1439
bestial(l) *adj.* of zodiacal signs: having the figure of an animal 7Pla/45,
7Pla/94, 7Pla/101; **beestial** pertaining to animals Bac/459
bicche *n.* a female dog, bitch
SW2/1341
biclippith *pr.3sg.* ~ *to* encloses, surrounds DHN/142
bie *inf.* buy 7Pla/164
bie, bien see **be**
bifore-comyth *pr.3sg.* acts in advance
CHP/129; **bifore-comen** *p.ppl.* pre-
vented, anticipated CHP/200
bifore-feelith *pr.3sg.* feels in advance
CHP/123

bifore-goeth *pr.3sg.* anticipates
CHP/117
bifore-past *ppl.adj.* preceding
CHP/532
bihoveful *adj.* suitable, necessary
CHP/479, Inst/76
bynd(e) *inf.* bind, tie CHP/23,
SW2/588, etc., *impv.* SW2/757,
SW2/1499, etc., **byndith** *pres.3sg.*
DHN/242, ~ *pres.1pl.* SW2/1776,
8Med/54, *pres.2sg.subj.* SW2/759,
pres.3sg.subj. 7Pla/138; **byndith**
pres.3sg. collects, draws together
Fle/50
binethfurth, bynethfurth see **benethfurth**
binote *impv.* examine, take note of
CHP/317
binotyng *vbl.n.* an examination of (sb.)
CHP/323
bion see **be**
birthen *n.* a burden, something carried, fetus SW2/1326
bitakith *pr.3sg.* leads, tends [L. *tendit*
'stretches, extends'] Coi/37
bitwen(e) *prep.* and *adv.* between
Age/578, Age/754, etc.; *be* ~ be present [L. *interesse*] Coi/116; ~ *long
space* at long intervals CHP/1062
bitwene-while *adv.* periodically Coi/177; at times, sometimes
CHP/178, CHP/188, CHP/1397; *it is
~ of* it concerns, it is a matter of [L.
interest 'it concerns'] CHP/137
biwerid *p.ppl.* used, spent [L. *perfrui* 'to
use up, fulfill'] DHN/304
blaase *n.* a blazing fire Plag/118
blac *adj.* black, dark, swarthy Age/79,
CHP/374, SW2/110, 7Pla/292, etc.,
blake Age/423, Age/1032, Age/1397,
SW2/111; ~ *coler* black choler, the
humour melancholy Age/934; ~
compas see **compas**; ~ *sope* a dark
soap used medicinally SW2/1572
bladder *n.* the urinary bladder
Age/1121, Age/1815, etc., **bladdir**
DHN/185, **bledder** Age/1151; ~ a
bag used for douching SW2/955

blaynes *n.pl.* sores SW2/1539
blake see **blac**
blakkith *pr.3sg.* blackens, darkens Age/1349
ble(e)che *adj.* pale, wan CHP/962, CHP/966, CHP/970, CHP/991
bler(e)-eyed *adj.* having rheumy eyes CHP/568, CHP/581, CHP/631
blerid *ppl.adj.* of eyes: rheumy, bleary Age/381, Age/1349, **blered** Bac/391
bleridnesse *n.* rheuminess, bleariness Age/513, **blerednes** Age/509
bocche *n.* a sore, an external ulcer CHP/963, CHP/966; a plague sore, bubo Plag/245, Plag/269, etc.
bochiers *n.pl.* butchers 7LA/570
bodieth *pr.3sg.* becomes incorporated Age/2091, Bac/118
boistous *adj.* rough, brutal 7LA/162; of flesh: ?coarse Age/868n
boistously *adv.* roughly, stiffly [L. *rigiditatem* 'stiffness, an erection'] Coi/37
bolis see Materia Medica, s.v. **bolis gall(e)**
bolkyng *vbl.n.* vomiting Fle/65
bolle *n.* ~ *of tree* a sawed-off tree trunk, carved into a seat 8Med/11, 8Med/12
boln *p.ppl.* swollen Fle/27
bolnyng *vbl.n.* swelling Age/1438, Fle/13, Coi/253, CHP/881, 8Med/22, etc.
boole *n.* a bull Bac/564, **boles** *pl.* SW2/624; *booles galle* see Materia Medica, s.v. **bolis gall(e)**
bo(o)rde *n.* a board, flat piece of wood Inst/84, Inst/308, Inst/328, Inst/939; a table (used *fig.* of the kidneys) DHN/213
bo(o)re *inf.* drill Inst/72, Inst/259, *impv.* SW2/1451
bord(o)ure *n.* a border, an outer edge Inst/282, Inst/1029, etc.
bore *p.ppl.* born 7Pla/235, 7Pla/314, etc.
bore *n.* a boar, male pig Bac/564, SW2/623, SW2/624, SW2/1805

bost *n.* boastfulness 7Pla/263
bostyng *pr.ppl.* boasting, boastful 7Pla/287
***bothor** *n.* a small pustule SW2/498n
boundis *n.pl.*(1) bonds Bac/162
boundis *n.pl.*(2) limits 7LA/256
bowe *impv.* cut an arc in (sth.) Inst/254; ~ *pr.3pl.* bend, curve 7LA/78, **bowyng** *pr.ppl.* DHN/93, SW2/1205, **bowid** *p.ppl.* SW2/1223, 7LA/93, **bowed** CHP/796, 7LA/91
bowe *n.* a bow 7LA/81; an arc of a circle 7LA/430, 7LA/541
bowel *n.* an intestine DHN/162, DHN/163, **bowels** *pl.* Age/1120, Age/1385, Age/1814, **bowellis** Age/1064; *bowels of th'erth* the innermost parts of the earth, the ground below the surface of the earth Age/9, Age/309, etc.; *xij* ~ the duodenum DHN/155
bowght *n.* ~ *of the arme* the inner angle of the elbow Plag/279
box *n.* a cupping glass (for bloodletting) Plag/274, Plag/281; *bloode boxes pl.* cupping glasses SW2/508
boxe *inf.* apply cupping glasses to (sb.) Plag/377, **boxed** *p.ppl.* Plag/373
bradder see **brode**
bray *inf.* chop or crush into small pieces SW2/610, *impv.* SW2/276, SW2/1836, **braied** *p.ppl.* Plag/300
brayn(e) *n.* the brain Age/396, Age/523, DHN/3, etc.; *first* ~ the forward ventricle of the brain Age/571
bras *n.* brass SW2/611, Inst/937
brasen *adj.* made of brass SW2/1559
breche *n.* ~ *of the peritoneon* a perineal breach or tear SW2/1754, SW2/1758
breed(e) *n.* breadth CHP/921, SW2/265, Inst/986, 7LA/405, etc., **brede** Inst/279, 7LA/556, etc.; ~ geographical latitude Inst/528, Inst/532; angular distance (from a celestial circle such as the ecliptic, equator, or the sun's apparent

diurnal path) Inst/538, Inst/568, Inst/586, etc.; distance Inst/1317; *in the* ~ within the breadth (of an instrument), i.e., on the instrument Inst/370

brekyng *vbl.n.* crushing Age/346; rupture, bursting CHP/1455, CHP/1463, etc.; destruction 7Pla/64; refraction (of a beam of light or of vision) Bac/100, 7LA/361

brenne *inf.* burn CHP/990, SW2/399, Plag/22, Plag/23, *impv.* SW2/446, **bren** SW2/447, *pr.1pl.* 8Med/48, **brent** *p.ppl.* SW2/477, SW2/570, etc., **ibrent** SW2/394, SW2/450, etc., **ibrend** SW2/368, SW2/401; **brennyth** *pr.3sg.* becomes hot with fever CHP/1081; **brennyng** *pr.ppl.* hot, feverish Age/1414, CHP/414, etc.; **brennyth** *pr.3sg.* causes a burning sensation SW2/480, **brenneth** SW2/965; **brennyng** *pr.ppl.* ardent, inflamed Coi/243

brennyng *vbl.n.* burning, destroying by heat Age/346, SW2/1546, 7Pla/60, etc.; alteration of humours by bodily heat CHP/411; a burning sensation CHP/836, CHP/1052, SW2/541, etc., **brynnyng** SW2/98

bries *n.pl.* eyelids SW2/73, SW2/95, SW2/106n, **bryes** SW2/102

brist *n.* the upper part of the torso, the breast CHP/1059

brode *adj.* (as *n.*) something broad, wide DHN/217n; **bradder** *comp.* broader, wider in diameter Inst/1119

brond *n.* a hot coal or some other burning substance SW2/101

broughtfurþ *n.* the product of multiplication Inst/1406

bruse *impv.* crush, mash SW2/991

brusyng *vbl.n.* bruising, crushing 8Med/33

buyle *inf.* boil SW2/177, SW2/1544, *impv.* SW2/1731, SW2/1736, etc., **buyled** *p.ppl.* SW2/1849, SW2/1881

buystes *n.pl. ventusyng* ~ cupping glasses SW2/804

bulles *n.pl.* papal or episcopal decrees or letters Bac/513

bullyeng *vbl.n.* a humoral disturbance or transformation by heat CHP/980

busy *adj.* busy, active CHP/38, CHP/263, Plag/351, etc.; ~ *puls* rapid pulse CHP/549

busyers *n.pl.* people engaged in negotiations 7Pla/90

busily *adv.* busily, constantly Age/1818, Age/1858; eagerly Plag/89; carefully, attentively SW2/1206, Inst/1126

busynes(s) *n.* interest, solicitation Age/728, Age/1652; labor, exertion Age/1679, Age/1832, SW2/1764, etc.; characteristic or proper activity CHP/241

calcyned *ppl.adj.* reduced to powder by heating Bac/110

canal *n.* a bodily channel or vessel DHN/139, **canals** *pl.* DHN/11, DHN/35, DHN/97, etc., **canels** DHN/125

Cancer *n.* the constellation and zodiacal sign Cancer Inst/476, Inst/526, **Cancri** 7Pla/142; *cercule (cercle, parilel) of* ~ the tropic of Cancer, the geographical parallel at 23° 33' N Inst/122, Inst/378, Inst/397

cancres *n.pl.* festering ulcers, tumors, cancers SW2/1537, **cankers** SW2/1525

cancres *adj.* ulcerated, having the qualities of "canker" SW2/1548 [see *MED,* s.v. *canker* n.(1); Norri 1992, 309]

cancryng *vbl.n.* festering, ulceration SW2/1535

canels see **canals**

cankretis *n.* ?cankered things, things affected by "canker" SW2/1525 [see *MED,* s.v. *canker* n.(1); Norri 1992, 309]

canon *n.* a rule or principle of practice CHP/493 [see also Persons, Places, and Works, s.n. **Avicen**]

cantarice *n.* a purgative [L. *catarticum* 'cathartic,' poss. confused with *cantharides* 'medicine made from cantharis beetles'] CHP/704

capax *adj.* susceptible (to sth.) 7Pla/261

Capricorn *n.* the constellation and zodiacal sign Capricorn Inst/475, Inst/478, Inst/1068, etc., **Capricornij** 7Pla/204; *cercle (cercule, circule, parilel) of ~* the tropic of Capricorn, the geographical parallel at 23° 33′ S Inst/105, Inst/122, Inst/378, Inst/397, etc.; *gree(s) of ~* degrees into the constellation Capricorn Inst/1048, Inst/1052, Inst/1055

captief *adj.* captive Age/1487

caput Arietis (L.) *phr.* the head or beginning of the zodiacal sign Aries Inst/535

carbuche *n.* a large boil CHP/967

carbucle *n.* a large boil CHP/960, **carbuncles** *pl.* SW2/1526

cardiac *n.* heart pangs, palpitations Age/1164, CHP/733

cardiacle *n.*(1) heart pangs, palpitations Age/933, Age/945, SW2/85, etc.

cardiacle *n.*(2) a vein in the arm thought to come from the heart Plag/258, **cordiacle** Plag/279

cardial *adj.* *~ fevers* fevers pertaining to or associated with the heart CHP/743

cardynal *adj.* *medicynes ~* , *~ medicynes* essential medicines, sovereign remedies Age/928, Age/992

careyn(e) *n.* carrion, a carcass Age/599, Age/602, CHP/828, etc.

carl(l) *n.* a peasant Bac/60, Bac/499, etc.

castigacioun *n.* correction, chastisement Age/1328

cataplasme *impv.* make a poultice (of) Fle/96

catataxim *n.* drawing blood from the side of the body on which a lesion or an illness occurs Fle/41, **cacatrisim** Fle/48 [L. *catecesin, catacarsim, cacatarsim*, Gr. *katarrexin*; see Gil Sotres 1994, 127: *kat'ixin* 'on the same side as the lesion']

cathaplasme *n.* a plaster or poultice made with herbs, applied directly to a wound 8Med/4, 8Med/14, etc.

catheria *n.* ?cachexia, general ill health Age/1059n

cawdroun *n.* a kettle or cauldron CHP/787, 8Med/10, 8Med/11

causatiefly *adv.* causally, through a causal relationship Plag/10

cause *n.* a cause (of sth.), an origin Age/105, Age/178, Age/242, Coi/144, Bac/65, etc., **causees** *pl.* Age/652; *causes accidental* incidental or non-essential causes Bac/371; *vj kyndes (gendris, gendirs) of causes, vj kyndes of necessarie (necessary) causes, vj kyndly causes, vj general causes, vj causis* the six "non-naturals" of medieval medicine Age/266n, Age/282, Age/958, Age/963, Age/1664, Age/1671, Age/1823, Age/1998; *~ laborious* a cause of distress or pain CHP/1076; *causes neccessary (necessarie) causes* that necessarily bring about their effects Age/187, Age/981; *primytief causis, primitief causes, causes (causis) primytief, prymatief causes (causis)* ultimate, non-corporeal causes CHP/491, CHP/495, CHP/679, CHP/658, CHP/688, Plag/60, Plag/61; *~ secundarie* a secondary cause Plag/62, Plag/63

causon *n.* a fever caused by putrefaction of choler in the veins CHP/303, CHP/1176

cautels *n.pl.* precautions Age/1503, CHP/1087

cenyth *n.* the celestial zenith, the point of the sky directly overhead

Inst/1116, Inst/1325; a part of an astrolabe representing the celestial zenith Inst/1006, Inst/1019; *cercle (of)* ~ a circle on a quadrant passing through the zenith Inst/839n, Inst/843, Inst/847; ~ *of our hede* the celestial zenith Inst/1096

centre *n.* the center of a circle or of an object Inst/33, Inst/41, 7LA/356, etc.; ~ *of the (that) sterre (sterris)* the center of the physical dot (of diameter proportional to magnitude) representing a star on a celestial globe or quadrant Inst/167, Inst/177, Inst/414, etc.

cephalargices *n.pl.* headache sufferers CHP/579

cephalargie *n.* a headache, pain in the head Fle/53

cephalic *n.* the cephalic vein, one of the major veins in the arm Fle/94, **cephalica** Fle/31, Plag/277, **chephalicon** Fle/28; ~ (as *adj.*) Fle/52

cercle *n.* a circle (*lit.* and *fig.*) Bac/275, Bac/619, Inst/15, 7LA/81, 7LA/356, etc., **circule** Inst/108, Inst/134, 7LA/463, etc., **cerculis** 7LA/435, **sercle** Inst/951; ~ a circlet, collar Age/923; course, (circular) path Age/166, Age/1645, Age/1791; orbit 7Pla/1, **sercles** *pl.* Plag/7; **sercle** the upper region or layer of a urine sample SW2/1009, SW2/1015; *cerclis of the firmament* the celestial spheres Plag/4; *right* ~ the right horizon, the horizon as seen by an equatorial observer Inst/542, Inst/869; *shamefast (secret)* ~ the anus DHN/166, DHN/253; one of various circles on the celestial or terrestrial sphere or their representations on astronomical instruments: ~ *(circule) antartik (artike, articus, of Cancer, of Capricorn, cenyth, equinoccial, equinoxial, meridional, oblique, zodiac), right (streight)* ~ Inst/110, Inst/113, Inst/108, Inst/397, Inst/397,

Inst/839, Inst/396, Inst/544, Inst/838, Inst/546, Inst/572, Inst/542, Inst/621, etc. [see modifying terms for definitions]

cered *ppl.adj.* impregnated with wax 8Med/43

certitude *n.* certainty 7LA/128, 7LA/586

chaffyng see **chauf(f)yng**

chaffith see **chauf**

chambre *n.* a room, chamber Plag/117, Plag/119, etc., **chamber** SW2/256; *prevy* ~ a toilet SW2/764; *chamber of sapience* treasury of wisdom [L. *thesaurus sapientie*] Age/27; *thorny* ~ ?a spiny vault, used *fig.* of the ?larynx [L. *spinosa camera*] DHN/141

charge *inf.* care, be solicitous Bac/345, **chargith** *pr.3sg.* Bac/384, 7Pla/127, 7Pla/196, **chargen** *pr.3pl.* Bac/601

charge *n.* a burden, weight (also *fig.*) Age/215, Age/217, CHP/823; responsibility Bac/190; care CHP/34

chauf *inf.* warm, heat DHN/289, **chaufith** *pr.3sg.* Age/1811, Coi/227, Coi/228, **chauffith** Age/1287, Fle/144, **chaffith** SW2/965, **chauffen** *pr.3pl.* Age/1265, **chaufed** *p.ppl.* Coi/280

chauf(f)yng *vbl.n.* heating Age/1264, Age/1425, Age/1846, DHN/214, **chaffyng** 8Med/49

chaunchyng *vbl.n.* changing Age/904

chekes *n.pl.* the cheeks SW2/906, **chekis** SW2/908, **cheekis** CHP/953

chest *n.* ~ *of the lyver* ?the liver as an 'ark' or container [error for L. *arte epatis* 'by the art or skill of the liver'] DHN/176

chewed *ppl.adj.* error for L. *chimus* or *euchimia* '(good) juices in foods' Age/756, Age/1125, *wel(e)* ~ Age/94n, Age/239, etc.

chewers *n.pl.* error for L. *euchimia* 'good juices in foods' Age/786, Age/818, Age/820 [see Age/94n]

chewyng *vbl.n.* error for L. *chimus* or *euchimia* '(good) juices in foods'

Age/198, Age/748, etc. [see Age/94n]

chieldith *pr.3sg.* gives birth, gives birth to DHN/264, CHP/962, SW2/1143, **chielden** *pr.3pl.* 7Pla/221, **chield** *pr.3sg.subj.* DHN/283

chieldyng *vbl.n.* child-bearing SW2/57, SW2/1723

chymeny *n.* ~ *of heete* the flow of heat through the body CHP/813

chynes *n.pl.* splits, chapping SW2/1516

cifre *n.* a cipher, the symbol for the number zero 7LA/198, 7LA/202

cymphon *n.* a kind of musical instrument 7Pla/326 [see *MED*, s.v. *simphonie* n.]

cinapisme see **synapisme**

cynorose *n.* error for L. *timorosos* 'fearful (men)' Age/946n

ciphac *n.* the peritoneum, the membrane lining the abdominal cavity CHP/1297, CHP/1420, CHP/1424

circuite *n.* in ~ all around, surrounding DHN/161

cirurgien *n.* a surgeon 7Pla/145

cistes *n.pl.* chests Age/1489

citee *n.* in the ~ error for L. *a vicinitate* 'from the closeness' Fle/79

citezenis *n.pl.* inhabitants of a city 7Pla/35

citryne *adj.* reddish or brownish yellow Age/1212, Age/1309, etc., **citryn** SW2/501

clarifie *impv.* remove impurities, refine SW2/1552, **clarifieth** *pr.3sg.* Age/239, Age/931, Age/1017, Age/2073, **(i)clarified** *p.ppl.* Bac/254, SWA/244, etc., *ppl.adj.* SW2/350, SW2/1734, etc.

claudicacioun *n.* lameness CHP/521

clensyng place *phr.* a location on the body through which poisons are eliminated Plag/227, Plag/229, etc.

clepe *pr.1pl.* call, name Inst/1099, **clepen** SW2/47, *pr.3pl.* SW2/513, Inst/1115, **clepid** *p.ppl.* SW2/43, Plag/177, Inst/420, etc., **cleped** SW2/1357, Plag/318, Inst/230, etc.

clepynges *vbl.n.pl.* names Age/551

clew *n.* a ball of yarn or thread SW2/571

cliftes *n.pl.* cracks, clefts SW2/1516

clymat(e) *n.* a region of the earth Inst/1094, Inst/1113, etc.

clymyng *vbl.n.* the astronomical ascendant, the degree of the zodiac rising in the east at a given time Inst/420

clippen *pr.3pl.* press, squeeze SW2/531

clister(ie) *n.* an enema Age/1077, Age/1079, Age/1080, 8Med/69

clodered *ppl.adj.* clotted DHN/246, Bac/390n

clog *n.* a weight that hampers movement 7LA/21

cloth *inf.* clothe, adorn [L. *induere*] Age/1625, **clothith** *pr.3sg.* Age/1499, **clothen** *pr.3pl.* Age/101, Age/499, Age/531

cloth *n.* a piece of fabric Age/1017, Age/1019, SW2/213, etc.; a membrane in the body [L. *pannus*] DHN/9, DIIN/18, etc.; a discoloration or pustulous outbreak of the skin Age/1572; **clothis** *pl.* fabrics, cloths Age/1531, SW2/794, etc.; bedclothes CHP/999, CHP/1017, CHP/1022; ~ *fantastic* the membrane in the forepart of the brain DHN/50

clowdis *n.pl.* clouds 7Pla/16; cloudy substances suspended in urine CHP/80

clowte *n.* a piece of cloth SW2/1755, SW2/1774, SW2/1788

clunes *n.pl.* the buttocks Coi/49

coaguled *ppl.adj.* thickened DHN/29

coart *inf.* hold (sth.) together 8Med/32, 8Med/35; **coartith** *pr.3sg.* restrains Fle/146, Fle/147

coct *ppl.adj.* boiled SW2/348; produced or processed by heating within the body Coi/63, Coi/194

cofre *n.* a cylindrical container used as a standard measure of volume Inst/1225, Inst/1245, Inst/1247

cogitacioun *n.* a thought, thinking Age/697, Age/704, Age/1537; ~ *fantastic* thought generated in the fore-part of the brain Coi/17

cognicioun *n.* knowledge Age/264, Age/894, Bac/257, etc.

coite *n.* coitus, sexual intercourse Plag/100

cokyng *vbl.n.* of humours: cooking, altering through bodily heat Age/99

colden *pr.3pl.* become cold Age/1010, CHP/628

coler *n.* the bodily humour choler, bile Age/1028, Age/1864, Fle/81, CHP/976, etc., **colre** SW2/500; *colre adust* choler that has been overheated or mixed with black bile SW2/1527; *blac* ~ black bile, the humour melancholy Age/934, Fle/111; *rede* ~ , ~ *rede* red bile, choler from the gall bladder DHN/189, Fle/112, CHP/981, etc.

colerik(e) *adj.* characterized by an excess of choler CHP/471, CHP/1097, SW2/101, etc., **coleryk** SW2/965, **col(e)ric** Bac/124, Plag/142, **colryke** Plag/223; ~ of persons: irascible, choleric 7Pla/164; *fever* ~ a fever caused by or associated with excess choler CHP/70, CHP/100

coleccioun *n.* an accumulation of a morbid substance in the body CHP/1289, CHP/1291, etc.; contraction of earlobes or skin CHP/436; synthesis, summary 7LA/138, 7LA/141

col(l)ik *n.* a disease involving severe intestinal pain, colic SW2/1829, SW2/1843

coluber *n.* a kind of snake Age/1367, Age/1422, Age/1432

colur(e) *n.* one of two great circles in the heavens or on a celestial globe, intersecting at right angles at the north and south poles Inst/93, Inst/124, etc.; ~ *equinoxial* the colure passing through the equinoctial points of the ecliptic Inst/93; ~ *solsticial* the colure at right angles to the equinoctial colure Inst/100, Inst/113, *Inst/115

combe *n.* the pubic bone and area [L. *pecten*] DHN/225

***combust** *n.* destruction by burning or heat 7Pla/61

comento(u)r *n.* a commentator CHP/951, CHP/1235, Plag/57, etc. [see also Persons, Places, and Works, s.n. **Comentor**]

comfortable *adj.* strengthening, invigorating SW2/228, SW2/375, SW2/413

comfortacioun *n.* relief, comfort Age/1414; **confortacioun** stimulation, strengthening Age/1715

comfortati(e)f *adj.* soothing, bringing relief Age/2100; stimulating, invigorating SW2/1483

comforte *inf.* comfort, soothe, strengthen Age/459, Age/1157, etc., **comfortith** *pr.3sg.* Age/75, Age/946, SW2/665, etc., **comforten** *pr.3pl.* Age/100, Age/144, CHP/478, etc., **comforted** *p.ppl.* Age/115, Age/362, Plag/282, etc.

commestible *adj.* edible Age/445, (as *n.*) an edible substance Bac/599

commestioun *n.* eating, consumption Age/1684

commixtioun *n.* mixing, an instance of mixing Age/1177, Age/1317, Age/2023, **commyxtioun** Age/591, **conmixtioun** CHP/411

commocioun *n.* disturbance, agitation Coi/275, Coi/278, etc.

comodites *n.pl.* benefits Age/481, Age/1255

compaccioun *n.* a framework, structure DHN/271

compact *n.* a framework, structure DHN/13, **compacts** *pl.* DHN/37

company see **cumpany**

comparisoned *p.ppl.* likened to CHP/159; *han* ~ error for L. *compereruerunt* 'have found' Age/1305

compas *n.* an instrument for drawing circles, a compass Inst/9, Inst/81, etc.; a circle Inst/938; ~ *of age* the course or path of old age Age/166, Age/1791; *blac* ~ a dark layer at the top of a urine sample Plag/410; *in* ~ in a circle (around sth.) Inst/958, 8Med/65; inside a circle Inst/1409; *just* ~ a perfect circle Inst/1120; *shame-fast cercle or* ~ the anus DHN/166; *without* ~ on the outside of a circle, inscribed around a circle Inst/1410

compassith *pr.3sg.* surrounds Age/157, **compassyng** *pr.ppl.* Age/178

competent *adj.* fitting, suitable CIIP/142, CHP/478, etc.

competently *adv.* successfully, satisfactorily Fle/77, CHP/208

complement *n.* completion CHP/1107

completief *adj.* causing completion, perfecting Age/1667, **completiefs** Age/268

complexioun *n.* physical make-up or nature of a person or thing, seen as a combination of the four humours or the four qualities (heat, cold, moisture, dryness) Age/437, Age/440, etc.; *high* ~ noble or vigorous nature SW2/30, SW2/40 [cf. *MED*, s.vv. *complexioun* n., 3a.(d), and *heigh* adj., 3(a)]

composicioun *n.* formation, construction DHN/250, DHN/257, DHN/267, Inst/242, Inst/273

compowne *inf.* create, fashion, compose Age/25, DHN/305, Inst/3, Inst/30; arrange Bac/231; **compowned** *p.ppl.* compounded, composed of diverse ingredients or qualities Age/1231, Coi/78, etc., **compovned** Age/1989, **compound** Age/95, Age/1461, CHP/1182, **compovnd** Coi/113

comune *n.* a community Bac/407, Bac/478

comune *adj.* ordinary, typical Bac/425, Bac/426, Bac/611, 7LA/564, etc.; shared CHP/14; of low rank Age/1996, CHP/797, 7Pla/97; public Age/306, Bac/236, 7LA/311, 7LA/312; (as *adv.*) commonly 7Pla/142; *of* ~ commonly CHP/367; *oile* ~ olive oil SW2/577, SW2/1035, SW2/1171; ~ *savour* usual pleasure DHN/224; ~ *werke* sexual activity DHN/220

concavyng *vbl.n.* a hollowness or depression Inst/190

concavite *n.* a hollowness Coi/14, CHP/1418, Inst/237, etc.

concorde *n.* harmony, concord 7LA/250

concours *n.* a coming together, concurrence Bac/191, CHP/196

concubyne *n.* intercourse Coi/115

concubyne *pr.3sg.subj.* should have intercourse Coi/244

concubith *pr.3sg.* has intercourse Coi/266

concupiscence *n.* inordinate desire Coi/244, 7Pla/191, 7Pla/232

condutes *adj.* prepared Plag/144

confeccioun *n.* a medicinal preparation, confection Age/1134, SW2/1513, Plag/69, etc.

confermyth *pr.3sg.* solidifies DHN/259; prevents Fle/164; **confermed** *p.ppl.* established Age/654, Plag/334

confessioun *n.* ?description, ?acknowledgment [error for L. *confectio* 'preparation'] Age/349n

confirmacioun *n.* support for an argument by appeal to authorities 7LA/170, 7LA/177

conformatief *adj.* conforming or similar to Bac/542

confortacioun see **comfortacioun**

confusif *adj.* confusing, obscure CHP/312

confusioun *n.* harm, ruin 7Pla/147

congel *pr.3sg.subj.* freeze, turn to ice Age/488; **congeled** *p.ppl.* clotted, solidified Age/935, CHP/412

congregacioun *n.* collection Bac/95, Bac/98, etc.

congrue *adj.* suitable, apposite Coi/85; correct, proper 7LA/62

congruyte *n.* correctness, propriety 7LA/39, 7LA/61, **congruite** 7LA/119

coniunccioun *n.* contact 7LA/97; the astronomical aspect having an angular distance near or equal to 0°, close proximity 7Pla/26, 7Pla/27, 7Pla/227

conmixtioun see **commixtioun**

connyng *n.* wisdom 7LA/22 [see also **konnyng**]

connyng *adj.* skillful, knowledgeable SW2/1229

consequence see **consequens**

consequens *n.* *bi ~* consequently [L. *per consequens*] Bac/590, CHP/583, etc., *per consequens* (L.) Inst/1137; *bi ~ (consequence) folowyng* consequently Bac/253, CHP/382, CHP/1232

consonauns *n.* harmony, consonance 7LA/188

consowde *inf.* make solid, knit (flesh) 8Med/32

constellacioun *n.* a configuration of heavenly bodies Bac/234, Bac/316, etc.; the influence of a heavenly body 7Pla/253, 7Pla/260, etc.

constriccioun *n.* constipation Age/1801; tightness CHP/927

constrict *ppl.adj.* of the windpipe: closed DHN/102, DHN/103; thickened, clotted DHN/247

construccioun *n.* syntactic structure 7LA/120; physical constitution *DHN/104

consules *n.pl.* governors, rulers 7Pla/34

consumpt *ppl.adj.* consumed Age/114, CHP/974, etc.

contentief *adj.* of humours: able to be contained CHP/472; of corporeal virtues: able to contain bodily substances CHP/633; (as *n.*) the corporeal virtue that contains bodily substances CHP/681

continence *n.* ?moderation 7Pla/97

contynuaunce *n.* continuity CHP/102; duration, length of time CHP/1455, CHP/1458

contrauersie *n.a* controversy, conflict 7LA/176

convey *impv.* draw (lines) Inst/43

convenient *adj.* suitable, appropriate Age/134, Age/441, etc., **convenyent** Age/1373, Age/2085, etc., **conuenient** Age/1074, Age/1362, etc., **conuenyent** Coi/202

conveniently *adv.* appropriately, suitably Age/500, Age/1838, etc.

convicten *pr.3pl.* ?declare [error for L. *ceruici* 'neck'] DHN/140; **convict** *ppl.adj.* ?demonstrated, shown [error for L. *coniuncto* 'joined'] DHN/241

copulacioun *n.* a coupling, joining Age/431n

cord(e) *n.* a cord, heavy twine (for hanging an object) Inst/224, Inst/297, Inst/307, Inst/341, etc.; *~* a chord (of an arc of a circle) Inst/784, Inst/791, **corda** (L.) Inst/789, Inst/814; *~ prima* the first chord found in a calculation (of two mentioned) Inst/862; *~ recte, corda recta* (L.) graduations on one side of a quadrant for calculating sine functions Inst/371n, Inst/788, Inst/796, Inst/860, etc.; *~ verse, corda versa* (L.) graduations on one side of a quadrant for calculating versine functions Inst/372n, Inst/795, etc.

cornerd *adj.* *vj houre ~* located at the sixth hour-angle (i.e., the meridian) Inst/1209

corner(e) *n.* a corner of a square or other polygon Inst/943, Inst/944, 7LA/596, etc.; *~ of þe erth* the degree of the zodiac directly below the observer at a given time Inst/423; *~ of the quadraunt* the rectangular corner of a quadrant Inst/408, Inst/901, 7LA/419, etc.; *right (streight)* ~ a right angle Inst/943, Inst/956

corosie *n.* corrosive destruction of tissue CHP/1457

corosief *adj.* associated with destruction of tissue by corrosion CHP/1441

corporale *adj.* pertaining to the body [error for L. *cordialis* 'strengthening the heart, stimulating'] CHP/479n

corrumptith *pr.3sg.* decays, causes (sth.) to decay CHP/1327, CHP/1480, **corrumpten** *pr.3pl.* CHP/235

corrupcioun *n.* infection, decay Age/332, Age/809, Bac/32, etc.; morbid matter SW2/1060, SW2/1253; impairment Age/645n

corrupt *ppl.adj.* infected, impaired, decayed Age/438, Age/463, Bac/29, etc.; of humours: unbalanced SW2/117, SW2/524, Plag/163, etc.

corrupte *inf.* become infected, decay Plag/29, **corruptith** *pr.3sg.* Age/417, Age/847, Plag/12, etc.; **corruptith** *pr.3sg.* infects, destroys Age/333, Age/436, Bac/355, etc., **corrupten** *pr.3pl.* Bac/31, Bac/354, **corruptid** *p.ppl.* Age/334, **corrupted** Bac/130

corruptible *adj.* subject to decay Bac/140, Bac/142, 7Pla/258; ~ *cause* something that can cause decay or harm Plag/22

cost *n.* expense, price Age/306, Age/1995; *of light* ~ inexpensive SW2/839

costis *n.pl.* countries, regions Plag/14

cotidian *adj. fevers* ~ fevers that recur at daily intervals SW2/666

cotidianly *adv.* every day, daily Age/1593, Age/1884, Age/1888; in relation to a cotidian fever CHP/303

cotis *n.pl. litel* ~ the tunicles or tissues of the eyes DHN/32

cours *n.* a course, path Age/164, Age/1646, Plag/181, etc.; of a heavenly body: the celestial path Inst/1089, 7LA/57; *natural ~, ~ nat-*

ural a natural process Age/142, Age/211, Age/1612, CHP/599; of blood: flow, flowing Fle/112

covenable *adj.* suitable Coi/85, Coi/177, Bac/211, etc.

covenably *adv.* appropriately Bac/552

covercle *n.* a cover for a pot, lid SW2/1805

coueryng *vbl.n.* a covering, protection Bac/170

covertour *n.* a cover for an instrument Inst/284; **couertour** a head covering Age/412

cracchyng *vbl.n.* scratching Age/381

craft *n.* a skill, an art Age/50, Bac/39, Inst/95, etc.; power 7LA/1; **craftis** *pl.* skilled trades 7LA/564, 7LA/570; *liberal* **craftes** liberal arts 7Pla/300; *mecanic craftes* mechanical arts, skilled trades 7Pla/300

crafti *adj.* of persons: skillful, learned CHP/179, **crafty** Age/1656; ~ of things: artful, skillful 7LA/179, **crafty** 7LA/206

craftily *adv.* skillfully, carefully Age/874, Inst/196, Inst/288

crasith *pr.3sg.* breaks, bursts CHP/1483

crepature *n.* a rupture, hernia CHP/1464, CHP/1482

creperith *pr.3sg.* ruptures CHP/1483

crepuscle *n.* dusk Inst/424, Inst/427

cresceth *pr.3sg.* increases Inst/797

cretik *adj. day* ~ *(cretic)* the day on which a disease appears or takes a turn for better or worse CHP/1141, CHP/1146, etc.

crisis *n.* the turning point in a disease CHP/152, CHP/1095, etc.

crisp *adj.* of hair: curly Age/1232, Age/1460; of serpents: ?undulating Age/1373

crispacioun *n.* wrinkling Age/484

cristallyne *adj.* ~ *humour* the material of the crystalline lens in the eye CHP/1008

croceat *adj.* saffron-colored Fle/111, Fle/119

cronikes *adj.* (as *n.pl.*) chronic sicknesses CHP/1126; *sikenessis of cronykes* chronic sicknesses CHP/1108
crosse *adj.* perpendicular Inst/1136
crul *adj.* of hair: curly Age/1232
crusel *n.* a crucible Plag/120
crustuls *n.pl.* scabs, crusts DHN/241
cubite *n.* a unit of measure equivalent to one and a half feet Age/822, 7LA/453, 7LA/455, etc.
cumpany *inf.* have sexual intercourse SW2/80, **company** SW2/139
cumpany *n.* sexual intercourse SW2/555
cumpanyng *vbl.n.* sexual intercourse SW2/555
cupped *p.ppl.* bled by use of a cupping glass SW2/148, SW2/328
curacioun *n.* healing, curing Age/1927
curious *adj.* solicitous, eager 7Pla/110, 7Pla/116, etc.
cursers *n.pl.* people who curse 7Pla/285
cursible *adj.* moving easily CHP/1400
cursour *n.* a sliding scale on an old quadrant Inst/1351, Inst/1365, etc., **cursure** Inst/1349; *cursure of the day* the point on the cursor corresponding to the current day Inst/1354
cutters *n.pl..* ~ *of *weynes* bloodletters 7Pla/56

damage *n.* harm, injury 7Pla/110, 7Pla/197
dar *pr.1sg.* dare CHP/256, *pr.1pl.* CHP/669, *pr.3sg.* DHN/205
dawyng *vbl.n.* dawn Inst/426
daungier *n.* power, control 7Pla/126
debilitacioun *n.* weakness CHP/521
debilite *n.* weakness Age/161, Age/169, Age/1875, etc.; ~ *of vertu* weakness of a physical power CHP/452, CHP/485, etc.
declynacioun the fourth and final stage of an illness CHP/41, CHP/53, etc.; the angular distance (of a heavenly body) from a celestial great circle such as the ecliptic

or equinoctial Inst/479, Inst/496, etc.; ~ *of eche (that) gree* the distance of a given point on the ecliptic from the equinoctial (i.e., from the celestial equator) Inst/517, Inst/522; ~ *of al the meridie* the maximum distance of the sun from the equinoctial Inst/376
decoc(c)ioun *n.* a medicine made by boiling selected ingredients Age/1568, SW2/245, SW2/685, SW2/1436, 8Med/27, etc., **decoctions** *pl.* SW2/1725; ~ the process of boiling medicinal ingredients 8Med/25; ~ a transformation through heat (e.g., in the body, in food or drink, etc.) Age/422, Age/1320, DHN/153, CHP/297, **deccocioun** Age/853, **deccocciouns** DHN/245
decoct *ppl.adj.* transformed by heat Age/1945, DHN/154, DHN/243
decoctith *pr.3sg.* cooks, heats DHN/158, DHN/163
decoracioun *n.* decoration, ornament Age/77n, Age/482, Age/1012, etc.
decrepite *n.* decrepitude Age/32, Age/166
decrepit(e) *adj.* worn out, feeble Age/522, Age/1769, Age/1940; ~ *age* advanced old age Age/168, Age/1691, etc.
dedly *adv.* like something dead SW2/1367
dedly lif *phr.* mortal life, life in this world Bac/205
deepe *adj.* deep 7LA/48, **diepe** CHP/569, CHP/655, **depper** *comp.* Inst/14; ~ *mesure* depth Inst/1403
deepe *adv.* deep, far (within sth.) SW2/212, SW2/219, **depe** SW2/1385
defaute *n.* default, failure, lack, defect Age/20, Age/158, etc.
defectief *adj.* defective, lacking Coi/39, Coi/41, Bac/393
defence *n.* protection, defense Age/249, Age/250, Plag/187, etc., **defense** Age/1766

defensed *ppl.adj.* defended Age/113

defensioun *n.* protection, defense Age/57

defie(n) *inf.* digest, break down physiologically SW2/914, SW2/1766, **defieth** *pr.3sg.* Plag/388

defieng *vbl.n.* digestion SW2/312, Plag/104

deformatief *adj.* deformed, misshapen Age/479

defoulyng *pr.ppl.* defiling Plag/100

degre(e) *n.* one of four gradations of heat, cold, dryness, moisture, or temperateness Age/1114, Age/1115, etc.; a degree of arc Inst/44, Inst/109, Inst/161, etc.; a unit of measure equal to two cubits 7LA/455, 7LA/456; *in the x (10)* ~ to the fullest extent [possibly due to an erroneous reading of the arabic numeral *4* as the roman numeral *x*] Age/2103, Age/952; error for L. *sensus* 'senses' Age/1348n

deieccioun *n.* loss of power or position, degradation 7Pla/37, 7Pla/49

dele *n.* a part SW2/1205

delectacioun *n.* sensual pleasure Coi/8, Coi/126, Coi/268, **dilectacioun** DHN/202, Coi/117

delicious *adj.* sensual, hedonistic 7Pla/327

demonstratief *adj.* revealing a present condition CHP/4, CHP/9; **demonstratiefs** (as *n.pl.*) things showing a present condition CHP/28

departyng *pr.ppl.* separating, dividing DHN/270, SW2/1213, Inst/980, **departing** DHN/277; ~ parting with 7Pla/276

departyng *vbl. n.* the act of separation, removal Age/358

departynges *vbl.n.pl.* divisions or regions of the brain DHN/7

depeynted *ppl. adj.* depicted Age/1633

depnes(se) *n.* the interior SW2/541, SW2/545, SW2/1000; depth CHP/425, Inst/277, 7LA/417, 7LA/449, etc.

depose *inf.* expel CHP/551; push aside CHP/998; ***deposen** *pr.3pl.* press down DHN/60

deposicioun *n.* expulsion, excretion Age/1102, Age/2101, CHP/298

depuryng *vbl.n.* cleansing, purifying CHP/1496

derrest see **diere**

descence *n.* descent Inst/581

descencioun *n.* declining astrological influence 7Pla/93

descendaunt *adj.* descending Inst/372, Inst/374, Inst/477, etc.

descendith *pr.3sg.* descends Coi/64, Coi/273, etc., **descenden** *pr.3pl.* Age/1852, DHN/109, Coi/46, **descendyng** *pr.ppl.* Coi/36; **descende** *pr.3sg.subj.* error for L. *distendat* 'should stretch, should be distended' CHP/1377

descendens (L.) *pr.ppl.* descending or turning (to a topic) CHP/375

desiccacioun *n.* drying Age/1113; dryness Age/1910, CHP/400

destitucioun *n.* lack, loss CHP/341

destitute *adj.* lacking, not present CHP/409; deprived Fle/80

determyne *inf.* terminate, reach a limit CHP/1358; **determyneng** *pr.ppl.* judging CHP/271; **determyned** *p.ppl.* defined, ascertained Age/1711, CHP/6, etc.; terminated CHP/1302, CHP/1389, etc.; *determyneth of* discusses CHP/267

detracciouns *n.pl.* slanders 7Pla/293

dever *n.* do his ~ of a medicine: achieve its purpose SW2/1420

diametrely *adv.* along the diameters Inst/39

diapason *n.* a musical octave 7LA/274, 7LA/277

diapent *n.* a musical fifth 7LA/274, 7LA/275

diasintastik *n.* the study of syntax 7LA/121

diatesseron *n.* a medicine with four ingredients SW2/193 [see Materia Medica, s.v.]; a musical fourth 7LA/273, 7LA/275, 7LA/277

diere *adj.* dear, beloved Age/79, Age/90, etc., **derrest** *sup.* Age/1165

diew(e) *adj.* due, fitting, appropriate Age/253, Bac/5, 7LA/149, etc., **due** SW2/64, SW2/92, Inst/170, 7LA/19, etc., **dewe** Plag/386

dieute *n.* ~ *of nature, natures diewte* the call of nature, relief of the bowels Age/174, CHP/299

differencen *pr.3pl.* differ Age/754, **diffirensen** 8Med/62

differre *inf.* defer CHP/190, **differred** *p.ppl.* CHP/194, CHP/562, **deferred** CHP/197, CHP/200

diffynicioun *n.* definition 7LA/138, 7LA/139

diffynisshith *pr.3sg.* defines Coi/54

diffugured *p.ppl.* disfigured CHP/342

diffuse *adj.* spread out, radiating CHP/1033

digest(e) *inf.* digest, assimilate nourishment Age/790, CHP/297, etc., **digested** *p.ppl.* Age/198, Age/757, Coi/196, etc., **digestid** Age/866, Coi/198; ~ *inf.* break down morbid matter or humour(s), transform CHP/300, CHP/1166, **digestith** *pr.3sg.* Age/1417, Age/2039, Age/2049, Age/2057n, **digested** *p.ppl.* CHP/68, CHP/1051, CHP/1493

digesti(e)f *adj. vertu* ~ the physiological power of digestion Age/220, Age/362, Age/546, CHP/302

digestioun *n.* assimilation of food Age/194, Age/367, etc.; *first (secunde, thrid, iiij)* ~ one of the four stages of digestion and conversion of food into flesh, in the stomach and intestines, the liver, the other organs, and in select specialized organs respectively Age/451, Age/451, Age/376, Age/449, etc.; *iiij digestiouns* the four stages of digestion Age/361; *of light (light of)* ~ easily digested Age/1944, Plag/103; *parfite* ~

completed digestion CHP/52; *signe of* ~ a symptom of the quality of digestion found in urine and other excreta CHP/51, CHP/60, etc.

dight *p.ppl.* prepared SW2/208

dightyng *vbl.n.* preparation 7LA/569

dilated *p.ppl.* expanded 7LA/294

dilectacioun see **delectacioun**

diminucioun *n.* decrease, diminution Age/252, Age/503, CHP/598, **dyminucioun** Age/715, Age/718, **dyminicioun** CHP/1432, **dymunyssioun** Age/160; *dyminucioun of blood(e)* blood-letting Age/498, Age/505, Bac/392; **dymunycioun, dyminucioun** error for L. *divisione* 'a division or category' Age/1027n, Age/1104

dymynusith *pr.3sg.* diminishes, decreases Coi/66, **dymunysshed** *p.ppl.* Coi/200

dyminute *ppl.adj.* diminished Age/1805

dymmy *adj.* discolored, livid CHP/721

dymnes(se) *n.* darkening of vision CHP/567, CHP/627, etc.

dindimes *n.pl.* parts of the male reproductive system between the testicles and the penis Coi/49n, Coi/50 [see Norri 1998, 335]

dipsni *n.* abbreviation for *dipsnia*, respiratory difficulty, a form of asthma [correctly *dispnia* or *disnia*] Fle/55

direccioun *n.* the west-to-east movement of planets through the zodiac Inst/592; instruction, guidance 7LA/49

directis *n.pl. in the (evene)* ~ *of* in line with Inst/323, Inst/566

dirivith *pr.3sg.* ~ *to the nakidnesse* error (possibly in translator's exemplar) for L. *Dinamidiarum* 'Dynamidia' Age/1879n

disceit *n.* ?gangrene CHP/912 [cf. *MED*, s.v. *deceit(e* n., 3(a)]

dischargith *pr.3sg.* relieves, releases CHP/948

disconuenyent *adj.* unsuitable 7LA/38
discouered *ppl.adj.* uncovered Age/411
discresen *pr.3pl.* decline Age/1174; **discresyng** *pr.ppl. discresyng the moone* when the moon wanes Age/1210
discrete *adj.* discerning Age/326; (?as *n.pl.*) ?things discerned Coi/97n
discribed *p.ppl.* inscribed 7LA/423
discrive *inf.* inscribe Inst/34, Inst/79, etc., *impv.* Inst/98, Inst/511, 7LA/505, 7LA/508, **discrivyng** *pr.ppl.* Inst/104, 7LA/499, **discrived** *p.ppl.* 7LA/430, **discryved** 7LA/210; **discryve** *inf.* determine Inst/935
discure *inf.* reveal, disclose SW2/18
discuryng *vbl.n.* disclosure SW2/11
disiunctief *adj.* having different meanings CHP/1234
disparagiþ *pr.3sg.* damages CHP/1316
disparplith *pr.3sg.* disperses Coi/66, **disparpled** *p.ppl.* Coi/15, SW2/542
dispise *inf.* despise SW2/22, 7Pla/140, **dispisith** *pr.3sg.* *SW2/19, SW2/21, **dispisyng** *pr.ppl.* 7Pla/288; **dispicith** *pr.3sg.* dissipates Age/1905n
disputacioun *n.* discussion, academic disputation, or an instance thereof DHN/234n, 7LA/141
dissentery *n.* dysentery 8Med/7, **dissintery** Age/1148
dissenterik *n.* a person with dysentery 8Med/11, **dissinterik** 8Med/34
dissymulyng *pr.ppl.* deceptive CHP/1212
dissolucioun *n.* dispersal (of a humour), disintegration Age/98, Age/297, etc.; weakening CHP/589; wasting away SW2/1274
dissolut(e) *adj.* dispersed Age/219, CHP/1051
dissolutes *adj.* (as *n.pl.*) things that have been dispersed Age/113
dissolve *inf.* dissolve, break up Age/1157, SW2/1843, **dissoluen** SW2/1363, **dissolue** *impv.* Fle/168, SW2/1569, **dissolvith** *pr.3sg.* Age/239, Age/1248, etc., **dissolueth** Age/2070, DHN/238,

dissolueþ Age/1158, **dissoluith** DHN/298, **dissoluen** *pr.3pl.* Age/217, **dissolued** *p.ppl.* Age/296, Age/926, etc., **dissolved** Age/58, Age/249, etc.
dissolvyng *vbl.n.* a rebuttal, negation 7LA/178
disteinte *adj.* distended, swollen CHP/1216
distemperat(e) *adj.* characterized by humoral imbalance or an excess of one of the primary qualities Age/943, Age/1240, Coi/74, Coi/76
distemperaunce *n.* an imbalance in the humours or qualities Age/160, Age/169, CHP/1118
distemperith *pr.3sg.* disturbs the humoral balance Age/1241
distencioun *n.* a distension, swelling CHP/1378
distendyng *pr.ppl.* stretching, expanding CHP/608
distinctith *pr.3sg.* distinguishes Age/1974, Age/1979
distreyneng *pr.ppl.* pressing, straining CHP/1346; **distreyned** *p.ppl.* compressed CHP/610, CHP/1183
dyuersite *n.* diversity, variety, difference Age/434, Age/1326, etc., **diuersite** Age/740, CHP/599, Plag/32, etc.; **dyuersitees** *pl.* distinguishing traits, circumstances Age/1656
diuersith *pr.3sg.* differs CHP/1223, **dyuersen** *pr.3pl.* Age/1258
dividaunt *adj.* dividing Inst/817
divyne *adj.* divine, of heavenly origin Age/317, Age/319n, Age/634, etc.; divinely inspired CHP/127, CHP/176
divulsif *adj.* ragged, heterogeneous CHP/80
doctrynall *adj.* pertaining to the principles of a discipline 7LA/183
dogflies *n.pl.* biting insects 7Pla/15
doyng *vbl.n.* action, deeds SW2/1387; *mannes ~* sexual intercourse with a

man SW2/1353; **doynges** *pl.* influ-
ences Bac/137
donward(e) *adv.* downward SW2/582,
SW2/693, etc., **dounvard** SW2/530
do(o)re *n.* a door, an entrance (also
fig.) DHN/25n; *at the* ~ imminent
CHP/696
dosis *n.pl.* doses, specific amounts of
medicine Age/527n
dough *n. soure* ~ sourdough SW2/1035,
*SW2/1050
draynt *p.ppl.* submerged, immersed
SW2/809
drames *n.pl.* drams, units of weight
equal to an eighth of an ounce
SW2/451 [usually abbreviated ʒ]
drapiers *n.pl.* clothiers, cloth-makers
7LA/577
draught(e) *n.* a drink Bac/60,
SW2/158, SW2/181, etc.; a line,
something drawn Inst/945,
Inst/958, **drawghtis** *pl.* Inst/950
dreame reders *phr.* prophetic dreamers
[L. *somniantes* 'dreamers'] Bac/261
dred(e)ful *adj.* frightening, threatening CHP/492; fearful 7Pla/340
dreede *inf.* fear, dread Age/700,
CHP/615, etc., *impv.* CHP/1263,
dre(e)dith *pr.3sg.* Age/700,
Bac/350, etc., **dreeden** *pr.3pl.*
CHP/1259, **dredyng** *pr.ppl.*
CHP/256; **dreeden** *pr.3pl.* error for
L. *tenuiter* 'sparingly' DHN/92
dresse *inf.* arrange, position SW2/1193,
impv. SW2/1167, *pr.ppl.* **dressyng**
SW2/1160, SW2/1186, SW2/1206,
(i)dressed *p.ppl.* SW2/1178,
SW2/1217, **dressid** SW2/1187;
dressed *p.ppl.* guided DHN/226
dried *p.ppl.* desiccated, dehydrated
Fle/69
drift *n.* sexual intercourse, co-
itus Coi/4, Coi/9, etc.; agitation
CHP/869, CHP/1227
dryve *inf.* have sexual intercourse
Coi/44, etc., **drive** Coi/272,
Coi/287, **dryvith** *pr.3sg.* Coi/184,

Coi/198, **drivith** Coi/270, **dryven**
pr.3pl. Coi/201, ~ *pr.3sg.subj.* Coi/178,
etc., **dryven** *p.ppl.* Coi/246, **drive**
Coi/246; ~ *inf.* drive, force, push
SW2/1022, **drivith** *pr.3.sg.* Coi/238,
Plag/192, **dryvith** Plag/187, **dryven**
pret.3pl. Bac/562, *p.ppl.* Bac/564,
driven Age/284, **dryve** CHP/639;
dryven *pr.3pl.* of the eyes: move
rapidly, show agitation CHP/639,
drivyng *pr.ppl.* CHP/568
drivyng *vbl.n.* sexual intercourse
Coi/218, Coi/228, etc.; growing,
thriving Plag/8
dropesy *n.* dropsy, a pathological accumulation of excess fluid, usually in the abdominal area Age/1859,
SW2/83, etc., **dropesie** Age/1432,
Age/2047, SW2/896, etc.; *colde
dropesies* dropsies caused by an excess of cold humours SW2/676;
dropesie of the matrice accumulation
of fluid (esp. blood) in the uterus
SW2/892, SW2/906, SW2/909 [see
also **idropesy**]
drownen *pr.3pl.* (?or *inf.*) overflow,
flood CHP/907; **drowned** *p.ppl.* immersed Age/1323; of eyes: sunken
CHP/655
drunk(e) *p.ppl.* imbibed, drunk
Age/78, Age/1004, SW2/871, etc.,
drunken SW2/722, Plag/51; *drunk-
en of* soaked in Age/428
due see **diew(e)**
duely *adv.* suitably, properly 7LA/60
dulnes(se) *n.* stupidity, mental dull-
ness Age/645, Age/995, etc.
dung(g)ed *ppl.adj.* manured Age/801,
Age/828, etc.
dunggy *adj.* containing dung or ma-
nure Age/798, Age/800
duplacioun *n.* doubling (of a number)
7LA/205, 7LA/215
duplicacioun *n.* of joints: bending
CHP/799, CHP/888
duratief *adj.* long-lasting SW2/1436,
8Med/59

dure *adj.* hard, solid 8Med/68
duretik *n.* a diuretic SW2/1725

eare *n.* an ear, the organ of hearing DHN/17, DHN/22, Fle/5, Plag/180, etc., **eeris** *pl.* CHP/399, CHP/403, etc., **eeres** CHP/372; ~ *of the herte* an auricle of the heart DHN/113, **earis** *pl.* auricles DHN/115; *after (the) earis* behind the ears Coi/23, Coi/26, Coi/46
easy *adj.* easy, not intense Age/125, SW2/253, etc.; ~ *fever* a low fever SW2/1018; ~ *fuyre* a low fire SW2/1837
e(a)sily *adv.* easily SW2/255, SW2/271, etc.; gently SW2/1194, SW2/1553, SW2/1753
ebullicioun *n.* heating, boiling, physiological transformation through heat CHP/66, CHP/983
ecliptik(e) *n.* the apparent orbit of the sun and the planets through the heavens Inst/1042, Inst/1044; the representation of the celestial ecliptic on an astronomical instrument Inst/121, Inst/379, Inst/646, etc., **ecliptic** Inst/1064
ecliptik(e) *adj.* ~ *lyne* the celestial ecliptic Inst/1049; the representation of the celestial ecliptic on an astronomical instrument Inst/1051, Inst/1061, etc.
econverso (L.) *adv.* conversely Inst/826, Inst/830, Inst/833
edder see **addir**
edificacioun *n.* building 7LA/435
educith *pr.3sg.* brings (out) Age/1924
eekyng *vbl.n.* increasing, extending DHN/194
eere *n.* an ear of grain Age/997, Age/1205n
effeccioun *n.* infection, contamination Bac/575
effectual *adj.* efficacious, successful Bac/151, Bac/219, Bac/532
effectual(l)y *adv.* in effect Coi/57n, Plag/10

effusioun *n.* expense, outflow Bac/602, CHP/1435, etc.; ~ *of seed(e)* emission of semen Coi/24, Coi/26, Coi/127
egal *adj.* equal Inst/314, Inst/362, 7LA/77
egest *inf.* defecate CHP/551
egestio(u)n *n.* feces DHN/199, CHP/56, SW2/1768, etc.; defecation CHP/550
eg(ge) *n.* an egg Age/1559, DHN/30, SW2/755, SW2/1503, etc., **egg** Age/1557, **egges** *pl.* Fle/99, SW2/1472, SW2/1475; *rere* ~ a softboiled egg Age/2090, Fle/135 [see also **ey**]
egge *n.* the edge (of the teeth) 7LA/102, 7LA/105
egre *adj.* bitter Plag/135
ey *n.* an egg SW2/936, SW2/1057, **eyren** *pl.* SW2/371, SW2/622, etc. [see also **eg(ge)**]
eye *n.* an eye Age/576, CHP/581, etc., **eyen** *pl.* Age/381, Age/509, etc., **eyn** CHP/552; *biholde at* ~ see with one's own eyes Bac/19
viij [i.e., **eight**] see **notis**
eyren see **ey**
eyshel-ful *n.* a unit of measure, the amount that fits in an eggshell SW2/1316
ey-shellis *n.pl.* eggshells SW2/401, SW2/450
ekith *pr.3sg.* increases Coi/102 [cf. **eekyng**]
elate *adj.* exalted, superior Coi/152
eld *n.* old age Age/1680
elder *adj.* older Age/2n, Age/167, Bac/377, etc. [see also Age/122n]
eldyng *vbl.n.* aging Age/44, Age/119
eleccioun *n.* selection, choice Age/323, Age/919, 7LA/301
elect *p.ppl.* selected Age/974, Age/1384
electuarie *n.* a compound medicine in a thick sweet substrate such as honey or syrup Age/772, Age/1105, SW2/360, etc., **electuary** Bac/536,

SW2/269, etc. [see also **lectuary** and Materia Medica, s.v.]

elegance *n.* refinement, precision CHP/1435, CHP/1436

elipered *ppl. adj.* boiled Age/1909n

eliquiteth *pr.3sg.* liquefies, generates (a liquid) Coi/21; **eliquit** *p.ppl.* liquefied, made liquid Coi/22

elnes *n.pl.* ells (units of varying length) Inst/1297

elongacioun *n.* drawing out or extraction of an essential property Age/344, Age/917; distance CHP/513; removal CHP/1431

emagoge *adj.* stimulating blood flow SW2/269

embosyng *vbl.n.* bulging, convexness Inst/190

emboton *n.* a small pipe for introducing medicinal smoke into the vagina SW2/791, *embotus* SW2/794

embrio(u)n *n.* an embryo *DHN/230, DHN/262, DHN/280, DHN/287, DHN/288, DHN/290, DHN/301

embrocacioun *n.* the sprinkling or bathing of a patient's face or wound with a medicinal liquid *8Med/5, 8Med/40

emerawdis *n.pl.* hemorrhoids SW2/84

emyspiere *n.* hemisphere Inst/1009

emplasme *n.* a poultice or wet compress applied on both sides of a wound 8Med/63, 8Med/66

emplaster *impv.* apply a medicinal plaster SW2/333, SW2/1304, **emplastred** *p.ppl.* SW2/410, SW2/840, **emplasterd** Age/1270

emplaster *n.* a medicinal plaster, poultice, or salve SW2/283, SW2/372, SW2/824, etc., **emplastres** *pl.* SW2/1043, *SW2/1723; ~ *diasinthy* a plaster containing a compound medicine based on quinces Fle/96

empostem(e), empostym see **apostem(e)**

empted *p.ppl.* emptied, delivered SW2/1097

emtymene *n.* an enthymeme, a partial syllogism 7LA/131, **emtyme** 7LA/134

emunctories *n.pl.* locations on the body through which poisons are eliminated Plag/177, Plag/178, etc.

enarke *impv.* bend Inst/254

enarkyng *vbl.n.* bending, curve Inst/255

encatisme *n.* an herbal bath for the buttocks of a dysenteric patient 8Med/4, 8Med/6

encheaso(u)n *n.* cause, reason SW2/64, SW2/523, Plag/12

encheasounyng *pr.ppl.* causing, occasioning SW2/1359, **encheasound** *p.ppl.* SW2/1351

enchewed *p.ppl.* error for L. *euchimia* '(good) juices in foods' Age/741 [see Age/94n]

enchewynges *n.pl.* error for L. *euchimia* '(good) juices in foods' Age/742 [see Age/94n]

encorpore *impv.* blend SW2/1129

encres *n.* an increase Age/1170, DHN/263

encresyng *pr.ppl.* ~ *the moone* while the moon waxes Age/1175

endiadym *n.* hendiadys, the rhetorical figure of using two nouns joined by *and* CHP/184

endlong(es) *adv.* lengthwise, from end to end Inst/1062, Inst/1081

enfast *impv.* fasten Inst/82

enfastnyng *pr.ppl.* fastening Inst/104, **enfastned** *p.ppl.* Inst/213

enfectyng *pr.ppl.* infecting Age/597, **enfect** *p.ppl.* Plag/319

enfigure *inf.* draw, depict Inst/187

enforke *inf.* make a fork in (sth.) Inst/288

enforme *inf.* teach, instruct, inform 7LA/59, **enformyth** *pr.3sg.* 7LA/39, 7LA/122, **enformeth** 7LA/116, **enformed** *p.ppl.* 7LA/41; **enformyth** *pr.3sg.* gives form to DHN/277

engyne *n.* device Age/937

enhaunce *inf.* raise Inst/311, Inst/314; **enhaunsith** *pr.3sg.* heightens the reputation of (sb.) CHP/26, CHP/28, CHP/228

enhaunsyng *vbl.n.* ~ *of the poole* altitude of the pole above the horizon Inst/1108

enigmate (L.) *n. in* ~ obscurely Bac/494

enjoynaunt *vbl.n.* combining Inst/723

enlarged *p.ppl.* expanded, dilated [errors for L. *debilitatus* 'weakened' and L. *illatus* 'carried'] Age/1612, DHN/202

*enoryme *n.* matter suspended in urine [L. *eneorima*] CHP/80

enplace *inf.* put in position Inst/168, Inst/173

enserchers *n.pl.* seekers, scholars 7LA/346

ensesyng *pr.ppl.* grasping, understanding Inst/917

ensigne *inf.* inscribe, draw Inst/15

ensure *impv.* make secure Inst/352

entierly *adv.* ~ *holl, holl* ~ pure, sound [L. *sincerus*] Age/749, Age/750 [see also **intierly**]

entre *inf.* enter Age/1324, SW2/796, Plag/216, Inst/259, ?8Med/49, etc.

entre *n.* entry, entrance Plag/301

entremeted *p.ppl.* introduced 8Med/68

epatic *adj.* pertaining to the liver: (as *n.*) the hepatic vein, one of the major veins in the arm Fle/28, Fle/45, Fle/56

epedemy(e) *n.* epidemic disease Plag/318, Plag/337

epedymal *adj.* epidemic, pestilential Plag/309

epedimia (L.) *n.* epidemic disease Plag/13

epilence *n.* epilepsy DHN/86, **epilensie** Fle/53

epilentices *n.pl.* persons afflicted with epilepsy Bac/260

epilentik *n.* epilepsy CHP/235

epithymye *n.* a plaster or poultice made with herbs, applied around a wound 8Med/4, **epithemy**

8Med/38, 8Med/65, **epithimy** 8Med/63, **epitym** Age/1636

epizotis *n.* the diaphragm DHN/133, DHN/143, **epizotos** DHN/141

equacioun *n.* ~ *of houses* the equal dividing of the sky into astrologically significant segments Inst/1023

equalite *n.* of humours or elements: an even balance Age/475, Age/1233, Bac/293, Bac/295, etc.; evenness (of physiological symptoms, qualities, etc.) CHP/293, CHP/1196, CHP/1210

equate *adj.* of balanced temperament Bac/156; **equat** equated, equally divided Inst/1262

equatour *n.* the equator on a celestial globe, the great circle halfway between the two poles Inst/95, Inst/105, etc.; ~ *of the day* the equator on a celestial globe, celestial equator ["equator" is a shortened form of the phrase "equator of the day"] Inst/87

equinoccial(l) *adj.* ~ *cercle, cercle* ~ *(equinoxial)* the celestial equator Inst/385, Inst/544, Inst/548, Inst/689, etc.; (as *n.*) the equinoctial circle, the celestial equator Inst/374, Inst/376, Inst/525, Inst/661, etc., **equinoxial** Inst/653, Inst/1325n; *colure equinoxial* the colure passing through the equinoctial points of the ecliptic Inst/93; *poole equinoxial* one of the poles on the axis of the celestial equator, the north or south celestial pole Inst/37, Inst/38

equite *n.* equality, parity DHN/311

erjatamyes *n.pl.* yieldith ~ ?error for L. *reiterato/a uice* 'a repeated time' DHN/286n

erried *pret.3sg.* plowed Bac/61

ersely *adv.* of birth presentation: with buttocks first SW2/1231

erth(e)ly *adj.* characterized by the qualities of the element earth Age/1322, 7LA/113; having to do

with this world Age/365, 7Pla/280;
~ *signe* a zodiacal sign associated
with the element earth 7Pla/12,
7Pla/59, etc.; ~ error for L. *tarda*
'slow' Age/1384n

erthly *adv.* like the element earth
Age/359

erupcioun *n.* the bursting or rupture of an aposteme CHP/1459,
CHP/1472, CHP/1473

estatis *n.pl.* conditions Plag/413

ested *pret.3pl.* of stars: were in the east
Bac/219

estyval *adj.* of summer, summer-time
Inst/477

estraunges *n.pl.* external things, for-
eign substances Age/113

et(h)ikes *n.pl.* hectic fevers Age/230,
Age/235, CHP/385

evacuacio(u)n *n.* evacuation of super-
fluous humours or waste Age/96,
DHN/118, Coi/258, Bac/23,
CHP/545, etc.

evened *p.ppl.* straightened, put into
proper position SW2/1240; made
even Inst/451

evenes(se) *n.* evenness, equality
DHN/240, Bac/585, CHP/293, etc.

evenyng *vbl.n.* ~ *of the *houses xij* the equal
dividing of the sky into astrologically
significant segments Inst/600

evenlong *adj.* oblong, egg-shaped
SW2/755

evenstandyng *vbl.n. tyme (age) of* ~ the
prime of life [L. *tempus (aetas) consistendi*; see Age/40n] Age/1648,
Age/1736, Bac/387, Bac/410, *age of
evenstanding Age/1781

evenstandyng *adj.* ?equidistant
Inst/963

eventyng *vbl.n.* venting CHP/932

euereither *pron.* either (of two)
CHP/1162

everywher *adv.* ~ *of londis* in all countries Inst/1224

everlastyng *adj.* eternal 7Pla/353

everlastyng *adv.* always, for all time
7Pla/351

exaltacioun *n.* the point in the sky at
which a planet has its greatest influence Bac/328

exces(se) *n.* excessive behavior, gluttony Plag/212; an amount left over
or in addition Inst/451, Inst/766,
Inst/1188, etc.; an increment
7LA/228

excoriacioun *n.* the removal of skin
Age/2041

experyment *n.* a remedy or treatment
Bac/89, Bac/300, SW2/1144; **exper-
imentis** *pl.* proofs, observational evidence Bac/366

experymental *adj.* based on observation Bac/309, Bac/339, etc., **experimental** Bac/8, Bac/286

expert *adj.* skilled, knowledgeable,
experienced Age/327, Age/1217,
Bac/453n; tried, proven Age/1198,
SW2/497

explete *ppl.adj.* complete, fulfilled
Coi/229

expulsi(e)f *adj.* able to expel Age/767,
Age/1814; *vertu* ~ the physiological
power of expelling waste, excess humours, or poisonous matter from the
body CHP/1453, SW2/1111; ~ (as *n.*)
an expulsive substance [error for L.
expulsio 'expulsion'] CHP/66

exquisite *adj.* ?sought out, ?extreme
CHP/517

exsiccacioun *n.* drying out Age/1425

exspiracioun *n.* breathing out
CHP/292; emanation (of hot matter), exhalation CHP/1331

ex(s)pire *inf.* breathe out CHP/291;
come to an end (?by giving off
heat) CHP/1315, **exspirith** *pr.3sg.*
CHP/1318, CHP/1386, CHP/1429

extinct *inf.* extinguish Age/202

extraxioun *n.* ~ *of the roote* extract-
ing the square root (of a number)
7LA/206, **extraccioun** 7LA/225

extremyte *n.* the tip (of the nose)
CHP/423, CHP/425, CHP/427;
extremytes *pl.* the extremities of
the body CHP/399, CHP/409,

CHP/858; the extreme points in a scale of measurement CHP/358; **extremyte(e)s** of an object: the ends Inst/259, Inst/1262, Inst/1276, Inst/1394; **extremite(e)s** the top and bottom of something measured Inst/1305; outer points *Inst/962

facciouns *n.pl.* ?constitutions, ?physical tendencies 7Pla/7 [cf. *MED*, s.v. *facioun* n., 1(a)]

face *n.* the face Age/1016, Age/1019, etc.; a surface Inst/219, Inst/263; **fface** a ten-degree portion of an astrological sign Bac/329; ~ *natural(l)* the face in the state of health CHP/366, CHP/513; *vpon the* ~ *holden* error for L. *superficietenus* 'superficially' DHN/242n

faculte *n.* a power of the mind 7LA/127; **facultes** *pl.* riches, resources 7Pla/330

facunde *adj.* eloquent 7Pla/261, 7Pla/302

fairith *pr.3sg.* makes beautiful Age/1767

fallible *adj.* unreliable, slippery Age/8

fallyng evil *phr.* epilepsy Bac/261, SW2/87, SW2/521

famuliarite *n.* intimacy, closeness 7Pla/166

famulier *adj.* intimate 7Pla/137; ~ *(famuliar) and friendly* beneficial, favorable CHP/751, CHP/776

fantastic *n.* the cerebral region that houses the faculty called *fantasie* [L. *fantasia*], associated variously with sensory perceptions and the formation of mental images DHN/8, DHN/9, **fantastik** CHP/1034, CHP/1037

fantastic *adj.* generated by the fantastic faculty Coi/17; *cloth* ~ a membrane associated with the fantastic faculty or its cerebral location DHN/50; ~ *spirite* a physiological fluid transmitting the products or effects of the fan-

tastic faculty DHN/13; ~ *testule* the cerebral region housing the fantastic faculty DHN/13

fantastical *n.* the cerebral region housing the fantastic faculty DHN/15, CHP/1032

farynacioun *n.* error for L. *farmacia* 'drugs' Age/1917n, Age/1925n

faryng *pr.ppl.* ~ *weele* convalescing Age/425n

farmacy *n.coll.* drugs Age/872, **farmacie** Age/877, *Age/1050n

fastyng *pr.ppl.* fasting, not eating Age/1093, Coi/185, SW2/1473, etc.; *al* ~ while fasting Plag/398; ~ *intestief* the jejunum CHP/1478

fastyng *vbl.n.* fasting, not eating SW2/68, SW2/229, etc.

fastyng *n.* the jejunum DHN/157, DHN/171

fat(te) *adj.* fat, well-nourished DHN/301, Coi/226, Bac/313, SW2/389, SW2/423; fatty, greasy, oily Age/1032, SW2/103, SW2/110

favour(e) *pr.1pl.* warm up, wipe (with a warming liquid) [L. *foveamus* 'let us warm, caress, nurture'] Fle/93, Fle/94 [see also **savoure**]

feders *n.pl.* feathers Age/789

feere *n.* *in* ~ together SW2/1310

feyneng *n.* feigning, pretending [error for L. *figens* 'fixing, holding in place'] CHP/762

felawly *adj.* companionable 7Pla/149, 7Pla/208, etc.

felawshippen *pr.3pl.* engage in sexual congress DHN/316

felt *n.* a piece of felt fabric SW2/568, SW2/738

feluns *n.pl.* abscesses SW2/1526

femynalte *n.* of embryos: femaleness Coi/145

fernes *n.* distance Inst/190, Inst/936

ferthynges *n.pl.* farthings, coins or monetary units equivalent in value to a quarter of a penny 7LA/460

fervence *n.* heat Plag/149

feruent *adj.* burning, feverish CHP/397, CHP/812, etc., **fervent** CHP/394, CHP/464, CHP/1183

feruour *n.* passion Coi/137; intense bodily heat CHP/66

festres *n.pl.* festering sores SW2/1535

fever *n.* a pathological increase in the body's heat Age/224, CHP/87, etc., **fevors** *pl.* SW2/888, **feuer(e)s** Age/1012, Fle/70, CHP/261; ~ *heete* the increased body heat of a fever CHP/379, CHP/632, CHP/1213; ~ *agwe (colerike, cotidian, flewmatik, malencoly, quartan, quarteyn, sanguyn, sharp, tercian)* one of various types of fever [see modifying terms for definitions] Plag/288, CHP/70, SW2/666, CHP/100, CHP/101, CHP/1109, 7Pla/8, CHP/101, CHP/1125, SW2/666, etc.

feverous *adj.* feverish CHP/473

ficche *impv.* fix, set, or hold in place Inst/663, **ficched** *p.ppl.* Inst/392, Inst/696, etc.; *sterre ficched, ficched sterre* a star whose relative position in the sky does not change Inst/435, Inst/527, Inst/582, etc.

figuracioun *n.* shape, shaping Bac/272, Bac/277

figure *n.* a shape or posture, an appearance CHP/795, CHP/796, etc.; a geometrical shape 7LA/73, etc.; physical constitution Age/1977; a diagram Inst/150, Inst/192, 7LA/47, etc; an arabic numeral 7LA/192, 7LA/198, etc.; *in* ~ as a metaphor, figuratively 7LA/12

figurith *pr.3sg.* ?shapes, forms CHP/1467; **figured** *p.ppl.* positioned CHP/845

filyng *pr.ppl.* cutting away, filing off DHN/269, Inst/251, Inst/288

filynges *n.pl.* filings, scrapings Age/1135

filth(e) *n.* infected matter, pus, bodily discharge Age/619, CHP/1329, SW2/1555

filthed *n.* foul or infected matter, pus, bodily discharge Fle/42, Bac/391, CHP/1383, etc., **filthhed(e)** CHP/812, CHP/1308, CHP/1434; **filthede** immoral behavior 7Pla/144

filthy *adj.* containing pus, infected matter Fle/43

fynaly *adv.* ultimately Inst/4

firmably *adv.* firmly Inst/83

fistulis *n.pl.* deep ulcers Age/595

fix(e) *impv.* set or hold in place, affix Inst/83, Inst/119, **fix** *p.ppl.* Inst/1059, Inst/1079, Inst/1118; **fixt** *p.ppl.* set, limited Bac/332; *sterre fix* a star whose relative position in the sky does not change Inst/741, Inst/1338, *fix sterris* Inst/153, Inst/156, etc.

flayn(e) *p.ppl.* flayed, excoriated, abraded SW2/963, SW2/964, 8Med/35; *the naile* ~ ?the abraded fingernail [error for *cutem decoratione* 'the skin with adornment'] Age/101n

flakeryng *vbl.n.* a throbbing or tingling sensation Plag/248 [see also **flikeryng**]

fleamatic see **flewmati(c)k**

flea(w)me *n.* the bodily humour phlegm Age/199, Age/497, Fle/81, Coi/213, Bac/125, SW2/103, etc., **fleaume** Age/191, Age/1159, **fleam** Age/1134, **flewme** Age/1138, CHP/1361

fleyng *vbl.n.* flaying, excoriacion, removal of skin Age/77n [error for L. *decorationis* 'adornment'], Age/1407, Age/2041, 8Med/7

fleobotomy(e) *inf.* let blood Fle/29, Fle/60, Fle/100, *pr.1pl.* Fle/4, Fle/32; **fleobotomyed** *p.ppl.* phlebotomized, having had a vein opened for blood-letting Age/1975

fleobotomy(e) *n.* the letting of blood Age/1802, Fle/2, Fle/78, etc.; a fleam, an instrument for letting blood Fle/34

fle(s)shly *adj.* fleshy, made of flesh CHP/439, SW2/1349, SW2/1356; ~

lunges error for L. *canales pulmonis* 'passage-ways of the lungs' Age/1204n

flewmati(c)k *adj.* characterized by the humour phlegm Age/1097, Age/1951, Bac/125, etc., **fleamatik** Plag/141; *fever* ~ a fever caused by or associated with excess phlegm CHP/86, *fevers flewmatic* CHP/100; *fleamatik(e) humours* bodily fluids composed of or containing phlegm SW2/895, SW2/914, SW2/926

flewme *n.* a fleam, blood-letting implement Plag/336 [see also **flea(w)me**]

flewmy *adj.* characterized by an excess of the humour phlegm Age/1129

flien *pr.3pl.* fly CHP/1019, **fleyng** *pr.ppl.* Bac/560

flikeryng *vbl.n.* a throbbing or tingling sensation Plag/153 [see also **flakeryng**]

flo(o)re *n.* the floor of a room Plag/154, 7LA/448, 7LA/523, etc.; area 7LA/536, 7LA/538, 7LA/545, etc.; cross-sectional area 7LA/555 [often difficult to distinguish the first and second senses]

flour *n.* a flower, the bloom of a plant Age/1173, Age/1212, Bac/534, Plag/139, etc.; **flour(e)** the finest part of ground grain or other meal SW2/193, SW2/215, etc.; **floures** *pl.* the menses, menstrual blood SW2/1808, SW2/1815

flux *n.* an excessive discharge of bodily fluids, such as nosebleed, diarrhea, etc. Age/1151, CHP/261, CHP/1333, SW2/411, etc.; *bloody* ~ dysentery SW2/335, SW2/422, etc.; nosebleed CHP/1335; ~ *of hir matrice* a flux from the uterus SW2/341; ~ *of (the) wombe* diarrhea CHP/348, CHP/454, SW2/884, etc.

folowyng *pr.ppl. bi consequence (consequens)* ~ consequently Bac/253, CHP/382, CHP/1232

fomentacioun *n.* washing or soaking an afflicted part of the body with an herbal decoction SW2/875, 8Med/4, 8Med/25, etc.

fomyte *n.* ~ *of synne* the innate tendency to sin inherited from Adam and Eve 7Pla/233n

foote of houres see **houre**

forblayned *p.ppl.* afflicted with sores, ulcerated SW2/967

forfaiture *n.* failure, error Plag/338

formab(e)ly *adv.* carefully, properly SW2/1153, SW2/1160

formaly *adv.* in an orderly way Inst/205

forn agenst *prep.phr.* opposite Inst/375

*fornemeþe *pr.3sg.* takes away SW2/669

forscalded *p.ppl.* severely burned SW2/964

forsey *inf.* foretell CHP/211; **forseide** *p.ppl.* aforesaid Inst/929

for-to *conj.* until SW2/175, Inst/1008, etc.

fortreatith *pr.3sg.* deals deceitfully 7Pla/344

fortunat(e) *adj.* astrologically favorable 7LA/306; in an astrologically favorable position 7Pla/22, 7Pla/47

forwhi *conj.* because, so that, on account of which, wherefore, etc. [often translating L. *quia, nam, quoniam,* etc.] Age/43, Age/70, etc., **fforwhi** Age/202, Age/304, etc., **forwhy** Age/24, Age/36, etc., **fforwhy** DHN/317, **forwhye** CHP/450

foundament see **fundament**

founde *p.ppl.* ~ *to* constructed to match (sth.) Inst/938n

iiij- [i.e., **four-**] alphabetized under *i*

fracciouns *n.pl.* refractions of beams of light Bac/100

frame *n.* the frame of a lathe Inst/17, Inst/18, etc.

frenesy *n.* madness Age/2063, CHP/616, etc., **frenesie** CHP/1044

friende *n.* a friend CHP/114, CHP/156, etc.; ~ *pacient* ?a friend who is a patient CHP/222

friendly *adj.* friendly, companionable Coi/7; beneficial Bac/525; *famulier and* ~ see **famulier**

friendly *adv.* amicably, willingly DHN/70

frivolis *n.pl.* frivolous things Bac/79n

front *n. first* ~ the end (of a gauging rod) Inst/1227

frote *inf.* rub SW2/1328, 8Med/38, *impv.* SW2/589, **froted** *p.ppl.* 8Med/30

frotyng *vbl.n.* rubbing Age/1018, Age/1816, Age/1915

frowardly *adv.* athwart, cross-wise [L. *in obliquum*] DHN/19, DHN/172; ?at cross purposes [translating L. *oblita* 'having forgotten'] DHN/317

fugaciouns *n.pl.* ?pursuits, chases 7Pla/8

fuyre *n.* a fire, the element fire Age/181, Bac/124, Plag/107, etc.; *wield fuyres* erysipelas, an inflammatory skin disease SW2/1526

fuyrie *adj.* fiery red CHP/75; **fuyry** characterized by the qualities of the element fire Age/1321

fullers *n.pl.* fullers of cloth 7LA/577

fume *n.* smoke, a vaporous substance, an exhalation Age/523, Age/616, Age/1020, etc.

fumygacioun *n.* suffumigation, the medicinal use of smoke inhaled or otherwise introduced into bodily orifices SW2/584, SW2/590, etc.

fumous *adj.* redolent, aromatic Age/591, Age/1290, etc.

fundament *n.* the anus or rectum CHP/547, SW2/187, etc.; foundation, basis CHP/769, Plag/184, **foundament** Age/1670; **fundament-is** *pl.* posterior parts Coi/71

furiosite *n.* madness CHP/1281

furlong *n.* an eighth of a mile 7LA/453, 7LA/456, 7LA/457, etc.

furthright *adv.* directly, in a forward direction Inst/47

G. = **Galien** Galen CHP/883 [see Persons, Places, and Works]

gall(e) *n.* the gall bladder Age/2062, DHN/189, etc., **gal** SW2/1012

garcen *inf.* draw blood or poison by making incisions in the skin SW2/951, **(i)garced** *p.ppl.* SW2/147, SW2/329, SW2/608

gargarsmes *n.pl.* mouth-gargles, liquids used for gargling [L. *gargarismata*] Age/1095

garnysshith *pr.3sg.* furnishes, adorns CHP/115, **garnysshed** *p.ppl.* 7Pla/267; error for L. *minuuntur* 'are diminished' Age/46n

gastful *adj.* ghastly CHP/475, CHP/664

gawge *inf.* measure Inst/1273, **gauge** Inst/1391; **gawgyng** *pr.ppl.* ~ *yerd* measuring stick Inst/1224, Inst/1408

gawgyng *vbl.n.* rod or yerd of ~ a measuring stick Inst/1290

geldynges *n.pl.* eunuchs Coi/271, Coi/274, 7Pla/84

gemancie *n.* geomancy, divination by means of patterns of dots 7Pla/200

gendre *inf.* produce, generate Age/461, Age/787, Age/794, **gendrith** *pr.3sg.* Age/192, Age/198, Coi/138, etc., **gendreth** Age/400, **gendrit** Coi/157, ~ *pr.3pl.* Age/1355, **gendren** Age/752, Age/794, SW2/326, etc., **gendryng** *pr.ppl.* Age/502, Age/778, etc., **gendrid** *pret.3pl.* Age/890, **gendred** *p.ppl.* Age/770, Age/1515, Coi/198, 7LA/88, etc., **gendrid** Age/955, 7LA/79; ~ *inf.* beget (sth.), beget offspring DHN/301, Coi/25, Coi/27, etc., **gendrith** *pr.3sg.* 7Pla/259, **gendren** *pr.3pl.* Coi/146, Bac/30, etc.; **gendryth** *pr.3sg.* grows Bac/545

gendryng *vbl.n.* generation Age/254

gendris *n.pl.* kinds, types Age/642, Age/1639, etc., **gendres** Age/1003, **gendirs** Age/1998

gendrure *n.* production of offspring Coi/45

generatif *adj.* generative Age/190, Age/1880, **generatiefs** CHP/1421, CHP/1425

genicules *n.pl.* ?knees Fle/26 [cf. Latham 1980, s.v. *genu*]

genitails *adj.* genital CHP/1426; (as *n.pl.*) **genitals** reproductive organs Age/1351

gete *inf.* beget, conceive Coi/155, **goten** *p.ppl.* DHN/235, DHN/293; ~ get, acquire SW2/1864, Inst/934, **goten** *p.ppl.* Plag/297

gibbous *adj.* curved 7Pla/293, 7Pla/309, 7Pla/320

gilty *adj.* guilty [error for L. *renum* 'of the kidneys'] DHN/213n

gyve *inf.* give 7LA/47, 7LA/161, etc., **gyven** SW2/603, ~ *impv.* SW2/455, SW2/713, etc., **gyvith** *pr.3sg.* 7LA/328, **gaf** *pret.3pl.* 7LA/352, **gave** 7LA/286, **gyven** *p.ppl.* 7LA/118, **gevyn** 7LA/121 [see also **yeve**]

glad(de) *adj.* merry, glad Age/1234, Age/1535, SW2/232, etc.; error for L. *letalibus* 'lethal' Age/1408n

glandules *n.pl.* tumors or scrofulous eruptions Fle/49

glas(e) *n.* the substance glass DHN/31, *SW2/442, 8Med/43; a mirror 7LA/394, 7LA/395, etc.; ~ (as *adj.*) made of glass Age/1323; *bloode* ~ a cupping glass SW2/566; *double* ~ a double boiler made of glass SW2/648

glasen *adj.* made of glass SW2/658

glatty *adj.* slimy Coi/213

glister *n.* a clyster, an enema SW2/975

glueth *pr.3sg.* clots, sticks together Fle/101, ?DHN/184

gnast(e) *inf.* of teeth: grind CHP/940, CHP/942, *pr.3sg.subj.* CHP/941, **gnasten** *pr.3pl.* Coi/289, CHP/951

gnastyng *vbl.n.* grinding (of teeth) Coi/254, CHP/943, CHP/949, etc.

gnawyng *vbl.n.* gnawing Age/1392; a gnawing or biting sensation SW2/835

goynges *vbl.n.pl.* passageways, orifices DHN/291

gomes *n.pl.* the gums SW2/306, **gummes** DHN/64, Fle/9, etc.

gosselynges *n.pl.* goslings Age/1946

gote *n.* a goat SW2/386, SW2/1452, **gotes** *gen.* SW2/380, SW2/405, SW2/855, **gotis** SW2/568, SW2/881, SW2/1116

goten see **gete**

gowtis *n.pl. colde* ~ attacks of gout caused by cold humours SW2/675

grayne *n.* a grain as a unit of measure (1/3 of an inch) 7LA/454, 7LA/459; **graynes** *pl.* grains, crops Age/427, Age/773, etc.; kernels, seeds SW2/599, SW2/872

grapes *n.pl.* grapes Age/1868; **grapis** error for L. *duarum* 'of two' Age/613n

gre(e) *n.* a degree of arc Inst/52, Inst/103, Inst/483, Inst/1183, etc.

gre(e)ne *adj.* green CHP/374, CHP/445, SW2/201, etc.; ~ *canals (poores)* the renal veins and ureters DHN/176, DHN/183 [see Norri 1998, 347]

gre(e)nes *n.* greenness Age/429, CHP/525

grenyng *pr.ppl.* ~ *tyme* springtime Age/1171

gres(e) *n.* grease, fat DHN/256, SW2/1055, SW2/1100, SW2/1847, **grece** SW2/870, *SW2/1036, SW2/1847

greuaunce *n.* suffering, illness, harm SW2/46, SW2/317, etc., **grevaunce** SW2/3, SW2/535, etc., **greuans** SW2/1746

grevith *pr.3sg.* pains (sb., the teeth, the heart), gives pain to CHP/947, SW2/84, SW2/519, **grewith** SW2/171, **greved** *p.ppl.* CHP/816, 7LA/331, **grevid** Plag/199; **greved** *pret.3sg.* harmed, troubled 7LA/9; *hym* ~ *impers.* he is angry 7Pla/187

grynde *n.* the groin SW2/1210, **gryndes** *pl.* the groin *SW2/1225, Plag/179; ~ *of the thies (thigh)* Plag/344, Plag/367

gryndyng *pr.ppl.* ~ *stone* grindstone
SW2/1568
gryntyng *vbl.n.* grinding (of teeth)
CHP/943, CHP/949, CHP/955;
gryndyng grinding Age/345
gristell *n.* cartilage Age/922, **gris-**
til DHN/52, **grustul** DHN/303;
gristels *pl.* cartilaginous parts
DHN/102, **gristils** DHN/56,
DHN/100, **grustules** DHN/276,
grustulis DHN/302
gristely *adj.* cartilaginous, gristly
CHP/398
groundly *adj.* well-grounded Plag/36
grovelyng *adv.* face down, prone
SW2/1238
guyrdel *n.* a belt SW2/1326
guyrden *inf.* gird (sb.), put a belt or gir-
dle on SW2/1326
gurgulioun *n.* the gullet DHN/99,
DHN/100, DHN/101

haaste, haasten, haastyng see **haste**
habitude *n.* customary disposition
CHP/751; *lasse* ~ *of proporcioun* a
smaller relation of proportion,
smaller proportion Inst/893
had *p.ppl. predicament* ~ the category of
habit [L. *habitus*] Bac/621n; *evil* ~
error for L. *habitus* 'habit' Coi/242n
hak *impv.* chop, hack SW2/1845
halfuendel(e) *n.* half as much, a half
part SW2/950, Inst/583, Inst/1341,
haluendel SW2/1877
half wal *phr.* ?the midriff Coi/120n
halkes *n.pl. purgyng* ~ locations on the
body through which poisons are
eliminated Plag/177
hand(e) *n.* the hand Age/318,
CHP/750, CHP/998, etc.; *at the lift*
(right) ~ at the left (right) side of an
arabic numeral 7LA/217, 7LA/218;
on the right ~ in the units position of
an arabic numeral 7LA/199; ~ *wer-*
kis manual crafts 7LA/564
handful *n.* a measure of volume, a
handful SW2/342, SW2/923, etc.; a
measure of length, a hands-breadth
Inst/1298

hard(e) *adj.* hard, difficult, unyielding
Age/8, Age/359, SW2/58, etc.; *in*
~ rigidly Coi/37; *of* ~ with difficulty 7Pla/344, 7Pla/345; ~ *appetite* see
appetit(e)
harded *p.ppl.* hardened Plag/254
hardenesse *n.* induration, pathological
hardening SW2/1086
hardy *adj.* resolute, courageous
7Pla/316
hardynes *n.* boldness, courage
Age/996, Age/1344, etc.
harras *n.* a kind of skin disease
Age/415n
hast(e) *n.* speed, haste Age/163,
Age/1719, Bac/19, Bac/369, etc.
haste *inf.* hasten Age/298, Age/1722,
haaste Age/1036, **hastith** *pr.3sg.*
Age/39, Age/161, Coi/126, CHP/428,
etc., **hasten** *pr.3pl.* Age/111, Age/138,
Age/1005, Bac/362, etc., **haasten**
Age/1000, **hastyng** *pr.ppl.* 7Pla/281,
haastyng Age/1001
haun(n)tyng *pr.ppl.* of breath: frequent, rapid CHP/147, CHP/1057,
CHP/1061; **haunted** *p.ppl.* prac-
ticed, engaged in Coi/220
hed(e) *n.* the head of a human being
or an animal Age/515, Age/559,
Age/1381, etc.; the beginning of
a zodiacal sign Inst/475, Inst/520,
Inst/526, etc.; the uppermost part
of a thing DHN/100, CHP/830,
etc.; the upper end of an aposteme
CHP/1448, CHP/1449; a protrusion
Inst/259; *swolowyng of the* ~ error for
L. *capiti gurgulionis* 'to the superi-
or part of the throat' DHN/64n; ~
veyne(s) see **veyne**
hedelyng *adv.* headfirst SW2/1156
he(e)ris see **her**
heire *n.* air 7LA/265, 7LA/267n
helply *adj.* helpful, adjuvant Plag/169
helth *n.*(1) health Age/18, Age/50,
etc., **helþ** Age/247, Age/268, etc.;
rule of ~ a regimen of health Age/49,
Age/122, Bac/21, etc.
helth *n.*(2) error for L. *saltus* 'sudden
motion' CHP/901n; error for L. *sa-*

nies 'pus' CHP/1109n, CHP/1310n, CHP/1385, CHP/1387, CHP/1427n, etc., **helthes** CHP/1478, CHP/1488

her *n.coll.* hair Age/1094, Age/1458, SW2/568, SW2/1788, **he(e)ris** *pl.* Age/78, Age/79, Age/141, DHN/198, Coi/105, etc.

herisiple *n.* the inflammatory skin disease erysipelas CHP/1046, *horispilatus* (L.) SW2/1526

hernes *n.pl.* the brain Plag/241, **hernys** Plag/231

hert *n.*(1) a stag, hart (*Cervus elaphus*) Bac/49, Bac/443, Bac/545, SW2/1055, **hertis** *gen.*: *hertis bon* cartilage from the heart of a stag [*I.. os de corde cerui*] CHP/480; *hertis horn(es)* antler(s) SW2/394, SW2/400, etc.; *hertis skynne* stag's skin SW2/1327

hert(e) *n.*(2) the heart of a human being or an animal Age/17, Age/110, Age/918, etc., **hertis** *gen.* Age/2074; *high (of)* ~ proud (of) heart 7Pla/125, 7Pla/186

hervest *n.* autumn Age/428, Age/1482, etc.

hestis *n.pl. Goddis* ~ the Commandments SW2/559

heve *impv.* lift, raise SW2/749

hevy *adj.* burdensome, difficult Age/1958, 7Pla/275n; painful, distressing SW2/232, SW2/1301; hard to digest Age/1129, SW2/1766; of eyelids: difficult to keep open CHP/552; (as *n.*) heaviness DHN/269, DHN/287

hevieth *pr.3sg.* afflicts CHP/947

hevynes(se) *n.* lassitude CHP/280; a sensation of heaviness SW2/70, SW2/1323, etc.; sadness SW2/232, 7LA/295, 7LA/297

hid *ppl.adj.* hidden, secret, not visible Age/21, Age/52, etc. [see also **huydith**]

high *adj.* high (*lit.* and *fig.*) Age/121, Age/323, etc., **hier** *comp.* SW2/749, SW2/1761, etc., **higher** DHN/108, Inst/524, **hiest** *sup.* Age/26,

Bac/237, etc.; ~ of the heart: proud 7Pla/125, 7Pla/186; **hye** superb, excellent Age/1262; *in* ~ at the top DHN/120; *on* ~ upward, to the heights Age/7; *at the **highest*** to the extreme, completely Age/913

higheth *pr.3sg.* raises DHN/245, **highing** *pr.ppl.* SW2/1220; **highed** *p.ppl.* enhanced, elevated Bac/243

highly *adv.* greatly, fully DHN/243, 7Pla/187; tightly DHN/147; **hily** especially CHP/365

highnes(se) *n.* as term of honor: highness Age/7, Age/25, etc.; **higness-es** *pl.* of the eyes: protuberance or sunkenness CHP/614

hilith *pr.3sg.* covers SW2/1209

hold *inf.* hold, grasp, contain SW2/803, 7LA/419, **holdith** *pr.3sg.* Coi/191, 7Pla/251, **holdyng** *pr.ppl.* CHP/709, SW2/1174, **holden** *p.ppl.* CHP/404; ~ keep (in one place or position) CHP/793; ~ *pr.3pl.* hold fast, continue CHP/1275; **holden** *pr.3pl. holden toguyder* keep (sth.) together SW2/533; *holdith to* tends to CHP/604; *holdith with* ?agrees with DHN/244; *vpon the face holden* error for L. *superficietenus* 'superficially' DHN/242n; *into mylky juce holdith* error for L. *in lacteum & tenacem succum* 'into a milky and sticky juice' DHN/218

holde *impv.* believe, consider 7Pla/294, **hold** *pr.1pl.* Bac/79, **holden** *p.ppl.* SW2/939

holy *adj.*(1) holy Age/1828n, 7Pla/314

holy *adj.*(2) porous CHP/396

holownes *n.* a concavity, an internal space Age/229, CHP/393, etc.

holsum *adj.* bestowing health Age/624, 7Pla/243, 7Pla/313; healthy Bac/193, CHP/325, etc.; of a disease: mild CHP/65; ~ *rule* a regimen of health Age/126, Age/1688, Bac/42, etc.

holsumly *adv.* safely, without harm DHN/236, DHN/283

honyly *adv.* with honey Age/784n

hope *inf.* expect, anticipate CHP/532, CHP/533, CHP/534; **hopith** *pr.3sg.* hopes, anticipates with confidence Age/701, **hopid** *p.ppl.* Age/702

horyng *vbl.n.* greying Age/1696

horispilatus see **herisiple**

horny *adj.* ~ *tunycle* the cornea CHP/1008

horoscopo (L.) *phr. in* ~ in the degree of the zodiac rising above the eastern horizon, in the ascendant Inst/1086

hosiers *n.pl.* makers of hose 7LA/577

hote *adj.* hot, characterized or affected by the elemental quality of heat Age/772, Age/928, etc.

hotith *pr.3sg.* promises 7Pla/344

hound *n.* a dog Bac/564, CHP/199, **houndes** *gen.* SW2/568

hour(e) *n.* an hour Age/1943, SW2/443, Plag/173, etc.; *houres equal(e), houres equals* the twenty-four equal parts of a day (or a subset of them), as measured from one sunrise to the next Inst/397, Inst/446, etc.; ~ *inequal(e)* one of the twelve equal parts of the artificial day (from sunrise to sunset) or night (from sunset to sunrise) Inst/417, Inst/437, Inst/439, etc.; *in the* ~ *of* at the time of CHP/901; *in the* ~ *and tyme(s) of reuolucioun, in tyme and* ~ *of (hir) reuolocioun (revolucioun)* see **reuolucioun**; *vj houre cornerd* see **cornerd**; *foote of houres* the end of an hour-line on a quadrant opposite the end at the quadrant's apex Inst/1182n; *holl houres* equal hours Inst/1187; *houres of the quadraunt* unequal hours Inst/1152n

hous(e) *n.* a dwelling place (also *fig.*) Age/565, Bac/395, CHP/165, 7LA/449, **howsis** *pl.* Age/1398; ~ one of twelve 30-degree divisions of the heavens beginning at the eastern horizon and moving counter-clockwise Inst/603, Inst/605, Inst/703, etc.; **howse** the zodiacal sign in which a planet has the most influence Bac/328

hoveful *adj.* necessary Age/1843

huydith *pr.3sg.* hides Age/1543, **hidden** *pret.3pl.* Age/1785, **hidde** *p.ppl.* Age/245, Age/1741, etc. [see also **hid**]

huythes *n.pl.* landing-places on rivers, hithes Age/1212

humydite *n.* moisture, fluid in the body Age/91, Age/93, **humyditees** Age/1144, etc.

humosite *n.* dampness, moisture Age/1379

humour *n.* a bodily fluid, esp. one of the four constituent humours blood, phlegm, choler, and melancholy Age/139, Age/193, Age/374, etc., **hvmours** *pl.* 7LA/294, ***umours** Age/1440, **umoris** Age/1415; *cold (hote, dry, moist)* ~ a humour characterized by the quality of cold (heat, dryness, moisture) CHP/1177, CHP/614, SW2/103, SW2/107, etc.; *cristallyne* ~ the crystalline lens of the eye CHP/1008; *raw humours* undigested humours or moistures Age/1808, CHP/1050; *straunge humour(s)* extraneous moisture Age/200, Age/1045, etc.; ~ *of veer* a humour with the hot moist quality of spring, blood Age/1844

hurlyng *vbl.n.* a whirling sensation SW2/313, SW2/835

ibrend, ibrent see **brenne**

icche *n.* itch [error for L. *ictericia* 'jaundice'] Age/2062n

icchyng *vbl.n.* itching, irritation Age/381, DHN/165, SW2/1539, **ichyng** SW2/969

iclove *p.ppl.* split SW2/306

icterice *n.* jaundice Fle/112

idel *adj.* idle, worthless (perhaps understood as 'foolish') CHP/645; (as *n.*) *in* ~ in vain [?misreading of L. *maniam* 'mania, madness'] CHP/941, CHP/1271 [see also **idelnes, voidenes**]

idelnes *n.* emptiness, nothingness CHP/646, **idilnes** [L. *maniam,*

?misread as *inaniam*] CHP/640n; madness (perhaps as a species of foolishness) CHP/1272; *idilnes of wit* foolishness or madness CHP/1269

ydols *n.pl.* false optical images CHP/1010

idressed see **dresse**

idropesy *n.* dropsy, a pathological accumulation of excess fluid, usually in the abdominal area SW2/938, SW2/1365, **idropesie** SW2/912; ~ *of the matrice* accumulation of fluid (esp. blood) in the uterus SW2/903 [see also **dropesy**]

*idropike *n.* a person suffering from dropsy 8Med/21, **idropicis** *pl.* CHP/385

igarced see **garcen**

ihet *ppl.adj.* heated SW2/874

iiij-square *adj.* of square cross-section Inst/1296; (as *n.*) a square Inst/1410

iij sandal see Materia Medica, s.v. **sandal**

il *adj.* bad, unhealthy Age/794

iliche *adj.* equidistant Inst/966; of distance: the same Inst/1106, **ilike** Inst/1111; identical Inst/1105

iliche *adv.* ~ *moche* the same amount of each SW2/565, SW2/1730, etc.

ilkon *pron.phr.* each one Plag/299

illynied *p.ppl.* rubbed with an ointment Age/1559

imagynacioun *n.* the mental faculty of forming images from sensory input or by remembering them Age/571, Age/646, etc., **ymagynacioun** Age/1659

imedled see **medle**

impedient *adj.* of a planet: impeding, obstructive 7Pla/50, 7Pla/68, etc.

impotens *n.* powerlessness CHP/971

impotent *adj.* powerless Bac/360

inanicioun *n. spasme of* ~ a spasm caused by pathological draining of bodily humours CHP/707, CHP/710, CHP/863

incedent *adj.* ~ *of* related to [error for L. *intellige* 'understand'] Age/651n

incensible *adj.* imperceptible Age/2040

incensioun *n.* a burning sensation CHP/832

incidentis *n.pl.* substances that dissolve phlegm Age/1913

incomodite(e)s *n.pl.* inconveniences, afflictions Age/116, Age/298, Age/1737, etc.

inconveniens *n.* harm, injury CHP/174

incorporatith *pr.3sg.* is assimilated Age/2091; **incorporat(e)** *p.ppl.* incorporated (into) Age/2087, SW2/1524, SW2/1563

indigence *n.* a lack, an absence Coi/41, Coi/43

indigested *ppl.adj.* undigested [error for L. *indigencia* 'lack, absence'] Coi/38n

indigestioun *n.* poor or unfinished digestion of food Age/192, Age/221, etc.

indignacioun *n.* ?swelling, ?irritation [?error for L. *inflationem*] Fle/26 [cf. *MED*, s.v. *indignacioun* n., 2]

induccioun *n.* an inductive argument 7LA/131, 7LA/132

induce *inf.* bring in, lead in, cause DHN/95, Bac/570, CHP/1377, **inducith** *pr.3sg.* Age/406, Age/1352, Fle/36, 7Pla/230, **inducit** *pr.3sg.* Age/1081, **inducen** *pr.3pl.* Age/149, **inducyng** *pr.ppl.* Age/400, Age/1042, **induced** *p.ppl.* Fle/106, **inducith** *?p.ppl.* CHP/193

indurith *pr.3sg.* hardens CHP/1319

inequal(e) *adj.* of humoral complexion: unbalanced, uneven Bac/147; **inequal(l)** of (an) unequal length 7LA/483, 7LA/484, 7LA/485; *signes inequal(s)* unequal divisions Inst/1234, Inst/1274, Inst/1393; *houre* ~ see **hour(e)**

infallible *adj.* unfailing Age/328

infeccioun *n.* contamination, infection Age/159, Age/1548; **infectioun** a pathological alteration SW2/72

infilyng *pr.ppl.* smoothing Inst/176
inflacioun *n.* swelling (of a body part) Fle/13, Coi/285, etc.
infrigidacioun *n.* chilling DHN/296
infuse *impv.* soak SW2/1511, SW2/1528
infuse *ppl.adj. ley (lai)* ~ soak, steep SW2/1399, SW2/1520, SW2/1556 [cf. *MED*, s.v. *infuse* adj.]
ingenie *n.* intelligence Age/303
Inglissh *adj.* English SW2/1735; (as *n.*) the English language 7LA/193
ingrossen *pr.3pl.* become coarse [error for L. *nigram* 'black'] Age/1551n
inleedyng *vbl.n.* an introduction Inst/927
inmortal *adj.* immortal Bac/11, Bac/13, etc.
inmortalite *n.* immortality Bac/595
innecte *inf.* fasten, connect CHP/23
innermore *comp.adj.* interior DHN/110, DHN/186, etc.
innewe *inf.* renew Age/868
inplanyng *pr.ppl.* planing, making smooth Inst/176
inquietacioun *n.* disturbance, distress Age/528
inshedith *pr.3sg.* pours (sth.) forth DHN/126; **insheede** *pr.3pl.* ?error for L. *infrigidant* 'chill' Fle/137
inspire *inf.* breathe in DHN/104
instaunt *adj.* immediately pressing, urgent CHP/19, CHP/43
*inster *?coll.n.* ?interior parts SW2/877n
instinctucioun *n.* impulse, tendency CHP/797
instrument *n.* a tool or implement (musical, astronomical, medical, etc.) Bac/184, SW2/790, Inst/3, Inst/31, 7LA/168 (*fig.*), etc.; **instrumentis** *pl.* organs or other bodily parts that carry out physical or mental functions (e.g., mind, breath, soul, etc.) Age/360, Age/368, Age/1650, etc.; means or agents

7LA/583; *instrumentis perspectief* optical instruments Bac/98
intentifly *adv.* attentively, closely CHP/144, CHP/623
intercept *p.ppl.* of an arc on a great circle: included (between two points) Inst/1116
interfeccioun *n.* killing 7Pla/9
*interpellaciouns *n.pl.* interruptions CHP/103
intestief *adj. fastyng* ~ the jejunum, a part of the small intestine CHP/1478
intestives *n.pl.* the intestines CHP/1476, **intestyves** CHP/1422; *grete* ~ the large intestine CHP/1479
intierly *adv.* purely, cleanly, without taint Age/753, Age/756, Age/818, etc.
into(u)rned *p.ppl.* of ears or eyelids: inverted CHP/444, CHP/449, CHP/689, CHP/692
introduct *ppl.adj.* introduced Age/1720
introite *n.* entrance Inst/624
invnccioun *n.* rubbing with oil, anointing Age/241, Age/1955, etc.
invencioun *n.* a finding, calculation, measurement Inst/1411, 7LA/219; **invenciouns** *pl.* things devised or discovered Age/569
involuciouns *n.pl.* envelopings, entanglements, ?ensnarings 7Pla/8
inward *adj.* inner SW2/1137, 7LA/98; (as *n.*) inner part 7LA/79; ~ *wittis* psychological senses, faculties 7LA/11
inward(e) *adv.* in, toward the center CHP/373, SW2/212, SW2/775, Inst/372, Inst/1063
inwrityng *vbl.n.* inscription Inst/153
ipissaried *p.ppl.* treated with a pessary, made into a pessary SW2/470
iplastred see **plaster** *inf.*
iplited *p.ppl.* plaited, braided Inst/303
ypocundr(i)e *n.* the lateral part of the abdomen just below the ribs, the hypochondrium CHP/1220,

CHP/1232, etc., *pl.* **ypocundrus** CHP/1181, CHP/1184, etc., **ypocundris** CHP/1226, CHP/1230, **ypocundries** CHP/1205, CHP/1212, **ypocundres** CHP/1217

ypocundrium (L.) *n.* the hypochondrium CHP/1186, CHP/1188, *pl. ypocundria, ypocondria* CHP/1185, CHP/1187

ipostasis *n.* sediment in the lower portion of a urine sample CHP/97, **ipostasie** CHP/300

ipostatat *adj.* of urine: containing sediment CHP/81

irn *n.* iron Age/1135, Age/1663

is see **be**

is *pron.* his SW2/1013

ysaphac *n.* the esophagus DHN/94, DHN/103

iscomed see **scomed**

ise *n.* ice Age/488, 7Pla/16

ishore see **shere**

isode(n) see **seeth(e)**

ysophagus *n.* the esophagus DHN/98, DHN/138

isperate ?*p.ppl.* ?reserved, ?stored SW2/1037 [cf. *MED*, s.v. *sparen* v., 5]

isshyng *pr.ppl.* coming forth Age/1370n

issue *inf.* go forth, flow out DHN/265, Coi/196, **issueth** *pr.3sg.* DHN/211, DHN/258, Coi/162, Bac/14n, ~ *pr.3sg.subj.* DHN/260, **issuyng** *pr.ppl.* CHP/1239

issue *n.* an outlet, a place to go out DHN/291, SW2/151, Plag/98, etc.; the act of going out Coi/127, Bac/120; discharge, that which goes out CHP/808, SW2/1746, etc.; **issues** *pl.* error for L. *existentibus* 'existing things' CHP/908

istrawed see **straw**

itende *p.ppl.* kindled, set on fire SW2/570

itered *p.ppl.* repeated Age/1568

itosed *p.ppl.* of cotton: teased SW2/1553

iwasshe *n.* ~ *of frankencence* see Materia Medica, s.v. **frankencens(e)**

iwrongen see **wryng**

janglyng *vbl.n.* garrulousness Age/529

joynctures *n.pl.* joints of the body Age/232, **joynturis** Age/469; **jointours** seams of a container SW2/1806

joyned *ppl.adj.* joined, added Age/356, DHN/121, etc., **ioyned** Inst/750, Inst/986; ~ of planets: in astronomical conjunction Bac/222, **ioyned** Inst/617

jointly *adj.* combined Coi/84

jointly *adv.* in combination, in union SW2/1164

jowes *n.pl.* the jaws CHP/884, CHP/953, CHP/956

juce *n.* plant sap or an herbal or floral extract Age/1484, SW2/225, SW2/932, etc.; broth Age/378; a bodily fluid of milky quality DHN/155, DHN/220, etc., ~ *of mylke, mylky* ~ DHN/151, DHN/218

just *adj.* exact Inst/1120; **iust** (as *n.*) that which is just or proper Age/14

iustly *adv.* exactly, accurately, precisely Inst/19, Inst/22, etc.; (as *adj.*) exact Inst/16

iuvamentis *n.pl.* helpful things Age/205

keele *inf.* cool CHP/860, SW2/339, etc., **keelith** *pr.3sg.* Age/219, Age/476, DHN/229, Fle/79, Coi/227, etc., **keelen** *pr.3pl.* Age/1009, CHP/399, **kelyng** *pr.ppl.* DHN/286, **keelid** *p.ppl.* Age/220, Age/223

ke(e)ne *adj.* sharp, spicy, sour SW2/160, SW2/965, SW2/1329

keenes *n.* sharpness, acridness SW2/355

kene *inf.* show, teach 7LA/13

keneship *n.* keenness, sharpness, acridness SW2/297

kerf *n.* a carved-out space Inst/290

kernel *n.* the inner part (of a nut or cherry stone) SW2/1442, SW2/1825, SW2/1834; ?a nucleus, core CHP/142n

kerve *inf.* extend (a line) Inst/1013; ~ *vpon* extend (a line) through (a point) Inst/1000, Inst/1005, etc.; ~ intersect, cross Inst/1189, **kervith** *pr.3sg.* Inst/113, Inst/115, etc., **kervyng** *pr.ppl.* Inst/127, Inst/1011

kydes *n.pl.* kids, young goats Age/771, Age/1853

kiene *n.pl.* cows Age/1856

kyndelen *pr.3pl.* blaze up Age/614

kyte *n.* a European kite (*Milvus milvus*) 7Pla/295

knyttyng *vbl.n.* combining, joining DHN/149, DHN/271

knocken *pr.3pl.* throb Fle/64

knockynges *n.pl.* error for L. *tonsillis* 'tonsils,' ?read as form of *tundere/tunsum* 'to knock/knocked' DHN/88; ?error for L. *texibiles* DHN/146

knowlachith *pr.3sg.* reveals, makes manifest CHP/1071; **knowlachen** *pr.3pl.* acknowledge Bac/404

konnyng *n.* knowledge Age/628, 7LA/153, 7LA/339, 7LA/341, etc., **kunnyng** 7LA/587 [see also **connyng** *n.*]

kunt *n.* the genitalia (of a female hare) SW2/1812

label *n.* a movable ruler on an astronomical instrument Inst/394, Inst/1028, etc.

lacert *n.*(1) a muscle DHN/105, CHP/390, CHP/1267, CHP/1298, etc.

lacert *n.*(2) a lizard Age/1638n

lackyng *vbl.n.* lack, absence SW2/1352

lai see **ley**

laise *adj.* ?of lesser rank, ?lay 7Pla/300n

lak *n.* lack, absence Age/1635n

lakkith *pr.3sg.* lacks, needs Age/957, CHP/1314, **lakken** *pr.3pl.* Age/857,

lakkyng *pr.ppl.* Age/222, **lacked** *p.ppl.* Age/1758

lanyfice *n.* working in wool, textile crafts 7LA/566, **lanefice** 7LA/575

larde *impv.* insert small pieces (of a substance) into a surface SW2/201

large *adj.* big, ample, broad Age/1369, DHN/38, etc.; generous 7Pla/315, 7Pla/333

lassyng *vbl.n.* reduction, diminution *Age/719, DHN/312, CHP/611; blood-letting Fle/3

lassith *pr.3sg.* lessens, grows less Age/1126, *Coi/62, **lassen** *pr.3pl.* Age/37, **lassed** *p.ppl.* CHP/510, CHP/603

latitude *n.* breadth Inst/63, Inst/73, Inst/143, 7LA/497, etc.; celestial latitude, the angular distance of a star or planet north or south of the ecliptic Inst/162, Inst/164, etc.; terrestrial latitude, the distance of a point or region above or below the equator Inst/1112, Inst/1115, etc.; ~ *meridional* (*septentrional*) celestial latitude south (north) of the ecliptic Inst/1079, Inst/1069

laton *n.* latten, an alloy of copper, tin, and other metals Inst/31, Inst/60, etc.

launcet *n.* a lancet, blood-letting implement Plag/336

lavaciouns *n.pl.* medicinal washes Age/448

laxatief *n.* a laxative Age/1060, SW2/250, SW2/291, Plag/162, etc., **laxatives** *pl.* Age/464, Age/1072

lb. *n.* abbreviation for *libra(e)* 'pound(s)' SW2/242, SW2/244, etc.

leche-craft *n.* the practice of medicine CHP/113

lechour *n.* a lecher, lascivious person 7Pla/105, 7Pla/151, 7Pla/175

lectuary *n.* a compound medicine in a thick sweet substrate such as honey or syrup SW2/733, Plag/379, **letuarie** Plag/144 [see also **electuarie**]

lede *n.* the metal lead SW2/1018

le(e)che *n.* a physician Age/971,
Age/1823, Coi/197, Bac/27, CHP/8,
CHP/777, CHP/778, CHP/1259,
etc., **lecchis** *pl.* Bac/346; ~ *fynger* the
ring finger Plag/366
le(e)dissh *adj.* of color: leaden
CHP/519, CHP/520
leefen *pr.3pl.* omit, fail to do Age/41
leer *n.* the face SW2/1318
le(e)sith *pr.3sg.* loses Age/540,
SW2/1067, 7Pla/346, etc., **leesen**
pr.3pl. DHN/86
leete *inf.* let (blood) Plag/415, **letith** *pr.3sg.* Plag/416, **lete** *p.ppl.*
Age/1975, Age/1981, Age/1985,
leeten Plag/358
leetyng see letyng
left see leve
legaciouns *n.pl.* diplomatic missions
7Pla/96
ley *inf.* apply (a medicinal substance)
SW2/1514, *impv.* SW2/725, SW2/738,
etc., **lei** SW2/1570, **lai** SW2/1520,
~ *pr.1pl.* SW2/1791, **laide** *pret.3sg.*
SW2/959, **leide** SW2/957, **laide**
p.ppl. SW2/283, SW2/285, etc.; ~
impv. lay (sth.), place Inst/1028,
Inst/1031, Inst/1122, **leyeng**
pr.ppl. SW2/1215, **laide** *pret.1sg.*
Inst/1056, Inst/1064, Inst/1079,
leide Inst/1059; ~ *doun* cause (sb.)
to recline Plag/122; ~ *(lai) infuse*
soak, steep SW2/1399, SW2/1520,
SW2/1556 [cf. *MED,* s.v. *infuse* adj.]
leinnes *n.* thinness SW2/346
*leis *n.pl.* lees, dregs, material that
settles to the bottom of a solution
SW2/661
lene *inf.* give, provide DHN/90,
le(e)nyth *pr.3sg.* Age/1344,
Age/2074, DHN/5, Coi/136, etc.,
lenyþ CHP/117, **leneþ** DHN/271,
leenyng *pr.ppl.* DHN/51
leng(g)er *comp. adj.* longer DHN/39,
CHP/481, etc.
leng(g)er *comp.adv.* longer Age/39,
Age/1899, DHN/194, Bac/106, etc.

length *n.* length, extent Age/1688,
Bac/228, Inst/640, etc., **lengþ**
Inst/1244; ~ *of a sterre* a star's ecliptic longitude, distance along the
ecliptic from the vernal equinoctial
point Inst/494; ~ *of resonable soule* error for L. *longitudinem a re non naturali* 'distance from the non-natural
thing' Age/1687n
lent *adj.* slow CHP/1145
Leonis *n.* the constellation and zodiacal sign Leo, the Lion 7Pla/150
lepyng *pr.ppl.* of the pulse: forceful,
bounding CHP/1229, CHP/1241,
etc.
lepyng *vbl.n.* strong pulsation
CHP/1242, CHP/1264
lepre *n.* leprosy or a skin disease
with similar symptoms Age/348,
Age/1352, Bac/116, etc.; **lepres** *pl.*
?leprous or similarly diseased areas
of the skin Age/2074
lesioun *n.* damage, harm Age/461,
Age/648
lesyng *vbl.n.* lying Bac/572
lesith see le(e)sith
lessen *inf.* lose SW2/678 [see also
le(e)sith]
letyng *vbl.n.* letting (of blood)
Age/1802, CHP/261, SW2/144,
etc., **leetyng** Plag/317, Plag/332,
Plag/386
lette *inf.* hinder, prevent, harm
Plag/73, 7LA/309, 7LA/322, **lettith** *pr.3sg.* Age/596, Age/620, etc.,
letten *pr.3pl.* Age/524, Age/644,
SW2/118, **lettyng** *pr.ppl.* 7Pla/50,
7Pla/68, **letted** *p.ppl.* Age/594,
Coi/12; (of a planet) obstructed
7Pla/35, 7Pla/98, **lettid** 7Pla/91
letter *n.*(1) a letter of the alphabet
7LA/64, 7LA/73, 7LA/83, etc., **lettris** *pl.* 7LA/66; ~ a version of a text
CHP/867, CHP/1208
letter *n.*(2) something that hinders
7Pla/4
letuarie see lectuary

lewk(e) *adj.* tepid, lukewarm Age/1097, Age/2100, Fle/91, CHP/851, CHP/857

leve *inf.* leave, allow to remain Inst/873, *impv.* Age/1567, *pr.2pl. subj.* Inst/258, **levith** *pr.3sg.* Coi/47, CHP/990, **left(e)** *p.ppl.* Age/301, Age/1222n, Inst/752, etc.; **levith** *pr.3sg.* ceases, leaves off DHN/310, ~ *pr.3sg.subj.* let (him) Age/1936, *pr.3pl.subj.* Age/1984, **left** *p.ppl.* Age/1982; ~ *inf.* remain, be left over Inst/445, **levith** *pr.3sg.* SW2/1157, SW2/1444, Inst/434, Inst/440, etc., **leven** *pr.3pl.* Inst/896, ?DHN/85; **levith** omits, fails CHP/1110, **leven** *pr.3pl.* Age/41, **left** *pret.3sg.* CHP/1089; **leften** *pret.3pl.* abandoned Age/1786

leve(y)ned *ppl.adj.* leavened, containing leaven Age/1508, Age/1852, Age/1946, **leveynd** Fle/136

levis *n.pl. lily* ~ a decorative metal device, shaped like four joined leaves, for suspending a celestial globe Inst/354, Inst/357

li. *n.* abbreviation for *libra(e)* 'pound(s)' SW2/275, SW2/290, etc.

liberal *adj.* generous 7Pla/117, 7Pla/180; appropriate for study by free men 7Pla/300, 7LA/30, 7LA/584

licour see **liquour(e)**

lieful *adj.* lawful, *fig.* granted [L. *licet* 'although, granting that,' *lit.* 'it is lawful'] Age/761, Age/938, Bac/439, CHP/860

liefully *adv.* lawfully, *fig.* admittedly [L. *licet*] Age/1258, Coi/244, Bac/86, CHP/42, etc.

liendis *n.pl.* the loins SW2/328

lifly *adj.* living, alive 7Pla/10, 7Pla/41; of physiological powers: pertaining to the animating faculty of the mind and body [L. *animalis*] Age/45, Age/145, Age/1626, CHP/398, CHP/756, Plag/214, etc., **lively** CHP/1131

liflode *n.* livelihood 7Pla/97

lift *adj.* left DHN/112, Coi/146, SW2/547, etc.

ligge *inf.* lie down, be recumbent, rest Age/1899, Bac/192, CHP/749, etc., **liggen** *pr.3pl.* SW2/87, SW2/522, SW2/777, ~ *pr.3sg.subj.* CHP/791, **liggyng** *pr.ppl.* CHP/623, CHP/755, SW2/750, etc., **leyn** *p.ppl.* SW2/385; *vnder have leyn* have been subject Bac/161

liggyng *vbl.n.* resting, lying (in bed) Age/1813, CHP/776, etc.

light *pr.3sg.subj.* descend, come to rest Age/1389

light *adv.* easily Age/280

lighten *inf.* ease, lighten Age/1622, *pr.3pl.* Age/1965, **lyghten** Age/1821

lighteneþ *pr.3sg.* eases, lightens Plag/389, **lightnen** *pr.3pl.* Age/1474

lighter *n.* a giver of light, that which illuminates 7Pla/255

lightlier *comp.adv.* more easily Inst/708, Inst/820

lightloker *comp.adv.* more easily SW2/192

lightned *p.ppl.* illuminated CHP/1009, 7Pla/271

lightnen see **lighteneþ**

lightnes *n.* softness, easiness Age/1815, CHP/279, CHP/427, CHP/1191

lik(e)nes *n.* similarity Age/329, Age/600, Age/1242; appearance, likeness Age/1809, DHN/241, CHP/754, etc.; essential nature or species Bac/12; **licknes** a visual or mental image Coi/128; *vpon his likeness* in a similar fashion Inst/508; ~ error for L. *spiritus* 'spirit' DHN/312; **liknesses** error for L. *species* 'spice' Age/1474

liklynes *n.* similarity Age/637, Age/652, CHP/281, CHP/324

lily *n.* a metal device in the shape of joined lily leaves Inst/363; *lily levis* see **levis** [see also Materia Medica, s.v. **lilie**]

lymbe *n.* a rim Inst/282, *Inst/283; a graduated border on a quadrant Inst/389, Inst/448, etc.

lymbum (L.) *n.* the circular edge of a quadrant Inst/959, Inst/968, Inst/978; *in lymbo* on the outer border of an astrolabe or quadrant Inst/454n, Inst/584n, Inst/645, Inst/974n

lyme *n.* birdlime (possibly made of mistletoe berries) SW2/994 [cf. *MED*, s.v. *lim* n.(2), 3(a)]

***lineares** *n.pl.* long thin nerves DHN/145, DHN/147

lyniament *n.* an ointment Age/1562; **liniamentis** *pl.* wipings or rubbings with ointments Age/1540, Age/1541, Age/1561

linied *p.ppl.* rubbed with an ointment Age/1557

lipotomy(e) *n.* faintness, fainting Fle/62, Fle/75, **liptomye** Fle/141

lippient *adj.* of eyes: inflamed CHP/635

lippitude *n.* inflammation of the eyes CHP/631, CHP/633, CHP/637, **lipputid** CHP/653

liptocozans *n.pl.* ?learned men Age/1652n

liquefac(c)ioun *n.* dissolution, melting away CHP/451, CHP/602

liquified *p.ppl.* dissolved, melted away CHP/432, CHP/603, **liquefied** CHP/632

liquite *n.* a liquid, liquid form 8Med/68

liquit(e) *adj.* liquid Age/1574, Coi/63, CHP/476; ~ *meatis* liquefied foods SW2/1762

liquour(e) *n.* a drink Bac/61, Bac/500, Bac/610; water in which medicinal ingredients are dissolved or boiled Age/353, **liquor** SW2/1838; **liquor** cooking liquid SW2/1574; **licour** the fluid component of semen Coi/66

lise *n.pl.* lice Age/1407, Age/2040

lissyng *vbl.n.* relief, easing Age/453

litargie *n.* a lethargy CHP/235

lively see **lifly**

lividite *n.* a bluish-grey or leaden color CHP/731

longaon *n.* the rectum DHN/169

longen *pr.3pl.* belong or are proper (to) 7LA/303

longitude *n.* length Inst/61, Inst/1241, Inst/1243, 7LA/431, etc.; celestial longitude, the angular distance of a star or planet eastward from the vernal equinoctial point of the ecliptic Inst/159, Inst/175, Inst/1043, etc.; terrestrial longitude, the angular distance of a point on earth from a fixed meridian Inst/1105, Inst/1110; *after the ~ of the armyl (armyl meridian), after the ~ meridional* following the (inner) circumference of the meridian ring of a celestial globe Inst/91, Inst/99, Inst/129, etc.

loosith *pr.3sg.* loosens, relieves, releases, dissipates Coi/242, Coi/256, etc., **loosed** *p.ppl.* Coi/236, Coi/237, CHP/1105, **loused** Fle/36

lordship *inf.* rule, have power Age/12, **lordshippith** *pr.3sg.* Age/1809

lottith *pr.3sg.* allots [?error for L. *sarcietur* 'is healed,' taken as *sortietur* 'casts lots'] Fle/101

loused see **loosith**

luce *n.* a freshwater fish, the pike (*Esox lucius*) Age/790

lump *n.* a shapeless mass SW2/1349, SW2/1356, etc.

luted *p.ppl.* sealed with clay SW2/1806

magnificence *n.* greatness of spirit 7Pla/212

May *n.* ~ *butter* unsalted butter made in May SW2/291, SW2/1171, SW2/1378

male *adj.* male, of masculine gender Age/1636; (as *n.*) a male child or person Coi/118, Coi/146, Coi/153, Coi/156, Coi/164, Bac/94, **mall**

Coi/102, **mals** *pl.* Coi/105; ~ error for L. *musculis* 'muscles' DHN/152

malencoly *n.* the bodily humour black bile Age/589, Age/770, etc., **malencolie** CHP/411; ~ sorrow, anger Age/2075, Coi/243

malencoly *adj.* pertaining to or generated by black bile CHP/982, CHP/1068; *fever* ~ a fever caused by or associated with excess black bile CHP/101

malencolik *adj.* dominated by the bodily humour melancholy Fle/107; angry, sorrowful 7Pla/148

malencolious *adj.* dominated by the bodily humour melancholy Fle/109, Fle/114, Bac/126; angry, sorrowful 7Pla/162

malfit *n.* an evil, something done wrong Fle/80

malici misreading of L. *malencolicam* 'caused by excess black bile' Age/1149n

malicious *adj.* of disease: harmful, dangerous CHP/468, CHP/667, etc.; hateful, wicked 7Pla/143, 7Pla/163, 7Pla/164

malivelous *adj.* ill-willed, malevolent, harmful 7Pla/244, 7Pla/284, **maliuolous** 7Pla/339, 7Pla/350

manaunt *n.* the mathematical result of subtraction, remainder Inst/726

mandibules *n.pl.* the jawbones CHP/746

mangier *n.* a manger, feeding trough SW2/859

maniac *n.* the large bowel, the colon and rectum DHN/164, DHN/166, DHN/170, **manic** DHN/170; *or myanic* upper mouth of the bowel DHN/168

mansif *n.* *vnto the* ~ error for L. *ad mensuram* 'to the measure,' poss. corrupt in original Fle/7

mansioun *n.* a daily position of the moon Inst/395, 7Pla/272

mansleer *n.* a manslayer, murderer CHP/221

marcial *adj.* ?fierce Plag/168n

margarit(e) *n.* a pearl or bead on the cord of a hanging celestial sphere Inst/342; a pearl or bead on a quadrant's plumb-line Inst/1158 [see **almury**]

mary *n.* marrow DHN/12, DHN/87, Fle/144, Coi/47, SW2/624, etc.

masculosite *n.* masculinity Coi/144

masor *n.* a drinking vessel Inst/277n

masticacioun *n.* chewing, mastication Age/1109, Age/1111

matrice *n.* the uterus DHN/221, DHN/287, Coi/150, CHP/1135, SW2/43, etc.

maturacioun *n.* of apostemes: coming to a head and forming pus, suppuration CHP/1498

mature *n.* maturity, maturation CHP/1363

maturizacioun *n.* of apostemes: coming to a head and forming pus, suppuration CHP/1323, CHP/1371

mawe *n.* liver [L. *iecur* 'liver'] Fle/110

meane *n.* the median cubital vein in the arm Fle/38, Fle/95

mean(e)ly *adv.* moderately Age/1840, Age/1898; by means of, through the mediation of 7Pla/257

meate *n.* a going forth, ?birth Coi/200n

mecanic *adj.* mechanical, manual 7Pla/300

medateresim *n.* ?corruption of L. *metacentesis* 'drawing blood from the side of the body on which an illness occurs' Fle/29

med(e)lyng *vbl.n.* the act of mixing, a mixture Age/1840, Bac/579; ~ *of reaso(u)n* mental confusion, madness CHP/890, CHP/939, CHP/1228

mediacioun *n.* halving (of a number) 7LA/205, 7LA/218

median *n.* the median cubital vein in the arm Age/1983

mediatly *adv.* being linked DHN/128; not directly, without direct contact CHP/393; ~ *with* by means of CHP/1342

medicynable *adj.* therapeutic Age/447, Age/1122, Plag/323, etc.

medle *impv.* mix, mingle, compound Age/1558, SW2/182, etc., **medil** SW2/179, SW2/1461, **medlen** *pr.3pl.* CHP/1006, **(i)medled** *p.ppl.* Age/850, Age/993, SW2/113, SW2/116, Plag/13, etc., **medeled** SW2/636, SW2/1033, **medlid** Age/1179, Age/1440; **medlith** *pr.3sg.* disturbs, agitates Age/610; causes confusion Age/613; **medled** *p.ppl.* joined, brought (to the mouth) DHN/66; ~ *impv.* ?deal with (a planet), concern oneself with 7Pla/51, 7Pla/68, 7Pla/79 [cf. *MED*, s.v. *medlen* v., 2a, 2c]; ~ *with* have sexual relations with SW2/121, SW2/128, *pr.3pl.subj.* SW2/135

medlith see also **mydlith**

meete *inf.* hinder, prevent, stand in the way of Age/204, CHP/21, **mete** Age/266, **meetith** *pr.3sg.* Age/1047, **meeten** *pr.3pl.* Age/130, Age/243, Bac/442, **meetyng** *pr.ppl.* Age/1048, **mette** *p.ppl.* CHP/17; ~ *inf.* meet, encounter (sb. or sth.) Coi/14, **meetith** *pr.3sg.* Age/1063, CHP/318, CHP/331, **met** *pret.3sg.* Age/985; ~ *pr.1pl.* counteract CHP/553; **metith** *pr.3sg.* of lines: intersects Inst/1174; *metith with* hinders, prevents Age/2071; *metyng agenst* hindering Age/1855; **metten** *pret.3pl.* error for L. *obseruauerunt* 'they observed, followed,' read as *obuiauerunt* 'they met' Age/670

meetyng *vbl.n.* obstruction, hindering (of sth.) Age/243, Age/260

megre *adj.* meager, emaciated CHP/346

mele *n. fynger (fyngres)* ~ the breadth of a finger SW2/825

melters *n.pl.* refiners of metals Age/490

membre *n.* a part of the body, an organ or limb Age/361, Age/416, DHN/85, etc., **member** CHP/620;

noble ~ an organ of higher physiological status CHP/972, CHP/1247, CHP/1312; *nutritief (norysshyng) membris* digestive organs DHN/134, CHP/1421; *prevy* ~ *(member)* the private parts, a genital organ SW2/71, SW2/774, etc.; *ij prevy membres* the vagina and the anus SW2/766; *principal membris (membres)* the brain, heart, liver, and sometimes the testicles Coi/70, CHP/462, Plag/175, etc.; *spiritual membris (membres)* respiratory organs CHP/1237, CHP/1419; the lungs and the heart DHN/133; ~ error for L. *embrionis* 'embryo' DHN/234n; *litel (smale) membris* error for L. *membranulis, -as* 'small membranes' DHN/127, DHN/210, DHN/214, *litil* **membro** DHN/215

membrely *adv.* error for L. *membranum* 'membrane' DHN/141n

membriculis *n.pl.* error for L. *membranulis* 'small membranes' DHN/127

membro see **membre**

memoratief *adj.* pertaining to memory, serving as memory aids Inst/1214

memorial *n.* the faculty of memory DHN/8, DHN/10, etc.

mendyng *pr.ppl.* amending, straightening SW2/1216

menge *impv.* mix, mingle SW2/380, SW2/471, **mengith** *pr.3sg.* Plag/234, **menged** *p.ppl.* Plag/221, Plag/322

Menours *n.pl.* Friars Minor, Franciscans Age/1

menstruat(e) *n.* the menstrual flow Age/2061, Fle/17, SW2/683

menstrues *n.pl.* the menstrual flow *SW2/1255, SW2/1466, 8Med/50

mensuracioun *n.* moderation Age/282, Age/290; measuring 7LA/371

menuse *inf.* bleed, phlebotomize Plag/153

mercers *n.pl.* textile merchants, members of the Mercers' Guild 7LA/581

meridian *n.* terrestrial longitude Inst/1103, Inst/1105, Inst/1107; **me-**

ridians *pl.* lines of terrestrial longitude Inst/1104; *height of the ~ = meridian height* Inst/849 [see **meridian** *adj.*]

meridian *adj.* of a star: southern, in the southern celestial hemisphere Inst/165; (as *n.*) south Inst/202; *ark meridiane* an arc along the celestial meridian marking the sun's position at midday Inst/1115; *armyl ~ (meredian), roundel ~* , *meredian armyl* a metal ring on a celestial globe representing the great circle passing through the observer's zenith Inst/29, Inst/57, Inst/69, Inst/221, etc.; *~ corde* a cord passing through the southernmost point along the horizon ring on a celestial globe Inst/346; *~ height, height ~* the altitude of the sun at noon Inst/467, Inst/470, Inst/484, Inst/661n, etc.; *~ height (of a sterre)* the altitude of a star when it crosses the celestial midline Inst/651, Inst/862; *~ hole* a hole at the southernmost point along the horizon ring on a celestial globe Inst/313, Inst/345; *lyne ~* the celestial midline, the great circle including the pole and the sun's noontime position Inst/415, Inst/432, etc.; *~ poole, poole ~* the south pole Inst/37, Inst/116

meridie *n.* the south Inst/514; the mid-heaven line or celestial midline, passing through the sun's position at noon and the pole, Inst/762, Inst/765, Inst/850, etc., **meredie** Inst/530; *declynacioun of al the ~* the maximum distance of the sun from the equinoctial (i.e., the celestial equator) Inst/376

meridional *adj.* midday, noontime, pertaining to the sun's position at noon Inst/1099; southerly, southern Inst/67, Inst/163, Inst/480, etc., **meridionall** Inst/677; *~ (as n.)* a circle on an astronomical instrument representing the celestial midline Inst/811, Inst/1166; **meridi-**

onals *pl.* the zodiacal signs from Libra through Pisces Inst/525; *cercle ~* a circle on an astronomical instrument representing the celestial midline Inst/838; *~ height, height ~* the altitude of a celestial body at the meridional line Inst/534, Inst/537, Inst/657; *lyne ~ , ~ lyne* the celestial midline, running through the pole and the sun's noontime position Inst/520, Inst/1030, Inst/1035, etc.; *longitude ~* the length of the (inner) circumference of the meridian ring of a celestial globe Inst/99

meridional-occidental *adj.* southwesterly Inst/501

mervously *adv.* marvelously SW2/682

mesels *n.pl.* lepers SW2/81

meson *n.* the median cubital vein in the arm Fle/28, Fle/38

messe *n.* a meal, an instance of eating food SW2/252, SW2/253

mesurably *adv.* in moderation SW2/1762, SW2/1764, Plag/288, 7LA/42, **mesurable** Plag/220, Plag/295

meth(e) *n.* mead *SW2/270, SW2/1060, SW2/1104, Plag/105

metrikly *adv.* metrically, in verse Age/87n

meve, mevyng see **moeve**

myanic see **maniac**

miche *adj.* ?great, sudden, continuous CHP/745

microcosme *n.* the microcosm, the human body as a reflection of the universe 7Pla/250

myd *adj.* *~ mure* ?the midriff Coi/120n

myd(de) *adj.* middle, mid- 7Pla/251, 7LA/483; *~ hevene* the mid-heaven point or zenith, directly above the observer Inst/869

myddil *n.* *~ (of, of the) hevene*, **middil** *(of) hevene* the mid-heaven point or zenith, directly above the observer Inst/39, Inst/422, Inst/468, Inst/491, Inst/518, etc.

mid(e)ref *n.* the diaphragm, midriff CHP/1053, CHP/1136, etc., **mydref**

CHP/1060, CHP/1076, **midrif** CHP/1248, **mydrif** SW2/1001

mydlyne *n.* the 45° line on a quadrant 7LA/378

mydlith *pr.3sg.* ~ *(the) hevene* crosses the mid-heaven line Inst/490, Inst/742, etc.

mygrayn *n.* an intense headache, a migraine CHP/605

mykelnesse *n.* size, measure Inst/941

miln *n.* a mill DHN/94n

milt(e) *n.* the spleen Age/1859, DHN/189, Fle/13, CHP/769, etc., **mylt** Fle/113, CHP/1296, etc.; **mylt** a disease of the spleen Age/2047

myne *n.* source, root, origin Age/2014, CHP/457; **mynes** *pl.* innermost parts, the heart CHP/464

myneral *n.* source, root, origin Age/533, Age/543, Age/2026, Age/2030

myneral *adj.* mineral, not living Age/744

mynere *n.* source, root, origin Age/1127, Age/1139, **mynier(e)** Age/313, Age/2080, **mineres** *pl.* Age/1177; **myncrs** *pl.* innermost parts, the heart, essence Age/1227, Age/2104, Bac/520n, **mynieres** Age/312

myng *n.* one of the two cerebral meninges DHN/6 [see **myringes**]

mynisterie *n.* a service, ministering DHN/152

mynistracioun *n.* administration, provision Age/1675, Age/1678, Age/1682

mynucioun *n.* bloodletting Age/1834, Age/1973, **mynusioun** Fle/3

mynush(e) *inf.* reduce, diminish Age/160, Age/213, **mynussh(e)** CHP/909, CHP/910, **mynush** *pr.1pl.* Age/505, **mynushen** *pr.3pl.* CHP/920, **mynushed** *p.ppl.* CHP/918, **mynusshed** CHP/433; **mynushed** *p.ppl.* bled, phlebotomized Age/1972

mynusith *pr.3sg.* reduces, diminishes Age/1022, Fle/146, Coi/103, **my-**

nusen *pr.3pl.* Age/36, Age/1832, **mynused** *p.ppl.* Age/125, Age/569, CHP/1479

mirach *n.* the anterior abdominal wall CHP/1424, CHP/1428

myringes *n.pl.* the cerebral meninges (dura mater and pia mater) CHP/609, CHP/1045

myscheuous *adj.* harmful SW2/1743

myschief *n.* harm, affliction, infirmity SW2/768, SW2/780, SW2/953

myscible *adj.* (?as *coll.n.*) (things) able to be mixed, miscible (things) Bac/579n

miserac *adj.* mesenteric, pertaining to the folds of the peritoneum DHN/171, **myserac** DHN/159 [see also **veync**]

mysfaren *pr.3pl.* fare ill, suffer SW2/1246

mystempered *ppl.adj.* out of balance, badly mixed Plag/16

mytigacioun *n.* easing Bac/418, CHP/811, etc.

mytigate *inf.* soften, relieve, Bac/299, Bac/468, **mytigat(e)** *p.ppl.* Bac/107, Bac/413

myxtioun *n.* a mixture, commingling Age/1898; ~ *(mixtioun) of reasoun* mental confusion, madness CHP/939, CHP/1227, CHP/1262

moder *n.* a mother, female parent (also *fig.*) Bac/396, SW2/43 [as an explanation of the next sense], SW2/681, etc.; the uterus DHN/263, ?DHN/291 [see appendix on Accidence, 739, n. 1], SW2/46, SW2/690, etc.; *his ~ wombe* his mother's womb Age/582, SW2/39, SW2/1260, etc.

modirly *adj.* uterine DHN/298

modulaciouns *n.pl.* melodies 7LA/272

moevable *adj.* movable, mobile Coi/136, Inst/954, etc.

moeve *inf.* move Age/1529, Bac/441, CHP/757, etc., *impv.* Inst/414, Inst/630, etc., **meve** Inst/627, **moevith** *pr.3sg.* Age/1516, DHN/250,

Coi/35, CHP/577, etc., **movith** Age/1499, CHP/1367, ~ *pr.3pl.* Inst/71, 7LA/265, **moeven** *pr.3pl.* Age/187, SW2/902, **moevyng** *pr.ppl.* Age/1888, CHP/279, etc., **mevyng** SW2/130, **movyng** CHP/592, **moeved** *p.ppl.* Age/1457, Age/1694, Coi/129, etc., **moevid** 7LA/304

moevyng(e) *vbl.n.* motion Age/146, Coi/218, SW2/902, 7LA/45, 7LA/250, 7LA/262, etc., **movyng** Age/186, **mevyng** 7LA/251

mola *n.* uterine mole, a growth in the womb SW2/1348, SW2/1357, SW2/1366, etc.

mola matricis (L.) *phr.* uterine mole, a growth in the womb SW2/279, SW2/1347, SW2/1348, etc., *molam matricis* SW2/1302

mole *n.* a spot, mark Inst/1128

mollificacioun *n.* an ailment thought to be caused by "softening" of nerves or muscles, causing paralysis or hernia CHP/727, CHP/761, CHP/1225

mollifie *inf.* soften SW2/258, **mollifieth** *pr.3sg.* Age/1295, **mollifien** *pr.3pl.* CHP/717, **mollifieng** *pr.ppl.* Age/536

monamac *n.* the caecum, the upper part of the large intestine DHN/162 [see Norri 1998, 371]

monapagie *n.* an intense headache CHP/605

moreyne *n.* pestilence, plague Plag/18; an instance of pestilence Plag/88

mormals *n.pl.* sores, abscesses SW2/1526

mornyng *n.* morning Age/1068, Age/1962, Coi/202, etc.

mornyng *vbl.n.* mourning, grieving SW2/1068

morphew *n.* a skin disease, morphea Age/415, Age/442, Age/1409, **morphews** *pl.* Age/364; *white morphews (morphues)* morphea originating in phlegm Age/353, Age/939

mortalite *n.* the state of being subject to death, transient earthly existence Bac/205

morter *n.* a bowl for grinding ingredients, mortar Age/1387, SW2/265, etc.

mortifie *inf.* of tissue or blood: become necrotic, be destroyed CHP/1067, **mortified** *p.ppl.* CHP/412

mow *inf.* be able to Age/1712, **mow(e)** *pr.3sg.* can, is able to SW2/576, SW2/1450, ~ *pr.1pl.* Age/1778, *pr.3pl.* SW2/1772, **mown** *pr.1pl.* CHP/21, CHP/22, CHP/683, *pr.3pl.* Age/125, Age/389, CHP/16, etc.

mountenaunce *n.* amount, size SW2/200

mowth *n.* the mouth Age/240, Age/1145, DHN/57, etc.; the opening of a container or concave space CHP/392, Inst/281, *Inst/283, **mouth** Inst/279; ~ *(mowthe) of the matrice* the cervix Coi/156, SW2/133, SW2/595, etc.; ~ *of the (that) prevy membre*, ~ *of the privitees* the external opening of the vagina SW2/812, SW2/1172, SW2/1182, SW2/1196; ~ *of the (þeir) stomac* the esophageal opening into the stomach CHP/833, CHP/836, SW2/74, etc.; ~ error for L. *os* 'bone' DHN/17n

movith, movyng see **moeve**

mundificacioun *n.* cleansing Age/495, Age/1504, Age/1625

mundifieþ *pr.3sg.* cleanses Age/1157, **mundifieth** Age/1500, **mundified** *p.ppl.* Age/458

mure see **myd**

muscilago (L.) phlegm or other thick bodily substances [misunderstood by translator as plant muscilage from marsh-mallow; cf. Norri 2004, 137, for further example of translators' difficulties with L. *muscilago*] Age/508

mvte *n.* a consonant other than *l, m, n, r, s,* or *x* 7LA/87, 7LA/98, 7LA/116, **mutis** 7LA/86

naddair *n.* the point on the celestial sphere diametrically opposite to another point or the representation of this point on an astronomical instrument Inst/733, Inst/1038, **naydar** Inst/609; ~ *solis* the point opposite the solar zenith Inst/778, Inst/872, **naddayr** *of the sonne* Inst/755, *naydar solis (of the sonne)* Inst/417, Inst/425, Inst/459; *naydar gree ascendyng* the point opposite the degree ascending Inst/607

nail(e) *n.* a human fingernail or toenail Age/1458, DHN/198, DHN/255, SW2/1450; a metal or wooden nail Inst/75, Inst/82, Inst/175, Inst/259, etc., **nayles** *pl.* Inst/984; ~ error for L. *cutis* 'skin' Age/101n, Age/149, Age/494, Bac/390n, CHP/1457, etc., **nayle** DHN/256n

nakidly *adv.* ?error for L. *crura* 'shins' DHN/269n

natheles *adv.* nonetheless SW2/27, SW2/30, SW2/554, etc.

nathycietica *n.* sense uncertain [?corruption of L. *plagiotomia* or *plagiostomo*, 'blood-letting instrument with a curved blade'] Fle/33

nativite *n.* birth, time of birth Bac/92, Bac/381, **natiuite** CHP/951; of the moon or a planet: influence at a person's birth 7Pla/278, 7Pla/307, *natiuite* 7Pla/291, 7Pla/318

navil *n.* the human navel Coi/120, CHP/1408, SW2/70, etc.

necessarie *adj.* necessary, required, indispensable Age/11, Age/82, Coi/17, etc., **necessary** Age/123, Age/1671, CHP/199, etc., **neccessary** Age/187

neck(e) *n.* the human neck DHN/270, DHN/301, SW2/72, SW2/673, etc., **nekke** *CHP/843, CHP/845, SW2/1860; **nekke** the neck of an animal Age/923, Age/1370; ~ *(nek) of the bladder* the outlet of the urinary bladder DHN/180, DHN/182; ~ *of the matrice* the cervix DHN/221

nedely *adv.* necessarily Inst/94, 7LA/137

nedil *n. quarel* ~ a needle, possibly of square cross-section SW2/772

neere *adj.* near, close (to) Coi/151, **nerrer** *comp.* CHP/359, CHP/360, **more neere** Age/71, Age/844, Age/1252, **more nerrer** Bac/310; ~ *of* closer to Bac/317

neere *prep.* near, close (to) Plag/246, 7LA/104

negocioners *n.pl.* people engaged in negotiations 7Pla/90

neither *adj.* lower, nether SW2/307, Plag/368, Inst/974, etc., **nether** Inst/958, 7LA/107; (as *n.*) 7LA/100

neither *conj.* neither, nor, and not Age/954, Age/1250, Bac/133n, Bac/345, etc.; ~ . . . *nor* neither . . . nor Age/38, Age/706, Coi/43, etc., ~ . . . *nor* . . . ~ Coi/32, ~ . . . *ne* Age/44, CHP/1081, ~ . . . ~ Bac/125, Inst/1180, *nat* . . . ~ Age/366, Bac/437, CHP/367, etc., *no* . . . ~ Age/1706; ~ *wounder* ?nor is it a wonder CHP/601 [see also **nother**]

nere *adv.* nearly Inst/980; **nerrer** *comp.* nearer, closer (to) Inst/1102 [see also **neere** *adj.* and *prep.*]

nerf *n.* a sinew or tendon DHN/77, Fle/36, Fle/46, Coi/272, **nerves** *pl.* Age/536, Age/539, Age/1146, Fle/16, CHP/738, etc., **nervis** Age/537, Age/2061, CHP/402, etc., **nerues** Age/575; **nerves** *pl.* nerves, fibers, or fine tubes transmitting physiological spirits or information through the body DHN/209, Coi/36, CHP/978, etc., **nervis** DHN/210, CHP/435; *ob(i)tic nerve* the optic nerve CHP/1032, CHP/1034, *nervis opticis* CHP/609 [the two principal senses are not always easy to distinguish]

nerrer see **neere** *adj.*, **nere** *adv.*

nerved *adj.* error for L. *(h)umeris* 'to the shoulders' DHN/302n

nervous *adj.* containing muscle fibers or tendons CHP/1218; related to the nerves CHP/1230

nessh(e) *adj.* soft SW2/489, SW2/771, etc.; gentle SW2/1130

nesshen *inf.* soften SW2/259

nether see **neither** *adj.*

netly *adv.* in the manner of a net DHN/147

newed *p.ppl.* renewed Age/881

*neumatic *adj.* respiratory DHN/98, ***newmatic canal** the trachea DHN/139

nygh *impv.* approach, draw near Inst/1304, Inst/1307, Inst/1309, **nygheth** *pr.3sg.* CHP/958

nygramansier *n.* a magician 7Pla/145

nyknamed *adj.* designated Age/334n

nyme *inf.* take SW2/795, *impv.* SW2/828

noyaunce *n.* harm, trouble Age/324

noye *inf.* do harm (to), hurt, trouble DHN/130, **noyeth** *pr.3sg.* Age/1331, Coi/171, CHP/810, *Plag/24, etc., **noyeþ** Coi/223, **noieth** CHP/1479; ~ *inf.* harm (sb.), trouble (sb.) Coi/231, 7Pla/107

noyful *adj.* harmful 7Pla/61, 7Pla/63

noyous *adj.* harmful CHP/595, Plag/186, 7LA/38, etc.

noisaunce *n.* harm, trouble, damage Age/449, Age/1560, CHP/574, etc., **noysaunce** CHP/1027, CHP/1134, etc., **nuysaunce** Age/572, Age/637, etc.

no(o)te *n.* ~ *kernel* the inner kernel of a nut SW2/1442; **nootis** *pl.* nuts DHN/245 [see also Materia Medica, s.v. **noote**]; **notis** error for L. *inice* 'inject' Age/1080n

nooten *pr.3pl.* ?use Coi/139n

norice *n.* a nurse Age/206n, SW2/43, Plag/395

northen *adj.* of the north, northern Inst/1333

nother *pron.* of two things: neither CHP/581, (as *adj.*) SW2/1803

nother *conj.* neither, nor, and not Age/1379, CHP/742; ~ . . . *nor* nei-

ther . . . nor Age/1313, ~ . . . *or* Age/345, ~ . . . *ne* Bac/27, *Plag/23, Plag/47, ~ . . . *neither* Bac/124, *neither* . . . ~ CHP/703, ~ . . . ~ SW2/1483, *nat* . . . ~ SW2/1245, *non* . . . ~ Inst/190 [see also **neither**]

notice *n.* information, knowledge DHN/43, Plag/413

notifie *inf.* ~ *to* signify Inst/818

notis *n.pl.* marks Inst/321, Inst/324; *viij* ~ a series of eight musical tones, an octave 7LA/280

noveltes *n.pl.* novelties 7Pla/303

nuysaunce see **noisaunce**

nutrencie *n.coll.* nourishing things Age/769n

nutribil *adj.* nourishing DHN/153, **nutrible** DHN/196

nutryment *n.* nourishment, nutriment Age/72, DHN/244, etc., **nutriment** Age/439

nutritief *adj.* nourishing Age/1284; ~ *membris* organs involved in digestion and nourishment CHP/1421

nutritives *n.pl.* nourishing things Age/94, Age/1263, Age/1835; organs involved in digestion and nourishment CHP/1419

ob. *n.* abbreviation for halfpenny (L. *obolus*) Plag/166

ob(i)tic *adj.* ~ *nerve* the optic nerve CHP/1032, CHP/1034, *nervis opticis* CHP/609

obiect *p.ppl.* objected to, argued against Bac/288

oblaciouns *n.pl.* offerings, food CHP/286

oblique *adj.* slanting Inst/1221; *cercle (orizont)* ~ the horizon of an observer not on the earth's equator Inst/546, Inst/692n, Inst/756, etc.

obliuioun *n.* forgetfulness Age/563, Age/565, Age/1347, etc., **oblivioun** Age/1650, Age/1659

oblivious *adj.* forgetful Age/1726

oblonge *adj.* *spiere* ~ the oblique sphere, the celestial sphere as seen by an observer between the earth's equator and one of the geographic poles Inst/772n, Inst/773, Inst/779

obtic see **ob(i)tic**

occasioun *n.* occasion, opportunity Age/383; hindrance, harm Age/418, CHP/322; cause Coi/251; *of ~* ?error for L. *decoctione* 'cooking, digestion' Age/1503n

occident *adj.* western Inst/416, Inst/426, etc.; (as *n.*) the west Inst/202, Inst/516

occidental *adj.* western Inst/430; (as *n.*) the west Inst/421

occidental-septentrional *adj.* northwesterly Inst/501

odorible *adj.* pertaining to smell DHN/47

odoriferaunt *adj.* fragrant Age/1507

offendith *pr.3sg.* causes offense 7Pla/344, **offende** *pr.2sg.subj.* 7Pla/130, **offended** *p.ppl.* 7Pla/118; **offenden** *pr.3pl.* strike against, encounter CHP/1036, CHP/1037; **offendith** *pr.3sg.* harms Age/1015, **offendyng** *pr.ppl.* CHP/292

office *n.* function, purpose Age/550, 7LA/30, 7LA/125, etc.

often *adj.* frequent Coi/218, Coi/225

oft-sithes *adv.* frequently SW2/764, SW2/904

oilet *n.* a device for drawing an arc Inst/1175n, Inst/1205, etc.; a small hole Inst/1227n, Inst/1228, Inst/1362, **oilettis** *pl.* Inst/1348n, Inst/1366, etc.

oynement *n.* an ointment Age/241, Age/1481, Age/1482, Age/1961, SW2/812, etc., **oignement** Age/1483, Age/1489, Bac/504, etc.

oyntement *n.* an ointment SW2/718

only *adv.* solely, only Age/40, Age/199, etc., **oonly** Age/548; error for L. *tamen* 'nevertheless' or *tum* 'then' Bac/15n, Bac/85, Bac/162, Bac/404n, Bac/414n, CHP/1268, etc. [an error that may also occur in other texts, such as 7Pla]

oone *inf.* coagulate, thicken Coi/82, **ooned** *p.ppl.* Age/933, Age/1807

oones *adv.* once Age/1941, Age/1942, Bac/67, etc., **oonys** SW2/615; *at o(o)nes* together SW2/278, SW2/451, Plag/30, etc.; *~ nature* error for L. *seminalis* 'seminal' Coi/38n

operacioun *n.* working, function Age/20, Age/278, Age/593, DHN/84, CHP/1469, 7LA/31, etc.; of heavenly bodies: influence on human affairs Bac/218, Bac/219

operatief *adj.* working, practical Age/738, Bac/90

oppynioun *n.* reputation Fle/104; **oppynion** belief, opinion 7LA/350

opposite *n.* an astronomical position or object diametrically opposed to a given point or object Inst/404, Inst/422, Inst/611, Inst/1025, etc.; of astronomical bodies: opposition, a relative separation of 180° Inst/617; a contrary belief or statement 7Pla/207; the reverse (of a situation or circumstance) Inst/599

opposit(e) *adj.* opposing, opposed (to), at a position 180° away from (sth.) Bac/223, Inst/8, Inst/612, etc.

opteyneth *pr.3sg.* acquires, obtains, holds DHN/72, **opteigneth** DHN/258, DHN/261, **opteynen** *pr.1pl.* Age/309, **opteyned** *p.ppl.* Age/6, Bac/64

opticis see **ob(i)tic**

or *conj.*(1) or Age/8, Age/45, etc.

or *conj.*(2) before, ere, until Age/1301, SW2/58, SW2/759, Plag/243, Plag/251; *~ than* before SW2/14, SW2/209, SW2/528, Plag/109, Plag/116, *ar than* Plag/137; *~ that* before SW2/1269

ordeyne *inf.* arrange SW2/1195, *impv.* Inst/566, **ordeyneth** *pr.3sg.* DHN/106, **ordeyneng** *pr.ppl.* 7LA/329, **ordeyned** *pret.3sg.* 7LA/24, **ordeyned** *p.ppl.* DHN/210, 7LA/85, **ordeigned** Bac/225; ~

impv. choose Inst/572; **ordeigned** *p.ppl.* commanded, decreed Age/632, Bac/7, Bac/38, Bac/194, etc.; **ordeyned** *p.ppl.* established 7LA/592, **ordayned** 7LA/51, **ordeigned** CHP/225; **ordeyned** *p.ppl.* devised, prescribed SW2/188; placed, situated SW2/819; marked, divided Inst/978

order *n.* of things: an orderly arrangement or disposition, a sequence Bac/364, CHP/154, Inst/239, 7LA/47, 7LA/53, 7LA/198, etc.; a row of figures 7LA/213, 7LA/214, 7LA/216, **ordres** *pl.* 7LA/209; ~ of breath: regularity CHP/1116, CHP/1124; ~ *and rule* of the diaphragm: evenness or similarity on both sides when palpated [L. *ordine* 'order, regularity'] CHP/1192; a religious order Age/1

orderith *pr.3sg.* gives structure to 7LA/348

orient *adj.* eastern Inst/415, Inst/427, etc.; (as *n.*) the east Inst/201, Inst/515

oriental *adj.* eastern Inst/455, Inst/506, etc.; (as *n.*) the east Inst/420; **Orientals** (as *n.pl.*) people of the Orient Age/607

oriental-meridional *adj.* southeasterly Inst/500

orientis see **semidiatrum**

orifice *n.* the opening of the vagina, the exit from the birth canal SW2/636, SW2/1161, SW2/1243, etc. **orificium** SW2/1221

orizont *n.* the horizon Bac/181, Inst/323, etc., **orisont** 7LA/383; ~ a circle on a quadrant representing the horizon Inst/469, Inst/493, etc., **orisont** Inst/697; ~ *(orisont) armyl, armyl of the* ~ , ~ *(orisont)* a metal ring on a celestial globe representing the observer's horizon Inst/195, Inst/213, Inst/243, Inst/280, etc.; ~ *oblique* the horizon of an observer not on the equator Inst/756; *right*

(riet, reetis) ~ the horizon of an equatorial observer Inst/674, Inst/698n, Inst/787, etc.

or myanic *phr.* see **maniac**

ornat *adj.* ornamented 7Pla/262

ornatly *adv.* handsomely, elegantly 7Pla/267

ortocon *adv.* orthogonally, at right angles Fle/40

***ortogonialiter** *adv.* orthogonally, at right angles Inst/311

ortographie *n.* correct spelling 7LA/62

ortomye *n.* a kind of asthma in which inhalation and exhalation are both difficult, orthopnea Fle/55 [see Norri 1992, 354]

ostensioun *n.* showing, appearance CHP/1072, CHP/1119

othe *conj.* ~ . . . *or* either . . . or SW2/694

other *adj.* other, remaining, different (from) Age/80, Age/100, Age/1947, etc., **oþer** Age/308, Age/760, SW2/144, etc., **oother** SW2/1063; ~ (as *pron.*) another thing or person Age/38, Age/244, etc., **ooþer** SW2/900, ~ *pl.* other things or people Age/92, Age/633, Age/1403, etc., **oþer** Age/934, Bac/470, SW2/657, etc., **oother** CHP/1138, SW2/901, SW2/902; ~ *pl.* some CHP/3; *either* ~ each other separately Age/759

other *conj.* or SW2/116, SW2/284, SW2/934, etc., **oþer** SW2/227, SW2/729, etc.; ~ . . . *or (. . .* ~*)* either . . . or (. . . or) Bac/101, CHP/208, CHP/1314, SW2/65, SW2/396, etc.; ~ . . . ~ . . . ~ . . . either . . . or . . . or . . . SW2/67; *outher* . . . ~ either . . . or CHP/1171 [use of **other** as *conj.* esp. common in SW2]

otherwhile *adv.* sometimes SW2/77, SW2/79, etc., **otherwhiles** SW2/84, SW2/114, etc.

oughwher *adv.* anywhere, in any way Coi/15, **owhere** SW2/1387

outcast *inf.* throw away, eliminate, reject Inst/1396, *p.ppl.* Inst/1270

outdrawyng *vbl.n.* drawing out, extension Inst/933

outher *conj.* or CHP/585, **owther** CHP/853; ?sometimes CHP/446 [L. *aliquando*]; ~ *(owther)* . . . *or* either . . . or Age/331, Bac/218, CHP/5, etc.; ~ . . . *other* either . . . or CHP/1171

outrage *n.* excess, overindulgence Plag/211

outrageous *adj.* excessive Plag/130

outsenden *pr.3pl.* secrete (a bodily fluid), emit, release Coi/27

outward *adj.* outer, external, away from the center Plag/271, 7LA/97, 7LA/101, 7LA/113; southward Inst/1082; ~ *wittis* physical senses 7LA/11, 7LA/365

outward(e) *adv.* out, away from SW2/607, SW2/1195, SW2/1279, 7LA/71

over *adj.* upper Inst/362, 7LA/81, 7LA/89, 7LA/412, etc.

over *adv.* over, beyond Age/271, DHN/78, Coi/259, CHP/382, SW2/767, Inst/258, etc., **ouer** Age/81, Age/272, Bac/119, CHP/314, etc.

over *prep.* above, over, more than SW2/156, SW2/177, Plag/251, Inst/165, etc.; around Inst/383n [prepositional sense only in second part of manuscript]

overcouered *p.ppl.* overcome CHP/1081

overhigh *adj.* of eyes: bulging CHP/654

overhille *inf.* cover SW2/1498

ouermoche *n.* an excess Age/1006

ouermoche *adj.* excessive Age/1006, **overmoche** Plag/96

ouermoche *adv.* excessively Fle/125, **overmoche** CHP/691, SW2/1479, Plag/148, 7Pla/264

over-part *n.* surface Age/1544

oversenden *pr.3pl.* send out, release Coi/72

ouersight *n.* error for L. *superficie* 'surface' Bac/273

*ouerthwert *adv.* transversely, crosswise DHN/146

overthwert *prep.* across, from one side to the other of Plag/264, Inst/1136

overwered *ppl.adj. wele* ~ of cloth: wellworn, soft SW2/1407

owhere see **oughwher**

owther see **outher**

oxio *n.* error for L. *tyro* 'viper' Age/1422n

paale *adj.* pale, pallid CHP/519, CHP/520, 7Pla/142, etc., **pale** 7Pla/279

paalenes *n.* paleness, pallidity Age/496

paas *n.* passage, going forth Age/1371, **pas** Bac/120

palasie *n.* shaking, palsy CHP/387, SW2/672, etc., **palasy** SW2/701, SW2/704, etc., ***palesye** SW2/1822

palat(e) *n.* the roof of the mouth DHN/57, 7LA/88, 7LA/90, etc.

pallidnes *n.* paleness, pallidity Age/380n, Bac/390

pallith *pr.3sg.* fades, decays Age/802

palues *n.pl.* bits of chaff CHP/1017

pan *n.* the skull CHP/745

pannycules *n.pl.* shreds, tatters CHP/995n

parfite *inf.* profit, be of use [L. *proficere*] Age/39

parfit(e) *adj.* perfect, completed Age/1637, Age/1933, DHN/153, etc.

parfo(u)rme *inf.* perform, carry out Coi/45, 7Pla/331, **parformyth** *pr.3sg.* Plag/33; ~ *inf.* complete, fulfill, bring to perfection Bac/128, Bac/139, Bac/204, **parformyth** *pr.3sg.* DHN/283, DHN/312, Bac/149, etc., **parformeth** Bac/47, **parformeþ** Bac/172, *p.ppl.* **parformed** DHN/256, Inst/111, Inst/196, Inst/355

parilels *n.pl.* parallel circles on the celestial sphere or their representa-

tion on an astronomical instrument
Inst/378

parolel *adj.* parallel Inst/316

particioun *n.* a rhetorical division of
an argument 7LA/138, 7LA/170,
etc.

particles *n.pl.* topics, parts of an argument Age/1690; qualities, features
CHP/471, CHP/474, CHP/483; **par-
ticules** divisions of a text CHP/441,
particulum (L.) *sg.* CHP/648,
CHP/783

particuliers *n.pl.* specific details
CHP/368, CHP/502; specific qualities 8Med/58

pas see **paas**

passe *n.* a measure of length, a 'pace'
7LA/456, *pl.* **passis** 7LA/456

passio(u)n *n.* a disease or affliction
DHN/86, Bac/261, etc.; the suffering of Christ 7LA/25; the state
of being acted upon Bac/580,
Bac/590; ~ *of age* a geriatric ailment Age/124, Bac/106, Bac/468,
Bac/550, etc.; *passiouns of the soule*
emotional and moral states Bac/24,
Bac/380

past *n.* dough SW2/928

pasted *p.ppl.* sealed with a paste
SW2/1806

pasture *n.* pasturage, feeding of animals Age/786, Age/838, Age/839;
pastures *pl.* pastures, grazing lands
7LA/568

pavyng *vbl.n.* a paved floor, floor tiles
Plag/154

pawme *n.* a unit of length, hands-
breadth SW2/820, SW2/1126;
pawmes *pl.* the palms (of the
hands) SW2/1328; *in breede of a litel*
~ a small handsbreadth SW2/1127

peased *p.ppl.* appeased 7Pla/116,
7Pla/170

peyntours *n.pl.* painters CHP/798

peire tablis *phr.* a pair of portable writing tablets hinged or tied together
Inst/1058

pellicules *n.pl.* membranes CHP/1420,
pelliculis CHP/1424

pellis *n.pl.* pills SW2/400

penaunce *n.* pain, suffering SW2/256,
SW2/765, etc.

penne *n.* ~ *fether* lobe (of the lungs)
DHN/111

penurie *n.* poverty Age/546; dearth,
lack 7Pla/13

perambulacioun *n.* a path, a distance
traversed (by the pointer on an astrolabe) Inst/633

perce *inf.* penetrate (*lit.* and *fig.*), enter deeply Age/1543, CHP/790,
percith *pr.3sg.* Age/437, Age/466,
DHN/142, DHN/215, **percen** *pr.3pl.*
DHN/12, **percyng** *pr.ppl.* Age/669,
Age/1288, DHN/37, CHP/577,
perced *p.ppl.* Inst/963

perche *n.(1)* a freshwater fish, the
European perch (*Perca fluviatilis*)
Age/790

perche *n.(2)* a measure of length, equal
to a rod 7LA/453 [see **rod(de)**]

per consequens (L.) *phr.* consequently
Inst/1137

perdicioun *n.* loss CHP/419, 7Pla/43;
waste Bac/591n, Bac/594n

perforate *adj.* pierced Inst/84, Inst/342

periplemenon *n.* an inflammation of
the lungs CHP/916, CHP/926, etc.,
periplemynon CHP/301, **peri-
plemon** CHP/993, **periplemo-
nia** CHP/914, **perriplemonis** *pl.*
CHP/900

peritoneon *n.* the perineum, the area
between the vagina and the anus
SW2/1746, SW2/1754

perle *n.* a pearl or bead Inst/343,
Inst/1158, etc.

permixtioun *n.* confusion CHP/1006;
~ *of (in) reason* mental confusion,
madness CHP/890, CHP/1063,
CHP/1251, etc., *permyxtioun of reasoun* CHP/1260

permutacioun *n.* mental confusion
Age/644, Age/716

perpendicle *n.* a plumb-line Inst/411, Inst/1353, etc., **perpendicule** 7LA/377

perpendicle *adj.* perpendicular 7LA/424, 7LA/426

perpetuall *adj.* everlasting Bac/104; *perpetuel assise* permanent position Inst/1356

perspectief *n.* the science of optics Bac/8, Bac/89, Bac/183, **perspectif** 7LA/354, 7LA/358, 7LA/363

perspectief *adj.* optical Bac/99

***pessaried** *p.ppl.* inserted by means of a pessary SW2/875

pestilence *n.* an infectious, epidemic disease, especially plague Bac/235, Plag/13, etc., **pestelence** Plag/73; *sikenes of ~* a pestilential disease Age/1250

pestilencial *adj.* pertaining to or caused by plague Plag/10, Plag/52, Plag/384, etc.

phiole *n.* a container, flask Bac/61 [see also **viole**]

phisik(e) *n.* medical science CHP/895, Plag/47, 7LA/566, etc.

picture *n.* a figure or diagram 7LA/382, 7LA/404, 7LA/428

pilers *n.pl.* pillars 7LA/25, 7LA/28, 7LA/337

piles *n.pl.* hair Age/408, Age/411, **pilis** Age/412, Age/420, Age/423

pillyng *vbl.n.* a peel or rind of a plant SW2/1023

pyniat *adj.* pointed, terminating in a point CHP/1451

pynnels *n.pl.* pinnules, sighting plates on an astrolabe or quadrant Inst/557n

pipe *n.* a pipe for applying medicine SW2/794, SW2/955; **pipes** *n.pl.* respiratory or circulatory vessels DHN/97n, Bac/392

piscinis *n.pl.* fishponds Age/1376

pissarie *n.* a pessary, vaginal suppository SW2/361, SW2/464, SW2/974, etc., **pissary** SW2/686, SW2/1062, etc., **pissory** SW2/1058

pistel *n.* an epistle, a text written in epistolary form Age/664, **pistil** Age/1534

plaas *n.* a place Age/836

plaate see **plate**

plagiatomye *n.* ?blood-letting by means of a plagiotome, a lancet with a curved blade [L. *plagiostomo, plagiotomo*] Fle/47

playn(e) *n.* a level area, plain Inst/640, Inst/877, 7LA/388, etc.; a smooth surface Inst/387

playn(e) *adj.* smooth Coi/110, CHP/372, Inst/308, 7LA/112, etc., **pleyne** Inst/939; *~* level 7LA/48, 7LA/394, 7LA/539; clear, obvious Bac/336; flat Age/1369

planymetrie *n.* plane geometry 7LA/372, 7LA/405

plantis *n.pl.* plants Age/339, Age/797, etc., **plantes** Age/320, Age/842, Age/1326, **plants** Age/826; **plantes** the palms of the hands DHN/78; *~* the soles of the feet Fle/87, Fle/93

plaster *inf.* apply a medicinal poultice or salve SW2/1057, *impv.* SW2/418, SW2/612, SW2/857, *p.ppl.* **plasterd** SW2/1337, **plastred** SW2/432, **iplastred** SW2/614

plaster *n.* a medicinal poultice or thick salve Age/1567, SW2/280, SW2/365, etc., **plastre** SW2/1790

plate *n.* a flat piece of metal or wood Inst/31, Inst/60, etc., **plaate** Inst/199, Inst/230, etc.

pley *inf.* engage in sex SW2/1816; use (a skill or science) Inst/1088

pley *n.* *~ of knyghthode* knightly sports, jousting Age/540; **pleyes** *pl.* dramatic performances 7LA/574

pleyeng *vbl.n.* recreation, entertainment, performance 7LA/574

pleynmetric *adj.* pertaining to plane geometry Inst/920, **pleynmetrik** Inst/922

plener *adj.* *~ and ful tyme* the fullness of time 7LA/24n

pleuresis *n.* pleurisy CHP/301,
  CHP/1120, **pleuresy** *CHP/166,
  CHP/239, **pleuresin** Fle/57
plom *adj.* plumb, straight down
  Inst/1124; (?as *adv.*) 7LA/377
podagre *n.* gout Fle/15, Fle/76
pointel *n.* a pointer Inst/213
poket *n.* a pouch SW2/265, SW2/808,
  etc.
policie *n.* government 7LA/311; **pollicie** wisdom, good judgment
  7LA/441
polite *adj.* polished, smooth 7LA/363
pollicie see **policie**
polluciouns *n.pl.* nocturnal emissions
  of semen Coi/125, Coi/128, etc.
ponders *n.pl.* weights 7LA/355, 7LA/429
poole *n.* the north or south pole of
  a set of coordinates in the celestial sphere Inst/374, Inst/1325, etc.,
  pooles, poolis *gen.* Inst/67, Inst/67;
  ~ *artik* the north terrestrial pole
  Inst/1114; ~ *equinoxial* on the meridian ring of a celestial globe: a point
  corresponding to an end of the axis
  perpendicular to the north-south
  axis Inst/37, Inst/38; ~ *meridian* the
  south celestial pole Inst/37; ~ *of the
  orizont* the zenith Inst/260; ~ *septentrioun the north celestial pole
  Inst/37; ~ *(pooles, poolis) of the zodiac*
  the end(s) of the axis of the celestial
  sphere perpendicular to the ecliptic
  Inst/114, Inst/118, Inst/130, etc.
poores *n.pl.* pores of the skin Age/620,
  Plag/348, **pooris** Plag/98, Plag/99,
  etc. **pores** Plag/233; ~ small passages in the body (for blood, urine,
  etc.) DHN/179, SW2/298, **poris**
  DHN/104; *greene* ~ the renal veins
  and ureters DHN/183 [see Norri
  1998, 347]
possibilit(i)e *n.* possibility Bac/46,
  Bac/151, Bac/382; *possibilites of craft*
  things that are possible through art
  Bac/603; ~ *of mesures (mesuris)* the
  capacity of the things that are to be
  moderated or balanced Age/283,

Age/293, Age/963, Age/982; *whan
  ~ be* if it be possible Coi/12
postem(e) see **apostem(e)**
potable *adj.* (as *n.*) a drinkable substance Bac/599
potage *n.* a soup or stew Age/1003,
  SW2/249, SW2/354, Plag/292, etc.
potel *n.* a unit of liquid measure equal to
  half a gallon SW2/337, SW2/343, etc.
pownce *n.* the pulse, pulsing of the
  blood SW2/1012
practique *n.* applied knowledge, practice (of medicine or geometry)
  Age/1396, Age/1405, Age/1518,
  practic Plag/37, Inst/920, **practik**
  Inst/916, Inst/918
precedent *adj.* preceding CHP/531;
  precendentis (as *n.pl.*) the preceding things, preceding sections
  CHP/1384
precessith *pr.3sg.* proceeds Coi/58
precipitacioun *n.* ~ *of the matrice (moder)* uterine prolapse SW2/53,
  SW2/690, etc.
predicament *n.* a category in logic
  Bac/618, Bac/621, 7LA/140 [see
  also Persons, Places, and Works,
  s.n. **Porphirie**]
preemynent *adj.* predominant Coi/155
prefocacioun *n.* choking Fle/58
preignant *adj.* (as *n.*) a pregnant
  woman Age/1714, DHN/283; **preig-
  nauntis** *pl.* ?error for L. *pterygoma-
  tibus* 'orifices of the tubes whereby
  a woman's seed enters the uterus'
  DHN/220
prelate *n.* that which is brought forward or aforementioned (referring
  to male and female seed) DHN/228
prelibate *adj.* mentioned previously
  Coi/53
preparat(e) *ppl.adj.* prepared Age/874,
  Bac/574, etc.; ready to use
  Age/1257, Age/2102
prepucie *n.* the prepuce, foreskin
  DHN/225
prerogatief *n.* a prerogative, privilege
  CHP/1175n

prescript *adj.* aforementioned DHN/41, DHN/45

prevy *n.* a privy, toilet SW2/100, SW2/104, SW2/286, SW2/1277

prevy *adj.*(1) trustworthy, able to keep secrets SW2/995, SW2/1514, 7Pla/132; hidden SW2/16, SW2/1745; ~ *chambre* a toilet SW2/764; ~ *membre (member, shap)* private parts, genitalia, vagina SW2/71, SW2/186, SW2/774, SW2/957, etc.; *the ij ~ membres, both ~ membris* the vagina and the anus SW2/766, SW2/1498; ~ *thynges (membris)* the private parts of men or women Plag/267, Plag/272, Plag/368; ~ *termes* menses SW2/958 [see also **priues**]

prevy *adj.*(2) proven, effective SW2/1565

previth *pr.3sg.* proves, demonstrates Bac/260, **preved** *pret.3sg.* Bac/315, *p.ppl.* Bac/572

prike *n.* a mark made as a reference point Inst/1055, Inst/1058, Inst/1066, etc.

prikyng *pr.ppl.* pungent, sharp Age/1338, Age/1864

prikyng *vbl.n.* a pricking sensation, a sharp pain DHN/166, SW2/98, etc., **prickyng** SW2/1071; *prickyng (of bloode)* agitation or stirring of the blood Plag/153, Plag/248, Plag/327

primytief *adj.* of causes, esp. causes of disease: originating, external to the body CHP/495, CHP/658, Plag/61, **primitief** CHP/679, CHP/688, **prymatief** CHP/491, Plag/60

principalte *n.* *obteynen the* ~ be superior Age/309

prively *adv.* gently, unobtrusively 8Med/41; secretly 7Pla/216

priuen *pr.3pl.* are deprived of [L. *priuantur*] Age/426, *p.ppl.* **prived** [L. *priuatur*] Age/656

priues *n.pl.* the private parts Age/947 [see also **prevy** *adj.*(1)]

privite *n.* a mystery [L. *archanum*] CHP/205; the female private parts,

vagina SW2/1381, **privitees** *pl.* SW2/18, SW2/813

probable *adj.* plausible 7LA/145

proces(se) *n.* course (of a disease), duration CHP/481; emission 7LA/359; a rhetorical discourse 7LA/175, 7LA/180

product *adj.* *nombre* ~ the number produced by multiplication Inst/844; (as *n.*) the number produced by multiplication Inst/813, Inst/861, etc.

proef *n.* proof, evidence SW2/1802

proeved *p.ppl.* proved, demonstrated, tested SW2/408, Plag/44, 7LA/132, etc., **proevid** 7LA/133, 7LA/443, 7LA/503, **proved** Age/1435, Bac/366, 7LA/507, etc.

prof(o)unde *adj.* deep Coi/14, Inst/1253

profundacioun *n.* of the eyes: a hollowing, deepening CHP/430

profundymetrie *n.* measurement of depth 7LA/372, **profundemetrie** 7LA/417

profundite *n.* depth Inst/1263, Inst/1287, 7LA/551, etc.

progres(se) *n.* the generation of a sequence of numbers 7LA/230, 7LA/232, etc.

progressioun *n.* a sequence of numbers 7LA/206, 7LA/228

proheme *n.* an introduction to a work Age/49, **prohcmne** Age/745, *prohemium* (L.) CHP/112

proiecciouns *n.pl.* projections of astronomical aspects (i.e., angular distances between positions on the zodiac) to the celestial equator Bac/330n

prompt *adj.* immediately available, ready Bac/336, Plag/21

pronosticacioun *n.* prognostication, foretelling CHP/2, CHP/9, etc.

pronostical *adj.* predictive CHP/5, CHP/1310, CHP/1360

pronostik *inf.* prognosticate, foretell CHP/1391, **pronostith** *pr.3sg.*

CHP/1409, *p.ppl.* **pronostikt** CHP/1397

prosodie *n.* the art of versification 7LA/123

prouerbe *n.* ?error for L. *pronostica* or *pronosticatio* [see CHP/352n] CHP/524, **proverbe** CHP/1016

provide *inf.* foresee, predict CHP/140, *p.ppl.* **provided** 7LA/322

providence *n.* foreseeability, predictability CHP/36, CHP/140

provisioun *n.* prognostication, foreseeing CHP/137, CHP/139, CHP/563, **prouisioun** CHP/244

provisour *n.* a prognosticator, predicter CHP/127

prouocacioun *n.* inducing (of a bodily fluid), eliciting Age/458, Age/767

provocatief *adj.* inducing blood flow SW2/272

provoke *inf.* induce, elicit Age/2061, CHP/553, 8Med/46, **prouoke** Age/1814, **provokith** *pr.3sg.* Age/1121, CHP/121, **provoken** *pr.3pl.* Coi/293, **provokyng** *pr.ppl.* Fle/88; **provokith** *pr.3sg.* stimulates (an anatomical organ) SW2/665

ptisi *n.* phthisic, a wasting lung disease Age/225, CHP/1110

publique *adj. thyng* ~ the common good [L. *res publica*] Bac/236

pulpis *n.pl.* the fleshy parts of the ears, earlobes CHP/372, CHP/401, CHP/432, **pulpes** CHP/405

puls *n.* the pulse, pulsing of the blood Age/374, CHP/293, CHP/295, etc.

pulsacioun *n.* the pulsing of the blood CHP/1227, CHP/1236, etc.

punchyng *vbl.n.* a pricking sensation Plag/153

pungitief *adj.* pungent, spicy Age/1864

purchace *inf.* acquire Age/1092, Bac/207, etc., *pr.3sg.subj.* 7Pla/212, **purchaceth** *pr.3sg.* Age/1117, **purchacith** Age/1147, **purchasiþ** CHP/246, **purchased** *p.ppl.* CHP/476; **purchasyng** *pr.ppl.* buying 7Pla/262,

purchacyng 7Pla/306, **purchaced** *p.ppl.* 7Pla/263

purchasour *n.* a buyer of land 7Pla/105

pure *adj.* uncontaminated Age/891, DHN/190, Coi/55, etc.; ~ *flessh* the flesh itself CHP/378

purgacio(u)n *n.* purgation, removal of excess bodily substances Age/463, Age/515, etc.; menstruation SW2/29, SW2/32, SW2/36, etc.

purpos *n.* intention, intended result Plag/47, Inst/1319

purpose *inf.* imagine, conceive of Age/693; **purposed** *p.ppl.* selected 7LA/221, 7LA/223; intended, sought for 7LA/226; error for L. *composito* 'composed' Age/887

quadra(u)ngule *adj.* quadrangular 7LA/464, 7LA/469; (as *n.*) a quadrangle 7LA/434, 7LA/491

quadrate *n.* a square or rectangle Inst/1292, 7LA/467, etc.

quadrat(e) *adj.* four-sided, square Inst/1283, Inst/1401, 7LA/464, 7LA/466

quadraunt(e) *n.* an instrument for surveying and making astronomical measurements, a quadrant Inst/271, Inst/369, Inst/379, etc., **quadrant** Inst/1218; ~ *of the altitude, altitude* ~ a quarter-ring on a celestial sphere, used for taking altitudes Inst/244, Inst/268, Inst/269, Inst/275 [see also Inst/242n]; *quadrant of the cercle* the squaring of the circle, finding the dimensions of a square with the same area as a given circle Bac/619; ~ *FA* the quarter-circle delimited by points F and A (on an unsupplied diagram) Inst/317, Inst/319

quadrupet *adj.* four-footed 7Pla/65

qualite *n.* nature, character, quality Age/269, Age/1233, etc.; manner, mode Age/204, Age/1048; *audible (visible)* ~ the faculty or sense of hearing (sight) DHN/23, DHN/33, etc.; *of tast the* ~ the faculty or sense of taste DHN/71; **qualit** error for L. *quantitate* 'quantity' Age/1345

quantite *n.* a measurable amount (of size, length, width, number, etc.) Age/269, Age/747, etc.; of stars: magnitude Inst/170, Inst/179

quarel nedil see **nedil**

quartan *adj.* of fevers: intermittent, recurring every third day CHP/1109, SW2/667, **quarteyn** 7Pla/8; **quarteyne** (as *n.*) a quartan fever Age/1378

quarter *n.* a quarter, one-fourth (of a circle, of the zodiac, etc.) Inst/50, Inst/132, Inst/912, etc.; **quarters** *pl.* the four quadrants of the earth Inst/399

quartern *n.* one-fourth of a unit of measure SW2/239, SW2/244, SW2/685, etc., **quarteron** SW2/491, **quater** SW2/487

quartile *adj.* (as *n.*) the astronomical aspect having an angular distance of 90° Inst/617

quarto canone (L.) *phr.* in the fourth book of (Avicenna's) *Canon* Plag/55

quasshyng *vbl.n.* bruising, breaking, smashing Age/539

quater see **quartern**

quatriple *n.* the number four (as part of a ratio) Inst/894

quenche *inf.* assuage by cooling Age/1157; *impv.* submerge (sth. hot in a fluid) SW2/386; **qwenche** *inf.* cool (sth.), extinguish Age/203, **(i)quenched** *p.ppl.* CHP/1082, SW2/571, **iquenchid** SW2/569; **quenchith** *pr.3sg.* is cooled, extinguished Age/173, Age/181

quenchyng *vbl.n.* extinguishing Age/180

quetir *n.* pus SW2/1489, **quetor** SW2/320, **quitour** SW2/1059

quik(e) *adj.* alive, living Age/743, SW2/281, etc.; ~ *coles* live coals Plag/120

quik(e)-siluer *n.* mercury Age/1020, SW2/1411, **quike-silver** SW2/1250

quikly *adj.* alive, free of decay Age/816; signifying or predicting survival CHP/270; *qwikly (quekly) vertu* the animal virtue, the power that controls movement and perception [L. *virtus animalis*] Age/68, Age/560; ~ error for L. *uvam* 'uvula' DHN/88

quyveryng *vbl.n.* tremor Coi/253

quiverith *pr.3sg.* trembles, quivers Fle/94, Fle/95, **quyver** *pr.3sg.subj.* Fle/97, **quiveryng** *pr.ppl.* CHP/654, CHP/1372, **quyveryng** CHP/1370

quocient *adj.* resulting from division of one number by another 7LA/392, 7LA/427, **quociens** Inst/782, Inst/815, etc.; (as *n.*) the result of division of one number by another 7LA/399

radical *adj.* fundamental, underlying CHP/450

raynes *n.pl.*(1) the kidneys Age/1860, SW2/71, etc., **reynes** Age/1120, Fle/15, DHN/176, etc.

raynes *n.pl.*(2) rains, rainstorms 7Pla/42, **reynes** 7Pla/18

rarefien *pr.3pl.* soften (flesh, muscles) Plag/97n

rathest *sup.adv.* most rapidly Age/465

rawnesse *n.* abrasion, laceration SW2/963, SW2/996

ravisshyng(e) *pr.ppl.* rapid, rushing Age/163n, Age/1788, Age/2082

reason *n. light* ~ a feeble mind CHP/1252

receit(e) *n.* a fastening, tether [L. *retinaculum*, poss. misunderstood] DHN/215; a medical recipe Plag/67

recheles *adj.* reckless, careless Plag/26

recours see **recurse**

recta see **cord(e)**, *scala*, **vmbre**

rect(e) *adj.* straight 7LA/62, 7LA/76, 7LA/409, 7LA/439, 7LA/462, etc.; ~ *angule* right angle 7LA/410, 7LA/473, etc.; *cord(e)* ~ see **cord(e)**

rectificacioun *n.* a correction Age/441; an improvement 7LA/50

rectifie *inf.* guide, correct 7LA/30, **rectifien** *pr.3pl.* Plag/41, **rectifie** 7LA/43, 7LA/337, **rectified** *p.ppl.* 7LA/269; **rectifieth** *pr.3sg.* restores (bodics, complexions) to health Age/1272, Bac/474, **rectifien** *pr.3pl.* Bac/449

rectis spiere *phr.* the celestial sphere as seen by an observer at the earth's equator Inst/724

recurse *n.* a return, returning CHP/980, CHP/989, **recours** DHN/45

recursed *p.ppl.* returned CHP/978

redditi(e)f *adj.* pertaining to the power of exhaling DHN/58, DHN/60

rede *adj.* red Age/78, Age/1231, etc.; *cliere ~* bright red Age/1402, SW2/96, SW2/1008; *dym ~* dull or pale red SW2/1008; *swart ~ , ~ swart* dark red SW2/102, SW2/141, SW2/1009

reduce *inf.* return, bring back Age/1269, Bac/317, *impv.* Age/2036, Inst/605, **reducith** *pr.3sg.* Age/943, Age/1272, Age/2025, **reduced** *p.ppl.* Age/460, Age/1569, etc., **reducid** Age/2084; *~ inf.* convert, change 7LA/491, 7LA/512, *impv.* Inst/705, **reduced** *pret.2sg.* Inst/767; *reduced equaly to the half (to the half evenly)* of two measurements: averaged Inst/1277, Inst/1395

reedis *n.pl.* muscle fibers [?error for L. *carnis* 'flesh'] DHN/65

reete *n.* a rotable star-map on the front of an astrolabe Inst/397, Inst/483, etc., **reetis** *pl.* Inst/485; a set of calendric circles on the back of an astrolabe Inst/388n, Inst/395

reetis *adj. ~ orizont* right horizon, the horizon of an equatorial observer Inst/698n; *~ spiere* right sphere, the celestial sphere as seen by an observer at the earth's equator Inst/713n

refreyneth *pr.3sg.* holds back, restrains itself CHP/65

regendre *inf.* regenerate Age/871, **regendrith** *pr.3sg.* Age/1630, CHP/1467, **regendryng** *pr.ppl.* Age/1506

reherse *inf.* report, state, describe 7Pla/236, **rehersith** *pr.3sg.* Coi/148, Coi/174, Bac/66, etc., **reherce** *pr.1pl.* [?error for L. *reperimus* 'we find'] Bac/16n, **reherced** *pret.3sg.* Bac/490, **rehersed** *p.ppl.* SW2/1281, 7LA/337

reynes see **raynes** *n.pl.*(1) and *n.pl.*(2)

reyneth *pr.3sg.* reigns Plag/210

reyny *adj.* rainy CHP/259, CHP/260, Plag/138

relinted *p.ppl.* softened SW2/1521

remembraunce *n.* memory Age/563, Age/567, Age/689

remembraunciers *n.pl.* people who remember, recorders Age/569

rememoratief *adj.* of signs: serving as a reminder CHP/3, CHP/7, CHP/26

remollith *pr.3sg.* softens CHP/1378

repaire *inf.* restore Age/1618, **repairith** *pr.3sg.* Age/1359, Age/1433, Age/2045, **repairen** *pr.3pl.* Age/147, Age/553, Age/1620, **repaired** *p.ppl.* Age/552; *~ inf.* mend, correct Bac/90, **repaired** *p.ppl.* Bac/105; *~ inf.* error for L. *repperi* 'I have found' Age/86n; **repairen** *pr.3pl.* error for L. *reperiuntur* or *reperiantur* 'are found, may be found' Age/755, Age/761; **repaired** *p.ppl.* error for L. *temperata* 'temperate' Age/2103n

repercussief *adj.* striking CHP/1034; **repercussyves** (as *n.pl.*) medicines to drive out excess humours SW2/1022

repleccioun *n.* overabundance (of humours, food, etc.), repletion Age/1977, CHP/619, Plag/96, etc.

reple(e)te *adj.* full or overly full Coi/197, CHP/508, **replet** Plag/16; *~* having an excess of humours CHP/624, SW2/550, SW2/1466, Plag/161

replied *p.ppl.* bent down Age/1171; repeated Inst/384n, Inst/1249, Inst/1264

reprehensioun *n.* criticism, blame CHP/230; in rhetoric: rebuttal of opposing views 7LA/170, 7LA/178

reprenten *pr.3pl.* re-impress (an image) CHP/1010

repressith *pr.3sg.* restrains CHP/897; **repressed** *p.ppl.* overcome SW2/1245

reproved *p.ppl.* rebuked, condemned DHN/306

repugneth *pr.3sg.* prevents, resists Age/1152, **repugnyng** *pr.ppl.* Plag/191; **repugnen** *pr.3pl.* are contradictory Coi/89, Coi/93

require *inf.* be requisite Bac/205; **requirith** *pr.3sg.* demands, calls for Inst/264, 7Pla/146, 7LA/316, **requireþ** Bac/190, **requireth** 7LA/438, **required** *p.ppl.* CHP/1147; ~ *impv.* inquire Inst/1213

reryng *vbl.n.* altitude, elevation above the horizon Inst/528n

reserve *inf.* keep in mind, retain Age/703; **reserved** *p.ppl.* preserved Age/124

residue *n.* the result of a calculation, remainder Inst/679, Inst/846, Inst/865

resolucioun *n.* the dispersal of bodily humours Age/143, Age/170, CHP/1330, etc.; *light of ~* of apostemes: easily brought to a head, dispersed CHP/1343

resolut(e) *adj.* dispersed, dissolved, broken up Age/110, Age/774, CHP/1238, etc.; (as *n.*) that which has been dispersed Age/1284; (as *n.*) a substance produced by resolution of humours CHP/1346

resolue *inf.* dissipate, loosen, soften (humours, apostemes, other bodily matter) CHP/1327, **resolvith** *pr.3sg.* Age/134, Age/782, CHP/1321, etc.,

resolueth Age/1593, CHP/1315, **resoluith** CHP/1386, **resolveþ** Age/746, **resolved** *p.ppl.* Age/92, Age/135, etc., **resolued** Age/1595, **resolvid** Age/134; ~ *impv.* dissolve SW2/600, SW2/1121, **resolued** *p.ppl.* Bac/528, SW2/573, SW2/1116, **resolved** Age/2022; **resolued** *p.ppl.* of fumes: given off SW2/542, SW2/545; **resolved** *p.ppl.* transformed SW2/125

resonable *adj.* reasonable, in accord with reason CHP/483; possessing the faculty of reason (esp. of the soul) Age/572, Age/654, Bac/13, etc.; *length of ~ soule* error for L. *longitudinem a re non naturali* Age/1687n

resownyng *vbl.n.* reasoning 7LA/127

respect *n.* (as) *to the ~ of* in comparison to Bac/294, CHP/332, CHP/1285; *~ agenst* effect on, power against Plag/70

respectives ?*n.pl. as ~* respectively, vice versa [L. *et respective*] CHP/662

rest *pr.3sg.subj.* attend (to sth.) 7Pla/348 [cf. *MED*, s.v. *resten* v.(3), (c)]

reteigne *inf.* retain, keep, hold Age/942, Age/979, **reteyne** Age/943, ~ *pr.3pl.* Age/1597, DHN/196, **reteignen** *pr.3pl.* Age/286, Age/904

retencioun *n.* retention of material in the body Bac/24, Bac/343, Bac/380; retention of blood (esp. menstrual blood) in the body SW2/1108, **retencio(u)n(i)s** *pl.* SW2/258, SW2/867

retrogradacioun *n.* of planets: an apparently reverse motion through the zodiac Inst/592

retrograde *adj.* of planets: moving backward through the zodiac Inst/598

rewme *n.* a catarrh or cold attributed to watery humours Fle/9, SW2/672

reuersioun *n.* a return of harmful humours to an aposteme CHP/971

revoke *inf.* call back, bring back [error for L. *renovare* 'renew'] Coi/5, **revoked** *p.ppl.* Coi/5

reuolucioun *n.* the orbit of a planet through the sky 7Pla/91; *in (the) houre(s) and tyme(s) of ~* at a particular time in a planet's orbit 7Pla/4, 7Pla/21, etc., *in tyme and houre of hir revolucioun* 7Pla/98

rib *n.* the side of a quadrangle 7LA/466, 7LA/467, etc., **ribbes** *pl.* 7LA/472; *grete ~* hypotenuse 7LA/518; **ribbes** *pl.* the ribs of the body CHP/820, **ribbis** CHP/1414; *tender ribbis* the lower ribs, just above the hypochondrium CHP/1186; **ribbes** ?error for L. *costo* ?costmary Age/1186n

riche *adj.* of an odor: strong Plag/104

riet *adj.* ~ *orizont* right horizon, the horizon of an equatorial observer Inst/674

rige-bon(e) *n.* the backbone, spine SW2/71, SW2/515, etc., **rigge-bon** DHN/87

rightwisnes *n.* righteousness 7LA/12

rigour *n.* pathological rigidity Coi/252, Coi/278, Coi/281

rynde *n.* bark, a piece of bark SW2/78, SW2/429, etc.; *myddil ~* the middle layer of bark SW2/342, SW2/883

rise *n.* rice SW2/379, SW2/390; *flour of ~* rice flour SW2/469

rismon n. a putative Greek word for 'number' [in a mistaken etymology for the word **algorisme**, properly derived from the name of the Islamic mathematician Muhammad ibn Mūsā al-Khwārazmī; but cf. Greek *arithmos* 'number'] 7LA/193

riveled *p.ppl.* wrinkled Age/491

rod(de) *n.* a staff or rod used for measuring Inst/1238, Inst/1390, 7LA/407, 7LA/408, etc.; a measure of length, equal to eighteen feet 7LA/453, 7LA/458; *Mercuries ~* the wand of Mercury as a symbol for the art of rhetoric 7LA/163; *vessel roddis* rods for measuring containers Inst/1408

rote *inf.* ?soak or steep, ?rot SW2/647; **roteth** *pr.3sg.* rots, decays Age/799

roten *adj.* rotten SW2/1363

rotened *p.ppl.* ?soaked or steeped SW2/195 [cf. *MED,* s.v. *roten* v.(1), 4]

rough *adj.* wrinkled Age/491, Age/1552; rigid, in spasm CHP/751, CHP/812

rowghith *pr.3sg.* grows stiff, becomes erect Coi/280

roughly *adv.* (held) rigidly, in spasm CHP/804

roughnes(se) *n.* wrinkledness, rugosity Age/117, Age/489, etc.; of meat: coarseness, toughness Bac/563; ~ *of nail(e)* roughness of the fingernails (an error for 'roughness of the skin') Age/151n, Age/493, Bac/390n, etc. [see also **nail(e)**]

roundel *n.* a metal ring attached to a celestial globe Inst/197; ~ *meridian* a ring representing the great circle passing through the observer's zenith Inst/29

rubifaccioun *n.* reddening CHP/617

ruggyng *vbl.n.* rumbling in the stomach [L. *rugitus* 'braying'] Coi/289

rule *inf.* govern, control Age/1731, Bac/200, etc., **rulith** *pr.3sg.* CHP/862, 7LA/315, **rulen** *pr.3pl.* Bac/399, Bac/401, **rulyng** *pr.ppl.* CHP/600, CHP/638, **rulid** *p.ppl.* Age/1845, CHP/29

rule *n.* a guide for behavior, regimen of health Age/42, Age/49, etc.; governance, control of self or others Bac/5, Bac/195, 7LA/311, etc.; a principle of action Age/250, Age/664, Inst/658, 7LA/339, etc.; a ruler or pointer, measuring tool Inst/219, Inst/403, etc.

rulyng *vbl.n.* the act of governing, controlling CHP/762

ruln *n.* a regimen of health Age/1589

sacellacioun *n.* the application of a poultice 8Med/5, 8Med/53, 8Med/61

saciatives *n.pl.* error for L. *sciaticis* 'people suffering from sciatica' Age/2063n

sadde *adj.* thick SW2/928; solid, three-dimensional Inst/925

saged *ppl.adj.* learned 7LA/346

Sagittarij *n.* the constellation and zodiacal sign Sagittarius, the Archer 7Pla/189

salsodes *n.pl.* a kind of blood vessel Fle/24 [cf. Latham 1980, s.v. *salsotes, vene* 'varicose veins']

sanguyn(e) *n.* the bodily humour blood Bac/124, CHP/976, CHP/981, CHP/985, 8Med/56

sangwyn(e) *adj.* characterized by an excess of the humour blood Bac/125, Plag/142; *fever sanguyn* a fever caused by or associated with excess blood CHP/101

sanies *n.* pus, a suppurating wound CHP/1490, CHP/1491

sapience *n.* wisdom, learning Age/27, Age/327, Bac/3, etc.

sapient *adj.* wise, learned Age/48, Age/85, Bac/44, CHP/136, 7Pla/133, etc.

sarce *inf.* sift SW2/1858

satournous *adj.* of wine: sweet, full-bodied SW2/627

sauf *adj.* healed, unharmed, safe CHP/1083, CHP/1190; error for L. *saluia* 'sage' Age/2060n

sauf *prep.* except Age/1074, Age/1722n, CHP/388, etc.; (as *conj.*) Age/1855, Plag/162

sawtry *n.* a psaltery, a stringed instrument 7Pla/326

savour *n.* taste, smell Age/807, Age/865, DHN/67, CHP/693, SW2/588, etc.; sexual pleasure DHN/224

savourde *ppl.adj.* scented SW2/744

savoure *pr.1pl.* warm up, wipe (with a warming liquid) [L. *foveamus* 'let us warm, caress, nurture'] Fle/87 [see **favour(e)**]; **savourith** *pr.3sg.* tastes CHP/694

savoury *adj.* tasty, delicious Age/811, Age/1300, DHN/66, etc.

scabbed *ppl.adj.* having scabs SW2/968

scala (L.) *n.* ~ *recta* the horizontal side of the shadow square on a quadrant Inst/886, Inst/905; ~ *versa* the perpendicular side of the shadow square on a quadrant Inst/884, Inst/902 [see **vmbre**]

scale *n.* a calibrated scale on a quadrant Inst/383, Inst/831

scalis *n.pl.* rinds, pods SW2/1309

scalpels *n.pl.* ?veins in the foot [L. *scalpellis*, perhaps a corruption of *salvatellis/salvaticis (venis)* 'veins of hand or foot'] Fle/19 [see Latham 1980, s.v. *salvatella*; MED, s.v. *salvatica* n.]

scarste *n.* scarcity 7Pla/37, 7Pla/40, 7Pla/42

sciatic *n.* sciatica Fle/15

sciatic *adj.* ~ *passioun* sciatica Fle/120

scomed *p.ppl.* skimmed, having had the scum removed SW2/350, **iscomed** SW2/1881

scotomy(e) *n.* a dimming of vision or the appearance of small flecks in the visual field, sometimes accompanied by vertigo Age/1437, CHP/1097, CHP/1335, etc., **scotayne** SW2/89

scourf *n.* a scaly skin disease often affecting the scalp, scurf CHP/744, **scurphes** Age/1427

scourged *p.ppl.* afflicted, burdened Age/987; whipped Bac/565

scourphi *adj.* afflicted with scurf CHP/741

scripule *n.* a unit of measure, one twenty-fourth of an ounce Age/922 [usually abbreviated ℈]

scrutacioun *n.* scrutiny Age/608

secret(e) *n.* hidden knowledge, a mystery Age/335, Age/911, Bac/229, etc.; a confidential matter 7Pla/109,

7Pla/133, etc.; the female genitals DHN/225

secret(e) *adj.* hidden, esoteric Bac/94, Bac/297, etc.; ~ *cercle* the anus DHN/253; ~ *genitals* the genitalia, private parts Age/1351

secundyne *n.* the afterbirth, placenta SW2/60, SW2/682, etc., **secundynes** *pl.* (with *sg.* sense) SW2/1254, **secondynes** SW2/1302

sedacioun *n.* relief, alleviation CHP/1320

see *inf.* see CHP/318, CHP/650, CHP/702, etc., **seene** SW2/697, ~ *impv.* Age/820, CHP/797, **seest** *pr.2sg.* Age/1725, CHP/1249, Inst/557, **seeth** *pr.3sg.* Age/692, DHN/184, CHP/693, etc., **seeþ** CHP/1039, ~ *pr.1pl.* Age/242, Age/793, etc., *pr.2pl.* 7LA/395, etc., ~ *pr.2sg.subj.* CHP/573, *pr.3sg. subj.* CHP/190, CHP/1461, **se(e)** *pr.1pl.subj.* Age/383, Age/1584, Age/1777, **seeyng** *pr.ppl.* 7LA/368, **sawe** *pret.1sg.* Plag/67, Inst/1066, **sigh** *pret.3sg.* Bac/215, Bac/508, CHP/164, **seen** *p.ppl.* Age/242, Age/352, etc.

seeche *impv.* seek, calculate Inst/539, Inst/760, *pr.1pl.* Inst/921, Inst/922, Inst/923

seeth(e) *inf.* boil SW2/209, SW2/277, etc., *impv.* SW2/175, SW2/337, SW2/1290, etc., **seeþ** SW2/737, **seth(e)** SW2/404, SW2/429, etc., **seeþ** *pret.3sg.* SW2/949, **(i)soden** *p.ppl.* Age/1203, Age/1386, SW2/157, SW2/158, etc., **(i)sode** Age/1003, SW2/432; **se(e)thith** *pr.3sg.* heats or cooks within the body DHN/114, DHN/116, etc., **seethiþ** DHN/177, **seeth** Age/1342, **seethen** *pr.3pl.* DHN/172, **soden** *p.ppl.* DHN/165, DHN/173, etc.

seeþing *vbl.n.* boiling, decoction SW2/924

seieng *pr.ppl.* saying CHP/1338

seienges *vbl.n.* teachings, sayings Age/667

seynt *n.* a saint Bac/469, SW2/644, Plag/315, etc.; *x seyntis* error for L. *x scientiis* 'ten sciences' Age/1828n

sellen *pr.3pl.* sell [error for L. *vindicat* 'claims,' read as form of *vendere* 'sell' or *venditare* 'try to sell'] DHN/148

semidiatrum (L.) *n.* ~ *orientis* the east horizon-line on an astrolabe Inst/543n

semynably *adv.* error for L. *similem* 'similar' Coi/57n

semyvowel(l) *n.* one of the consonants *l, m, n, r, s,* and *x* 7LA/86, 7LA/87, 7LA/111

sensible *adj.* perceptible to the senses Age/709, Inst/595, Inst/919; capable of sensation, sensitive DHN/79, CHP/834; ~ *organs* the sensory organs Bac/391; ~ *wittis* the senses, sensory faculties Age/554, Age/635, etc.

sensitief *adj.* sensory CHP/1010

septentrional *adj.* northern, northerly Inst/162, Inst/236, etc., **sempten-trional** Inst/590; ~ (as *n.*) the north Inst/202, Inst/514; ~ *poole* the north pole Inst/67, Inst/114

septentrional-oriental *adj.* northeasterly Inst/500

*****septentrioun** *adj. poole* ~ the north pole Inst/37

sequestrith *pr.3sg.* separates DHN/107

serche *inf.* ?mistrans. of forms of L. *significare* 'signify': CHP/593, **serchith** *pr.3sg.* CHP/600, CHP/601n, CHP/618, etc., **serchen** *pr.3pl.* CHP/619; **serchid** sought for, scrutinized *p.ppl.* Age/9

serche *n.* the act of investigating, scrutinizing Age/609, CHP/558; *in* ~ *of* searching through, undertaking inquiries in Age/83; ?mistrans. of a form of L. *significare* [see **serche** *inf.*] CHP/594

serchyng *vbl.n.* searching for, scrutinizing CHP/369

sercle see **cercle**

serene *adj.* of weather: clear, serene Age/609

sermo(u)n *n.* a part of a treatise Age/564, Age/624, etc.; a written discussion, treatment of a subject CHP/259, CHP/641, etc.; a term or phrase CHP/1092, CHP/1469

serue *inf.* maintain, hold to Bac/87

setelid *p.ppl.* settled, calmed down SW2/1776

seth(e), sethith see **seeth(e)**

setil *n.* a seat 8Med/6

sextile *adj.* (as *n.*) the astronomical aspect having an angular distance of 60° Inst/616

shamefast *adj.* ~ *cercle* the anus DHN/166, DHN/253

shameful *adj.* ashamed SW2/2

shaply *adj.* shapely, handsome 7Pla/325

shap(pe) *n.* form, shape Age/279, Age/711, Age/997, SW2/755, etc.; *prevy* ~ genitalia, genital area SW2/957

share *n.* the crotch, pubic area SW2/284, SW2/366, etc.

sharp(e) *adj.* bitter, pungent, sharp-tasting Age/590, Age/770, etc.; pointed, narrow DHN/120, CHP/371, CHP/1448, etc.; of fevers and other illnesses: acute CHP/36, CHP/261, CHP/263, etc.; of tools or fasteners: keen of edge or point Inst/13, Inst/84, Inst/174; of words: narrowly defined CHP/1092n, CHP/1101; error for L. *cutis* 'skin' DHN/199n

sharpith *pr.3sg.* becomes sharper CHP/423; makes (sth.) sharper or keener Fle/146, 7LA/348, **sharpiþ** Plag/389

shedyng *vbl.n.* pouring Age/1013

sheede *impv.* pour Age/1558; **she(e)dith** *pr.3sg.* diffuses, issues forth CHP/1478, CHP/1480, **shediþ** DHN/218, **shede** *pr.3sg.subj.*

CHP/1312, **shed(de)** *p.ppl.* Age/472, DHN/209, Coi/15, etc.

shere *inf.* cut across, intersect Inst/848; **ishore** *p.ppl.* shorn SW2/726

shermen *n.pl.* shearmen, shearers of the nap of woolen cloth 7LA/577

shetten see **shit**

sheweres *n.* a female revealer 7Pla/272

shevyng *pr.ppl.* ~ *fynger* the index finger, "showing finger" Plag/376

shynynges *n.pl.* flashes of light 7Pla/17

ship-brechis *n.pl.* shipwrecks 7Pla/19

shire *adj.* ?clean, ?fine SW2/1521

shit *inf.* shut, close CHP/886, **shittith** *pr.3sg.* DHN/154, **shetten** *pr.3pl.* CHP/875, ~ *p.ppl.* DHN/103, **shitte** SW2/793, SW2/1183

shittyng *vbl.n.* shutting, closing Age/595

short *inf.* shorten Bac/29, **shorteþ** *pr.3sg.* CHP/745, **shorten** *pr.3pl.* CHP/391, **shorted** *p.ppl.* Bac/17, Bac/33, CHP/119, etc.

shrewd(e) *adj.* wicked, malicious, harmful Age/217, CHP/936, 7Pla/285; of reputation: negative Fle/104

shuldistow *pr.2sg.* should you Plag/54

shulder *n.* shoulder SW2/1186, **shuldre** Plag/374, **shuldres** *pl.* SW2/1152, SW2/1190, Plag/281, etc.; ~ *bladis* shoulder blades SW2/75

siccite *n.* dryness CHP/523

siege *n.* a seat SW2/792, SW2/1786, SW2/1787

sield *adj.* ?thin CHP/397

sield *adv.* seldom Age/1254

sielden *adj.* infrequent Age/1015, CHP/1062

sielden *adv.* seldom, infrequently Age/504, Coi/217, Bac/347, etc.; *of* ~ rarely, infrequently CHP/675

sigh see **see**

sighynges *vbl.n.pl.* ~ *of sikenessis* labored breathing or groaning caused by sickness CHP/906

signator *n.* a planet symbolizing particular persons, activities, or things 7Pla/89

signe *inf.* set a mark (on sth.), inscribe (a mark) Inst/1299, *pr.2sg.subj.* Inst/1226, **signed** *p.ppl.* Inst/1395; **signes** *impv.* [a Northern form] mark with a dot Inst/1174, Inst/1183n, Inst/1191, etc.

signe *n.* a sign, an indication, a symptom Age/131, Age/613, Age/1400, CHP/3, etc.; a mark, esp. for purposes of measurement Inst/324, Inst/1228, Inst/1233, etc.; *pl.* the number of digits on the shadow scales of a quadrant Inst/815n; a zodiacal sign or its representation on an astronomical instrument Inst/126, Inst/144, 7Pla/47, etc.; *signes inequal(s) (equals)* gradations of unequal (equal) distance on a measuring rod Inst/1234, Inst/1274, Inst/1280, etc.; *air(e)ly (erthly, watery) ~, ~ airly* a zodiacal sign associated with the element air (earth, water) 7Pla/15, 7Pla/12, 7Pla/18, 7Pla/41, etc.; *bestiall (mannes) ~* a zodiacal sign in animal (human) form 7Pla/45, 7Pla/56; *signes of (a) man, signes (signis) of mankynd(e)* zodiacal signs in human form 7Pla/6, *7Pla/36, 7Pla/72, 7Pla/86, 7Pla/93; *northen (northern) signes, signes septentrional* the zodiacal signs from Aries to Virgo Inst/524, Inst/1333, Inst/1369; *~ quadrupet* a zodiacal sign in the form of a four-footed animal 7Pla/65; *southren (southern) signes* the zodiacal signs from Libra through Pisces Inst/1334, Inst/1370

signeres *n.* a female signifier (i.e., a planet symbolizing particular persons, activities, or things) 7Pla/96

significatief *adj.* *~ of* signifying CHP/276

signifior *n.* a planet symbolizing particular persons, activities, or things 7Pla/2

sikelith *pr.3sg.* becomes ill, sickens Age/621, Age/656, Age/1240, **siklith** CHP/1103

sikernes *n.* certainty 7LA/353

sikly *adj.* sick Age/1677; **sikeliest** *sup.* most conducive to illness Plag/414

siklith see **sikelith**

similitude *n.* likeness, similarity Age/329, Age/334, **simylitude** DHN/141; *~ comparison* CHP/1445

symulith *pr.3sg.* dissembles, lies 7Pla/343

synapisme *n.* the sprinkling of a stiptic or drying powder on a bruised or wounded member 8Med/4, **cinapisme** 8Med/31 [cf. Latham 1980, s.v. *sinapisma* 'mustard plaster'; *MED*, s.v. *sinapizen* v.]

sincopim *n.* fainting CHP/1158, **sincops** CHP/1160

synewy *adj.* containing tendons CHP/859

synewe *n.* a nerve or tendon Age/575, Fle/36, CHP/738, etc.

singul(i)er *adj.* individual, particular Age/709, CHP/115, CHP/180, CHP/310; **singuliers** (as *n.pl.*) particular instances 7LA/133

synne *n.* a sin, moral transgression Bac/10, Bac/359, etc.; *actual ~* a sin committed by an individual (in contrast to original sin) 7LA/24; *fomyte of ~* see **fomyte**

synneth *pr.3sg.* is at fault Age/456; sins Coi/193, Coi/202, **synned** *p.ppl.* Bac/598

sinochus *n.* a steady fever CHP/304, CHP/1176

sinthomates *n.pl.* symptoms CHP/233, **sinthomatis** CHP/541, **sinthomyes** CHP/1175

sith *adv.* afterward Inst/859

sith *conj.* since 7LA/291, 7LA/335

sithes *n.pl.* times Inst/384, Inst/892

skies *n.pl.* the heavens Age/1824

skyn(ne) *n.* the skin of an animal, an animal skin Bac/455, CHP/996, SW2/1327, 7LA/576; the human skin Age/1458, CHP/373, Plag/98, etc.; a membrane CHP/80, SW2/44, SW2/1440, etc.; ~ *that is betwixt the ij prevy membres* the perineum SW2/766

skynners *n.pl.* sellers and preparers of animal skins 7LA/577

sle(e) *inf.* slay, kill CHP/458, SW2/1247, Plag/185, Plag/235, **sleeth** *pr.3sg.* CHP/668, CHP/1306, *SW2/1447, etc., **sleen** *pr.3pl.* CHP/728, CHP/1413, **sleyng** *pr.ppl.* Age/1391, CHP/714, **slayne** *p.ppl.* Bac/566, SW2/681, SW2/1185

sleeve *n.* ?the caecum of the large intestine DHN/162; the large bowel DHN/164, DHN/170 [see **maniac, monomac**]

slek *inf.* slake, relieve Plag/220

slugges *n.pl.* lazy people 7LA/161

smered *p.ppl.* rubbed with an ointment Age/1560

smert *pr.3sg.subj.* experience pain SW2/933

smertyng *vbl.n.* pain SW2/303, SW2/307

smythes *n.pl.* blacksmiths Age/490; *gen.* SW2/810, **smethis** SW2/1568; ~ *shoppe* a smithy 7LA/282

smoke *n.* smoke SW2/425, etc.; an emanation of vapor, fumes, or vaporous corporeal substance Age/523, SW2/514, SW2/518, etc.

smokyng *vbl.n.* a fumigation, the application of medicinal materials by means of smoke SW2/990

smoth *inf.* make (sth.) even Inst/31

smoth *adj.* smooth, polished 7LA/109, 7LA/363, **smoþ** CHP/722n

smothenes *n.* smoothness CHP/747

smulder *n.* smoke Plag/119

sode, soden see **seeth(e)**

soeffren *inf.* allow, permit Age/433n

soft *adj.* soft, gentle Coi/111, Bac/188, etc.; receptive, amenable 7Pla/261

soft(e)ly *adv.* gently Fle/91, SW2/309, SW2/749, Inst/86, etc.

solsticial *adj.* pertaining to the solstices Inst/100, Inst/113, *Inst/115; (as *n.*) one of the solstices Inst/479, Inst/488; ~ *estyval (of somer)* the summer solstice Inst/476, *Inst/1148; ~ *hiemal (of wynter)* the winter solstice Inst/475, Inst/1140

solucioun *n.* purgation, a purging Age/1081, CHP/704, CHP/717, etc.; a rupture in the continuity of the flesh CHP/1455, CHP/1458; ~ *of (the) wombe* loosening or purging of the bowels Age/205, Age/469, CHP/554, etc.

solutief *adj.* causing softening, loosening, or relaxation CHP/873, SW2/283

solutives *n.pl.* laxative medicines Age/467

solue *inf.* disperse, dissipate Coi/81; loosen, purge Coi/226, **solueth** *pr.3sg.* Coi/241, **solvith** Coi/284, **solued** *p.ppl.* CHP/1105; **solve** *inf.* dissolve Age/351, **solued** *p.ppl.* Bac/110

somme *n.* an arithmetical sum 7LA/240, 7LA/242, etc.

son *adj.* ~ *argument* ?sound argument 7LA/130

sonner see **soon(e)**

sookyng *pr.ppl.* of fire: gentle, slow SW2/1848

sooles *n.pl.* the soles (of the feet) Bac/505, Bac/506, SW2/1234, **soolis** Bac/67, SW2/589, SW2/1328

soon(e) *adv.* soon, quickly Age/57, Age/333, DHN/40, etc., **sonner** *comp.* Age/411n, Age/414, CHP/1344, etc.

soote *adj.* sweet, fragrant Fle/89

sophen *n.* the saphenous vein, located below the ankle Plag/274n

sophister *n.* one who uses sophistical reasoning 7LA/150 [see also Persons, Places, and Works, s.n. **Sophister**] sophisticat *ppl.adj.* adulterated Bac/543

sophistorie *n.* sophistry, specious wisdom CHP/225

sowde *inf.* heal by knitting (veins, flesh) together SW2/352, **sowden** SW2/362, **sowdith** *pr.3sg.* SW2/382, **sowdyng** *pr.ppl.* SW2/1548

sowen *p.ppl.* sown, planted (*fig.*) Coi/8; of diseases: ?spread about, disseminated CHP/260

sowkyng *ppl.adj.* of an animal: suckling Age/1853, SW2/398, **soukyng** Age/771

soule *n.* soul, spirit, mind Age/11, DHN/279, Coi/179, Bac/13, etc.; *litel* ~ error for L. *adminiculo* 'by the support' DHN/174

soulyng *pr.ppl.* bringing in the soul DHN/279

souped *p.ppl.* sipped, consumed in small amounts Age/1004

soupyng *n.* soft or liquid food Age/2090; ?a potion DHN/199n

souple *adj.* supple SW2/1753

souplyng *vbl.n.* softening Age/1908

south lyne *phr.* meridional line, the midline of the sky Inst/1138 [see **meridional**]

spacith ?*p.ppl.* measured DHN/156

spadouns *n.pl.* eunuchs 7Pla/83

span *n.* a unit of measure equivalent to a handspan, handsbreadth SW2/265

spargith *pr.3sg.* spreads, disperses Age/426

sparyng *pr.ppl.* protective, merciful 7Pla/323

sparlier *n.* the calf of the leg SW2/148, **sparlyuer** SW2/609

sparpled *p.ppl.* spread, dispersed Age/681

spatil *n.* spittle Coi/62, CHP/301

speche *n.* the faculty of speech Age/706

spechis *n.pl.* kinds, species Inst/920

special *adj.* ~ *sciences* the liberal arts 7LA/28, 7LA/336, etc.

speculacioun *n.* theorizing, abstraction Plag/36, Inst/917, 7LA/476

speculatief *adj.* having theoretical knowledge Age/326; **speculatif** theoretical Age/738

spered *p.ppl.* blocked, confined Plag/240

sperik see **spierike**

sperma cete *phr.* ambergris Bac/541

sperme *n.* semen, the male or female reproductive seed DHN/232, Bac/541, SW2/630, etc.

spetomy ?*n.* sense uncertain Fle/152

spewe *inf.* vomit *SW2/286, SW2/827

spice *n.* kind, species Age/231, Age/637, Age/1473, DHN/68, CHP/1158, 7LA/150, etc.

spicers *n.pl.* spice-sellers Plag/299

spices *n.pl.* spices Age/2083, Bac/94, etc., **spicis** Age/527, Age/1441, etc.

spier(e) *n.* a sphere Bac/276, 7LA/537, etc.; a globe showing the positions of stars and various celestial great circles Inst/25, Inst/83, etc., **spire** Inst/274; a treatise on making a celestial globe 7LA/357; **spier-is, spieres** *pl.* the celestial spheres, the concentric spheres revolving around the earth in Aristotelian cosmology Plag/4, Inst/149; ~ *oblonge* the oblique sphere, the celestial sphere as seen by an observer between the earth's equator and one of the geographic poles Inst/772, Inst/773, Inst/779; *right (rectis, reetis)* ~ , *right spire* the celestial sphere as seen by an observer at the earth's equator Inst/699, Inst/713, Inst/719, Inst/724, etc.

spierike *adj.* spherical Inst/35, **sperik** Inst/8, **spirek** Inst/80

spindel *n.* ~ *of the bak* the spine DHN/12, Coi/47

spirit(e) *n.* a physiological fluid that carries or transmits various bodily functions and faculties Age/498, Age/1543, DHN/5, Coi/18, etc.; breath CHP/290, CHP/1052,

CHP/1066, etc.; **spiritis** *pl.* respiratory organs CHP/920; ~ *animal* the animal [L. *animalis*] spirit, the physiological fluid carrying the animating principle of the mind and body Fle/79; ~ *of divyne sapience* the essential principle of divine wisdom or the Holy Spirit Age/633, Bac/471; *fantastic* ~ the physiological fluid that carries the fantastic or image-making faculty DHN/13; *lifly* ~ , ~ *of lif* the animal spirit Age/506, Coi/64, CHP/398, CHP/428, Plag/214; *treatable* ~ the physiological fluid transmitting the sense of touch DHN/77; *visible* ~ , ~ *visible* the physiological fluid that transmits visual images CHP/575, CHP/583, CHP/1031, CHP/1036, etc.

spiritual *adj.* respiratory, pertaining to respiration DHN/98, DHN/133, CHP/857, etc.; (as *n.*) the respiratory system DHN/100, DHN/104, **spirituals** *pl.* CHP/917; ~ error for L. *spinalem* 'spinal' DHN/213n

spiritualy *adv.* with respect to respiration DHN/102; spiritually 7Pla/317

spleen(e) *n.* the spleen DHN/189, SW2/547, **splcne** Fle/113; a disease of the spleen Age/1433

spongious see **spungious**

spreynt see **spreng**

spreng *impv.* sprinkle 8Med/31, **sprenit** *p.ppl.* Age/681, **spreynt** Plag/155

spumous *adj.* frothy Coi/59

spungious *adj.* spongy DHN/65, **spongious** DHN/159

sqwamous *adj.* scaly SW2/115

square *impv.* divide (a circle) in quarters Inst/200

squat *pr.3sg.subj.* squash, crush SW2/1168

stacioun *n.* a position Age/47; a point to or from which measurements are taken Inst/880, Inst/1307n, Inst/1316, etc.

stande *inf.* stand upright CHP/911, **stonde** Bac/191, CHP/816, etc.,

standyng *pr.ppl.* Bac/492, **stonde** *p.ppl.* CHP/900; **standith** *pr.3sg.* is, exists, is located CHP/461, **stant** SW2/1013, **stond** *p.ppl.* Age/291; **standith** *pr.3sg.* consists (in sth.) Age/907, Bac/378, CHP/226, 7LA/188, etc., **stondith** Bac/22, Bac/359; **stonde** *inf.* be left undisturbed SW2/277, SW2/1799, SW2/1849, ~ *pr.3sg.subj.* Age/1301, **stonde** SW2/661; **stond** *p.ppl.* stopped, caused to stop changing Bac/491; **standyng** *pr.ppl.* remaining in place, fixed Inst/91, Inst/98, Inst/947; **stond** *inf.* of finely powdered substances: float (in a sunbeam) Age/2081; ~ *even(e)* be in the prime of life Age/1734, Bac/398, *evene standyng* being in the prime of life Age/1757

standyng *vbl.n.* the act of standing upright 7LA/380; *hath an high* ~ ? is elevated SW2/1176

state *n.* a condition of being, situation Age/15, Bac/63, etc.; the third of four stages of an illness, when the climax is reached CHP/41, CHP/82, etc. [see also **astate**]; ~ *of comune livyng* the usual lifespan Bac/426

stature *n.* height Inst/898, Inst/902; *right* ~ erect posture 7LA/13

steyne *inf.* color, dye Age/1607, **steyneth** *pr.3sg.* Age/1526, **steynen** *pr.3pl.* Age/141, **steyneng** *pr.ppl.* Age/1095

stellifien *pr.3pl.* make star-like Bac/102

stepils *n.pl.* steeples 7LA/438

steppe *inf.* follow the trail of (sth.), investigate Age/29n

steppyng *vbl.n.* pursuit, investigation Age/629n

steppis *n.pl.* traces CHP/990, Plag/15; skin-blemishes Age/1572n

steriometric *adj.* pertaining to solid geometry Inst/921, Inst/923

sterre *n.* a star or planet Bac/186, Inst/159, Inst/496, 7Pla/323, 7LA/304, etc.; ~ *ficched* (*fix*), *ficched* *(fix)* ~ a fixed star, a star whose celestial position remains constant Inst/153, Inst/435, Inst/527, Inst/582, Inst/741, etc.

stiches *n.pl.* sharp pains SW2/852

stide *n.* a place, position SW2/786, SW2/789, Inst/403, Inst/477, **stiede** Inst/985; *in (the)* ~ *of* instead of Age/1256, SW2/369, etc.

stied *pret.1sg.* climbed Age/7

stiewes *n.pl.* bath-houses Plag/97

stil *impv.* distill SW2/1868, **stilled** *p.ppl.* Age/1915, Plag/284, Plag/382

stile *n.* ~ *shewed* ?error for L. *plaustri sterilis* 'of a barren wagon' Age/684n

stillatories *n.pl.* stills, distilling apparatuses SW2/1869

stillen *pr.3pl.* are silent about Age/1275

stynche *n.* a foul odor, stench Coi/283, CHP/1498, SW2/802, SW2/868, **stinche** CHP/1392

stiptik *adj.* astringent Age/1413, CHP/479, 8Med/35, etc., **stiptic** Age/1441, 8Med/8; ?error for L. *constipatus* 'constipated' *Age/1934

stith *n.* an anvil 7LA/283

stok *n.* a tree stump or a block of wood Inst/1122; **stokk** lineage Age/4

stond(e), stondith see **stande**

stone *n.* a piece of rock SW2/1473, Inst/1121, **stones** *pl.* Age/321, Bac/47, etc.; stone as a material 7LA/436; ~ a gemstone Age/341, SW2/478, SW2/1339; the pit of a fruit SW2/242; *the* ~ a kidney stone attack Age/1121, SW2/1823, etc.; **stones** *pl.* the testicles Age/1859, SW2/526, SW2/623, etc.; *gryndyng* ~ a grindstone SW2/1568

stony *adj.* like stone, containing stones Age/1377, Age/1635; ~ *aposteme* the hardened part of an aposteme CHP/1321

stonyeng *vbl.n.*(1) amazement, astonishment Bac/492; vertigo, mental disorientation SW2/89; tingling, numbness Fle/16

stonyeng *vbl.n.*(2) being hit by a stone 8Med/33

stoppe *inf.* block, stop up (bodily organs or secretions) SW2/321, SW2/1324, SW2/1768, **stoppith** *pr.3sg.* Age/588, Age/619, **stoppeth** SW2/1268, **stoppying** *pr.ppl.* Age/597, Age/1547, **stopped** *p.ppl.* Age/360, SW2/152, etc., **istoppid** *p.ppl.* SW2/113; **stop** *inf.* seal, put a stopper in (a container) SW2/443, **stopped** *p.ppl.* 8Med/43; **stopped** *p.ppl.* of a lute-string: pressed down 7LA/279, 7LA/281; (as *n.*) a person suffering a blockage Age/934; *stoppyng the tung* styptic, astringent DHN/69

stoppyng *vbl.n.* a blockage, an obstruction (of bodily organs or secretions) Age/1151, Age/1859, CHP/809, SW2/48, etc.

strayneng see **streyneng**

straite *adj.* constrained CHP/280, CHP/718; taut CHP/437; constricted CHP/569, SW2/1183; narrow, not wide *SW2/1176; *most straitest* *sup.* most ominous, most threatening CHP/850

straitly *adv.* tightly DHN/154

straitnes *n.* constriction CHP/613, CHP/864, Plag/395, **straitenes** DHN/90, CHP/928, **straitissnes** Age/517

strangle *inf.* suffocate Age/203; **stranglith** *pr.3sg.* quenches Age/2076

stranglyng *vbl.n.* suffocation Age/1047, CHP/915

strangurie *n.* strangury, the blockage of urine Fle/165

straw *impv.* sprinkle (a powder) SW2/198, SW2/776, etc. **istrawed** *p.ppl.* strewn SW2/1314

straunge *adj.* extraneous, excess, external (esp. of humours or augmentation of humours) Age/99n, Age/173, etc.; unfamiliar, unknown Bac/141, 7Pla/208, 7Pla/304

straungiers *n.pl.* external things Age/2094; unfamiliar people, strangers 7Pla/217, **straungiors** 7Pla/215

streight *adv.* directly Plag/353

streight(e) *ppl.adj.* stretched, taut CHP/372, CHP/374, CHP/444, CHP/690; straight, not curved CHP/794, Inst/824, Inst/943, 7Pla/309, etc., **strei3t** CHP/796; of planets: moving forward through the zodiac (in contrast to **retrograde**) Inst/598; ~ *cercle* right horizon [see **orizont**] Inst/621; ~ *corner* a right angle Inst/943; ~ *mesuryng* linear measure Inst/924

streyne *impv.* strain, pass through a sieve or cloth SW2/1837, **strayne** SW2/1883; ~ constrain, restrict 8Med/50, **streyneth** *pr.3sg.* Fle/145; **streyned** *p.ppl.* contracted CHP/439, CHP/1203; stretched, extended CHP/1245, 7LA/92, 7LA/262, 7LA/279

streyneng *vbl.n.* constriction of flow (of the bladder) Age/1151; stretching, extending 7LA/89; **strayneng** contraction CHP/1347

streng(g)er *comp.adj.* stronger Age/837, Bac/400, CHP/1143; (as *n.*) the stronger one 7Pla/31; **strengest** *sup.* strongest CHP/1131, SW2/1863

strictories *n.pl.* constricting or styptic medicines SW2/1484

striff *n.* strife, conflict 7LA/176, **strives** *pl.* 7Pla/293

strike *n.* a line, stroke Inst/1134

studiauntis *n.pl.* scholars Bac/625

stue *inf.* bathe in a hot bath or a steam bath SW2/180

stuphe *inf.* cause (sb.) to inhale medicinal vapor SW2/923

stuphe *n.* a herbal decoction for use in a hot-air or steam bath SW2/149, SW2/714, SW2/734, etc.; a hot-air or steam bath SW2/258, SW2/1468, etc.

suasioun *n.* *to the* ~ at the encouragement Age/1652

subfumed *p.ppl.* fumigated from below SW2/677

subfumygacioun *n.* the therapeutic introduction of smoke into the body, usually from below Age/1838, SW2/790, 8Med/4, **svbfumygacioun** 8Med/47

subfumygate *n.* smoke used in subfumigation SW2/683

subiect *ppl.adj.* ~ *to* dominated by, subordinate to Plag/21, **subiett** Bac/10; ~ *of membris* ?determined by the functions of bodily members Age/550

substancial *adj.* derived from the substance of the body Coi/257, CHP/449; of a voice or sound: full, loud 7LA/70

subtil(e) *adj.* thin, refined, not dense Age/1142, CHP/439, CHP/472, 7LA/362, etc.; fine-ground Age/342, SW2/1523; sophisticated, penetrating Age/278, Age/607, etc.; gentle, careful Age/1540, Age/1541; of an instrument: skillfully made Inst/1049; of a line: fine, narrow Inst/945, Inst/953; of wine: light Age/1298, Age/1897; precise, exact Inst/1252, **subtilior** *comp.* Inst/854, **subtiliest** *sup.* Inst/9

subtily *adv.* finely Age/1566, DHN/184, SW2/1134, etc.; carefully, attentively Age/104, Age/665; ingeniously Bac/569; elaborately Age/1370; gently Age/1501; **subtilier** *comp.* more precisely Inst/854

subtilite *n.* thinness SW2/298; ?ingenuity, cleverness 7Pla/49

subtilith *pr.3sg.* thins, makes less dense, dissolves Age/612, Age/932, Age/1915, CHP/91, **subtiled** *p.ppl.* Age/1335, Age/1929

succeden *pr.3pl.* follow after [error for L. *sincerant* 'purify'] Age/111

successivily *adv.* gradually Age/212; **successively** afterward Age/1211

succide *n.* ?unhealthy thinness (of blood) SW2/374n

succuren *pr.3pl.* aid, support Age/900

suerte *n.* confidence, a sense of security Age/51, Age/248, CHP/1087, etc.

sufficience *n.* fulfillment of needs Bac/175

sufficiente *n.* a sufficiency 7Pla/178

suffocacio(u)n *n.* constriction or hindrance of breath CHP/612, CHP/809, CHP/915; ~ *of the matrice* compression of heart and lungs believed to be caused by upward movement of the uterus SW2/52, SW2/510, etc.

suffrable *adj.* able to bear suffering CHP/560

Sinty *n.* Cynthia, the moon 7Pla/241n

sumdel *adv.* somewhat SW2/4, SW2/489, SW2/1561

superfice *n.* a surface Age/1099

superficial *adj.* two-dimensional, pertaining to a surface Inst/925

superflu(e) *adj.* superfluous Age/96, Age/545, Age/1008, DHN/318, etc.

superfluly *adv.* excessively Coi/270

suppose *inf.* expect, anticipate CHP/533, *pr.1sg.* 7LA/548; **supposith** *pr.3sg.* places (sth.) beneath CHP/787; **supposed** *p.ppl.* (being) posited Inst/796

surculis *n.pl.* twigs CHP/995

suscepcioun *n.* the act of taking in, receiving DHN/3

sustentacioun *n.* support, sustenance Age/722, Age/944, Age/1742

swagith *pr.3sg.* assuages Age/1297, Age/2010

swart *adj.* dark SW2/102, SW2/132, etc.

sweete *n.* sweetness (of a harp) 7LA/167

sweete *adj.* sweet Age/1313, Age/1440, DHN/68, etc., **swetter** *comp.* CHP/1142; ~ of milk: fresh Age/1566

swetheles *n.* a swaddling band SW2/757, SW2/759

swolowyng *vbl.n.* that which swallows, the throat DHN/64n

swoune *pr.3sg.subj.* faint SW2/1327

swoun(e) *n.* a faint, swoon SW2/87, SW2/522

swounyng *vbl.n.* fainting SW2/445

table *n.* a list of information laid out in tabular form Age/720, Age/1633, Inst/158, Inst/182, Inst/708, etc., **tabulis** *pl.* Age/722; ~ a plate of metal on an instrument Inst/255, Inst/257, etc.; *in tables* on a table or board Inst/1235n; ~ *of the declynacioun* a table showing the sun's declination from the equinoctial at every degree of the zodiac Inst/1367n; ~ *men* pieces in a board game such as chess, backgammon, or draughts SW2/1299; *a peire tablis* a pair of portable writing tablets hinged or tied together Inst/1058

tablettis *n.pl.* thin metal plates attached to a quadrant Inst/961

tail(e) *n.* the tail of an animal Age/1370, Age/1395; ~ *of the dragon* the point on the ecliptic at which the moon crosses to the south of the ecliptic [L. *cauda draconis*] 7Pla/26; ~ *ende* buttocks SW2/1386

tailours *n.pl.* tailors, clothes-makers 7LA/576

talis *n.pl.* tales, stories Bac/79n

tarie *inf.* delay, retard Age/35, Age/941, Bac/106, etc., **tarieth** *pr.3sg.* Age/926, Age/955, CHP/959, etc., **tarien** *pr.3pl.* Age/120, Age/135, Age/197, etc., **taryeng** *pr.ppl.* Age/1077, Bac/417, etc., **taried** *pret.3sg.* Age/1167, **tarieden** *pret.3pl.* Bac/298, **taried** *p.ppl.* Age/118, Age/121, Bac/107, Plag/332, etc.; **tarieth** *pr.3sg.* remains Fle/68

taryeng *vbl.n.* retardation, delaying DHN/173, Bac/414, CHP/22, **tarieng** Age/1; ~ lingering, resting Age/766, Age/847; *degre of the* ~ the degree in which a celestial object (e.g., the sun) is located Inst/1366

tarre *n.* tar SW2/1757, SW2/1758

tawen *impv.* soften SW2/770

Tauri *n.* the constellation and zodiacal sign Taurus, the Bull 7Pla/121

tauerners *n.pl.* owners of taverns 7LA/570

teatis *n.pl.* the breasts SW2/149, etc.; teat-like or nipple-like parts of the body DHN/227

techyng *vbl.n.* teaching, instruction Bac/210, Plag/305; **techynges** *pl.* ?error for L. *mucos* 'mucus secretions' DHN/198

teene *inf.* harass, annoy SW2/1424

temper *inf.* mitigate, cool, put into balance Plag/283, **temperith** *pr.3sg.* Age/1294, **tempereth** Plag/387, **temperyng** *pr.ppl.* Age/1288, **tempred** *p.ppl.* 7LA/270; **tempre** *inf.* mix SW2/973, ~ *impv.* SW2/371, SW2/689, etc., **tempre** SW2/396, **tempered** *p.ppl.* Age/927, Age/1301, etc., **tempred** Age/1287

temperament *n.* balance Coi/181

temperat(e) *adj.* balanced (esp. between qualities or properties) Age/69, Age/71, Age/927, Coi/70, etc.; moderate Age/1957, Age/1967, 7Pla/324, etc.; of wine: tempered, mixed with water Age/1897

temperatly *adv.* moderately, in moderation Age/1239, Age/1816, etc.

temperaunce *n.* balance, moderation *Age/631, Age/905, Age/943, Bac/345, etc. **tomperaunce** Age/71

tempestuously *adv.* ?profusely, ?mistrans. of L. *tempestive* 'seasonably, on time' Coi/105

tempre, tempred see **temper**

tempre *n.* a balance of humours DHN/116

tenden *pr.3pl.* incline, tend Age/1742, Age/1772

tender *adj.* soft CHP/396; ~ *ribbis* the lower ribs, just above the hypochondrium CHP/1186

tendernes *n.* sensitivity CHP/336; softness CHP/422, **tendirnes** CHP/1185; ~ *of the ribbes* the

cartilaginous parts of the lower ribs CHP/820

tensioun *n.* tightening CHP/1225

tephan see **veyne**

tercian *adj.* of fevers: intermittent, recurring every other day SW2/666, **tercians** (as *n.pl.*) tercian fevers 7Pla/58

term(e) *n.* a set period of time or the end of that period Age/27, Age/1710, Bac/6, etc.; a period in which a planet's influence is heightened Bac/329; a limit or boundary Bac/415, Inst/900, etc.; **termes** *pl.* terminology proper to a discipline Bac/373; terms, words CHP/1187; ~ *of deth* the specific time of death CHP/220, CHP/222; *grete* ~ the conclusion to a phase of a disease CHP/908; ~ *of lif* the span or length of life Bac/40, Bac/108, Bac/382; *prevy termes* menses SW2/958; *termes* error for L. *tinnitus* 'sound' DHN/26; *to the* ~ error for L. *ad ter* 'three times' Age/1981n

termyne *inf.* determine, calculate Inst/1315, **termyned** *p.ppl.* Inst/1199; **termyneth** *pr.3sg.* concludes Inst/1193, **termyned** *p.ppl.* CHP/1452, Inst/1197; **termyneng** *pr.ppl.* marking, indicating Inst/1194, **termyned** *p.ppl.* CHP/266

testicle *n.* a testicle Coi/48, Coi/75, etc., **testicules** DHN/218, Coi/23, etc.; *wymmens testiculis* ovaries DHN/226

testimonial ?*adj.* bearing witness, ?*n.* guarantor, witness 7Pla/32

the *pron.*(1) thee (*2sg.*) CHP/263, CHP/544, Inst/445, 7Pla/52, etc.

the *pron.*(2) a rare form of *thei* 'they' (*3pl.*) DHN/196, Bac/298, Bac/449, ?CHP/49

theatrik *n.* drama as a craft, theatre 7LA/566, *7LA/573; a theatre, a place for performing plays and for sports *7LA/574

thenasmon *n.* an unsatisfiable urge to defecate 8Med/54, 8Med/57

theorik(e) *n.* theoretical knowledge of a subject CHP/224, Inst/916, **theoric** Plag/36, Inst/916

theorike *adj. sermon* ~ the theorctical part of Haly Abbas's *Liber regalis* Age/564

thighes *n.pl.* the thighs SW2/76, SW2/189, Plag/230, Plag/266, **thies** SW2/589, SW2/930, SW2/1230, Plag/345

thigh-hoolis *n.pl.* the junctions of the thighs with the groin Plag/231

thilke *dem.adj.* this, that SW2/1184; *pl.* these, those SW2/1499, Inst/445, Inst/768

thyn(ne) *adj.* of bodily fluids, egg white: thin, not dense DHN/30, DHN/216, Coi/89, SW2/109, etc., **thynner** *comp.* DHN/175, DHN/208, **thynnest** *sup.* DHN/66; ~ of solids: thin, not having great depth SW2/826, SW2/1099, Inst/198; ~ of bodily tissues, vessels, or membranes: thin, fine, narrow: DHN/11, DHN/34, DHN/145, etc., **thynnest** *sup.* DHN/65; ~ (as *n.*) a thin substance produced in the duodenum DHN/158

thynnes(se) *n.* thinness, fineness, softness [L. *tenuitas*] DHN/37, DHN/290, Fle/75, etc.

thomul-too *n.* the big toe Plag/268

thorny see **chambre**

thought *n.* the faculty of reason Age/704, Inst/917; **thoughtis** *pl.* thoughts Age/697; *grete* ~ a state of anxiety, excessive brooding SW2/1265; *hevy thoughtes* sorrowful feelings SW2/232

iij [i.e., **three**] see Materia Medica, s.v. **sandal**

thre(e)d(e) *n.* a thread used for anchoring a suppository or for surgical sewing SW2/189, SW2/772, SW2/1755; a thread used as part of

an instrument Inst/411, Inst/662, Inst/674, etc., **thridde** Inst/645n; *wulle* ~ yarn 7LA/575 [see also **yerde** *n.* (2)]

thrid(de) *adj.* third (sometimes as *n.*) Age/22, Age/920, DHN/31, etc., **third** SW2/1861, 7LA/120, etc., **therde** 7LA/483; ~ *digestioun* the stage of digestion in which nourishment is converted from blood into flesh in the tissues of the body Age/376

thrillyng *pr.ppl.* piercing, penetrating Plag/99

thristen *inf.* push, press SW2/532, **thristeth** *pr.3sg.* SW2/707

thriveth *pr.3sg.* grows Age/311, **thrivith** Age/514

thrivyng *ppl.adj.* ~ *thynges (pinges)* vegetation Age/743, Age/830

throwes *n.pl.* uterine contractions during childbirth SW2/1150; *after* ~ pains or contractions following childbirth SW2/1309

tikelyng *vbl.n.* a tickling or tingling sensation CHP/11, SW2/637

til *prep.* up to Inst/49, Inst/254, 7LA/198, etc.

til *conj.* until, up to the time that Age/1335, Age/1343, CHP/908, SW2/35, etc.; while, as long as Age/43, Age/654, Age/905, etc.

tilied *p.ppl.* cultivated, plowed [?mistrans. of or corrupt in orig. L.] DHN/165n

tilieng *vbl.n.* plowing 7LA/566, 7LA/567

tilier *n.* a farmer, plowman Age/682, 7LA/334; *erth* ~ plowman Age/984, 7Pla/3; *vyne* ~ a cultivator of vines Age/804

tymber *n.* wood Inst/5, 7LA/436, etc.

tyme *n.* a period of time, a point in time, etc. Age/10, Age/12, Age/290, etc.; *to withstonde* ~ the prime of life [L. *tempore consistendi*] Age/40n, ~ *to be withstonde* Age/296, ~ *to (be)*

withstand(e) Age/159, Age/386,
etc., ~ *of withstandyng* Age/164,
Age/388, Age/1645, ~ *of evenstandyng* Age/1648, Bac/387, Bac/410, ~
evene withstandyng Age/741; *mannes*
~ human lives [error for L. *humanis
corporibus*] Age/681

tympanyt *n.* drum-like distension of
the abdomen by gas SW2/1360

timplis *n.pl.* the temples of the head
CHP/395, CHP/431, **tymplis**
Age/412, CHP/956, **timples** Fle/8,
CHP/443, CHP/690, **tymples**
CHP/372

tincturis *n.pl.* dyes Age/1217

tire *n.* a snake whose venom is both
poisonous and curative Bac/555,
Bac/568, **tirus** Bac/547, **tired**
Age/325n

tisik *n.* phthisic, a wasting lung disease
Age/1119, **tissic** Age/2064

***titilacioun** *n.* sensory stimulation, a
tickling sensation DHN/165

tofore *adv.* before, previously Inst/667,
Inst/718, etc.

tofore *prep.* in front of SW2/858,
Inst/212

tokener *n.* an astrological signifier
(i.e., a planet that symbolizes particular people, activities, or things)
7Pla/2

tomperaunce see **temperaunce**

topical *adj.* pertaining to widely-held
but unproven assumptions 7LA/147

tortuosite *n.* contortion CHP/590

totrode *p.ppl.* trodden, packed down
SW2/859

touche *inf.* discuss, deal with Bac/311,
touchith *pr.3sg.* Bac/408, **touched**
pret.3sg. CHP/213, **touched** *p.ppl.*
Bac/247, Bac/504; ~ *inf.* make
physical contact with (sth.), touch
Age/1009, Inst/256, **touchen**
Inst/954, **touchith** *pr.3sg.* Inst/411,
Inst/827, 7LA/234, etc., ~ *pr.2pl.*
Inst/22, *pr.3sg.subj.* 7LA/89,
7LA/94, etc., **touchyng** *pr.ppl.*

Inst/121, **touched** *p.ppl.* SW2/1360,
7LA/253, 7LA/259, **touchid**
7LA/253; *as touchyng* concerning Inst/59, Inst/299; *touched inequal* marked at unequal intervals
Inst/1230; **touches** *pr.3sg.* [Northern] *touches out* extends beyond
Inst/406

touch(e) *n.* physical contact, touch
Age/1238, Bac/457; the act of
touching or feeling CHP/1380,
CHP/1399; *vnder* ~ to the touch
CHP/1379

touchyng *vbl.n.* physical contact,
touch Bac/119, 7LA/88, 7LA/100,
7LA/101, 7LA/261; intersection (of
lines of sight) 7LA/361; a point of
contact Inst/790

towaile *n.* a towel SW2/1428, SW2/1768

tracis *n.pl.* tracks Plag/14

transible *adj.* ~ *vertu* a power that enables light to pass into the eye
DHN/29

transmutaciouns *n.pl.* physical changes 7LA/302

transmute *ppl.adj.* changed, transmuted Age/870

transumpt *ppl.adj.* of a field of learning: adopted, embraced [error for
L. *transmutatoria* 'transmutative, alchemical'] Age/87

transuertid *ppl.adj.* turned upside
down Inst/357

travaile *inf.* work SW2/7, **trauail** *pr.3pl.*
SW2/34; ~ *inf.* move, walk, travel
SW2/163; **travailith** *pr.3sg.* labors,
gives birth (to a child) SW2/1138,
SW2/1175, SW2/1210, **trauailen**
pr.3pl. SW2/781, ~ *pr.3sg.subj.*
SW2/1412

trauaile *n.* work, exertion SW2/1764

travailyng *vbl.n.* labor, childbirth
SW2/1308, SW2/1314, SW2/1744,
trauailyng SW2/1748, **travalyng**
SW2/1272, **traualyng** SW2/57

treble *impv.* triple, multiply by three
7LA/529

tremble *inf.* tremble, quiver SW2/1870, **tremelith** *pr.3sg.* 7LA/265, **tremelen** *pr.3pl.* Age/614, **tremelyng** *pr.ppl.* Age/948

tremelyng *vbl.n.* trembling, quaking, vibration Age/994, Age/1348, Coi/282, 7LA/91, etc., **tremulyng** CHP/1275

trem(o)ure *n.* quaking, quivering CHP/640, CHP/643, CHP/1278

tremuly *adj.* of eyes: twitching, rolling CHP/569

tretable *adj.* accommodating, tractable CHP/327; **treatabil, treatable, treatible** errors for L. *tactabilis* 'tactile, pertaining to the sense of touch' DHN/75, DHN/77, DHN/80

trewe see **tr(i)ew(e)**

triacle *n.* a medicine used against poison or other ailments Bac/548, SW2/595, Plag/140, etc.; ~ *diatesseron* a kind of triacle, originally compounded from four ingredients SW2/193

triangle *n.* a three-sided polygon, triangle 7LA/71, 7LA/73, etc., **triangule** 7LA/423, 7LA/477, etc., **triangulis** *pl.* 7LA/432, 7LA/491, **tryangulis** 7LA/434

triangule *adj.* triangular 7LA/464, 7LA/477, etc.

triduan *adj.* of an illness: lasting three days CHP/48

tr(i)ew(e) *adj.* true, accurate, exact, veracious, trustworthy, etc. Age/455, Age/808, etc.; of diseases: properly so called (in contrast with *nat triewe*) CHP/1045, SW2/1357, etc.; (?*as adv.*) truly, indeed [L. *vero* 'indeed'] Bac/523

triplicite *n.* a set of three astrological signs associated with the same element and each 120° from the others Bac/329

tristy see **trusty**

trosciscy a medicated lozenge, a troche SW2/1295n, **trociscy**

SW2/1376, **trocisces** *pl.* Age/1388, SW2/1401, etc., **trocissis** SW2/686, **trocisses** SW2/1110, **troscisses** SW2/1106, **trosikes** SW2/278, *trocisci* (L.) SW2/1601

troden *p.ppl.* ?squeezed, crushed [?trans. L. *constringitur* 'it is bound, constricted'] DHN/109

tropik *adj.* metaphorical, as a turn of speech [L. *tropice* 'figuratively, by means of a trope'] CHP/1093, CHP/1101

trouble *n.* disturbance, agitation Age/611

trouble *adj.* of urine: turbid, murky CHP/93

troubled *ppl.adj.* of air, weather: murky, stormy Age/606, Age/612, Plag/108, **troublid** Age/609, Age/610; of persons: disturbed, agitated 7Pla/125; ~ harmed Age/1459

troubly *adj.* of urine: turbid, murky SW2/1014

trowe *inf.* believe CHP/1011, *pr.1sg.* Bac/76, CHP/666, **trowest** *pr.2sg.* CHP/8, **trowith** *pr.3sg.* Age/700, CHP/270, etc., **trowen** *pr.3pl.* Coi/226, **trowid** *pret.3sg.* CHP/166, **trowiden** *pret.3pl.* Bac/445, **trowed** *p.ppl.* Age/701, Bac/324, 7Pla/245

trussyng *vbl.n.* building with trusses, supporting with trusses 7LA/438, 7LA/441, 7LA/443

trust *inf.* have confidence in (sb.) CHP/214, 7Pla/117, 7Pla/153, **trustith** *pr.3sg.* CHP/161, 7Pla/198, ~ *pr.2sg.subj.* 7Pla/134, **trusted** *p.ppl.* CHP/120; ~ *inf.* entrust CHP/121; *impv.* believe Inst/1102

trust *n.* reliance CHP/28; *his* ~ ?by his trust Age/1532n; *in verray* ~ ?absolutely steadfast or reliable Bac/338n [see also **trusty**]

trusty *adj.* firm, strong Age/1976; **trusti** ?steadfast, true Bac/473n, **tristy** Bac/535n

trustily *adv.* confidently 7Pla/109

tuicioun *n.* protection CHP/972

tumorie *n.* a tumor, swelling Age/2069

tumour *n.* swelling or an instance thereof, a tumor Fle/54, CHP/1280, etc.

tumous *adj.* of lips: swelling, full 7Pla/267

tvne *n.* a musical note or sound 7LA/276, *pl.* **tunys** 7LA/273, **tunes** 7LA/274

tunicle *n.* one of several membranes of the eye DHN/28, DHN/36, **tunycles** *pl.* DHN/32, DHN/41, DHN/49; *horny* **tunycle** cornea CHP/1008

tunsil(i)s *n.pl.* the tonsils DHN/88, DHN/92

turne *inf.* move (from or toward sth., sth. from or toward sth. else) Age/492, **torne** CHP/788, CHP/791, ~ *impv.* Inst/663, etc., **turn** Inst/454, **tornyth** *pr.3sg.* CHP/779, ~ *pr.3sg. subj.* CHP/176, *pr.1pl.* Coi/293, **turnyng** *pr.ppl.* CHP/836, **turned** *pret.1sg.* Inst/1083, **torned** Inst/1065, **turned** *p.ppl.* SW2/1182, SW2/1191; **tourne** *inf.* convert, change Age/875, **torne** Age/320, CHP/1443, **turnyth** *pr.3sg.* Age/422, Age/1241, etc., **tornyth** Age/438, CHP/1308, CHP/1396, **torneth** Age/431, CHP/1304, **turneth** CHP/1383, **tournyth** Age/440, **tournen** *pr.3pl.* Age/420, **turn** CHP/1389, **turned** *p.ppl.* Age/1343, DHN/150, etc., **torned** Age/375, DHN/174, etc., **tourned** CHP/19, CHP/1391, **turnd** CHP/965; ~ *impv.* rotate or bend (sth.) around a point Inst/86, Inst/104, etc., **turnyng** *pr.ppl.* Inst/141, **turned** *p.ppl.* CHP/373, Inst/10, etc., **torned** CHP/401, CHP/405, etc.; ~ *impv.* reverse 7Pla/47, 7Pla/77, **tournyth** *pr.3sg.* SW2/90, **turned** *p.ppl.* Inst/1288, 7LA/75; ~ *pr.3pl.* return 7LA/257; ~ *a square (circle) in a circle (square)* construct a square having the same area as a circle or vice versa 7LA/601, 7LA/603

turne *n.* a frame for turning wood Inst/20

turnyng *vbl.n.* change CHP/524, 7Pla/30; rotation Inst/14, Inst/17; **tornyng** inversion, twisting CHP/726

twies *adv.* twice Age/1872, SW2/722, etc., **twyes** Age/822

vlk *n.* a sore CHP/963, CHP/966

vmbre *n.* a shadow Inst/510; a side of the shadow square or shadow scales marked on a quadrant, used for calculating heights and distances Inst/829, Inst/1221, **vmbra** (L.) Inst/821, Inst/824; *vmbra recta* (L.) the horizontal side of the shadow square or the units marked thereon Inst/807n, Inst/815, etc.; *vmbra versa* (L.) the perpendicular side of the shadow square or the units marked thereon Inst/807n, Inst/819, etc. [cf. *MED*, s.v. ombre n., 3]

umoris, umours see **humour**

vncciouns *n.* anointings, oil-rubs Age/448, Age/1472

vnce *n.* an ounce Fle/129, SW2/1836, SW2/1857, Plag/123, **vncis** SW2/1511, SW2/1838 [usually abbreviated ℥]

vncoct *ppl.adj.* raw, uncooked Coi/62

vncomodious *adj.* troublesome Age/1693

vncomoditees *n.pl.* troublesome things Age/1732

vncon *n.* ?error for L. *non convenit* Fle/48

vnconuenient *adj.* unsuitable CHP/232

vnctuous *adj.* oily, greasy CHP/477

vndefied *ppl.adj.* not assimilated, not converted SW2/299

vndefouled *ppl.adj.* of earth: pure, good Age/828n

vnder- see also **vndir-**

vnder-citryne *adj.* yellowish CHP/96

vnderdrawith *pr.3sg.* draws away DHN/160, **vndirdrawen** *pr.3pl.* DHN/172

vnderfonge *inf.* apply (a medication) SW2/981, **vnderfange** *pr.3sg.subj.* SW2/209; **vnderfong** *p.ppl.* received SW2/8

vndergon *pr.3pl.* succumb to, suffer Age/1748, Age/1762

vnderjoyneth *pr.3sg.* appends CHP/1234

vnderlifted *ppl.adj.* supported DHN/141

vnder-rede *adj.* reddish Age/1399, CHP/991, 7Pla/319

vndir- see also **vnder-**

vndir-blac *adj.* blackish Age/1153

vndircome *pr.1pl.* ~ *to* support, assist Fle/91

vndirlith *pr.3sg.* is subject (to sth.) Age/879, Age/960, **vnderlith** Age/973, **wndirlith** Age/954, **vndirlyn** *pr.3pl.* Age/875, Age/972, **vnderlyne** Age/967; **vnderlith** *pr.3sg.* yields to (sth.), feels soft under CHP/1380, **vndirlye** *pr.3sg.subj.* CHP/1380

vndirput *inf.* suppose, take as an example CHP/501, *p.ppl.* CHP/503 [both instances trans. L. *supposita* 'supposed, assumed, hypothesized']; **vnderputtith** *pr.3sg.* rests upon, is placed upon DHN/17, DHN/139; ~ *p.ppl.* placed beneath DHN/100; **vnderput** *impv.* insert (a medicine), apply (a medicine to the lower part of the body) SW2/677, *pr.1pl.* 8Med/55, *p.ppl.* SW2/664, SW2/868

vndirstande *inf.* understand, comprehend 7LA/452, **vndirstonde** CHP/488, Plag/339, etc., **vnderstande** 7LA/495, **vnderstonde** SW2/25, 7LA/445, 7LA/559, **vndrestande** 7LA/536, ~ *impv.* Age/69, Age/1246, CHP/294, etc., **vndirstonde** CHP/276, **vnderstande** SW2/499, **vnderstonde** *pr.1sg.* CHP/64, SW2/977, **vndirstondith** *pr.3sg.* Age/887, CHP/85, CHP/1056, **vndirstandith** Age/1926,

Bac/264, **vndirstonden** *pr.3pl.* Age/235, **vndirstondyng** *pr.ppl.* 7LA/60, **vndirstode** *pret.3sg.* 7LA/15, 7LA/282, **vndirstonde** *p.ppl.* Age/84, CHP/101, **vndirstande** Bac/26, **vndirstanden** 7LA/126; **vndirstonde** *inf.* subsist, survive DHN/296n; **vnderstondith** *pr.3sg.* conceives SW2/1351; *this (it) is to ~ (vndirstonde)* this means Age/1060, Age/1085, CHP/469, etc.

vndirstandyng *vbl.n.* intelligence, reason, understanding Age/454, Age/625, etc., **vndirstondyng** Age/682, Bac/176, etc., **vndirstondinge** DHN/86, **vnderstandyng** Bac/569, 7LA/17; *derk* ~ secret meaning Age/21

vneven(e) *adj.* unfair, wicked [L. *iniquo*] Age/14; irregular 7Pla/319; **vnevyn** of complexion: unbalanced Bac/147

vnyformaly *adv.* in the same way 7LA/237

vnyte *n.* a numerical unit, the number one 7LA/194, 7LA/229, etc., **vnite** Inst/895, **vnitees** *pl.* 7LA/194, 7LA/222, etc.

vniuersite *n.* entirety 7Pla/96; **vniuersites** *pl.* universities Plag/314

vnkynd(e) *adj.* unnatural DHN/109; harsh, unkind 7Pla/124, 7Pla/179; ~ *he(e)te* excessive heat in the body SW2/543, Plag/219

vnkynd(e)ly *adj.* unnatural, against the natural course of events Age/172, SW2/1149, etc.

vnlawfully *adv.* wrongfully CHP/566 [error for L. *involuntarie* 'unwillingly, involuntarily'; see also **vnvoluntarily, vnwilfully**]

vnlikly *adj. among hemsilf* ~ dissimilar to each other CHP/1183

vnmedled *ppl.adj.* unmixed, consisting of a single element Plag/12

vnparfite *adj.* imperfect, incomplete Age/19, DHN/294, etc.

vnpower *n.* powerlessness Bac/403
vnresonable *adj.* of animals: without
    reason Age/1243, Bac/51, etc., **vn-**
    resonabil Bac/171
vnsufficiently *adv.* inadequately Bac/377
vntyme *n.* the wrong time, an unsea-
    sonable time SW2/50, SW2/294
vnvoluntarily *adv.* involuntarily CHP/636
vnwarely *adv.* carelessly 7Pla/274
vnwerily *adv.* tirelessly 7Pla/349
vnwilfully *adv.* involuntarily CHP/585,
    CHP/672
vnwitty *adj.* foolish, naïve 7Pla/194
vpon-set *ppl.adj.* placed, positioned
    DHN/114
vpper *comp.adj.* higher, top DHN/59,
    DHN/134, etc.; (as *n.*) the upper
    part (of a shadow scale) Inst/1219;
    ~ *browes* the eyebrows [L. *supercilia*]
    DHN/254
vpright *adj.* supine, flat on the back
    CHP/803, CHP/804, etc.; upright,
    perpendicular to a flat surface
    Inst/825, Inst/1123, Inst/1124
vptaken *ppl.adj.* of a field of learning:
    adopted, embraced Age/87 [cf.
    transumpt]
vryne *n.* urine Age/767, Age/1122,
    etc.; ~ *wey* the path of the urine, uri-
    nary vessels Coi/50
vrynous *adj.* like urine CHP/100
vse *n.* use, consumption Age/75,
    Age/190, etc., **wse** Age/1858; ~ *and*
    nature human activity and the nat-
    ural world 7LA/336; *natures* ~ na-
    ture's activity 7LA/303
vtilite *n.* value, usefulness Age/1763,
    Bac/480, CHP/20, CHP/25, 7Pla/20
vtter *comp.adj.* outer CHP/381,
    CHP/463, **vtterest** *sup.* outer-
    most CHP/1485; ~ *circumference* the
    length of the outer edge of a metal
    ring Inst/228, Inst/278; *to the vtter-*
    est to the extreme, as much as possi-
    ble Age/916
vttermest *adj.* outermost, furthest
    Bac/6, Inst/316

vttirly *adv.* entirely, completely Age/33,
    Age/56, etc., **vtterly** DHN/80

vagabunde *adj.* wandering 7Pla/273
vailable *adj.* useful, effective Age/724
vailith *pr.3sg.* avails, is effective
    Age/1163
vayne see **veyne** *n.*(1), *n.*(2), *adj.*
vapour *n.* water vapor Age/488,
    Age/608; a gaseous or gas-like
    substance produced and trans-
    ported within the body CHP/623,
    CHP/1004, etc.; **vapours** *pl.* fumes
    Age/284, Age/597, etc.; gaseous
    substances in the atmosphere
    Plag/13
vapourith *pr.3sg.* evaporates Coi/65
variaunce *n.* variety Plag/31
variole *n.* a pustule or a disease caus-
    ing pustules Fle/151, Fle/157
veer *n.* the season of spring Age/1372,
    Age/1483, Fle/72, etc., **ver**
    Age/1171, Age/1175
vegetacioun *n.* growth, growing Plag/8
veyne *n.*(1) a blood vessel Age/229,
    CHP/1334, SW2/302, etc., **vayne**
    SW2/147, SW2/735, etc., **vein-**
    is *pl.* DHN/227, *weynes 7Pla/56,
    7Pla/59; *basilic* ~ the basilic vein in
    the arm Age/1984; *body* ~ the medi-
    an cubital vein in the arm Plag/278;
    cephalic ~ , *hed(e)* ~ the cephalic
    vein in the arm Fle/52, Plag/277,
    Plag/278, Plag/375; *herte(s)* ~ the
    cardiac vein, the median cubital
    vein in the arm Plag/258, Plag/358;
    myddil ~ the median cubital vein
    in the arm Plag/375; *miserac (my-*
    serac) veynes blood vessels from the
    intestines to the liver DHN/159,
    DHN/171; *puls* ~ , *grete* ~ *pulsatief*
    a pulmonary vein CHP/1244,
    CHP/1247; ~ *tephan* the cephalic
    vein in the arm [error for L. *cephali-*
    cam venam] Age/1983
veyne *n.*(2) *in* ~ *(vayne)* without effect,
    futile(ly) Bac/455n, 7Pla/32

veyne *adj.* idle, empty Bac/444n, **vayne** 7Pla/328

velocite *n.* rapidity Age/1190

venemousite *n.* poisonousness, virulence Age/1419

venery *n.* the craft of hunting 7LA/566, 7LA/568

venyal *adj.* of sin: venial, lesser 7LA/27

venymeth *pr.3sg.* poisons, infects Plag/264, **venymed** *p.ppl.* Plag/261, Plag/264, Plag/302

ventosite *n.* gassiness or gaseous build-up within the body Age/1070, Age/1142, etc.

ventre *n.* a region of the brain Age/561, Age/570

ventriculis *n.pl.* regions of the brain Age/579, Age/662, etc., **ventricules** Age/588

ventuses *n.pl.* windy things Age/710n

ventusyng *pr.ppl.* drawing blood by means of cupping glasses SW2/804, **ventused** *p.ppl.* Plag/274, Plag/281

ventusyng *vbl.n.* the drawing of blood by cupping glasses SW2/786

Venus *n.* the planet Venus DHN/281, Inst/1047, 7Pla/239, etc., **Uenus** 7Pla/83, 7Pla/323; ~ *werkis* sexual activity Age/1006, Coi/104; *love of* ~ error for L. *more utris* [varr. *ventris, veneris*] Coi/37n

veray *adj.* true Age/484, 7Pla/133, 7LA/8, etc., **verray** 7LA/1, **ueray** Fle/2; ~ precise, exact Inst/1099; *in verray trust profite* trans. of L. *ineffabilis utilitas* 'inexpressible utility' Bac/338n; *nat* ~ of diseases: not properly so called [see also **tr(i)ew(e)**] SW2/1362

veray *adv.* very, completely 7Pla/154; ~ *triew(e)* absolutely true, most reliable Age/808, Age/2002, Bac/627; ~ *tristy* trans. of L. *ineffabilis* 'inexpressible' Bac/535n

vermicle *adj.* of blood containing an abundance of phlegm: vermilion-colored Fle/115 [see Latham 1980,

s.v. *vermiculus* subst. and adj. 'vermilion']

versa (L.) *adj.* perpendicular: see **scala, vmbre**; pertaining to versine mathematical functions: see **cord(e)**; *ark* ~ see **ark(e)**

verse *adj.* *corde* ~ see **cord(e)**

vertu(e) *n.* power, force Age/76, Age/147, Age/1391, CHP/296, etc.; a physiological power or faculty: ~ *appetief* the faculty of appetite or desiring food Age/546; ~ *digesti(e)f* the digestive faculty Age/220, Age/362, Age/546, CHP/302; ~ *expulsief* the excretory faculty CHP/1453, SW2/1111; ~ *odorible, smellyng* ~ the sense of smell DHN/47, DHN/51; *transible* ~ a power that enables light to pass into the eye DHN/29; *treatabil (treatible)* ~ the sense of touch DHN/75, DHN/80; ~ *visible* the sense of sight Age/1429; a power of the mind or soul: *natural* ~ , ~ *natural* the power that controls the senses Age/1622, DHN/174, CHP/768, etc.; *qwikly (quekly, lifly, lively)* ~ the animal virtue, the power that controls movement and perception [L. *virtus animalis*] Age/68, Age/145, Age/560, CHP/775, CHP/1131, etc.; ~ *vital* the power that animates the body, the vital force CHP/408; *mo(e)vyng (moevable)* ~ a physiological or mental power controlling movement CHP/884, CHP/948, Coi/136

vertuous *adj.* strong, powerful Age/358, Bac/181, Bac/279

vessel(l) *n.* a container Age/986, Age/1214, Inst/1258, etc.; **vessels** *pl.* blood vessels and other anatomical passageways DHN/257, DHN/309; ~ *roddis* measuring sticks for vats Inst/1408

*uicinite *adj.* nearby DHN/85n

vicious *adj.* improper, invalid Coi/86, Coi/88

viij notis see **notis**

vilidite *n.* ?error for L. *vtilite* or *virilite* Coi/138n

vyne *n.* a grapevine [L. *vinea*] Age/759, Age/806, Age/845, etc.; prob. error for L. *vinum* 'wine' Age/846n, Age/858; ~ *tilier* see **tilier**

vynous *adj.* of wine: strong, heady Age/850, Age/852

viole *n.* a container, flask 8Med/43 [see also **phiole**]

violence *n.* force, power Age/2022, Bac/107, etc.

violent *adj.* extreme, severe CHP/858, SW2/984, SW2/1011

vipera (L.) *n.* a venomous snake, viper (in the title of a chapter in Avicenna's *Canon*) Age/1366

viscous *adj.* thick, sticky Age/1032, Coi/213, *SW2/1110, etc.

visible *adj.* pertaining to vision Age/576; able to be seen DHN/40; ~ *qualite (spirite, spirites), spirites* ~ the substance that carries the faculty of vision DHN/33, DHN/38, CHP/575, CHP/583, CHP/1031, etc.; *vertu* ~ the sense of sight Age/1429

visory *adj.* *yerd* ~ a measuring rod Inst/1224

voidaunces *n.pl.* bodily excretions SW2/1747, SW2/1769

voide *inf.* let blood Fle/125

voide *adj.* of a vein: empty, having little or insufficient blood Fle/39, Fle/124; lacking, not full Coi/182, etc.; ?empty of natural humidity Age/484

voidenes *n.* emptiness [?misreading of L. *mania*, read as *inania*] CHP/642 [see also **idelnes**]

voidyng *vbl.n.* purgation or an instance thereof Age/97, Age/871, CHP/545

voidith *pr.3sg.* evacuates, removes, empties Coi/217, Coi/267, Coi/268, **voiden** *pr.3pl.* Age/139, Age/1133, Age/1608, **voided** *p.ppl.* Age/876, Bac/314, CHP/429, Plag/357

volubil *n.* the length of the **voluel** (q.v.) on a measuring rod, treated as a unit to be marked off along the length of the rod Inst/1300n

voluel *n.* a moving pointer on a quadrant Inst/388; the rete on an astrolabe Inst/431; a moving cross-piece on a measuring rod Inst/1297n, Inst/1315, etc. [see Headnote to chap. 13, 618]

voluyng *pr.ppl.* turning Inst/107

vomyte *inf.* regurgitate Age/934

vomyte *n.* regurgitation or an instance thereof Age/97, Age/1051, CHP/608, etc., **vomite** Age/1049; **vomytis** *pl.* emetics SW2/1142; ~ ?error for L. *sonitum* 'sound, noise' Age/1371n

vulua *n.* the vagina SW2/1776, SW2/1784, *vulue* (L.) *gen.* SW2/1756, *vuluam* *acc.* SW2/1590, SW2/1594

wacche *n.* waking, being awake, lack of sleep Age/285, Bac/23, CHP/454, SW2/1276, etc.

waite *impv.* watch, notice Inst/1377; ~ *aboute* wait until Inst/1126; **waityng** *on* waiting for Inst/1129

wakyng *vbl.n.* wakefulness, the state of being awake SW2/67, SW2/230, SW2/631, 7Pla/273; **wakynges** *pl.* periods of being awake Age/692, Age/712

walk(e) *inf.* walk, move on one's feet Age/1968, Bac/68, SW2/163; **walkith** *pr.3sg.* moves SW2/901, SW2/1095

wanyng *pr.ppl.* ~ *the moone* when the moon is waning Age/1174

wannes *n.* paleness CHP/732, CHP/733, CHP/734

wannyssh *adj.* pale SW2/79

want *inf.* be lacking Inst/1350n; **wantith** *pr.3sg.* requires Inst/1374; ~ *pr.3pl.* desire Fle/130

ware *adj.* wary, careful 7Pla/133, 7Pla/286; *be (bien)* ~ *of* avoid (sth.) [L. *vitare* 'avoid'] Age/283,

Age/525, Age/1023, etc.; *be (bien)*
~ *of* beware (sth.) [L. *cavere* 'beware (sth.)'] Age/1389, Age/1863,
CHP/539, etc.

wasshynges *n.pl.* ~ *of flessh* water in
which meat has been washed or
soaked Fle/50

wast *inf.* destroy, consume SW2/630,
SW2/679, **wastith** *pr.3sg.* SW2/630,
wasten *pr.3pl.* Age/92, **wasted** *p.ppl.*
CHP/397, CHP/813, etc.

wast *n.* depletion, consumption
DHN/239, CHP/378; destruction
DHN/318

watred *p.ppl.* of bodily vessels: irrigated,
provided with water DHN/227

watrynes *n.* excess moisture SW2/388

webly *adv.* like a web DHN/147

we(e)ke *n.* a wick, piece of wicking
SW2/364, SW2/570, **wike** SW2/618

weery *inf.* cause to become weary
Age/369; **weerieth** *pr.3sg.* becomes
weary Age/357, **werieth** Age/467,
weried *p.ppl.* Age/366

wegge *n.* wedge Inst/267

wey *n.* way, path Age/118, Age/216,
etc., **weis** *pl.* Bac/600; *weyes of the
matrice* the passageways of the uterus, the vagina SW2/259 [cf. *MED,*
s.v. *wei* n.(1), 1a.(e)]; ~ *of the sonne* the
sun's path through the sky Inst/586

weyeth *pr.3sg.* weighs, has weight
Age/922, **weieng** *pr.ppl.* SW2/1300,
weyed *pret.3sg.* 7LA/290

weik(e) *adj.* thin [L. *tenuis* 'thin,
weak'] DHN/11, DHN/18, etc.,
weiker *comp.* DHN/175, DHN/208;
~ weak Bac/47; lukewarm CHP/849,
CHP/851

weikenes *n.* thinness DHN/290,
CHP/383, CHP/1224; weakness,
susceptibility 7Pla/7

weikith *pr.3sg.* weakens Age/1158,
DHN/310, **weikyng** *pr.ppl.* DHN/288,
weiked *p.ppl.* Age/483, CHP/397,
CHP/1221

*****weynes** see **veyne**

weis see **wey**

wel(e) chewed see **chewed**

welfare *n.* well-being Age/1714n

welke *inf.* wither 7LA/309

wende *inf.* go, enter SW2/1371, **went**
pret.3sg. Bac/483

wesaunt *n.* the esophagus DHN/94

wested *pret.3pl.* of stars: were in the
west, moved west, set Bac/220

westyng *vbl.n.* the setting (of stars),
moving to the west Bac/182

wete *inf.* wet, soak in a fluid SW2/364,
impv. SW2/618, SW2/737,
SW2/1554, *pr.3sg.sbj* SW2/635, **wet**
p.ppl. SW2/570, 8Med/29

wex *inf.* grow, become CHP/909,
SW2/1030, **wexith** *pr.3sg.* SW2/768,
SW2/1350, SW2/1749, **wexeth**
CHP/904, SW2/1366, **wexen** *pr.3pl.*
CHP/606, SW2/79, ~ *pr.3sg.subj.*
SW2/1752, **woxen** *p.ppl.* SW2/1045,
SW2/1260, **waxen** SW2/1030

wex *n.* wax SW2/437, SW2/719, etc.;
rede ~ red sealing wax SW2/1056

wexed *pret.1sg.* covered with wax
Inst/1057

what *pron. any* ~ anything Coi/27n

whicc *rel.pron.* which [poss. a spelling
error] Age/2043

whiten *pr.3pl.* become white Age/411,
Age/420, Age/425

wield(e) *adj.* wild Age/922; of plants:
growing in the wild SW2/761,
SW2/942, etc.; ~ *fuyres* erysipelas, an
inflammatory skin disease SW2/1526

wike *n.* a week, seven days Age/1941,
SW2/167, Plag/113, etc.

wike see **we(e)ke**

wikked *adj.* harmful, evil CHP/625,
CHP/630, CHP/701; diseased, un-
healthy Plag/216, **wiked** CHP/599,
SW2/1348

wil *pr.3sg.* wants, wishes, wills Coi/164,
Bac/286, etc., **willith** DHN/14,
wilt *pr.2sg.* Age/1928, Age/2035,
etc., **wiln** *pr.1pl.* Bac/101, Bac/231,
Bac/278, **wiln** *pr.3pl.* CHP/163,
~ *pr.2pl.subj.* Inst/25, Inst/253,
etc., **willyng** *pr.ppl.* Coi/3, Coi/32,

Bac/511, **willed** *p.ppl.*. Bac/373; ~ means, intends, says [L. *vult*] Bac/432, CHP/339, etc., **willith** Bac/130, **wiln** *pr.3pl.* Age/869; as modal auxiliary expressing futurity, intention, etc.: ~ *pr.1sg.* SW2/16, Inst/641, *pr.3sg.* Age/703, Bac/345, SW2/39, etc., *pr.1pl.* SW2/1536, Inst/1379, *pr.2pl.* Inst/3, *pr.3pl.* SW2/93, SW2/910, **wiln** *pr.3pl.* SW2/95, SW2/224, Plag/380, etc., **wold** *pret.3sg.* SW2/207, SW2/220, SW2/1794, Plag/262, **wold** *pret.3pl.* 7Pla/107; ~ *they nil they* whether they want to or not SW2/1773

wilfully *adv.* willingly 7Pla/336

wil(le) *n.* will, intent, desire Age/343, Coi/260, Bac/268, etc.; *goode* ~ benevolence 7Pla/129, 7Pla/332; *bi his goode **will*** of his own accord 7Pla/277; *to* ~ as one wishes, at one's command Coi/42

willed *adj. evil* ~ malevolent, of evil influence 7Pla/244, 7Pla/339; *wele* ~ benevolent, of favorable influence 7Pla/243

wynd(e) *n.* wind Age/284, Age/412, etc.; gas, flatulence CHP/898, SW2/125, etc.; breath SW2/1002

wynden ?*n.pl.* ?fibers Plag/97n [cf. *MED*, s.v. *wrapping(e* ger., (d)]

wyndy *adj.* windy Age/836; characterized by or causing gas in the body CHP/1242, SW2/861

wyndynesse *n.* gassiness in the body or in parts thereof, distention as if by wind SW2/909, **wyndenes** SW2/1359

wyng *n.* ~ *of the lunges* a lobe of the lungs DHN/112

wipe *impv.* wipe or rub (sth.) in order to cleanse or soften it SW2/203, SW2/1752, **wipen** *pr.3pl.* Age/1016; **wipith** *pr.3sg.* wipes, rubs Age/1500, **wipen** *pr.3pl.* Age/1541; **wipith** *pr.3sg.* cleanses Age/1120

wipyng *vbl.n.* cleansing by rubbing Age/1017, Age/1501, Age/1540, Age/1541

wissh(e) *pret.3sg.* washed Bac/502, SW2/962

wit *n.* intelligence, reason Age/44, Age/76, etc.; *idilnes of* ~ madness [L. *mania*] CHP/1269 [see CHP/640n]

wite *inf.* know Inst/435, Inst/570, Inst/651, etc., **witen** SW2/537, SW2/1796, ~ *impv.* Age/79, Age/726, CHP/1250, Inst/474, etc., **wist** *p.ppl.* Bac/9, SW2/1795, Plag/195, etc.; *it is (for) to* ~ it is to be understood Coi/145, CHP/710, etc.; *that is to* ~ namely, that is to say Plag/176, Inst/1348

withdrawe *inf.* slow, retard Age/35, Age/1775, **withdrawen** *pr.3pl.* Age/197, **withdrawen** *p.ppl.* Age/118; ~ *inf.* draw away Age/1064, SW2/329, SW2/1757; ~ *inf.* contract CHP/729, **withdrawen** *p.ppl.* CHP/405, CHP/430, etc.; ~ *impv.* move away from Inst/1304, Inst/1308, Inst/1309, **withdrawith** *pr.3sg.* Age/852, ~ *pr.3sg.subj.* CHP/830, **withdriew** *pret.3pl.* Bac/292, **withdrawen** *p.ppl.* Bac/331; ~ *impv.* take away, subtract Age/2034, Age/2037, Inst/433, etc., **withdraw** Inst/768, Inst/774, Inst/1335, **withdrawith** *pr.3sg.* Age/1069, DHN/171, **withdrawen** *pr.3pl.* Age/2027

withdraught *n.* withdrawal Bac/332

withynfurth *adv.* within, on the inside Age/65, Age/240, etc., **withynfurþ** DHN/60, DHN/197, SW2/664, **withynnefurth** CHP/335, CHP/854, **withinfurth** Age/345, Age/450, etc., **wiþinfurth** CHP/1473, SW2/968; ~ of a passage in a text: below Age/67, Age/191, **withinfurth** Age/493 [both senses usually trans. L. *interius* or *inferius*]

witholde *inf.* retain, keep, hold SW2/301, *impv.* 7Pla/289, **witholdith** *pr.3sg.* Age/927, SW2/1268, **with(h)olden** *pr.3pl.* Age/286, Age/904, SW2/531, **witholde** *pr.3pl.* Age/1597, **withold** *pr.3sg.*

subj. Age/1493, **witholdyng** *pr.ppl.*
DHN/211, **withold** *p.ppl.* DHN/116,
witholden SW2/1352
witholdyng *vbl.n.* retention (of bodily
tissues or fluids) SW2/60, SW2/91,
etc., **withholdyng** SW2/97
withoutfurth *adv.* outside, on the outside [usually trans. L. *exterius*]
Age/64, Age/447, etc., **withoutfurþ** Age/66, CHP/382, CHP/577,
CHP/654, **withoutforth** CHP/576,
withoutforþ Age/455, **wiþoutfurth
Age/470
withstande *inf.* stand firm, resist
Age/47 [and see Age/40n],
Age/213, Bac/467, CHP/251, etc.,
withstonde Age/40n, CHP/326,
withstandith *pr.3sg.* Age/43,
Age/1745, Coi/268, CHP/687,
withstode *pret.3sg.* Age/1728,
withstand(e) *p.ppl.* Age/160,
Age/162, **withstonde** Age/297
withstandyng *vbl.n.* standing firm
Age/164, Age/388, etc. [see also
Age/40n]
witty *adj.* wise Age/303
wndirlith see **vndirlith**
womb(e) *n.* the abdomen Age/871,
Age/1438, Age/1908, Fle/69,
Bac/455, etc.; the uterus Age/582,
Coi/23, SW2/36, etc.; a ventricle
or region of the brain Age/561,
Age/570, Age/662; *solucioun (flux)
of (the)* ~ purging of the intestines, excretion, diarrhea Age/205,
CHP/348, etc.; ~ *of chieldhod* ?error
for L. *inicio pubertatis* Coi/119n
woneth *pr.3sg.* is customary DHN/315,
CHP/1336, **wonyth** DHN/300;
wont *p.ppl.* accustomed Age/21,
DHN/319, Coi/273, Inst/277, etc.
wont *n.* habit, custom CHP/852
wontly *adv.* habitually, customarily
Coi/180
woode *n.* a forest, woods Age/924,
Age/1490; the substance wood
Age/1490

woode *adj.* mad, insane Coi/246,
Coi/275, CHP/685, 7Pla/188
woodenes *n.* madness Age/645,
DHN/203, Coi/243, etc.
woodith *pr.3.sg.* becomes insane
DHN/205
word(e) *n.*(1) a word, an utterance,
a statement Age/26, Age/29,
Coi/250, Plag/91, 7Pla/123, etc.;
~ *absolute, absolute* ~ strictly speak-
ing, in absolute terms CHP/1101,
CHP/1112; *from* ~ *to* ~ verbatim
Bac/283; ~ *hid* cryptic language
Age/308, Age/314
word(e) *n.*(2) see **world**
wordy *adj.* talkative, voluble 7Pla/186
wore see **be**
world *n.* world Age/4, Age/155, etc.,
word(e) 7LA/56, 7LA/185; *the
lasse* ~ the microcosm, a human being as the microcosm reflecting
the macrocosm Age/37, Age/1363,
7Pla/250
wormes *n.pl.* worm-like shapes
DHN/248, DHN/275; insect lar-
vae or other worm-like creatures
breeding in stored urine SW2/1801,
SW2/1803; worms or caterpillars
that destroy trees 7Pla/14
worship *n.* high esteem, respect, wor-
thiness 7Pla/119, 7LA/15
worte *n.* a plant, an herb SW2/644;
wortis *pl.* prepared greens, a salad Age/526, Age/1003, Fle/138,
SW2/940, etc., **wurtis** SW2/391
worthe *pr.3sg.subj.* ~ *iholpen* may be
helped SW2/1387
worthy *adv.* in a deserving way
7Pla/352
wo(u)nder *adv.* marvelously, very
CHP/396, Plag/125, 7Pla/122, etc.
woxen see **wex** *inf.*
wrappe *inf.* wrap, envelop SW2/434,
SW2/1378, **wrap** *impv.* SW2/1084,
wrappyng *pr.ppl.* CHP/1424,
wrapped *p.ppl.* DHN/49, SW2/952,
SW2/1422, **wrappid** DHN/211;

wrappid error for L. *volenti* 'wanting' Age/12n

wrappynges *vbl.n.pl.* ?entanglements 7Pla/9

wrath *n.* anger Age/382, Age/516, etc.

wrathful *adj.* angry 7Pla/189, **wrothful** 7Pla/187

wrathith *pr.3sg.* grows angry DHN/205, **wrothith** 7Pla/187; ~ *refl.* grows angry CHP/935

wryng *impv.* wring, squeeze SW2/1098, **iwrongen** *p.ppl.* SW2/719; **wronng** *p.ppl.* twisted, contorted CHP/699, CHP/723, **wrongen** CHP/566, **wrongon** CHP/590

wrynggyng *vbl.n.* contraction, cramping 8Med/55, 8Med/57

wrong *n.* a wrong, an injustice 7Pla/49

wrongen, wrongon, wronng see **wryng**

wroth *adj.* angry SW2/159, 7Pla/116, etc.

wrothful see **wrathful**

wrothith see **wrathith**

wse see **vse** *n.*

wullen *adj.* woolen Age/1017; ~ *clew* a ball of woolen thread SW2/571

yaate *n.* a gate, an opening DHN/152; *in the yaatis* immediately impending CHP/696; ~ *of the wombe* the vulva Coi/22

yalow *adj.* yellow Age/1461, Fle/123, SW2/305, **yalew** Age/1373; *swart* ~ dark yellow SW2/132, SW2/135, lead-colored SW2/1017

ye *interj.* indeed, yes CHP/467n

yelkis see **yolkes**

yerd(e) *n.*(1) the penis DHN/186, Coi/22, SW2/526, etc., **yeerd** Coi/50; a rod or stick Inst/1226, Inst/1296, etc.; ~ *visory, gawgyng* ~ a measuring rod Inst/1224, Inst/1224, Inst/1408

yerde *n.*(2) a thread SW2/929n

yesen see **yisen**

yeve *inf.* give Bac/84, Bac/376, CHP/72, etc., **yeven** *SW2/1340, SW2/1483, ~ *impv.* SW2/170, SW2/228, etc., **yef** SW2/1471,

yevith *pr.3sg.* Age/248, Age/657, etc., ~ *pr.1pl.* Bac/142, **yeven** *pr.3pl.* Bac/268, Bac/437, ~ *pr.3sg.subj.* 7Pla/168, **yevyng** *pr.ppl.* Age/50, DHN/22, **yaf** *pret.3sg.* Age/908, **yaven** *pret.3pl.* Bac/440, **yeven** *p.ppl.* Age/366, Age/1203, Bac/626, etc., **yoven** Bac/51, Bac/557, Plag/45, etc. [see also **gyve**]

yield(e) *inf.* give, render, return Age/18, Age/973, DHN/155, etc., **yieldith** *pr.3sg.* Age/429, Age/479, DHN/75, CHP/1486, etc., **yielden** *pr.3pl.* DHN/79, DHN/132, 7Pla/124, **yieldyng** *pr.ppl.* DHN/282; **yieldith** *pr.3sg.* produces, gives rise to DHN/189, Coi/81, etc.; **yold** *p.ppl.* of a statement or report: rendered, given CHP/895; ~ *helth into helth* give health to a healthy person Age/18

yif *conj.* if DHN/129, *Plag/130, Plag/137

yiftes *n.pl.* gifts 7Pla/137, **yiftis** 7Pla/138

yisen *ppl.adj.* passed, gone by Inst/632n, **yesen** Inst/636n

yocsynges *n.pl.* hiccups [L. *syncopim* 'loss of consciousness, fainting,' poss. confused with *singultum* 'hiccup'] CHP/417

yold see **yield(e)**

yolkes *n.pl.* yolks SW2/622, SW2/889, etc., **yolkis** SW2/885, SW2/1475, **yelkis** SW2/1472

yonglynges *n.pl.* young people, adolescents [L. *adolescentes*, distinguished by the translator from "yong men," L. *iuvenes*] Age/389, **yonglyngis** Age/730

yowthith *pr.3sg.* becomes young [error for L. *adolescit* 'grows'] DHN/272

yoven see **yeve**

zodiac *n.* the band of the sky through which the sun and planets move, as represented on a celestial sphere or other astronomical instrument Inst/114, Inst/116, Inst/393, etc.

zodiac *adj.* zodiacal Inst/145, Inst/573

MATERIA MEDICA IN TCC R.14.52

The following glossary has been compiled with the help of Monica Green, who generated an extensive word-list of *materia medica* in *Sickness of Women* (by far the largest source of such terminology in the manuscript) on which the glossary is based, and of Bryan VanGinhoven, who assisted in locating the definitions for the words in that list. Both English and Latin terms are included; Latin words are italicized and given in their nominative case, whether or not that form actually appears in the text. A word has been classified as Latin when it occurs in running Latin text or appears in a Latin oblique case within otherwise English text. In a few thoroughly macaronic sentences and in cases where a Latin nominative form occurs in otherwise English text (and may thus be a naturalized loanword), the assignment of a word to a particular language is necessarily arbitrary.

Common names of plants and animals are usually followed by scientific genus and species classifications, which are deeply indebted to Hunt 1989, Getz 1991, Green 2001, and the *MED*. Those familiar with medieval scientific nomenclature will know that names of plants and sometimes of minerals can often have more than one referent; we have therefore sought to err on the side of inclusiveness in giving alternative identifications, separated by semicolons, of the plants and other materials listed below. Alphabetization and other formatting conventions follow the principles of the General Glossary (vocalic *y* and *v* treated as *i* and *u*, etc.; use of italic and bold fonts; punctuation; and so on). Entries for terms representing categories of *materia medica*—*bark(e), folia, juce, levis, oile, oleum, powder, radix, rynde, ro(o)te, ro(o)tes/-is, seede, semen, succus, water*—contain complete listings of all phrases related to the category. The abbreviation "spp." stands for "species" (*pl.*).

abrotanum southernwood (*Artemisia abrotanum*) SW2/1344, SW2/1599

absinthium wormwood (*Artemisia absinthium*) SW2/1652, SW2/1678

acalar, rede dragante of a form of vitriol, a metal sulfate [L. *dragantum rubeum abacalay; abacalay* may be a corruption of an Arabic word for vitriol, such as the (latinized) *alcalcadis, alcolcotar,* and *alcalcantum* for white, yellow, and green vitriol in Avicenna's *Canon* 2.2.48] Age/1198n

acarus see *achorus*

acasie acacia (*Acacia arabica*) SW2/798, *acasia* SW2/331, SW2/459, SW2/462, SW2/486

acedula acetula, wild garlic (*Allium ursinum*): **semen acedule** acetula seed SW2/1698

aceros a kind of mirabolans [L. *citrinos*] Age/1074

acetum vinegar SW2/1682

achory sweet flag; yellow flag (*Acorus calamus; Iris pseudacorus*) SW2/1394, **achorus** SW2/1602, **attory** SW2/208, ?*acarus* SW2/214

acornes acorns SW2/431, **acornys** SW2/369; ~ *cuppes* acorn caps SW2/493

aduelane assate roasted hazelnuts (*Corylus avellana*) SW2/1669

affadil wild garlic; sweet woodruff (*Allium ursinum; Asperula odorata*) SW2/1049, **affodil** SW2/155

agaricus larch agaric, bracket fungus (*Polyporus officinalis*) SW2/1390, SW2/1586, SW2/1601

aglienter eglantine; briar rose (*Rosa rubiginosa; Rosa canina*) Fle/154

agnus castus the chaste tree; St. John's wort (*Vitex agnus-castus; Hypericum androsaemum*) SW2/633, SW2/1642, SW2/1670

agrippa a medicinal ointment, possibly associated with Agrippa, king of the Jews SW2/724 [see Getz 1991, 312]

agrista verjuice, juice of sour or unripe fruit Plag/135

aisel vinegar Fle/90, Plag/323

albedo ouorum the white of eggs SW2/1683

alcalies, rede an alkaline substance derived from the ashes of plants Age/78

alcamy ?alcanna, the alkanet plant (*Alkanna tinctoria*) SW2/1518

ale ale, drunk with medicines SW2/407, SW2/452, SW2/1827, Plag/293, Plag/300

alisaunder alexanders, horse-parsley (*Smyrnium olusatrum*) SW2/1832, SW2/1835

allium garlic (*Allium sativum*) SW2/1702

almaundis almonds, the nuts of the almond tree (*Amygdalus communis*) Age/1868, SW2/363, SW2/625; *bitter* ~ a variety of almond SW2/876; *mylke of* ~ , **almaunde** *mylke* almond milk (produced by steeping finely ground almonds in boiling water) SW2/379, SW2/380, SW2/386; *potage of* ~ almond soup Plag/292; *swe(e)te* ~ a variety of almond Age/1565, Age/1573

aloe(s) the aloe tree (*Aquilaria agallocha*) Bac/543; the drug aloes Age/1054, Age/1061, SW2/1557; ~ *citrini* a kind of aloe, aloe citrine SW2/1581, *aloue cicotryn* Plag/164; ~ *of the lyver*, ~ *epatic* a kind of aloe,

aloe epatica Age/1061, Age/1637; *lignum* ~ wood of the aloe tree SW2/587, SW2/651, SW2/1585, SW2/1694, SW2/1701, Plag/124; *exiol* ~ lignum aloes Age/1638

*altea marsh mallow (*Althaea officinalis*) SW2/1645

altees marsh mallow plants Fle/98

alum of plume feather or plume alum, naturally occurring aluminum sulfate SW2/496

amatiste see **ematiste**

ambra ambergris Bac/540, Bac/541

ambre amber SW2/655, SW2/660, **amber** Age/2016 [prob. understood as 'ambergris'], **aumber** SW2/586; *lapis ambree* SW2/1641

ambrose wild sage, wood sage (*Teucrium scorodonia*) SW2/948

ameos one of several plants of the family Umbelliferae, such as cowbane; cow parsley; goutweed; wild angelica; hemlock (*Cicuta virosa; Anthriscus sylvestris; Aegopodium podagraria; Angelica sylvestris; Conium maculatum*) SW2/687, SW2/1434, SW2/1583

*amydoun crushed hulled grain, grits Age/1857

amigdala almond (*Prunus amygdalus*) SW2/1670

amomum poppy; cardamom; grains of paradise (*Papaver* spp.; *Amomum cardamomum; Aframomum meleguetta*) SW2/1701, ~ *interius* SW2/1702; **amomi semen* poppy or cardamom seed, or grains of paradise SW2/1602

anacardi see **theodoricon**

*anamonie poppy, anemonia (*Papaver* spp.) SW2/1835

anathasia athanasia, tansy (*Chrysanthemum vulgare*) SW2/464, SW2/465, *anathasia* SW2/506

anceris see **axungia**

anete dill (*Anethum graveolens*) SW2/263, SW2/687, SW2/839, SW2/864

anise anise (*Pimpinella anisum*)
Age/1479, Age/1956, SW2/263,
SW2/839, SW2/948, SW2/1396,
SW2/1855, **anyse** SW2/274,
SW2/332, SW2/1077, SW2/1469

anisum (= **anise**) SW2/1591,
SW2/1596, SW2/1603, SW2/1700;
semen anisi aniseed SW2/1582

antere the anther of a rose SW2/807

antos rosemary (*Rosmarinus officinalis*)
Bac/534

apen-ers the medlar tree, the "open-
arse" (*Mespila germanica*) SW2/429

apium wild celery, smallage (*Apium
graveolens*) SW2/214, SW2/840,
SW2/1595, SW2/1609

applis, wyne of an alcoholic drink
made from apples Age/760

aqua ardif distilled spirits SW2/1842

aqua pilosella water of hawkweed (*Hieracium pilosella*) SW2/1657

aqua rosarum rose water SW2/1519

aqua vite brandy, distilled spirits
SW2/1861, SW2/1862, SW2/1863

arage orache SW2/391

aragon the ointment arrogon
SW2/1286, SW2/1459, SW2/1784
[see Green 2001, 193]

archimesie see **arthemesia**

argent vief quicksilver, mercury
SW2/1294

argilla a styptic herb 8Med/9 [?poss.
error for *ardillus/-a, argentilla*, or *ar-
tillus*: see Hunt 1989, 33, 34, 37]

arian a kind of wine Age/1402,
Age/1403, **arean** Age/1403

aristologia birthwort, aristolochia
(*Aristolochia* spp.) SW2/878; ~ *longum* long aristolochia SW2/1603; ~ *rotunda*, **aristolochia** *rotunda* round aristolochia SW2/1695, SW2/1119, *rounde
aristologium* SW2/1508; ~ *rotunda &
longa* *SW2/1393, SW2/1600

armoniac, armoniak see **bo(o)le armoniac**

arnoglossa plantain (*Plantago major*)
8Med/9

arrellis crushed grape seeds Age/789n

arthemesie artemisia, mugwort
(*Artemisia vulgaris*) SW2/1121,
SW2/1123, **archimesie** SW2/879,
archimisie SW2/270, *arthemesia* SW2/1604, SW2/1658, *arthe-
misia* SW2/1578; *succus arthemesie*
(*archimesie*) mugwort sap or juice
SW2/1658, SW2/886

asa asafoetida (*Ferula assa-foetida*)
SW2/1398, *SW2/1600

asorum hazelwort (*Asarum europaeum*)
SW2/263, ?**asorie** SW2/1134, ?**asarie** SW2/1395

as(s)afetida asafoetida (*Ferula assa-
foetida*) SW2/592, SW2/807,
SW2/814, SW2/816, etc.

assh, rynde of the bark of the European ash tree (*Fraxinus excelsior*)
SW2/431

asshis ashes SW2/730, **asshen** SW2/1454

athanasia tansy (*Chrysanthemum vulgare*) SW2/376 [see also **anathasia**]

atriplex orache (*Atriplex* spp.)
SW2/1603

attory see *achorus*

aumber see **ambre**

avence wood avens, herb bennet
(*Geum urbanum*) SW2/250, **avons**
SW2/1872

***axungia** fat, grease SW2/1690; ~ *ance-
ris* goose grease SW2/1645

babilony see **bawme**

bacce lauri berries of the laurel tree or
spurge laurel (*Laurus nobilis; Daphne laureola*) SW2/1660, **bacce laure*
SW2/1695, *bucce lauriis* SW2/1391

bay a berry of the laurel tree (*Laurus
nobilis; Daphne laureola*) SW2/760,
baies SW2/1829; *oile of baie* a medicinal oil made from laurel berries
and leaves SW2/564, SW2/1459, *oile
de baye* SW2/1094

balaustia pomegranate (*Punica granatum*) SW2/369, **balaustie** SW2/470,
SW2/799, SW2/822

bal(le) a ball-shaped suppository
SW2/755, SW2/756, *SW2/783,
SW2/980, SW2/1405, SW2/1423;
a pill SW2/1299, SW2/1403,
SW2/1410

balsamum, oile (= **bawme, oile of**)
Age/1194

bardana burdock; cleavers (*Arctium lappa; Galium aparine*) SW2/1689

bark(e) the bark of various plants:
~ *of cassy fistule* cassia bark (a cinnamon-like spice) SW2/1132; ~ *of
citre* bark of the citron tree (*Citrus medica*) Age/1419, Age/1449,
~ *citre* Age/2054, Age/2065; *inward ~ of canel* cinnamon, the inner bark of the tree *Cinnamomum
zelanicum* SW2/1137; ~ *of sloue trees*
blackthorn (*Prunus spinosa*) bark
SW2/987

barly barley SW2/947; ~ *mele* barley
meal SW2/488, SW2/1034; *wyne of
~* an alcoholic beverage made from
barley Age/760

barowes grece boar's grease SW2/1846

bawme the balsam plant (*Commiphora
opobalsamum*) or the medicinal resin
derived from it SW2/225, SW2/587,
SW2/599, SW2/1093, etc., *herbe ~* ,
herbe baume SW2/1372, SW2/240;
~ , oile of ~ an ointment made
from the balsam plant Age/1388,
Age/1488, Age/1575; ~ *babilony* medicinal ointment from Babylon
Age/1636; ~ *certic* medicinal ointment from Crete Age/1636

bdellium a gum from an Asian or Af-
rican tree (*Commiphora africana;
Balsamodendron* spp.) SW2/1391,
SW2/1584

beane mele bean meal Age/1565,
SW2/960, SW2/1571

beanes beans SW2/862; *oile of *benen*
SW2/626

bech, first a kind of tanning liquor
[poss. from ME *bach, beche* 'stream';
see *MED*, s.v. *bach* n.(1)] SW2/473

beetis beets (*Beta vulgaris; Beta cicla*)
or beet leaves SW2/354, SW2/391,
Plag/146

benedicta (= **benet**) SW2/252,
SW2/253, **benedicte** SW2/248, *benedicta* (L.) SW2/1840

benedictum see *oleum*

***benen** see **beanes**

benet *herbe ~* hemlock, herb bennet;
cowbane; wood avens (*Conium maculatum; Cicuta virosa; Geum urbanum*)
SW2/1854

berberis barberry (*Berberis vulgaris*): se-
men ~ barberry seed SW2/1699

betayne betony (*Betonica officinalis*)
SW2/942, SW2/1088, SW2/1875,
Plag/298, **beteyne** Plag/284; *water
of ~* water infused with betony leaves
Plag/397

betonica (= **betayne**) SW2/1577,
SW2/1659

bicche see **mylke**

bismalow marsh mallow (*Althaea officinalis*) SW2/1036

bistorte knotgrass; snake-root (*Polygonum aviculare; Polygonum bistorta*)
SW2/798, *SW2/806, SW2/814

ble(e)te beet (*Beta vulgaris*) Age/1483,
Fle/96, Fle/167

bloode glas a cupping glass SW2/566

bodegarynum ?derived from bedegars
(galls) from rosebushes or eglantines SW2/1519

boles, stones of bulls' testicles SW2/623

bolis gall(e) bull's gall SW2/292,
SW2/685, SW2/1251, etc., *booles galle*
SW2/194

bones, rost see **rost bones**

bo(o)le a red earth used as a styp-
tic SW2/358, SW2/369, SW2/467,
SW2/1507, SW2/1518, *bolus*
SW2/1693, ~ *armoniac (armoniak)*
SW2/454, *SW2/457, SW2/492,
SW2/993, SW2/1791, Plag/298

bo(o)n bone: ~ *pat gendryth in the herte
of the hert, hertis ~* gristle from the
heart of a stag Bac/545, CHP/480;

hors bones ibrent burned horse bones SW2/569

borace sodium borate, used for treatment of leprosy, open sores, etc. SW2/1518

borage borage; bugloss (*Borago officinalis; Anchusa arvensis*) Age/1203, SW2/250, SW2/348, SW2/504, SW2/1462, SW2/1520, SW2/1874, Plag/146

borax (= **borace**) SW2/1293, SW2/1391, SW2/1399

bore boar: *brawne of a* ~ boar meat SW2/623; *stones of a* ~ , *stones of bores* boar's (boars') testicles SW2/1805, SW2/623

***bothon** rosemary; corn marigold; ox-eye daisy (*Rosmarinus officinalis; Chrysanthemum segetum; Chrysanthemum leucanthemum*) SW2/1119

bouinus see *fimus*

bouis see *fel*

brayne brain (as a fatty meat that increases production of sperm) SW2/625

braket bragot, a drink of ale and honey CHP/165

bran(ne) bran, ground wheat husks Age/1568, Age/1857, SW2/1798

braunche ***vrsyne** bear's breech, brancursine (*Acanthus mollis*) SW2/1374

braunchis of arrellis *lit.* branches of crushed grape seeds (L. *arillis racemorum* 'crushed seeds from bunches of grapes') Age/789n

braunchis of iuniper tree juniper branches Plag/118

brawne flesh, meat SW2/623

bred(e) bread Age/755, Age/756, Age/1507, etc.; ~ *wele leveyned* well-leavened bread Age/1852, Age/1945

briddes, smale small birds Age/1854

brymston brimstone, sulfur Age/1020, SW2/574

brome, myddil rynde of the the inner bark of the broom plant (*Saro-*

thamnus scoparius; Valeriana celtica) SW2/342

broth of rede chiches a broth of red chick-peas or peas (*Cicer arietinum; Pisum sativum*) SW2/1133

bucce lauriis see *bacce lauri*

butter butter SW2/768, SW2/1286, SW2/1751; *fressh* ~ *(buttur)* newly made butter SW2/222, SW2/982, SW2/1032, SW2/1035, SW2/1458; *May* ~ unsalted butter made in May SW2/291, SW2/1171, SW2/1378

cacabre ?a corrupt vernacularized form of *cantabrum/cancrabum* 'bran, husks of wheat or other grains' or ?a form of *cacabulum* 'black nightshade, petty morel' (*Solanum nigrum*) SW2/492

cakes pancakes SW2/1099

calamynt(e) calamint (*Calamintha* spp.) SW2/155, SW2/174, SW2/240, SW2/578, SW2/642, SW2/714, Plag/124, etc., **calmynt** SW2/654, *calamyntum* SW2/1591, SW2/1596

culamus aromaticus sweet flag, sweet myrtle, sweet sedge; sweet gale, bog myrtle (*Acorus calamus; Myrica gale*) SW2/579, SW2/586, SW2/652, *SW2/653

calf a calf: *mary of a* ~ calves' marrow SW2/982, SW2/1055; *sowkyng* ~ a suckling calf SW2/398; *flessh of soukyng (sowkyng) calves* tender veal Age/771, Age/1853

camamyl camomile (*Chamaemelum nobile; Anthemis nobilis*) SW2/263, SW2/641, SW2/1373, **camomyl** Age/1478, Age/1956, SW2/1529; *succus camamil* camomile sap or juice SW2/1655

camfre see **camphore**

camphore camphor, an aromatic derivative of the camphor tree (*Camphora laurus; Dryobalanops camphora; Cinnamomum camphora*) Age/1449, SW2/370, SW2/654, SW2/655,

SW2/657, SW2/660, **camphory**
SW2/656, SW2/1083, SW2/1090,
SW2/1518, SW2/1564, **camphour**
Age/1010, *camphora* SW2/1627,
*SW2/1628, **camfre** Plag/140; *ro.
camphorie* ?camphorated roses
CHP/479

canel cinnamon; cassia (*Cinnamomum
zeylanicum; Cinnamomum
cassia*) SW2/456, SW2/776,
SW2/864, SW2/1137, SW2/1760,
Plag/148

caparis, radix honeysuckle root
(*Lonicera caprifolium*) or caper
bush roots (*Capparis spinosa*)
SW2/1611

capree see *vesica capree*

cardamomum cardamom (*Elettaria car-
domomum*) Age/2063

careway caraway (*Carum carvi*)
SW2/1824, **carewey** SW2/1834

carlokes charlock, wild mustard (*Sinapis arvensis*) SW2/1866

carpobalsamum fruit of the balsam
plant (*Commiphora opobalsamum*)
SW2/652, *SW2/1393

carter trans. of L. *carnis tyri* 'viper's
flesh' Age/2065n

carui caraway (*Carum carvi*) SW2/687,
SW2/840, SW2/864, etc., **caruie**
SW2/454

cassatyne a medium-grade white sugar, in loaf or lump form SW2/506

cassia fistula cassia, bastard cinnamon
(*Cinnamomum cassia*) Age/1521,
SW2/503, SW2/1309; *barke of cassy
fistule* cassia bark SW2/1132, *cortex
cassie fistule* SW2/1596

cassia lignea the cinnamon-like bark
of the cassia tree (*Cinnamomum cassia*) Age/1419, *cassia liggnij (ligni)*
SW2/1393, SW2/1604

castory the perineal glands of the
European beaver (*Castor fiber*)
and their secretions SW2/573,
SW2/593, SW2/865, SW2/1134,
SW2/1136, SW2/1391, SW2/1529,

SW2/1856, SW2/1867, **castorie**
Fle/165, SW2/1335, SW2/1585,
castora SW2/653

caule cabbage and other plants of
the genus *Brassica* Age/1866,
SW2/1087

caulis cabbage (*Brassica* spp.); charlock (*Brassica oleracea; Sinapis arvensis*): *radix callium* root of cabbages
SW2/1683

celidoyne greater celandine (*Chelidoni-
um majus*) SW2/1043

cene see **sene**

centory the greater or lesser centaury; yellow-wort (*Centaurium erythraea;
Blackstonia perfoliata*) SW2/1043,
SW2/1506, *centauria* SW2/1394,
centauria maior SW2/1605, *centaurea* SW2/1585, *centaurea *minor*
SW2/1604

cera wax SW2/815, SW2/886,
SW2/1673

ceremountayne sermountain (*Laserpiti-
um siler; Siler montanum; Seseli montanum*) SW2/241, SW2/262

cerfolium chervil (*Anthriscus cerefolium*)
SW2/1709

certic see **bawme**

ceruse white lead SW2/363,
SW2/1519; *washe of ~* water in which
white lead has been submerged or
rinsed SW2/1557

ceruus see *os*

cesaryne, oignement a medicinal ointment based on three ingredients:
sandalwood (*Santalum album; Pterocarpus santalinus*), ?hemlock [L. *emleg*; see *MED*, s.vv. *emlege* n., *sandal(e*
n.], and the juice of "emablot"
[poss. a corruption of L. *emleg* and
succus herbe que dicitur bleta in *Secreta
secretorum*] Age/1483

cheri stones kernels the meat within
cherry stones SW2/1825, *kernels of
chery stones* SW2/1834

chervoile chervil (*Anthriscus cerefolium*)
SW2/251, SW2/922

chestayne chestnut (*Castanea sativa*) SW2/430; error for *oleum costiuum/ costinum* costmary oil Age/1188n

chiches, rede chick-peas or peas (*Cicer arietinum; Pisum sativum*): *decoccioun (broth) of ~* a broth in which chick-peas or peas have been boiled SW2/245, SW2/1133, SW2/1134

chikemete chickweed; scarlet pimpernel (*Stellaria media; Anagallis arvensis*) SW2/1738

chykens chickens Fle/135, **chikens** Plag/290; *flessh of ~ (chikens)* chicken meat Age/771, Age/1853, Age/1946

***chine *macedonicorum** sprouts or tips (var. of *cime*) of alexanders/ horse-parsley (*Smyrnium olusatrum*) SW2/1709

ciclamen cyclamen; sowbread or pignut (*Cyclamen hederifolium; Conopodium majus*) SW2/1314

ciclamia (= **ciclamen**) SW2/287

ciconii see *citonii*

cicotryn see **aloe(s)**

cicuta hemlock, herb bennet (*Conium muculatum*) SW2/1582

ciminum cumin (*Cuminum cyminum*) SW2/886, **cuminum** SW2/1700 [see also **comyn**]

cinamum cinnamon (*Cinnamomum zeylanicum*) Age/2062, **cynamum** Fle/166, **cynamun** SW2/1529, **cinamon** SW2/441, *cinamom* SW2/1702, *cinamon* SW2/1611

cinapium mustard (*Sinapis* spp.) SW2/1583

cyndres of irn crushed iron slag or rust scrapings Age/1135

cineres ashes SW2/1689

ciperus galingale; sweet flag (*Cyperus longus; Acorus calamus*) SW2/239, SW2/579, SW2/1394, SW2/1608, **ciprus* SW2/652

cipres(se) cypress (*Cupressus sempervirens*) SW2/1077, *cipressus* SW2/653; *nux cipressi* cypress cone ('nut') or seed SW2/799, SW2/817, SW2/821;

shavyng of ~ cypress shavings SW2/578, SW2/642

cirus see **syrus**

citeris of lupyne error for *farinam ciceris, lupini* Age/1565n

**citonii* quinces, fruits of the quince tree (*Cydonia oblonga*) SW2/1706, *ciconii* SW2/1704

citre, bark (of) bark of the citron tree (*Citrus medica*) Age/1419, Age/1449, Age/2054, Age/2065

citryn see **mirabolans**

citronade candied citron or orange peel Plag/144

clarre spiced, sweetened, and clarified wine SW2/246, *wyne ~* SW2/722

classa not identified SW2/1609

clawes hooves (of a goat) SW2/1452

clote burdock (*Arctium lappa*) SW2/723, SW2/952, SW2/953; *oyntement of clotes* SW2/718

clowte a piece of cloth: *lynnen ~* a piece of linen cloth SW2/1755, SW2/1774; *clowtis of wul and her* pieces of woolen cloth and hair-cloth SW2/1788

clowes cloves (*Eugenia caryophyllata*) SW2/579, SW2/752, SW2/990, SW2/1075, SW2/1727, SW2/1855, **cloves** Age/1526, SW2/1471, SW2/1475

cocanidium seed or berry of the laurel (*Daphne gnidium; Daphne laureola*) SW2/288

cokil corn cockle; darnel (*Agrostemma githago; Lolium temulentum*) SW2/865, SW2/934; *flour of ~ (cokel), cokel (cokle) floure* ground cockle, cockle meal SW2/193, SW2/215, SW2/217, SW2/927

cok a cock, rooster Age/1073n, Fle/135; *flessh of cokkis* chicken meat SW2/622

cole, quike a burning coal SW2/571

coliandrum coriander (*Coriandrium sativum*) SW2/458

colophony turpentine distilled to a resin, Greek pitch SW2/426, **colophonie* SW2/729, **colophonia* SW2/331, **colofony** Fle/99

coloquintida colocynth, a vine bearing a bitter fruit used as a purgative (*Citrullus colocynthis*) SW2/1120, SW2/1651, SW2/1841, *colloquintida* **SW2/287, SW2/1581, **colloquintide** SW2/1129

columbyne columbine (*Aquilegia vulgaris*) SW2/1739, *herba columbina* SW2/1633

comyn cumin (*Cuminum cyminum*) SW2/155, SW2/607, SW2/632, SW2/737, SW2/760, etc. [see also *ciminum*]

confery comfrey (*Symphytum officinale*) SW2/357, SW2/431, SW2/715, SW2/776, SW2/1759

consowde, pety daisy (*Bellis perennis*) SW2/1759

coost see **cost**

cophyns see **pigra**

coral the precious stone coral Age/341; *rede* ~ red coral SW2/454, SW2/475, SW2/492, ~ *rede and white* red and white coral SW2/457

corallus rubius et albus red and white coral SW2/1699, *corallus albus* **and rubie** SW2/358

cortex bark: ~ *cassie fistule* cassia bark, a cinnamon-like spice SW2/1596, ~ *lauri* laurel bark SW2/1660

cost costmary (*Chrysanthemum balsamita*) SW2/598, SW2/641, **coost** SW2/745, **costy** SW2/260, SW2/1380; *rootis (rotes) of* ~ poss. costus root (*Saussurea lappa*) SW2/1288, SW2/1290

costa ?ribwort (*Plantago lanceolata*), ?costmary (*Chrysanthemum balsamita*): *semen coste* ?ribwort or ?costmary seed SW2/1698

costy see **cost**

coton cotton SW2/195, SW2/216, SW2/468, SW2/618, SW2/664, etc.

cow(es) mylke cow's milk SW2/387, SW2/980, **cow milk** Age/1214, **kow mylke** SW2/973

cowslippes cowslips (*Primula veris*) SW2/1866

crasses see **cresses**

cream cream [error for L. *ceram* 'wax'] Fle/99

cres-seede cress-seed SW2/840

cresses cresses, various plants in the mustard family, such as water cress; garden or town cress; etc. (*Rorippa nasturtium-aquaticam; Nasturtium officinale; Lepidum sativum*) SW2/729, SW2/941, **crasses** SW2/161, **cressis** SW2/715

crocus saffron, crocus (*Crocus sativus*) SW2/652, SW2/1396, SW2/1580, SW2/1582, SW2/1655, SW2/1701, SW2/1702

croppes parts of medicinal herbs (buds, shoots, leaves, etc.), excluding the roots SW2/921, SW2/1874, **croppis** SW2/1098

cruddes curds Age/1866

cucuba cubeb, Java peppercorn (*Piper cubeba*) SW2/441, SW2/1394, SW2/1702

cucumbres cucumbers (*Cucumis sativus*) Plag/145

cucurbites gourds of various plants, esp. *Lagenaria vulgaris* Age/1867

culver dirt dove's dung SW2/854

cuminum see *ciminum*

cuscutis dodder (*Cuscuta* spp.) SW2/1581

cuzanton ?theriac or ?bole armeniac Age/474n

daates see **datis**

daisie daisy (*Bellis perennis*) SW2/357, SW2/431, **daisy** SW2/352

datis dates SW2/625, **daates** Age/1868

dauke wild carrot; wild parsnip (*Daucus carota; Pastinaca sativa*) SW2/1041, **dawke** SW2/172, *daucus* SW2/263, SW2/1605

dewte a medicinal salve SW2/1053, *SW2/1286, *SW2/1459

diaciminum a compound medicine based on cumin SW2/838

diacynamum a compound medicine based on cinnamon [error for *diaciminum*] Age/1861

diacitonicem a compound medicine based on quinces SW2/1705 [see also *diatoniden*]

diacodion a compound medicine based on poppies SW2/377

diacostory a compound medicine based on the dried perineal glands of the beaver Fle/163 [see castory]

diagredium a compound medicine based on scammony SW2/218, SW2/1585

dialtea a compound medicine based on marsh mallow SW2/1377

diamargarit a compound medicine based on pearls SW2/1841

diambra a compound medicine based on ambergris Plag/110

diamusca a compound medicine based on musk Plag/110

dianisum a compound medicine based on anise, or = *dionisium*, a compound medicine based on aloes and tansy SW2/838

diantos a compound medicine based on rosemary Bac/536, Plag/111

diapapauer a compound medicine based on poppies SW2/392, SW2/501, diapapaure SW2/414

diaquilon a compound medicine based on various plant juices Fle/95

diasinthy a compound medicine based on quinces Fle/96

diaspermaton a compound medicine based on various seeds SW2/235, SW2/838

diatesseron see triacle

diatoniden possible error for *diacitonicem* SW2/376

diptayne dittany of Crete; white dittany (*Origanum dictamnus; Dictam-

nus albus*) SW2/226, SW2/274, SW2/688, SW2/957, SW2/1249, etc., dipteyne Plag/382

diptanus (= diptayne) SW2/1345, SW2/1395, SW2/1578, SW2/1598, SW2/1694

dirt dung: culver ~ dove's dung SW2/854, sheepes ~ sheep's dung SW2/855

dockes, rede red-veined dock (*Rumex sanguineus*) SW2/1549

doder dodder (*Cuscuta* spp.) SW2/261

dough, soure leaven, sour-dough SW2/1035, *SW2/1050

draconis see *sanguis*

dragance a tree resin, tragacanth (from the tree *Astralagus gummifer*) SW2/978, dragans Age/1566, *dragantum* SW2/1517; *gummi (gumme) dragantum (album, whit)* SW2/1504, SW2/1511, SW2/1517, SW2/1520, SW2/1555, *gumme of draganti* SW2/482; *muscillage of dragantum (draganti)* *SW2/935, SW2/1560 [see muscillage]

dragante of acalar, rede see acalar, rede dragante of

dragaunce dragonwort, dragon arum (*Dracunculus vulgaris*) SW2/406; dragonwort or ?tragacanth [see dragance] SW2/366

drastis dregs SW2/873

dunge, gotis goat's dung SW2/881

duretik a diuretic, having diuretic effect SW2/1725

ebul, ebulis corruptions of *kebulus*, black or indic myrabolan (a prune-like fruit, *Terminalia chebula*) Age/1074, Age/1106, Age/1112

ebule danewort, dwarf elder (*Sambucus ebulus*) Age/1079n

ebulus (= ebule) SW2/1588, SW2/1678, 8Med/19; *succus ebuli* sap or juice of the dwarf elder SW2/1672

eele an eel SW2/423

eeris, hevenly error for *spica celtica* 'Celtic spikenard' (*Valerian celtica*) Age/1205n

eg(ge) egg: *rere* ~ soft-boiled egg Age/2090, Fle/135; *white of an egg(e)* Age/1557, Age/1559, SW2/1503, *white of egges* Fle/99; *yelkis (yolkis) of raw egges* raw egg yolks SW2/1472, SW2/1475 [see also **eyren**]

egipsium gypsum SW2/368

egremoyne agrimony (*Agrimonia eupatoria*) SW2/1142

eyren eggs SW2/1099; *white of ~* SW2/371, SW2/1551, *yolkes (yolkis) of ~* SW2/622, SW2/885, SW2/889

ey-shellis egg-shells SW2/401, SW2/450

elebor, blac black hellebore (*Helleborus niger*) Age/1088, Age/1090 [see also *el(l)eborum*]

electuarie a compound medicine in a thick sweet substrate such as honey or syrup Age/2017, Age/2089, Bac/539, SW2/233, SW2/360, SW2/421, SW2/837, SW2/838, **electuary** SW2/287, **lectuary** SW2/733, **letuarie** Plag/144, *electuarium* SW2/502, SW2/1705; *cold (hote) (e)lectuaries* electuaries characterized by the elemental qualities of cold (heat) Age/772, Plag/283, Plag/379; *comfortatief (comfortable) electuaries* electuaries with strengthening effect Age/2100, SW2/375; *electuary diantos* an electuary whose main ingredient is rosemary Bac/536; *electuary emagoge* an electuary to stimulate the flow of blood SW2/269; *electuarie of mirabolans* an electuary whose main ingredient is myrabalan Age/1105; *mirre electuarie* an electuary whose main ingredient is myrrh SW2/1584; *~ of succo rosarum* a electuary containing juice of roses SW2/971

eleryn see **ellern**

elfhame "elf-cloak, elf-skin," a medicinal plant SW2/962 [cf. *MED,* s.vv.

elf-thung n. 'hellebore,' *tunsing-wurt* n. 'white hellebore']

el(l)eborum hellebore: ~ *nigrum* black hellebore (*Helleborus niger*) SW2/287, *SW2/1118, SW2/1582, SW2/1605; ~ *album* white hellebore (*Helleborus foetidus; Veratrum album*) SW2/1417, SW2/1582; *radix *elleboris* hellebore root SW2/1649

ellern the European elder (*Sambucus nigra*) SW2/1098, **eleryn** SW2/264, **eldren** SW2/1573

emablot an ingredient in **oignement cesaryne** [L. *enablet*] Age/1484

ematicis, lapis hematite SW2/378

ematiste amethyst SW2/462, SW2/478, **amatiste** SW2/492

emboris, rasura ivory shavings SW2/1654

emboton a small pipe for introducing medicinal smoke into the vagina SW2/791, **embotus** SW2/794

empericon see **theodoricon**

emplaster a thick salve, a medicinal plaster SW2/283, SW2/372, SW2/494, SW2/824, SW2/887, etc., **emplastres** SW2/1043, *SW2/1723

emplastrum (= **emplaster**) SW2/1588, SW2/1590, SW2/1649, SW2/1679, SW2/1708

encens(e) incense, frankincense, SW2/416, SW2/728, **encence** SW2/720

endyve endive, wild lettuce, sow-thistle (*Sonchus oleraceus*) SW2/1028

enula campana elecampane, scabwort, horseheal (*Inula helenium*) SW2/336, SW2/1041

epatic see **aloe(s)**

epithemy thyme dodder, a parasitic growth on thyme (*Cuscuta epithymum*) Fle/166

epithemum (= **epithemy**) SW2/1581

erbis, bath of hote a bath containing herbs with the elemental quality heat SW2/606

erth, sealid see *terra sigillata*

erth that is tofore a beestis mangier that is totrode with the beestis feete and beperisshed packed earth from a stable SW2/858

eruca garden rocket, white rocket (*Eruca sativa*) SW2/1642

esula spurge (*Euphorbia* spp.) SW2/1585

euforbie spurge (*Euphorbia resinifera*) or a gum derived from it SW2/1406, SW2/1417, **euforby** SW2/594, **euforbe** Fle/166, *euforbium* SW2/1382, SW2/1585

exilocassie bark of the cassia tree (*Cinnamomum cassia*) SW2/586 [see **cassia lignea**]

exiol aloes lignum aloes, wood of the aloe tree Age/1638

exizacres sugar mixed in vinegar Age/1914

farina fabarum bean meal SW2/1672, SW2/1683, SW2/1684

farina ordij barley meal SW2/1675

farine ground grain, flour SW2/1405

fecches seeds of the legume vetch (*Vicia* spp.) SW2/862

fel(l) gall, liver bile SW2/1256; ~ *bouis* bull's gall SW2/1120, SW2/1122, *SW2/1256

feltes ibrent burned pieces of felt or of pressed wool fibers SW2/568

femygreke see **fenygreke**

fenel fennel (*Foeniculum vulgare*) SW2/155, SW2/250, SW2/262, SW2/643, SW2/839, SW2/948, Plag/146, etc.; *raddish of* ~ fennel root SW2/172; *rede* ~ a form of fennel with red or brown seeds SW2/1870

feniculum fennel (*Foeniculum vulgare*) SW2/1393, SW2/1588, SW2/1697

fenygreke fenugreek (*Trigonella foenum-graecum*) SW2/261, SW2/1033, SW2/1036, SW2/1282, SW2/1372, SW2/1456, SW2/1528, **femygreke** SW2/405

fesaunt pheasant (*Phasianus colchicus*) Age/771, Age/1854

fetherfoy feverfew; lesser or common centaury (*Chrysanthemum parthenium; Centaurium erythraea*) SW2/643

fethers brent burned feathers SW2/570

figges figs (*Ficus carica*) Age/858, Age/1868, Age/1878, Age/1880, Age/1881, SW2/625, SW2/1049, Plag/69

filynges of irn iron filings or scrapings of rust Age/1135

fillicia fetida stinking fern (*Polypodium vulgare; Pteridium aquilinum*) SW2/1580

fimus dung: ~ *bouinus* cow-dung SW2/1661; ~ *murum* mouse-dung SW2/1690

fissh fish Plag/290

flos marini flower of rosemary (*Rosmarinus officinalis*) Bac/534

flos populi poplar-flower (*Populus* spp.) SW2/1629

flos salicis willow-flower (*Salix* spp.) SW2/1629

flour flower Age/1173, Age/1174, Age/1212, Age/1974n [error for *flebotomia*], Bac/534, Bac/536, Bac/537, SW2/243, SW2/263, SW2/577, Plag/139

flour(e) flour, meal: ~ *of beane mele* finely ground bean meal SW2/1571; *cokle (cokel)* ~ SW2/193, SW2/217; ~ *of cokel (cokil)* SW2/215, SW2/927; ~ *of rise* rice flour SW2/469

folefoote coltsfoot (*Tussilago farfara*) SW2/1845

folia leaves: ~ *absinthij* leaves of wormwood SW2/1678; ~ *agni casti* leaves of the chaste tree SW2/1670; ~ *cene* senna leaves SW2/1390; ~ *galbani* ?leaves of the plant *Ferula galbaniflua* SW2/799 [see **galbanum**]; ~ *jusquimani* leaves of henbane SW2/1676, SW2/1688, SW2/1707; ~ *lauri* laurel leaves SW2/1577,

SW2/1605; ~ *malue* (*maluarum*)
mallow leaves SW2/1676,
SW2/1677; ~ *porry* leek leaves
SW2/1588; ~ *rute* rue leaves
SW2/1707

frankencens(e) frankincense (*Boswellia thurifera*) SW2/586, SW2/990,
SW2/1791, Plag/122; *iwasshe of
frankencence* water in which frankincense has been submerged or
rinsed SW2/1557

frenssh sene see **sene**

fumeterre fumitory (*Fumaria officinalis*) SW2/1693, **ffumytere** Plag/382,
fumetory Plag/166

furfur bran SW2/1632

furmente frumenty, a dish of hulled
grain boiled with milk and sweetened SW2/380

*****fursis** furzes (*Ulex europaeus; Ruscus
aculeatus*) SW2/210

galanga (= **galingal[e]**) SW2/440,
SW2/653, SW2/799, SW2/817,
SW2/1701

galangale see **galingal(e)**

galbanum a resin derived from the
plant *Ferula galbaniflua* SW2/289,
SW2/573, SW2/598, SW2/600,
SW2/1115, etc., **galbany** SW2/1435,
galbanum SW2/799, SW2/1390,
SW2/1583, etc.

galingal(e) galingale (*Cyperus longus*)
Age/2054, SW2/456, SW2/1075,
SW2/1855, Plag/136, **galyngale**
Age/2065, **galangale** SW2/864

gall(e) the bile secreted by the liver
and stored in the gall bladder: *bolis* (*booles*) ~ bull's gall SW2/194,
SW2/292, SW2/685, SW2/1251,
SW2/1291, etc.

galle oak galls SW2/822

galle muste ?a resinous medicine
containing musk SW2/752, *gallia*
SW2/357, *gallia muscata* SW2/585,
gallia mustice SW2/377 [cf. *MED*, s.v.
galle n.(3), (c)]

galli see ***testiculi***

gallis oak galls SW2/352

ganders, gres of grease from male
geese, ganders SW2/1055, *grece of
gandres* SW2/870

gariofil cloves; clove pink; ?wood avens (*Eugenia caryophyllata; Dian-
thus caryophyllus; Geum urbanum*)
Age/2016, Age/2054, Age/2065,
gariofilum SW2/653, SW2/1580,
SW2/1611, *gariofullum* SW2/1701

garlik garlic (*Allium sativum*) SW2/160

Gascoyne, wine of wine from Gascony
SW2/275

gees geese Age/1854

genciana gentian (*Gentiana* spp.)
SW2/1394, SW2/1695

gilofre cloves; clove pink; ?wood avens (*Eugenia caryophyllata; Dian-
thus caryophyllus; Geum urbanum*)
Age/1448, Plag/112

gyng(i)er ginger (*Zingiber officinale*)
Age/1526, Age/1914, SW2/607,
Plag/148

gladen one of various species of
iris (*Iris pseudacorus; Iris foetidis-
sima;* etc.) SW2/273, SW2/1248,
SW2/1415, **gladyn** SW2/1733

gladiole yellow flag; sweet sedge
(*Iris pseudacorus; Acorus calamus*)
SW2/1344

gold the metal gold Age/325, Age/348,
Age/1137, Bac/116, Bac/142,
Bac/146, Bac/164, Bac/524,
CHP/480; ~ *calcyned and solued* gold
reduced to a powder by high heat and
put into solution Bac/110; *litarge of* ~
yellowish-red lead oxide SW2/1558

goldes marigolds (*Calendula officinalis*)
SW2/948, **gooldis** SW2/942

goorde a gourd (esp. of *Lagenaria vulgaris*) SW2/1540, **gourdes** Plag/145

gosselynges, flessh of meat of goslings
Age/1946

gote a goat SW2/386, SW2/1452; *gotis
dunge* goat's dung SW2/881; *flessh
of gootis* goat meat Age/1856; *gotis*

her goat's hair SW2/568; *gotes myl-ke* goat's milk SW2/380, SW2/405, SW2/855, *gotis mylke* SW2/1116

grayne (= **greyne parice**) Plag/148

grana grains, seeds: ~ *lauriole* seeds or berries of spurge laurel (*Daphne laureola*) SW2/1119; ~ *(grane) paradisi* grains of paradise (seeds of *Aframomum meleguetta*) SW2/1580, SW2/1703

granosum see *terebentum*

grapes grapes Age/1868

gras grass Age/832; *v-levid* ~ creeping cinquefoil (*Potentilla reptans*) SW2/1495

grece fat, grease *SW2/1036, **grese** SW2/1100; *barowes* ~ boar's grease SW2/1846; ~ *(gres) of hennes or (and) of gandres* chicken fat or (and) goose grease SW2/870, SW2/1055; *sow gres* sow's grease SW2/1847

greyne parice grains of paradise (seeds of *Aframomum meleguetta*) Plag/136n

gres(e) see **grece**

gromel gromwell (*Lithospermum officinale*) SW2/1739, SW2/1824, SW2/1832, SW2/1834

groundeswilly European groundsel (*Senecio vulgaris*) SW2/1087

gumme a botanical gum or resin SW2/1402; ~ *arabik (arabic)* gum from an acacia plant SW2/458, SW2/978, SW2/1517, ~ *of arabie* SW2/1560; ~ *of dragantia* tragacanth gum SW2/482; ~ *draganti albi* white tragacanth gum SW2/1555

gummi (= **gumme**): ~ *of arabie* gum from an acacia plant, gum arabic SW2/1556, ~ *arabicum* SW2/1504, SW2/1511, ~ *aromaticum* an aromatic gum SW2/1120, SW2/1121, SW2/1298, SW2/1398, SW2/1435, *gummy aramatici* SW2/1390; ~ *dragantum* tragacanth gum SW2/1504, SW2/1511, SW2/1520

hare a hare: *kunt of an* ~ the vulva of a hare SW2/1812; *matrice of an* ~

the uterus of a hare SW2/1812; *sowkyng* ~ a suckling hare SW2/398; *stones of an* ~ the testicles of a hare SW2/1814

hemlocks hemlock plants (*Conium maculatum*) SW2/1789

hemp hemp (*Cannabis sativa*) SW2/261; *inmost pillyng of* ~ inner layer of bark or skin of hemp SW2/1023

henbane henbane (*Hyoscyamus niger*) SW2/921

hennes hens SW2/389; *grece (gres) of* ~ chicken fat SW2/870, SW2/1055; ~ *rosted* roasted hens SW2/437; *juce of* ~ chicken broth Age/378

herbe a medicinal plant Age/1208, Age/1483, Bac/47, Bac/93, Bac/103, Bac/448, SW2/153, etc.; ~ *baume (bawme)* the balsam plant (*Commiphora opobalsamum*) SW2/240, SW2/1372, ~ *pat is clepid bawme* SW2/1092; ~ *benet* hemlock, herb bennet; cowbane; wood avens (*Conium maculatum; Cicuta virosa; Geum urbanum*) SW2/1854; ~ *John* St. John's wort (*Hypericum perforatum*) SW2/644; *herba portulaca* purslane (*Portulaca oleracea*) SW2/1674

hermodactilis ramsons, wild garlic; crow garlic; meadow saffron (*Allium ursinum; Allium vineale; Colchicum autumnale*) SW2/1841

hert a hart, the stag of the red deer (*Cervus elaphus*): *the boon pat gendryth in the herte of the* ~ , *hertis bon* gristle from the heart of a stag Bac/545, CHP/480; *guyrdel of an hertis skynne* a belt made of hart's skin SW2/1326; *hertis horn(es) (i)brent (wele ibrend)* burnt hart's horns SW2/394, SW2/400, SW2/450, SW2/569, SW2/728; *mary of an* ~ hart's marrow SW2/1055; *hertis tung* hart's-tongue fern (*Phyllitis scolopendrium*) SW2/1875

hevenly eeris see **eeris**

hockis mallows (*Malva sylvestris;
Althaea officinalis*) SW2/846,
SW2/1087, SW2/1282, SW2/1317,
SW2/1456, **hockes** SW2/354,
SW2/1073, SW2/1090, SW2/1093

holy-hocke the marsh mallow (*Althaea
officinalis*) SW2/1783

hony honey Age/70, Age/1023, Fle/50,
Bac/56, SW2/177, Plag/69, etc.

horn horn, antler: *hornes of a gote* goat's
horns SW2/1452; **hertis horn(es)**
see **hert**

hors see **bon**

houndes her hair of a dog SW2/568

yera electuaries, sweet compound medicines Age/1065

ierapigra a purgative based on aloes (poss. misread as prop. name)
Age/1054

Ynde, exiol aloes of lignum aloes of
India Age/1638

ipericon St. John's wort (*Hypericum perforatum*) SW2/884 [see also **theodoricon**]

ipia minor chickweed (*Stellaria media*)
SW2/722, SW2/1710

ypoquistides a medicine made from
rose-galls (*Cytinus hypocistis*)
SW2/331, SW2/486, **ypoquistidos**
SW2/462

iris Florentine iris; yellow flag
(*Iris florentina; Iris pseudacorus*)
SW2/687, SW2/1394, SW2/1598,
yris SW2/1344, SW2/1549, **yres**
SW2/677, SW2/678; *radix ~ (yris)*
iris root SW2/1591, SW2/1714

irn see **filynges of irn**

iroes Florentine iris; German iris (*Iris
florentina; Iris germanica*) SW2/1251

isop(e) hyssop (*Hyssopus officinalis*)
SW2/155, SW2/226, SW2/251,
SW2/578, SW2/611, SW2/631,
SW2/642, etc., **ysop(e)** CHP/165,
SW2/273

isopus (1) (= **isop[e]**) SW2/1345,
SW2/1592, SW2/1598

isopus (2) a stone used to ease childbirth, *iaspis* 'jasper' SW2/1339n

jusquimanus jusquiamus, henbane (*Hyoscyamus niger*): *folia jusquimani* leaves
of henbane SW2/1676, SW2/1688,
SW2/1707; *succus jusquimani* juice of
henbane SW2/1639

ivy ivy (*Hedera helix*) SW2/154,
SW2/869, SW2/1547

jacynct jacinth, a blue (rarely red
or purple) gemstone Age/341,
Age/349, **jacinct** CHP/480

jeate jet, a black organic gemstone
SW2/1738

juce juice or sap (of plants), or a liquid extract made by boiling herbs
SW2/348, SW2/507, etc., **juse**
SW2/463; *~ of hennes* chicken broth
Age/378; for the underlying herbs
of the following juices, see the entries for the individual plants: *~ of
archimesie* SW2/879, *~ (of) arthemesie* SW2/1121, SW2/1123; *~ of bleete*
Fle/167; *~ of borage* SW2/1462;
~ of centory SW2/1506; *~ of clotes*
SW2/723; *~ of daisy* SW2/351; *~
of diptayne* SW2/225, SW2/1294,
SW2/1316, SW2/1410; *~ of elfhame*
SW2/962; *~ of emablot* Age/1484; *~ of
iroes* SW2/1250; *~ of isope* SW2/225;
~ of leeke SW2/1316, SW2/1460;
~ of mersh SW2/1036; *~ of mylfoile*
SW2/436; *~ of mynt(e)* SW2/350,
SW2/396; *~ of moleyn* SW2/360;
~ of mugwede SW2/396, SW2/410,
SW2/1125, SW2/1332; *~ of nept*
SW2/1377; *~ of percely* SW2/1460;
~ of pervynke SW2/459; *~ of pety
morel* SW2/1024; *~ of plantayne*
*SW2/350, SW2/360, SW2/396,
SW2/417, SW2/436, etc., *~ of planteyne* SW2/451; *~ of popie* SW2/350;
~ of puliol roial SW2/954; *~ of purslane* SW2/1503; *juse of roses, ~ of rede
roses* SW2/463, SW2/487; *~ of rewe*
SW2/1128, SW2/1332, SW2/1377,

SW2/1397, ~ of rue SW2/1401; ~ of
sanguinarie (*sanguynarie*) SW2/470,
SW2/881; ~ of saturey SW2/1335;
~ of savayne SW2/1382; ~ of sither Age/1516; ~ of sloue SW2/464,
SW2/465; ~ of veruayne SW2/1310,
SW2/1315; ~ of violet *SW2/935; ~ of
the water of betayne Plag/397; ~ of wormode SW2/1413

iuniper juniper (*Juniperus communis*):
braunchis of ~ tree juniper branches Plag/118

juniperus (= iuniper) SW2/1107,
SW2/1301, SW2/1392, SW2/1602

jusquimanus alphabetized under *i*

kernel the inner meat of a fruit-stone
or nut SW2/1825, SW2/1834

ker-seede cress-seed SW2/760 [see
cres-seede, cresses]

kerslokis rocket; charlock, wild mustard (*Eruca agrestis*; *Sinapis arvensis*)
SW2/1495n [see **carlokes**]

kydes kids, young goats Age/771,
Age/1853, **kids** Age/1946

kiene, flessh of cows' flesh, beef
Age/1856

knowholme butcher's broom, knee hol-
ly (*Ruscus aculeatus*) SW2/238

kow mylke see **cow(es) mylke**

kunt the vulva SW2/1812

lacert, toorde of lizard dung Age/1638n

lactica lettuce (*Lactuca virosa*) SW2/287;
semen *lactuse* lettuce seed SW2/1638

lamb(es), flessh of lamb Age/771,
Age/1853, Age/1946

lang de boef bugloss, ox-tongue (*Anchusa arvensis*) Plag/146

lapdanum see **laudanum**

lapis a stone of medicinal value: ~ ambree amber or ambergris SW2/1641;
~ ematicis hematite SW2/378; ~ ematiste (*amatiste*) amethyst SW2/462,
SW2/492; ~ sulpicis an unidentified
stone SW2/1636; ~ tophasius topaz
SW2/1639

laudanum a botanical resin or
gum, derived from a plant of the
genus *Cistus* SW2/1078, **lapdanum**
Plag/123

laurer the laurel tree; spurge laurel (*Laurus nobilis*; *Daphne laureola*) Age/1573, Age/1575, Age/1637,
SW2/1871, **lorer** SW2/578; baies of
pe ~ laurel berries SW2/1829

lauriol spurge laurel (*Daphne laureola*)
SW2/1415

lauriola (= lauriol) SW2/1119

laurus (= laurer): *folia lauri* laurel
leaves SW2/1577, SW2/1605; cor-
tex lauri & eius bacce laurel bark and
berries SW2/1660; *bacce laure* laurel berries SW2/1695, buccarum lauriis SW2/1391

lavender lavender (*Lavandula officinalis*) SW2/262, SW2/641, SW2/715,
SW2/1577, SW2/1873, **lavendre**
SW2/920, **lauender** SW2/1865,
lauende SW2/808

lectuary see **electuarie**

leeke leek (*Allium porrum*) SW2/226,
SW2/931, SW2/1316, SW2/1461

leer see **water**

lepus hare: *pili leporis* hairs of a hare
SW2/1662, sanguis leporis hare's
blood SW2/1692

lether leather, used to hold medicines on the body SW2/1126, **lethir**
SW2/857

letuarie see **electuarie**

letuse lettuce (*Lactuca virosa*)
Age/2028, SW2/355, **letuze**
Age/526, SW2/1028

leveyned leavened, containing yeast
or some other leavening agent
Age/1852, Age/1946

levis leaves, foliage of a plant
Age/1208, Bac/536, SW2/173;
(rede) rose ~ (red) rose petals
SW2/805, SW2/990; for the identity
of the following types of leaves mentioned in the texts, see the entries
for the individual plants: ~ of the

herbe þat is clepid bawme SW2/1092;
~ *of bletis* Fle/96; ~ *of calamynt*
SW2/173, SW2/577; ~ *of chike-*
mete SW2/1738; *clote* ~ , ~ *of clot-*
is SW2/952, SW2/953; ~ *of costy*
SW2/260; *eldren* ~ SW2/1573; *fenel~*
SW2/250, SW2/1374; *folefoote* ~
SW2/1845; ~ *of isope, isope* ~ SW2/577,
SW2/1576; *ivy* ~ SW2/1547; *laurer*
(lorer) ~ SW2/1871, SW2/578, *lorel*
~ SW2/155, SW2/210, SW2/921,
SW2/1073, SW2/1726; ~ *of malues*
SW2/260; ~ *of marygoolde* SW2/1738;
~ *of mersh* SW2/406; ~ *of mershe-*
malowe SW2/260; ~ *of mugwede*
SW2/173; ~ *of nept* SW2/577; ~ *of net-*
til SW2/868; ~ *of origanum* SW2/173,
SW2/577; ~ *of pastinake* SW2/260;
~ *of peritorie* SW2/1738; *pollipodie*
~ SW2/154; ~ *of pulegij* SW2/577;
rewe ~ *dried,* ~ *of drie rewe* SW2/1297,
SW2/1433; ~ *(grene) of rosemary*
SW2/243, SW2/577; ~ *of savyne*
SW2/173; ~ *of savoray* SW2/577;
strawbury ~ SW2/1845; ~ *of *tym*
SW2/577;~ *of wielde mynt* SW2/1433;
~ *of woderove* SW2/1433
licium a powder made from the residue of evaporated plant juices
SW2/973 [see *MED,* s.v. *licium* n.]
lye the alkaline solution lye SW2/1033,
SW2/1034
lignum, lignea a medicinal wood: see
aloe(s), cassia
lilie lily (*Lilium* spp.) SW2/814,
SW2/1373, **lily** Age/1573; **water lil-**
ies (*Nymphaea* spp.) SW2/633; ~ *me-*
sue not identified SW2/1159
lilium (= **lilie**): *oleum liliorum* oil of lilies, oil in which lily flowers have
been heated SW2/1378
lyme birdlime (possibly made of mistletoe berries) SW2/994 [cf. *MED,*
s.v. *lim* n.(2), 3(a)]
lynices a bark-bearing plant Fle/161
lynse(e)de linseed, the seed of flax
(*Linum usitatissimum*) SW2/261,

SW2/365, SW2/404, SW2/1282,
SW2/1374, **lyneseede** SW2/1036;
mele (made) of ~ ground linseed
SW2/1032, SW2/1048
liquericia (= **liquorice**) SW2/1606
liquorice the dried root of the
plant *Glycyrrhiza glabra* SW2/241,
SW2/459
litarge lead monoxide SW2/1519;
~ *of gold* yellowish-red lead oxide
SW2/1558, *litargium aurei* SW2/994
[see *MED,* s.v. *litarge* n.]
liver see **pigge**
lof sugre sugar in loaf form SW2/244
lollium corn cockle; darnel (*Agrostem-*
ma githago; Lolium temulentum)
SW2/1646
lorel the laurel tree (*Laurus nobilis*)
SW2/155, SW2/205, SW2/210,
SW2/760, SW2/921, SW2/1073, etc.
[see also **laurer**]
lorer see **laurer**
loveache lovage (*Levisticum officina-*
le) SW2/611, SW2/840, SW2/922,
SW2/1824, **louache** SW2/1834
lupyne lupin (*Lupinus* spp.) Age/1565,
lupines SW2/199
lupinus (= **lupyne**) SW2/1296,
SW2/1391, SW2/1433, SW2/1606

macedonisum alexanders, horse-parsley (*Smyrnium olusatrum*) SW2/1607,
*macedonici SW2/1709
macis mace, the ground rind of
the nutmeg (*Myristica fragrans*)
SW2/1856, Plag/112, **mac-**
es SW2/476, SW2/651, *macis*
SW2/579, SW2/1394, SW2/1701,
SW2/1702
macon (= ?**macis**) SW2/441
mader madder (*Rubia tinctorum*)
**SW2/154, SW2/1434, SW2/1437,
madder SW2/179; *Inglissh* ~
?madder indigenous to England
SW2/1735; *litel* ~ poss. *rubia minor,*
cleavers (*Galium aparine*) SW2/238
[see *rubia*]

maioran marjoram; sweet marjoram (*Origanum vulgare; Majorana hortensis*) Age/1208

maythes stinking camomile (*Anthemis cotula*) SW2/743

mal error for *violarum* 'of violets' Age/2030n

malba see *malua*

malowe mallow; marsh mallow (*Malva agrestis; Althaea officinalis*): **malowes** SW2/1372, **malues** SW2/251, SW2/261, **white malues** SW2/1872; *water of malowes* water infused with mallow leaves SW2/1783

malua (= **malowe**) SW2/1644, *malbe* (= **malowes**) SW2/1588; *folia malue (maluarum)* mallow leaves SW2/1676, SW2/1677

maluesy(n) malmsey, a sweet white wine SW2/645, SW2/647, SW2/1299, **maluesyne** SW2/671

maratrum fennel (*Foeniculum vulgare*) SW2/1603

marciaton a medicinal ointment SW2/1054, SW2/1785

margarites pearls Age/1522, Bac/532, **margaritis** Age/352

mary bone marrow SW2/624; ~ *of a calf* calves' marrow SW2/982; ~ *of an hert* hart's marrow SW2/1055

marygoolde marigold (*Calendula officinalis*) SW2/1738

marubium white horehound; black horehound (*Marrubium vulgare; Ballota nigra*): *succus marubij* horehound sap or juice SW2/1653

mastik the resin from the tree *Pistacia lentiscus*, gum mastic Age/1054, Age/1566, SW2/394, SW2/439, SW2/720, SW2/728, SW2/807, etc., **mastic** SW2/416, SW2/1543; *oile of* ~ oil containing powdered mastic or derived from the fruit of the mastic tree SW2/814

mastix (= **mastik**) SW2/358, SW2/440, SW2/652, SW2/816, SW2/1518, SW2/1529

mawe the stomach, liver, and other abdominal organs: ~ *of a sowkyng hare or of a sowkyng calf* the liver or stomach of a suckling hare or calf SW2/398

mel honey SW2/288, SW2/1397, SW2/1597, SW2/1611, SW2/1661, SW2/1679, etc.

melancium black cumin, fennel flower (*Nigella arvensis*) SW2/1606

mele meal, flour: *beane* ~ bean meal Age/1565, SW2/960, SW2/1571; *barly* ~ barley flour SW2/488; *whete* ~ wheat flour SW2/1031, SW2/1046, SW2/1048, SW2/1099; ~ *(made) of lynseede (other of fenygreke)* ground linseed or fenugreek seed SW2/1032, SW2/1048

melilote honeysuckle, melilot; clover, trefoil (*Melilotus* spp.; *Trifolium* spp.) Fle/98

melons melons (*Cucumis melo*) Age/1867

menta mint (*Mentha* spp.) SW2/1684, SW2/1700

merche see **mersh**

mercurie (1) quicksilver Age/1020

mercurie (2) dog's mercury (*Mercurialis perennis*) Age/1079, **mercury** SW2/251

mersh wild celery, smallage (*Apium graveolens*) SW2/406, SW2/1036, SW2/1040, SW2/1052, ***merche*** SW2/172

mersh(e)-malow(e) marsh mallow (*Althaea officinalis*) Age/508, Age/515, SW2/261

mesue, lilie not identified SW2/1159

meth(e) mead *SW2/270, SW2/1060, SW2/1104, Plag/105

miced not identified SW2/241

mile millet 8Med/53

mylfoile milfoil, yarrow (*Achillea millefolium*) SW2/436, SW2/942

mylke milk SW2/388, SW2/1117, SW2/1840, **mylk** Age/378, **milk** Age/1003, Age/1517; *almaunde* ~ , ~ *of almaundis* almond milk SW2/379,

SW2/380, SW2/386, ~ *of a bicche med-led with hony* dog's milk mixed with honey SW2/1341; *cowes (cow, kow)* ~ , *cow milk* cow's milk SW2/387, SW2/973, SW2/980, Age/1214; *gotes (gotis)* ~ goat's milk SW2/380, SW2/405, SW2/855, SW2/1116, ~ *of a gote* SW2/386; *sheepis* ~ sheep's milk SW2/404; *milk sweete* fresh or sweetened milk Age/1566; *wommans* ~ woman's milk SW2/482, SW2/1056, SW2/1343, SW2/1530

millefolium (= **mylfoile**) SW2/1588

mynced gynger minced ginger Age/1914

mynt(e) mint (*Mentha* spp.) Fle/89, SW2/350, SW2/355, SW2/396, SW2/416, SW2/431, SW2/761, etc.; *rede myntis* ?water-mint (*Mentha aquatica*) SW2/1726

mirabolans myrabolan, a prune-like fruit (*Terminalia chebula*) Age/1073, Age/1105, Age/1111, Age/1113, Age/1520, **myrabolans** Age/1109; **blac myrabolans** black or indic myrabolan Age/1103; **myrabolans citryn** yellow myrabolan SW2/500 [see also **ebul, ebulis**]

mirra (= **myrre**) SW2/579, SW2/653, SW2/1595, SW2/1601, etc.

myrre myrrh (*Commiphora myrrha*) Age/1482, SW2/194, SW2/276, SW2/878, SW2/991, SW2/1076, SW2/1128, SW2/1136, Plag/165, etc., **myre** SW2/275, **mirre** SW2/1433; *trosciscy (trocisces, troscisses) of (the)* ~ , *trocisces of mirre* medicated lozenges containing myrrh SW2/1106, SW2/1295, SW2/1432, SW2/1725, *trocissis of* **murs** SW2/686

myrte the European myrtle (*Myrtus communis*) SW2/799, SW2/806

myrtief (*adj.*) based on or made from myrtle (*Myrtus communis*) Fle/99

myrtil the European myrtle as an ingredient in medical recipes [see *MED*, s.v. *mirtille* n.] SW2/486, SW2/492,

SW2/814, SW2/817, SW2/1507, SW2/1519, etc., **mirtil** SW2/458

myscelyn see **muscelyn**

moleyn(e) mullein (*Verbascum thapsus*) SW2/360, SW2/471, SW2/806, SW2/987, **molen** SW2/461

morel, pety black nightshade (*Solanum nigrum*) SW2/1024

mores mulberries, fruits of the mulberry tree (*Morus nigra*) Age/1867

morien not identified SW2/1119

moton mutton SW2/388

mountaign origanum see **origanum**

mo(u)ntayne, puliol see **puliol**

mugwede mugwort (*Artemisia vulgaris*) SW2/155, SW2/158, SW2/173, SW2/182, SW2/239, SW2/259, SW2/396, etc., **mugwed** SW2/687

mugwort mugwort (*Artemisia vulgaris*) SW2/1283, SW2/1729, SW2/1732, SW2/1735

mulsa (= **mulso**) SW2/1659, *SW2/1675

mulso a honey drink, mead Age/61, Age/65, Age/69, Age/70, **mulse** Age/1517, **muls** Bac/495

mumie mumia, a resinous exudate from embalmed bodies *SW2/394, SW2/447

murs see **myrre**

murum see *fimus*

muscat see **noote**

muscata, gallia see **galle muste**

muscatelinos heavy sweet wines, muscatels Plag/139

muscelyn of a medicinal oil: compounded with musk and other spices SW2/1775, **myscelyn** SW2/268, **muscelon** SW2/1159, **muschilyng** SW2/639, **mushilyng** SW2/636

muscelon, mus(c)hilyng see **muscelyn**

muscillage a thick, sticky substance derived from various plants SW2/363, SW2/365, SW2/481, SW2/1524, etc.

muscus (= **musk[e]**) Plag/111; ~ *bonus* good musk SW2/654

musk(e) a glandular secretion of male musk deer (*Moschus moschifer-*

us) Age/993, Age/994, Age/1180, Age/1449, Age/2014, SW2/586, SW2/654, etc.

mustard the mustard plant (*Sinapis* spp.; *Brassica* spp.) or its seed SW2/161; **grete ~** ?black mustard (*Brassica nigra*) SW2/1868

muste, *mustice* see **galle muste**

narde nard, spikenard, an ointment derived from *Nardostachys jatamansi* Fle/165, *nardus* SW2/441, SW2/652, SW2/1601, SW2/1701, *SW2/1395

nastarcium garden cress (*Lepidium sativum*) SW2/1583

nemyfore, floures of flowers of the white or yellow water-lily (*Nymphaea alba; Nuphar lutea*) Plag/139

nep(i)ta (= **nept**) SW2/1598, SW2/1650; *succus nepitus* catnip juice SW2/1612

nept catnip, cat-mint (*Nepeta cataria*) SW2/156, *SW2/240, SW2/274, SW2/577, SW2/1377, SW2/1395, SW2/1468, etc.

nettil nettle (*Urtica* spp.; *Lamium* spp.) SW2/868, SW2/871; **rede nettlis** red dead-nettles (*Lamium purpureum*) SW2/1874

nigell black cumin (*Nigella sativa*) Fle/166, ***nigella** Age/1186

nymphee the white or yellow water-lily (*Nymphaea alba; Nuphar lutea*): *water of* ~ water infused with water-lilies 8Med/42

no(o)te a nut Age/1868, SW2/625; *nootis muscat* nutmegs (*Myristica fragrans*) Age/2054, Age/2069; *oile of notes* nut oil SW2/718

notemuges nutmegs (*Myristica fragrans*) SW2/752, SW2/1075, SW2/1855, Plag/112, **nootemugis** Age/1449

nuchium ceresorum pith of cherries, ?kernels of cherry stones SW2/1392 [cf. **cheri stones kernels**]

nux cipressi see **cipres(se)**

oignement see **oynement**

oile a medicinal oil (depending on the source of the oil, it may be prepared either by pressing or as an infusion of the source substance in olive oil) Age/64, Age/66, Age/325, Age/1193, SW2/583, etc.; *~ benedictum* a medicinal oil made with brick fragments Age/1195n; *~ comune* olive oil SW2/577, SW2/1035, SW2/1171; *drastis of ~* dregs of an oil SW2/873; *~ of lilie* oil in which lily flowers have been heated SW2/814; *~ of mastik* oil containing powdered mastic or derived from the fruit of the mastic tree SW2/814; *mete ~* vegetable oil SW2/205, SW2/222, SW2/640, SW2/1251; *~ muscelyn* an oil containing musk and other spices SW2/1775, *~ myscelyn* SW2/268, *~ muscelon* SW2/1159, *~ mus(c)hilyng* SW2/635, SW2/639; *~ of notes* nut oil SW2/718; *~ of roses* oil in which rose petals have been heated SW2/221, SW2/564, etc. *~ of rosis* SW2/824, SW2/934, *hote ~ of rosen* SW2/1476, *~ of rose* Age/477; *~ sambuc* elder-flower oil Age/1010. For the essential ingredients of the following oils, see the entries for the source of the oil: *~ of baie* SW2/564, SW2/1459, *~ de baye* SW2/1094; *~ balsamum* Age/1194, *~ of bawme* Age/1388, Age/1488, *~ of bawme myxt with ~ laurer* Age/1575; *~ of *benen and peson* SW2/626; *~ of ipie minoris* SW2/722; *~ of isope* SW2/1249; *~ of laurer* Age/1573, *~ laurer* Age/1575, Age/1637, *~ of lorel* SW2/205, SW2/1091; *~ of lilie mesue* SW2/1159; *~ of myntis* SW2/414; *~ myrtief, ~ of myrtils* Fle/99, SW2/1512; *~ of olive* Age/1189, SW2/1046; *~ of puliol* SW2/635, SW2/753, SW2/1084, SW2/1091, SW2/1158, SW2/1775, SW2/1785; *~ of violet* SW2/934, SW2/1026

oynement an ointment, a salve Age/241, Age/1481, Age/1482, Age/1961, *SW2/596, SW2/735,

SW2/812, SW2/1382, etc., **oignement** Age/1486, Age/1489,
Age/1491, Age/1571, Bac/504, **oyntement** SW2/718; *oignement cesaryne*
see **cesaryne, oignement**
oynon onion (*Allium cepa*) Age/1493,
SW2/888
oke oak (*Quercus* spp.) SW2/369,
SW2/430, SW2/431; *myddil ryndes
of an* ~ the inner bark of an oak
SW2/883; ~ *tree that no lyme comyth
nygh* ?oak on which no mistletoe
grows SW2/994
oken ryndes oak bark SW2/370
oleum oil SW2/886, SW2/1256,
SW2/1627; ~ *benedictum* a medicinal oil SW2/1391, SW2/1584 [see
also **oile benedictum**]; ~ *bodegaryni*
?oil made from or infused with flowers or bedegars (galls) from rosebushes or eglantines SW2/1519;
~ *commune* olive oil SW2/1672,
SW2/1674; ~ *liliorum* oil of lilies, oil
in which lily flowers have been heated SW2/1378; ~ *rosarum* oil of roses,
oil in which rose petals have been
heated SW2/1682, SW2/1689
olibanum frankincense Fle/162,
SW2/1077, SW2/1544, **olibany** SW2/807, *olibanum* SW2/394,
SW2/493, SW2/817, SW2/821,
SW2/1513, SW2/1519, SW2/1700;
white ~ ?a paste of frankincense
and water Plag/123 [see *MED*, s.v.
olibane n.]
olive the European olive (*Olea eu-
ropaea*): Age/1189, Age/1192,
SW2/1046, **olyves** Age/858
oote an oat (as a measure of weight;
Avena fatua) Age/1213; **otis** oats
8Med/53; *wyne of the* ~ an alcoholic
drink based on oats Age/760
opibalsamy the sap of the balsam
plant (*Commiphora opobalsamum*)
SW2/1289, **opobalsami**
SW2/1330

opie opium Fle/165
opopanak a gum derived from the
juice of plants in the genus *Opopanax* SW2/1435
opopanax (= **opopanak**) SW2/1298,
*SW2/1390, SW2/1584
ordium barley (*Hordeum* spp.)
SW2/1675
origanum marjoram; pennyroyal;
wild thyme (*Origanum vulgare; Mentha pulegium; Thymus serpyllum*)
SW2/154, SW2/174, SW2/578,
SW2/643, SW2/714, SW2/920,
SW2/955, etc.; *origanum* SW2/875,
SW2/1395, SW2/1414, SW2/1457,
etc.; *mountaign* ~ a wild form of marjoram, etc. SW2/1470
os de corde cerui gristle in the heart of a
stag SW2/1699 [see Headnotes to
chap. 6, 140–41, and chap. 9, 339–40]
osey wyne a sweet wine SW2/1736
oua eggs: *albedo ouorum* egg whites
SW2/1683; *vitelli ouorum* egg yolks
SW2/1688
oxdirt ox dung SW2/744
oximel a drink of vinegar and honey
SW2/712

panchristum an electuary used to relieve retention of the menses, typically containing opium, sugar,
ginger, henbane, etc. *SW2/234,
SW2/270 [cf. Berg 1917, 113-15]
papauer albus & niger varieties of opium poppy (*Papaver somniferum*)
SW2/458
paradisus see *grana, grane*
paris a medicine for jaundiced urine
SW2/1653
partriche a partridge (*Perdix perdix*):
flessh of ~ partridge meat Age/1854,
flessh of partriches (**pertriches**)
SW2/622, Age/771; *partriches irosted*
roasted partridges SW2/437
pastinake parsnip (*Pastinaca sativa*)
SW2/260, SW2/626

paulyni, powder of ?powder made from the compound medicine *Paulinum* SW2/684 [see Green 2001, 197-98]

peleter common pellitory; pellitory of the wall (*Parietaria officinalis; Parietaria diffusa*) SW2/1415; ~ (*peletir*) *of Spayne* pellitory of Spain (*Anacyclus pyrethrum*) SW2/201, SW2/217, SW2/1383, SW2/1406, SW2/1854; *litel* ~ little pellitory, ?serpillum, ?pellitory of Spain (*Anacyclus pyrethrum*) [see Hunt 1989, 236-37] SW2/217 [see also **peritory**]

pelow(e) a pillow containing herbs, on which a patient sits in a medicinal bath SW2/257, SW2/1717

penthaphilon creeping cinquefoil (*Potentilla reptans*) SW2/431; *radix pentafilon* cinquefoil root SW2/1666

peper pepper (*Piper* spp.) Age/1526, Age/2064, SW2/161, SW2/1335, Plag/136, **pepir** SW2/593, SW2/599, Plag/148; *long* ~ long pepper (*Piper longum*) SW2/1857; **pepercornes** peppercorns SW2/1740

percely parsley (*Petroselinum crispum*) SW2/172, SW2/262, SW2/687, SW2/922, SW2/942, SW2/948, SW2/1040, etc.

peritory common pellitory; pellitory of the wall (*Parietaria officinalis; Parietaria diffusa*) SW2/840, SW2/846, SW2/848, SW2/1283, SW2/1374, SW2/1468, SW2/1730, **peritorie** SW2/1738, **pereter** Fle/166

persenepe of the fielde wild parsnip (*Pastinaca sativa*) SW2/1733

persiles peaches (*Prunus persica*) Age/1867

pertriches see **partriche**

pertulake purslane (*Portulaca oleracea*) SW2/1027

pervinca periwinkle (*Vinca* spp.) SW2/471, **pervynke** SW2/460

pesen peas (*Pisum sativum*) SW2/862, **peson** SW2/626

petrolion petroleum SW2/575

petrosilium (= **percely**): *semen petrosilij* parsley seed SW2/1392

peusadanum hog's fennel (*Peucedanum officinale*) SW2/574, SW2/598

phelipendula dropwort; meadow-sweet (*Filipendula vulgaris; Filipendula ulmaria*) SW2/1825, SW2/1832

pic(c)he pitch, wood tar Age/1493, SW2/729, *SW2/773, SW2/774, SW2/856, SW2/1792

pigge piglet: *liver of a ~ that is delivered of sow alon* liver of a young pig born without litter-mates SW2/1818

pigra a purgative based on aloes Age/1056, Age/1059, Age/1060, Age/1061, Age/1072; ~ *frigida cophyns* a cold purgative associated with Copho of Salerno Plag/144

pili leporis hair of a hare SW2/1662

pillyng a layer or peeling (of inner bark) SW2/1023

pillule (= **pillules**) SW2/1586; ~ *rosarum* medicinal pills containing roses or rose derivatives Plag/158

pillules medicinal pills Age/1054, Plag/164, Plag/166, Plag/167

pilosella, aqua water of hawkweed (*Hieracium pilosella*) SW2/1657

pyment spiced wine SW2/246

pimpernel scarlet pimpernel; burnet saxifrage; great burnet (*Anagallis arvensis; Pimpinella saxifraga; Sanguisorba officinalis*) SW2/1693, **pympernel** Plag/284, Plag/298, Plag/382

pyne applis pine cones, fruits of the pine [L. *poma pini*] Age/1114

pionea (= **piony**) SW2/1392, SW2/1610

piony peony (*Paeonia* spp.) SW2/872, SW2/1736

piper pepper (*Piper* spp.) SW2/1659; ~ *nigrum* black pepper (*Piper nigrum*) SW2/1608, SW2/1703; ~ *lon-*

gum long pepper (*Piper longum*)
SW2/1703

piretrum pellitory of Spain (*Anacyclus pyrethrum*) SW2/1582, SW2/1607, **pyretrum** SW2/594

plantayne great plantain (*Plantago major*) *SW2/350, SW2/354, SW2/356, SW2/360, SW2/396, SW2/436, SW2/1531, etc., **planteyne** SW2/332, SW2/452; *rynde of ~* outer bark or skin of the plantain SW2/429; *succus ~* plantain juice or sap SW2/377; *water of ~* water infused with plantain leaves SW2/438

plicus a kind of spinach or beet (*Atriplex hortensis; Beta vulgaris*) Age/1908n

pliris an electuary Plag/111 [see Latham 1980, s.v.]

plomtre, blac a plum tree; a blackthorn or sloe tree (*Prunus domestica; Prunus spinosa*) SW2/429

plume see **alum of plume**

polipodium (= pol[l]ipodie) SW2/1374, SW2/1392, SW2/1578

politricum maidenhair fern (*Adiantum capillus-veneris*) SW2/1686

pol(l)ipodie the fern polypody; oak fern (*Polypodium vulgare; Thelypteris dropteris*) SW2/154, SW2/158, SW2/183

pome d'oranges oranges Plag/143

pomegarnad pomegranate (*Punica granatum*) SW2/469, **pomegarnettis** Plag/143

pomes citrinis condutes prepared citrus fruits, citron Plag/143

pomum ambre a perforated ball containing spices and perfumes, esp. ambergris Plag/115n [see *MED*, s.v. *pomendambre* n.]

popie the opium poppy (*Papaver somniferum*) Age/526, SW2/350; *white ~* a variety of poppy with white flowers SW2/978

populus the poplar tree (*Populus* spp.) SW2/1629

porcinas see *sotulares porcinas*

porrum leek (*Allium porrum*): *folia porry* leaves of leeks SW2/1588; *semen porri* leek seed SW2/1595; *succus porri (porry)* leek juice SW2/1586, SW2/1645

portulaca, herba purslane (*Portulaca oleracea*) SW2/1674

powder a finely ground or pulverized form of a solid substance Age/936, Age/2018, SW2/331, SW2/1120, SW2/1562, Plag/121, etc.; for the content of the following powders, see the entries for the material powdered: *~ of anathasia (anathasie)* SW2/464, SW2/465, SW2/505; *~ of anete* SW2/863; *~ of bay, of baies of þe laurer* SW2/760, SW2/1829; *~ of canel* SW2/775, SW2/1759; *~ of carui* SW2/863; *~ of castory (castorie)* SW2/573, SW2/593, SW2/1334, SW2/1867; *~ of cloves* SW2/1471, SW2/1475; *~ of colloquintide* SW2/1129; *~ of comyn* SW2/736, SW2/863, SW2/889; *~ of confery* SW2/1759, *~ of the rote of confery* SW2/775; *~ of coral that is fyne and right rede* SW2/475; *~ of cresses* SW2/729; *~ of egipsium ibrend* SW2/368; *~ of ey-shellis ibrent* SW2/450; *~ of encence* SW2/720, SW2/728; *~ of euforby (euforbie)* SW2/593, SW2/1417; *~ of the flour of rise* SW2/469; *~ of galangale* SW2/863; *~ of gallis that men make ynk of* SW2/352; *~ of hertis hornes ibrent and of ey-shellis ibrent* SW2/450, etc.; *~ of jeate* SW2/1738; *~ of ker-seede* SW2/760; *~ of lorel* SW2/760; *~ of mastik (mastic)* SW2/720, SW2/1543, etc.; *~ of oke tree that no lyme comyth nygh* SW2/993; *~ of paulyni* SW2/684; *~ of pepir (peper)* SW2/593, SW2/1334; *~ of pety consowde* SW2/1759; *~ of pomegarnad* SW2/469; *~ of psilium ibrend* SW2/368; *~ of pyretrum* SW2/593; *~ of scanomy* SW2/198; *~ of wield myntis* SW2/760; *~ of zedewale* SW2/863

powdred ground to a powder, finely ground: *ciminum* ~ finely ground
cumin SW2/886; *myrre* ~ finely
ground myrrh SW2/1128
poundgarnatis pomegranates (*Punica
granatum*) Age/858
primerol the common primrose, cow-
slip (*Primula veris*) SW2/1373,
SW2/1844, **prymerols** SW2/1873,
primerollis SW2/1866
prymeroses common primroses, cowslips (*Primula veris*) SW2/715
propoleos a tree resin collected by bees
and found in bee hives Age/1574
prunes plums or prunes, the fresh
or dried fruit of *Prunus domestica*
SW2/625
psidie the rind of pomegranate or
bark of the pomegranate tree (*Punica granatum*) SW2/369, SW2/798,
SW2/822, **psidia** SW2/331, *psidium*
SW2/1699
psilium fleawort (*Plantago indica*)
SW2/365, SW2/368, SW2/481, *psilium* SW2/363, SW2/574
ptisana a tisane, barley water
SW2/1667
pulegium (= **puliol**) SW2/578,
SW2/1610, SW2/1652, SW2/1694
puliol pennyroyal; wild thyme (*Mentha pulegium; Thymus serpyllum*)
SW2/240, SW2/635, SW2/753,
SW2/1084, SW2/1091, SW2/1158,
SW2/1297n, etc., **puliole** SW2/155,
pulliol SW2/1414; ~ *mo(u)ntayne* wild
thyme (also pennyroyal) SW2/920,
SW2/1730, SW2/1866; ~ *roial* pennyroyal (also wild thyme) SW2/210,
SW2/641, SW2/920, SW2/954,
SW2/1072, SW2/1469, SW2/1866
pulpe pulp or pith of a plant: ~ *of cassia
fistula* pulp of cassia fistula (*Cinnamomum cassia*) *SW2/503; *pulpa coloquintide* pulp of colocynth (*Citrullus
colocynthis*) SW2/1119
*puluis *dominicus ?some kind of
medicinal powder SW2/1841

purslane purslane, a salad herb (*Portulaca oleracea*) Age/2028, SW2/355,
SW2/1503

quaile the European quail (*Coturnix coturnix*): *flessh of* ~ quail meat
SW2/622
quik-siluer mercury Age/1020, **quike-
silver** SW2/1250, **quike-siluer**
SW2/1411
quynces fruits of the quince tree (*Cydonia oblonga*) SW2/482

raddish root: ~ *of fenel, percely, dawke, and
merche the roots of fennel, parsley,
wild carrot, and wild celery SW2/172
raddissh radish (*Raphanus sativus*)
SW2/179, SW2/1041, SW2/1872,
radissh SW2/1831
radix the root, rootstock, or rhyzome
of a plant: ~ *callium* root of cabbages
SW2/1683; ~ *caparis* root
of the honeysuckle or the caper
bush SW2/1611; ~ **elleboris* root of
hellebore SW2/1649; ~ *iris (yris)* iris
root SW2/1591, SW2/1714; ~ *pentafilon* cinquefoil root SW2/1666;
~ **rafani* radish root, a radish
SW2/1665
*rafanus radish (*Raphanus sativus*): *radix *rafani* radish root, a radish
SW2/1665
rapes turnips; rapes; radishes (*Brassica
rapa; Brassica napus; Raphanus sativus*) SW2/626, **rapis** SW2/849
raspaice a sweet wine SW2/809
rasura emboris ivory shavings
SW2/1654
reyne water rain water SW2/438
reiso(u)ns raisins SW2/242, SW2/1049
reptil a reptile Bac/518, Bac/556
rere eg a soft-boiled egg Age/2090,
rere egges Fle/135
resta bouis restharrow (*Ononis repens*)
8Med/9 [cf. **rost bones**]
reubarbium (= **rubarbe**) SW2/501,
**SW2/1395, SW2/1583

rewe rue; meadow rue; lesser meadow rue (*Ruta graveolens; Thalictrum flavum; Thalictrum minus*) SW2/195, SW2/273, SW2/631, SW2/643, SW2/1128, SW2/1297, SW2/1377, SW2/1434, etc.; *plaster of ~* a salve based on rue SW2/1051

ribwort ribwort, English plantain (*Plantago lanceolata*) SW2/431

rynde bark, outer husk SW2/78; *~ of assh* bark of the European ash tree (*Fraxinus excelsior*) SW2/431; *~ of the blac plomtre* plum-tree or blackthorn bark SW2/429; *oken ryndes* oak bark SW2/370; *~ of plantayne* bark or outer skin of the great plantain SW2/429; *~ of roses* bark of rose bushes SW2/429; *myddil ~* inner bark SW2/342, SW2/883

rise rice: *powder of flour of ~* finely ground rice flour SW2/469

ro. camphorie ?camphorated roses CHP/479

romanici see **wyne**

ro(o)te root, rootstock, or rhizome of a plant; for the identities of the following roots, see the entries for the plant in question: *~ of attory* SW2/207; *~ of ciperi* SW2/239; *~ of confery* SW2/775; *~ of enula campana* SW2/336; *~ of yres* SW2/677; *~ of lupines* SW2/199; *mersh-malow ~* Age/508; *~ of peletir of Spayne* SW2/201; *~ of smalache* SW2/200;

ro(o)tes, ro(o)tis: *~ of affadil* SW2/1049; *~ of alisaunder* SW2/1832; *~ of bistorte* SW2/798, *SW2/806, SW2/814; *~ of cost* SW2/1288, SW2/1290; *~ of diptayne* SW2/1383; *~ of dragaunce* SW2/406; *egremoyne with his ~* SW2/1142; *fenel ~*, *~ of fenel* SW2/1040, SW2/1831; *~ of gladen (gladyn)* SW2/273, SW2/1733; *~ of gromel* SW2/1832; *yres ~*, *~ of yris* SW2/678, SW2/1549; *~ of knowholme* SW2/238; *~ of lily* Age/1573; *~ of litel mader* SW2/238; *~ of moleyn*

SW2/806; *~ of mugwede* SW2/1290; *~ of percely, percely ~* SW2/947, SW2/1576, SW2/1732, SW2/1831; *~ of persenepe of the fielde* SW2/1733; *~ of phelipendula* SW2/1825, SW2/1832; *~ of radissh* SW2/1831; *~ of rede dockes* SW2/1549; *~ of rewe* SW2/273; *~ of savayne* SW2/273; *~ of savery* SW2/273; *~ of saxfrage* SW2/1832; *~ of smalache* SW2/1831; *sperage ~* SW2/239; *~ of stanmarche* SW2/947; *~ of vynes* SW2/208

rose a rose plant or flower (*Rosa* spp.) Age/1171, Plag/138; *juse of roses, juce of rede roses* a liquid extract of rose petals produced by boiling them SW2/463, SW2/487; *(rede) ~ levis* (red) rose petals SW2/805, SW2/990; *oile of roses (rosis)* oil of roses, oil in which rose petals have been heated SW2/221, SW2/564, SW2/824, etc., *oile of rosen* SW2/1476; *rynde of roses* bark of rose bushes SW2/429; *~ water* rose water, water in which rose petals have been infused Age/1010, SW2/463, SW2/1520, 8Med/42, 8Med/45, *water of roses (rosis)* SW2/438, SW2/440, SW2/487, Plag/156, etc.

rose rose plants or flowers (*Rosa* spp.) SW2/441; *aqua rosarum* rose water SW2/1519, SW2/1704; *conserua rosarum* conserve of roses SW2/359; *oleum rosarum* oil of roses, oil in which rose petals have been heated SW2/1682, SW2/1689; *pillule rosarum* medicinal pills containing roses Plag/158; *rose rubee* red roses SW2/1703; *succus rosarum* a liquid extract of rose petals produced by boiling them SW2/502, SW2/971; *sucrum rosarum, zuccarum rosarum* roset sugar, sugar mixed with macerated rose petals SW2/733, SW2/392, etc.; *water of rosarum zuccarum* ?dissolved roset sugar SW2/442

rosemary rosemary (*Rosmarinus offici-nalis*) Bac/534, SW2/154, SW2/243, SW2/577, SW2/641, SW2/1577, SW2/1726, SW2/1865, **rosemaryn** SW2/264, SW2/1469, *rose marinus* SW2/1591

roset see **zucre roset**

rost bones error for *resta bouis*, restharrow (*Ononis repens; Peucedanum offici-nale*) SW2/461, SW2/471

rote see **ro(o)te**

rotunda see **aristologia**

rubarbe rhubarb (*Rheum rhaponti-cum*) Age/1066, SW2/348, **ruberbe** Age/1068

rubia rubia maior, madder; *rubia mi-nor*, cleavers (*Rubia tinctorum; Gali-um aparine*) SW2/1396, SW2/1598, SW2/1694, SW2/1700, SW2/1709

rubias red sandalwood Plag/139

rue rue; meadow rue; lesser meadow rue (*Ruta graveolens; Thalictrum fla-vum; Thalictrum minus*) SW2/1043, SW2/1401, Plag/69

ruta (= **rewe, rue**) SW2/1345, SW2/1394, SW2/1578, SW2/1642, SW2/1694; *folia rute* ruc leaves SW2/1707; *semen rute* rue seed SW2/1608; *succus rute* rue sap or juice SW2/1396, SW2/1651

saf(f)ron the herb or the spice saf-fron; bastard saffron (*Crocus sati-vus; Carthamus tinctorius*) Age/993, Age/1278, Age/1526, Age/2015, SW2/305, SW2/476, Plag/165, etc., **safroun** Age/1180

salatry black nightshade; deadly night-shade (*Solanum nigrum; Atropa bella-donna*) SW2/1503

sal-gemme rock salt SW2/617

salgia (= **sauge**) SW2/1709

salix the willow tree (*Salix* spp.): *flos sal-icis* willow flower SW2/1629; *semen salicis* willow seed SW2/1641

sal-nitri prob. sodium carbonate SW2/617

salt salt SW2/1454, Plag/69; ~ *water* SW2/618; *vynegre and* ~ SW2/590, SW2/1329

sambuc the European elder (*Sambucus nigra*): *oile* ~ elder-flower oil Age/1010; *water of* ~ water infused with elder flowers Age/1010

sambucus (= **sambuc**) 8Med/19

sambus (= **sambuc**) Age/1080

sandal white sandalwood; red sandal-wood (*Santalum album; Pterocarpus santalinus*): iij ~ triasandal, a com-pound medicine containing three kinds of sandalwood CHP/479 [see **triasandis**]

sandalus (= **sandal**) SW2/1694, SW2/1699, Plag/139

sandragon the spice dragon's-blood, the sap of the dragon tree (*Dra-co dracaena*) SW2/357, SW2/416, SW2/447, SW2/457, SW2/994, SW2/1792, **sandragan** SW2/1507, SW2/1558, **sandragoun** SW2/369

sanguinarie shepherd's purse; knot-grass (*Capsella bursa-pastoris; Po-lygonum aviculare*) SW2/883, **san-guinary** SW2/882, **sanguynarie** SW2/470

sanguis blood: ~ *draconis* (= **sandrag-on**) SW2/1518; ~ *galli* rooster's blood SW2/1637; ~ *leporis* hare's blood SW2/1692

sarcocol gum sarcocolla; white bryony; agrimony (*Astragalus fasciculifolius; Bryonia dioica; Agrimonia eupatoria*) SW2/1528, **sarcocolla** SW2/1585

saturey summer savory; winter savory (*Satureia hortensis; Satureia montana*) SW2/879, SW2/1335

satureia (= **saturey**) SW2/1345, SW2/1592, SW2/1598

sauge sage; wood sage (*Salvia officina-lis; Teucrium scorodonia*) SW2/643, SW2/715, SW2/717, SW2/1855, SW2/1865, SW2/1877; **wield(e)** ~ wood sage SW2/942, SW2/1844, SW2/1865

saundres white sandalwood; red sandalwood (*Santalum album; Pterocarpus santalinus*) SW2/485

savayne savin; ?dwarf elder (*Juniperus sabina; Sambucus ebulus*) SW2/273, SW2/684, SW2/849, SW2/876, SW2/1137, SW2/1383, SW2/1437, SW2/1871, **saveyne** SW2/209, SW2/240, **sauayne** SW2/1248, SW2/1414, SW2/1735, **savyne** SW2/154, SW2/174, SW2/182, SW2/195, **sawine** SW2/1394

sauine (= **savayne**) SW2/1344, SW2/1609

saverey summer savory; winter savory (*Satureia hortensis; Satureia montana*) SW2/251, SW2/688, SW2/920, SW2/957, SW2/1414, SW2/1437, **saveray** SW2/1468, **savery** SW2/273, **savoray** SW2/578, SW2/1411, **savorey** SW2/642, **savory** SW2/260, **saueray** SW2/1577

sauine, savyne, sawine see **savayne**

saxfrage saxifrage; burnet saxifrage; spleenwort (*Saxifraga* spp.; *Pimpinella saxifraga; Asplenium* spp.) SW2/1824, SW2/1832, SW2/1834, **saxifrage** SW2/1086

scabious field scabious; small scabious; devil's-bit scabious; greater or lesser knapweed; elecampane (*Knautia arvensis; Scabiosa columbaria; Succisa pratensis; Centaurea iacea/scabiosa; Inula helenium*) Plag/285, Plag/298, Plag/382

scamone scammony (*Convulvulus scammonia*) SW2/1383, **scamony** SW2/1406, **scanomy** SW2/198

scarliol prickly lettuce; sow-thistle (*Lactuca serriola; Sonchus oleraceus*) SW2/949

seede (1) the seed or seeds of plants; for the identities of the following medicinal seeds mentioned in the texts above, see the entries for the individual plants: *alisaunder* ~

SW2/1835; *anyse (anise)* ~ SW2/274, SW2/948; *carewey* ~ SW2/1834, *caruie* ~ SW2/454; ~ *of ceremountayne* SW2/241; *cres-seede* SW2/840; *fenel* ~ SW2/262, SW2/274, SW2/839, etc.; *gromel* ~ SW2/1834; *hemp* ~ SW2/261; *ker-seede* SW2/760; *lavender* ~ SW2/262; *louache* ~ SW2/1834; *nettil* ~ SW2/871; *percely* ~ SW2/262, SW2/687, SW2/1833; *saxfrage* ~ SW2/1834; *smalache* ~ SW2/1833; ~ *of white popie* SW2/978;

seedis: SW2/276, SW2/1823, 8Med/58; ~ *of careway* SW2/1823; ~ *of columbyne* SW2/1739; ~ *of fenel* SW2/1823; ~ *of gromel* SW2/1739, SW2/1823; ~ *of letuse* Age/2028; ~ *of loveache* SW2/1823; ~ *of myrtil(s)* SW2/817, SW2/1507; ~ *of percely* SW2/1823; *percely and mersh with their* ~ SW2/1040; ~ *of purslane* Age/2028; ~ *of quynces* SW2/482; ~ *of saxfrage* SW2/1823; ~ *of smalache* SW2/1823; ~ *of stanmarche* SW2/1823; *duratief* ~ ?long lasting seeds, ?error for *duretik* ('diuretic') ~ SW2/1436

seede (2): ~ *of a beest that is cald castory* secretions of the perineal gland of the beaver SW2/1856 [cf. **castory**]

Seynt John worte see **worte, Seynt John**

semen (= **seede** [1]): ~ *acedule* wild garlic seed SW2/1698; **amomi* ~ poppy or cardamom seed, or grains of paradise SW2/1602; ~ *anisi* aniseed SW2/1582; ~ *berberis* barberry seed SW2/1698; ~ *cicute* hemlock seed SW2/1582; ~ *coste* ?ribwort or ?costmary seed SW2/1698; ~ *lactuse* lettuce seed SW2/1638; ~ *petrosilij* parsley seed SW2/1392; ~ *porri* leek seed SW2/1595; ~ *rute* rue seed SW2/1608; ~ *salicis* willow seed SW2/1641

sene powdered senna leaves or pods (*Cassia acutifolia; Cassia augustifolia*) SW2/348, SW2/1582; *frenssh* ~

French senna SW2/1856; *folia cene* senna leaves SW2/1390

serapin the gum of a plant related to galbanum (prob. *Ferula persica*) SW2/1298

serapinum (= serapin) SW2/1390, SW2/1399, *serepinum* SW2/798, *serapium* SW2/1434, SW2/1583

sermyny ?corruption of *cinnamoni* SW2/1297n

serpent a serpent, a snake (used in medicinal preparations) Age/1361, Age/2055, Bac/547, etc.; *serpentis flessh, flessh of serpentis* snake meat Age/75, Age/1423

seruicia ale or beer SW2/1654, SW2/1710

shavyng a shaving or scraping SW2/578, SW2/642

sheepe a sheep SW2/726, SW2/738; *sheepes dirt* sheep dung SW2/855; *sheepis mylke* sheep milk SW2/404; *sheepis talow* sheep tallow SW2/1542

shone shoes SW2/570

sigillata sce **terra sigillata**

silken threde silk thread (used for suturing) SW2/772, SW2/1755

siluer silver Age/348

simphite comfrey (*Symphytum officinale*) SW2/370

sinopide mustard Fle/98

sirie, flessh of the flesh of a viper, snake meat [L. *carnes tyrie*] Age/1405n, *flessh of cirus* Age/2054

sirup a thick liquid, usually sweet, often used as a base for medicines SW2/236, SW2/237, SW2/247, SW2/254, **syrup** Age/1913, Age/2017, **syrub** SW2/244, **surip(e)** Plag/166, SW2/1039

syrus a viper [L. *tirus*] Age/1366, **cirus** Age/2055

sither chick-pea [L. *cicereum*] (*Cicer arietinum*), poss. understood as a form of *sider* 'cider' Age/1516n

skynne, hertis a hart's skin SW2/1327

skirwhittes skirrets; wild parsnip; wild carrot; white-pepper plant, rocket (*Sium sisarum; Pastinaca sativa; Daucus carota; Eruca sativa*) SW2/1495n

sloue the sloe tree or its fruit (*Prunus spinosa*): *juce of* ~ sloe-juice SW2/464, SW2/465; *barke of* ~ *trees* sloe-tree bark SW2/987

smalache smallage, wild celery (*Apium graveolens*) SW2/200, SW2/1824, SW2/1831, SW2/1833; *croppes of* ~ *SW2/922

smethis trough, that lieth in the waste material from blacksmithing SW2/1568

smirinis ?a substance coming from Smyrna SW2/1609

smythes water water used by a blacksmith for quenching hot metal SW2/810 [see *MED*, s.v. *water* n. 5b., (b)]

smolent ?error for mullein (*Verbascum thapsus*) SW2/432

snailes snails: *plaster of* ~ a salve made with snails SW2/1047; *water of* ~ water in which snails have been soaked or cooked SW2/1037

solatrum (= salatry): *succus solatri* juice of nightshade (*Solanum nigrum; Atropa bella-donna*) SW2/1656, SW2/1682

solsequium marigold (*Calendula officinalis*) SW2/1875

solsequium (= solsequium) SW2/1598

so(o)te soot SW2/611, SW2/614, SW2/842

sope, blac a dark-colored soap SW2/1572

sorel common sorrel; wood sorrel (*Rumex acetosa; Oxalis acetosella*) SW2/356

sothernwoode southernwood (*Artemisia abrotana*) SW2/644, SW2/1283, SW2/1373, **soþernwoode** SW2/1248

sotulares *porcinas* pigskin shoes SW2/1668

sow a female pig: ~ *gres* sow's grease
SW2/1847

soukyng of a young animal: suckling Age/771, **sowkyng** Age/1853,
SW2/398

sowthistil sow-thistle (*Sonchus oleraceus*) SW2/948, **southistils**
SW2/941, **sowth thistil** SW2/941

sparowes sparrows Age/24; *flessh of
sparowis* sparrow meat SW2/622

sperage asparagus; cranesbill; spurge
(*Asparagus officinalis; Geranium* spp.;
Euphorbia spp.) SW2/239

sperma cete ambergris Bac/541,
sperme of the whale Bac/541, *sperma ceti* Bac/540

spigeanil spignel; campion (*Meum atha-
manticum; Silene* spp.) SW2/1842

spikenard the spikenard plant or the
ointment nard derived from it; gal-
ingale (*Nardostachys jatamansi;
Cyperus longus*) SW2/752, SW2/864,
SW2/1075, SW2/1288, SW2/1380,
SW2/1529, **spikenarde** SW2/241,
spicanard Age/2068, **spicaner**
Age/2061

spikenardus (= **spikenard**) SW2/1596,
SW2/1608

spynache spinach (*Spinacia oleracea*)
Age/1908

spodie a powder based on ashes of
elephant bones or ivory SW2/486,
SW2/979

squinantum camel's hay, squinant (*An-
dropogon schoenanthus*) SW2/1395,
SW2/1596, SW2/1609

stafisacre stavesacre (*Delphinium sta-
phisagria*) SW2/1119, SW2/1405,
staphisacre Fle/166

stanmarche horse-parsley, alexanders
(*Smyrnium olusatrum*) SW2/923,
SW2/948, SW2/1824, SW2/1855,
stanmariche SW2/251

stepcerea ?lavender (*Lavendula officinalis*)
SW2/1607 [cf. Hunt, s.v. *stipteras*]

stercus dung: ~ *hominis* human dung
SW2/1685; ~ *caprinum* goat's dung
SW2/1686

sterenices see **trifer**

stewe of herbis a decoction of herbs
SW2/153

sticados houseleek; ?French lavender (*Sempervivum tectorum; Lavandula latifolia* or *stoechas*) SW2/264,
SW2/1586; ~ *arabike* ?a kind of leek
or lavender SW2/243

stone a gemstone: ~ *of ematiste* amethyst
SW2/478; ~ *that hight isopus* jasper
SW2/1339n

stones rocks SW2/384; the pits
of fruits SW2/242, SW2/1825,
SW2/1835; testicles SW2/623,
SW2/1805, SW2/1814, SW2/1818

storax a gum derived from the storax
tree, commonly semifluid (*Styrax
officinale*) SW2/416, SW2/657,
SW2/659, Plag/123; *storax* SW2/653,
SW2/1136; ~ *liquida* a semifluid
form of storax SW2/586

strawbury the wild strawberry (*Fragrar-
ia vesca*) SW2/1845

suc juice (of a plant) Age/1079

succus (= **juce**): for the sources of the
following juices, see the entries for
the individual plants: ~ *archimesie*
SW2/886; ~ *arthemesie* SW2/1658;
~ *camamil* SW2/1655; ~ *ebuli*
SW2/1672; ~ *jusquimani* SW2/1639;
~ *marubij* SW2/1653; ~ *nepitus*
SW2/1612; ~ *plantayne* SW2/377; ~
porri SW2/1645, ~ *porry* SW2/1586;
~ *rosarum* SW2/502, SW2/971; ~
rute SW2/1396, SW2/1651; ~ *solatri*
SW2/1656, SW2/1682; ~ *titinmale*
SW2/288; ~ *veruene* SW2/1634; ~ *vrtice rubie* SW2/1653

sucrum rosarum roset sugar SW2/733
[see **zucre roset**]

sugre sugar Age/1203, Age/2018,
Age/2032, SW2/244, SW2/338,
SW2/344, **suger** Age/1106,
Age/1527, SW2/415, SW2/1838

sulpicis, lapis an unidentified stone
SW2/1636

sumac the European sumac (*Rhus cori-
aria*) SW2/370, SW2/486

suppositorie a solid medication introduced into a non-oral body cavity SW2/185, SW2/192, SW2/196, SW2/200, SW2/332, SW2/865, etc., **suppository(e)** SW2/216, SW2/221, SW2/271, SW2/364, 8Med/68, etc.

surip(e) see **sirup**

swetheles a cloth bandage, swaddling band SW2/757, SW2/759

swyne, flessh of pork SW2/622

talow tallow, rendered animal fat SW2/1542

tan-water tanning liquor SW2/988

tarre tar SW2/1757, SW2/1758

terbentyne the resin of the terebinth tree (*Pistacia terebinthus*) SW2/822, SW2/865, SW2/875

terbentynum (= **terbentyne**) SW2/288

terebentum album granosum grainy white terbentyne SW2/1581

terra sigillata sealed earth, earth shaped into a lozenge and stamped with a seal, used medicinally Age/473, SW2/493, SW2/993, Plag/299

testiculi galli cock's testicles SW2/1637

testitudo a snail SW2/1697 [see Latham 1980, s.v.]

theodoricon a purgative compound medicine: ~ *ipericon* (*empericon*) a compound medicine based on St. John's wort (*Hypericon perforatum*) SW2/233, SW2/713; ~ *anacardi* a compound medicine based on *anacardus*, the marking nut or anacard (*Semecarpus anacardium; Anacardium orientale*) SW2/234

theotic ?a kind of lizard Age/1638n [see Little and Withington 1928, 217 n. 177]

thistil, sowth see **sowthistil**

thus album white incense, frankincense (*Boswellia thurifera*) SW2/1647

tym thyme (*Thymus serpyllum*) *SW2/578, SW2/1469

timiama incense Plag/124

tire, flessh of viper's flesh, snake meat Bac/555, Bac/567

tired error for **tire** 'a snake whose venom is both poisonous and curative' Age/325n

tirobus unidentified SW2/1607 [Rowland (1981, 155) translates this as 'carob,' but we have not been able to confirm that identification]

tirus a viper, the flesh of which is used in the making of theriac Bac/547

tisan a tisane, barley water Plag/222, Plag/292, **tysan** SW2/947, Plag/323

titinmala spurge or houseleek (*Euphorbia* spp.; *Sempervivum tectorum*): *succus titinmale* sap or juice of spurge SW2/288

toorde a piece of dung Age/1638

tophasius topaz SW2/1639n

tormentil see **turmentil**

tormentillis (= **turmentil**) *SW2/1694, SW2/1700

tow tow, raw flax Fle/99

toun-cres garden cress, 'town-cress' (*Lepidium sativum*) SW2/226

triacle theriac, a compound medicine of many purposes, esp. as an antidote to poison Bac/548n, SW2/595, SW2/716, Plag/113, Plag/140, Plag/142; ~ *diatesseron* a medicine originally based on four ingredients SW2/193

triasandis triasandal, a compound medicine containing three kinds of sandalwood Plag/144

trifer a compound medicine with purgative effect Age/1103, Age/1113; *trifera magna* the great trifera SW2/234 [see Green 2001, 201-2]; *triferes more and lasse* the greater and lesser trifera Age/1107; *triferes sterenices* Saracen trifera Age/1520 [see Green 2001, 202-3]

trociscy a medicated lozenge, a troche SW2/1376, **trocisces** Age/1388, Age/1401, Age/2056, Age/2066, Age/2069, SW2/1389, SW2/1435, **trocisses** SW2/1110, **trosikes**

SW2/278; **trosciscy of myrre** a
troche containing myrrh
SW2/1295, **trocisces (trocissis,
troscisses) of (the) myrre (mirre,
murs)** SW2/686, SW2/1106,
SW2/1432, SW2/1725
trocisci (= trocisces) SW2/1601
turion a shoot of a vine or briar, vine-
crop Fle/154 [see Hunt 1989, 255]
turmentil common tormentil (*Potentilla erecta*) SW2/460, SW2/471,
SW2/798, SW2/806, SW2/815,
SW2/1495, SW2/1667, **tormentil**
Plag/284, Plag/298, Plag/382
turtil a turtle dove (*Streptopelia turtur*)
SW2/446

vnguent an ointment or salve
SW2/1720
vrsyne see **braunche vrsyne**
vrtica nettle (*Lamium* spp.; *Urtica* spp.)
SW2/1663; *succus vrtice rubie* juice
of red nettle (*Lamium purpureum*)
SW2/1653

v-levid gras creeping cinquefoil (*Potentilla reptans*) SW2/1495
valerian valerian (*Valeriana officinalis*)
SW2/240
ventusyng drawing blood with a cupping glass SW2/786; ~ *buystes* cupping glasses SW2/804
verious verjuice, juice of sour or unripe fruit Plag/135
veruayne vervain (*Verbena officinalis*)
SW2/1311, SW2/1315
veruena (= veruayne) SW2/1630; *succus veruene* vervain sap or juice
SW2/1634
vesica capree a goat's bladder
SW2/1668
vyne, asshen of a ashes of a vine
SW2/1454
vynegre vinegar SW2/175, SW2/176,
Plag/106, Plag/134, etc.
vinum wine SW2/1592, SW2/1597,
SW2/1647; ~ *album* white wine
SW2/1345, SW2/1578, SW2/1665,

*SW2/1675, SW2/1677; ~ *album
aromaticum* white aromatic wine
SW2/580; ~ *aromaticum* aromatic
wine SW2/1397; ~ *decoccionis* wine
in which ingredients have been
boiled SW2/1650, SW2/1657
violarie violets [L. *violarum*] (*Viola odorata*) Plag/146
violet the sweet violet (*Viola odorata*) Age/1956, SW2/250, SW2/354,
SW2/416, *SW2/935, SW2/1374,
SW2/1876, **violettis** Age/2016,
Age/2027, Age/2034, Plag/138;
oile of ~ oil infused with violet
flowers SW2/221, SW2/934,
SW2/1026; *syrup (of)* ~ syrup in
which violets are boiled Age/1914,
Age/2017
virga pastoris teasel, "shepherd's rod"
(*Dipsacus fullonum*) SW2/471,
SW2/883
vitelli cocti ouorum cooked egg yolks
SW2/1688
vitriole a metal sulfate SW2/477

walnotis walnuts, the nuts of the wal-
nut tree (*Juglans regia*) Plag/69
water water, used medicinally in a variety
of ways: ~ *of betayne* water infused with
betony leaves Plag/397; *lewke* ~ *aromatic*
tepid, sweet-smelling water Age/2100;
~ *of malowes* water infused with mallow
leaves SW2/1783; ~ *of mannes leer* the
water in which a man has washed his
face SW2/1318; ~ *of nymphee* water infused with water-lilies 8Med/42; ~ *of
plantayne* water infused with plantain
leaves SW2/438; *rose* ~ rose water,
water in which rose petals have
been infused Age/1010, SW2/463,
SW2/1520, 8Med/42, 8Med/45, ~
of roses (rosis) SW2/438, SW2/440,
SW2/487, Plag/156, etc.; ~ *of rosarum zuccarum* ?dissolved roset sugar
SW2/442; *salt* ~ salt water SW2/618; ~
of sambuc water infused with elder
flowers Age/1010; *smythes* ~ water
used by a blacksmith for quenching

hot metal SW2/810; ~ *of snailes* water in which snails have been soaked or cooked SW2/1037; ~ *stilled* a distilled herbal water Plag/284, Plag/381

watercresses watercresses (*Rorippa nasturtium-aquaticum*) SW2/250, **waterkersen** SW2/1876

we(e)kc a wick, piece of wicking SW2/364, SW2/570, **wike** SW2/618

wex wax SW2/437, SW2/719, SW2/1542, SW2/1558, SW2/1560; *rede* ~ red sealing wax SW2/1056

whay, white white whey SW2/504

whete, wyne of an alcoholic drink made from wheat Age/760

wyne wine Age/755, Age/762, Age/859, Age/1303, Coi/100, SW2/158, Plag/104, etc.; ~ *of applis* an alcoholic drink made from apples Age/760; ~ *arian (arean)* a red wine Age/1402, Age/1403, Age/1403; *bastard* ~ SW2/1737 spiced wine; ~ *clarre* SW2/722 spiced and clarified wine; *fumus, fumous* ~ strong, aromatic wine Age/1285, Age/1290, etc.; ~ *of Gascoyne* wine from Gascony SW2/275; ~ *of the oote* an alcoholic beverage made from oats Age/760; *osey* ~ a sweet white wine SW2/1736; *rede* ~ red wine Age/1312, Age/1332, SW2/432, etc.; ~ *romanici* ?aromatic wine SW2/1436; *strong swete* ~ *and satournous* a heavy sweet wine SW2/627; *temperat* ~ tempered wine, wine mixed with water Age/1897; ~ *of vyne* wine made from grapes Age/759, *vynous* ~ , ~ *vynous* Age/850, Age/852; ~ *watery* thin wine Age/851; ~ *of whete* an alcoholic drink made from wheat Age/760; *white* ~ white wine Age/1298, Age/1310, SW2/688, Plag/134, etc.; *white* ~ *of the Ryne* white Rhine wine Plag/294

woderof sweet woodruff (*Asperula odorata*) SW2/687, SW2/688, SW2/1297n, **wooderof** SW2/642, **woderove** SW2/1434

woose, tanners tanning liquor SW2/472

wormeton error for **wormode** SW2/993

wormode wormwood (*Artemisia absinthium*) SW2/611, SW2/615, SW2/643, SW2/746, SW2/947, SW2/1082, SW2/1090, etc., **wormoode** SW2/1282

worte, Seynt John St. John's wort (*Hypericum perforatum*) SW2/644

wortis prepared greens, a salad Age/526, Age/1003, SW2/252, SW2/940, SW2/943, SW2/945, **wurtis** SW2/391

wulfis, stones of wolves' testicles SW2/623

wul(l) wool SW2/726, SW2/738, SW2/1788

wullen woolen: ~ *clew* a piece of woolen thread SW2/571

xilobalsamum bark or wood of the balsam plant (*Commiphora opobalsamum*) SW2/652, *SW2/1393, SW2/1610

yelkis see **yolkes**

yolkes yolks SW2/622, SW2/889, SW2/1472, **yolkis** SW2/885, SW2/1475, **yelkis** SW2/1472

zedewar setwall, turmeric (*Curcuma zedoaria*) or its aromatic root Age/1419, Age/1449, Age/2054, Age/2065

zedoaria (= **zedewar, zedwale**) SW2/1701

zedwale (= **zedewar**) Plag/112; *powder of zedewale* ground turmeric SW2/863

zinziber ginger (*Zingiber officinalis*) SW2/454, SW2/1581, SW2/1702

zona potus ?a kind of ale [?poss. 'yeasty drink'; cf. ML *zyma, zomus* 'leaven' in Latham 1980] SW2/1710

zuccara water sugar water SW2/1041

zuc(c)arum sugar: ~ *album* white sugar SW2/359, SW2/1704; ~ *atrum* a dark sugar SW2/376, SW2/377; ~ *cassatyne* a medium grade white sugar, in loaf or lump form SW2/506; ~ *rosarum, rosarum* ~ sugar roset, a combination of sugar and macerated rose petals SW2/392, SW2/414, SW2/442, SW2/505

zucre roset sugar roset, a combination of sugar and macerated rose petals SW2/1727

PERSONS, PLACES, AND WORKS CITED IN THE TEXTS

The names of people, places, and works mentioned in the texts edited above, or in the marginal notes by the original scribe, are alphabetized below under the most common Middle English form found in the texts, followed by variant Middle English spellings and Latin forms (the latter mainly in the nominative case and drawn primarily from the scribe's marginal apparatus). Alphabetization and other formatting conventions follow the principles of the General Glossary above. References are by text and line and usually include all occurrences of the names and titles in the texts, except for extremely common names such as *Aristotil, Avicen, Galien,* and *Ipocras,* where additional instances in a particular text are indicated by "etc." A plus sign (+) before a form indicates that it occurs in a marginal note. An asterisk before a form or a line reference indicates that the form or instance of the name results from emendation.

Accidentis of Age, Booke of prob. the pseudo-Baconian *De retardatione accidentium senectutis* Bac/65, Bac/496, *Booke of Passiouns of Age* Bac/629

Adam Adam, the first man Bac/160, Bac/292, Bac/461, Bac/475, Bac/589, Bac/597, Bac/598, +*Adam* Bac/472

Afforismes, Afforissmes, Afforismus, +*Afforissimes,* +*Afforismi* see **Damascene, Ipocras**

Alexa(u)nder, +*Alexander,* +*Alexandrynus* see **Alisaunder**

Algo putative Indian inventor of Arabic numerals 7LA/192 [cf. General Glossary, s.v. *rismon*]

Alisaunder Alexander the Great (356–323 B.C.) Age/675, Age/909, Age/1035, Age/1330, Age/1534, Age/1828, **Alisaundre** Age/316, Age/1068, Age/1480, Age/1949, **Alysaunder** Age/1960, **Alexa(u)nder** Age/211, 7LA/318, +*Alexander* Age/314, Age/673, Age/907, Age/1067, Age/1479, Age/1533, Age/1827, Age/1947, Age/1959, +*Alexandrynus* (*sic*) Age/209

Alysaunder see **Alisaunder**

Alkamye, Booke of the More see **Avicen**

Almagest, +*Almagestus* see **Rasy**

Almayne Germany Age/845, Bac/77

Almaser, Booke of see **Rasy**

Almosorum see **Rasy**

Alnot ?title or incipit of an astronomical text Inst/386n

Amforismus, Booke of see **Galien, Ipocras**

+*Anima, De* see **Aristotil, Avicen**

+*Animalibus, (Liber) de* see **Aristotil, Avicen, Plinius, Solinus**

+*Animalium, Liber* see **Aristotil**

Arabie Arabia Age/885, SW2/1556, SW2/1560

Arabiens Arabians, Arabic writers Age/85

Archepius putative authority on longevity Bac/452, Bac/483, Bac/487, Bac/608, Bac/614, Bac/629, **Archephius** Bac/71, Bac/214, Bac/239, +*Archephius* *Bac/71; **philosophie, (booke of)** treatise on longevity attributed to Archephius Bac/452, Bac/488, Bac/629

Aristotil Aristotle (384–322 B.C.) Age/210, Age/351, Age/404, Age/410, etc., Bac/130, Bac/150, Bac/177, etc., CHP/241, 7LA/147,

7LA/318, etc., +*Aristoteles* Age/401, Age/410, Age/485, etc., Bac/339, Bac/406, Bac/464, +*Aristotiles* Age/677, Age/960, Age/1033, etc., Bac/176, Bac/200, Bac/553, etc., +*Aristotilles* Bac/129, +*Aristotillus* Age/314, +*Aristotilus* Age/350, CHP/240, +*Aristotolus* Age/209;

Booke(s) of Beestis On Animals Age/404, Age/486, Age/1193, Bac/177, +*liber Animalium* Age/402, Age/1192, +*liber (libri) de Animalibus* Age/485, Bac/177;

Dividyng of Problemes error for *(in primo Topicorum)* in dictione probabilis Bac/408n, +*In divisione problematis* Bac/406;

Elynkes the *Elenchi*, or *Sophistical Refutations* 7LA/151;

Methamorphice error for *Metaphysics* Bac/579n, Bac/581n, +*Methamorphice* Bac/581;

Methamorphoseos error for *Metaphysics* Bac/130n, +*Methamorphoseos* Bac/129;

predicamentis the *Categories* Bac/618n, +*(Aristotiles in) predicamentis* Bac/616;

Of the Soule On the Soul Bac/201, +*De Anima* Bac/200;

Topikes the Topics 7LA/148;

Epistel to Alexaunder/Alisaunder (Pseudo-Aristotle) *The Epistle of Aristotle to Alexander* (= *Secreta secretorum)* Age/211, Age/908, **booke that (whiche) he made at the praiers of Alisaunder (Alisaundre, Alysaunder)** Age/1827, Age/1948, Age/1960, **the booke the whiche he made in his age for the state of Alisaunder** Age/1034, **a pistil to Alisaunder** Age/1534, +*Epistola ad Alexandrynum/Alexandrum*, +*Epistola Alexandro* Age/209, Age/907, Age/1533, +*liber Alexandri* Age/1947, Age/1959, +*liber quam fecit ad preces Alexandri* Age/1826,

+*liber quem fecit in sua senectute* Age/1034;

Booke of Secretis (Pseudo-Aristotle) *Secreta secretorum* Age/627, Age/961, Age/1096, Age/1480, Bac/464, Bac/554, Bac/628, 7LA/318, *Booke of Rule of Lif* Bac/341, +*liber Secretorum* Age/627, Age/960, Bac/464, Bac/553, +*liber De regimine vite* Bac/339;

*De *causis* (Pseudo-Aristotle) *Liber de causis* (= *Liber de essentia purae bonitatis*) Plag/64n

August, Octovian Caesar Augustus, Roman emperor (Octavian; 63 B.C. – A.D. 14) Bac/490, **Lord August** Age/62, **Octoviam** Bac/58, +*August* Age/61

Augustinus unidentified medical authority SW2/1420n

Averoys the Arabic philosopher Averroës (Abu 'l-Walīd Muḥammad ibn Aḥmad ibn Muḥammad ibn Rushd, 1126–1198) Bac/578, +*Averoys* Bac/577;

in the x *Methamorphice* [*sic*] Averroës' commentary on Aristotle's *Metaphysics*, bk. 10 Bac/578n

Comentor super secundum *Phisicorum* Averroës as commentator on Aristotle's *Physics*, bk. 2 Plag/57

Avicen Avicenna (Abū 'Alī al-Ḥusayn ibn 'Abd Allāh ibn Sīnā, 980–1037) Age/49, Age/174, Age/184, Age/197, etc., Bac/144, Bac/168, Bac/434, Bac/451, Bac/621, SW2/497, SW2/805, SW2/1136, Plag/54, +*Avicen* Age/48, Age/171, Age/182, Age/194, Age/199, etc., Bac/144, Bac/434, Bac/450, Bac/620, +*Avicenna* Age/440, Bac/167, Bac/176;

Booke of the More Alkamye (Pseudo-Avicenna) *De anima in arte alkimia* Bac/144n, *Of the Soule* Bac/169, +*liber maioris Alkamie* Bac/144, +*De Anima* Bac/167;

Prescian the Latin grammarian Priscian (fl. A.D. 500) 7LA/63, 7LA/121, **Precian** 7LA/118;

his **more volume** either Priscian's *Ars major,* or the first sixteen books of his *Ars minor (Institutiones grammaticae),* known as "Priscianus major" 7LA/63n, **the grete volume** 7LA/119n;

the **lasse booke** poss. the *Institutiones grammaticae,* or *Ars minor,* or its last two books, known as "Priscianus minor" 7LA/121n

Priest, Edmond see **Edmond Priest**

prince, the sone (soone, sones) of the (a) Avicenna (often in the phrase "the sone of the [a] prince Obelay [Obealus]," occasionally simply "the prince" or "the prince Obolay") Age/74, Age/576, Age/689, Age/721, Age/744, Age/913, Age/1279, Age/1435, Age/1472, Age/1491, Age/1705, **the prince (Obolay)** Age/840n, Age/947, Age/1141, Age/1196, +*Obealus princeps* Age/688, +*Filius *principis* Age/1705, +*Princeps* Age/838n, Age/1140 [see also **Avicen, Obolay**]

prince of medicyne Avicenna Plag/54

Problemes, Dividing of, +*In divisione problematis* see **Aristotil**

Pronosticaciouns see **Ipocras**

Prouerbis, (Of/In) see **Bernard of Gordien, Galien**

Ptholome see **Tholome**

Quyntilian Marcus Fabius Quintilianus, Roman rhetorician (ca. 35 – ca. 95) 7LA/155

Raymund error for Rhazes Age/1027, +*Raymundus* Age/1026

Rasy Rhazes (Abū Bakr Muḥammad Zakariyyā' al-Rāzī, 860–932) Age/1104, Age/1189, Age/1537, Age/1562, Age/1781, Age/1798, Age/1830, Age/1895, Age/1972, Ra-

sis Age/1052, Age/1106, SW2/1106, SW2/1296, SW2/1432, SW2/1600, *Rasis SW2/1376, **sone of Zacharie** Age/951, +*Rasy* Age/1534, Age/1562, Age/1797, Age/1895, Age/1972, +*filius Zacharie* Age/951;

Booke of Almaser Liber ad Almansorem Age/1053, Age/1106, Age/1189, Age/1896, *Booke of Almosorum* SW2/1432, *Almagest* prob. error for *Almaser/Almansor* Age/1537, +*liber Almaser* Age/1895; +*Almagestus* Age/1534;

in his canon *Liber ad Almansorem* 4.14, "De iuuamentis & nocumentis flobotomie," and 4.31, "Summa de regimine aliarum etatum" Age/1972, +*in canone* Age/1972

Regaly, Regalis see **Haly** (1)

Remygius Remigius of Auxerre (ca. 841–948) 7LA/67

Richard, the grete Ricardus Anglicus, 12th-c. medical writer CHP/39, +*Ricardus magnus* CHP/39

Rogerus, Rogier see **Bacon**

Rome Rome CHP/164

Ruffus Rufus of Ephesus, Greek medical writer (fl. ca. 25 B.C. – A.D. 50) Coi/241, +*Ruffus* Coi/241

Rule of Age, Booke of prob. the *De universali regimine senum et seniorum* associated with the *De retardatione accidentium senectutis* Bac/515, *Booke of the Rule of Elder Men* Bac/553, **treatice** *Of Age and Rule of Elder Men* Bac/630n

Rule of Life, Booke of, +*liber De regimine vite* see **Aristotil**

Rule Sharpe see **Ipocras**

Salamon (1) Solomon, king of Israel (r. 974 – ca. 937 B.C.) Age/1276, 7LA/320, +*Salamon* Age/1273

Salamon (2) father of Isaac Israeli Age/931; +*Salamon* Age/930

Secretis, Booke of, +*liber secretorum* see **Aristotil**

BIBLIOGRAPHY

Abelson, Paul. 1906. *The Seven Liberal Arts: A Study in Mediaeval Culture.* Columbia University Teachers' College Contributions to Education 11. New York.

Africa, Thomas W. 1961. "The Opium Addiction of Marcus Aurelius." *Journal of the History of Ideas* 22:97–102.

Albertson, Mary. 1932. "London Merchants and Their Landed Property during the Reigns of the Yorkists." PhD Diss., Bryn Mawr College.

Albertus Magnus. *On Animals.* See Kitchell and Resnick 1999.

Albucasis (Abu 'l-Qāsim Khalaf ibn 'Abbās al-Zahrāwī). 1541. *Methodus medendi.* Basel.

Alonso Almeida, Francisco, ed. 1997. "Edition and Study of a Middle English Gynaecological Treatise: Yale Medical Library, MS 47, ff. 67r–71v." M.A. thesis, Facultad de Filologia, University of Las Palmas de Gran Canaria.

———. and Alicia Rodríguez Alvarez. 1996 [appeared 2000]. "The 'Sekenesse of Wymmen' Revised." *Manuscripta* 40:157–64.

Anthiaume, A., and J. Sottas. 1910. *L'Astrolabe-quadrant du Musée des Antiquités de Rouen: Recherches sur les connaissances mathématiques, astronomiques et nautiques au moyen âge.* Paris.

Aristotle. 1962. *Opera cum Averrois commentariis.* Facs. repr. of Venice 1562–1574 ed. 9 vols. Frankfurt am Main.

———. *Works.* See Barnes 1984.

Arnaldus of Villanova. 1504. *Opera.* Lyons.

Arrizabalaga, Jon. 1998. *The "Articella" in the Early Press c. 1476–1534.* Articella Studies 2. Cambridge and Barcelona.

Articella seu Opus artis medicine. 1487. Venice.

Articella seu Opus artis medicine. 1493. Venice.

Articella nuperrime impressa cum quamplurimis tractibus pristine impressioni superadditis. 1515. Lyons.

Articella nuperrime impressa cum quamplurimis tractibus pristine impressioni superadditis. 1534. Lyons.

Artis cuiuslibet consummatio (with OF trans. *Praktike geometrie*). See Victor 1979.

Ascelin of Augsburg. *Compositio astrolabii.* See Burnett 1998.

Austin, H. D. 1913. "Accredited Citations in Ristoro d'Arezzo's *Composizione del Mondo.*" *Studi medievali* 4:334–82.

———. 1937. "Artephius-Orpheus." *Speculum* 12:251–54.

Averroës (Abu 'l-Walīd Muḥammad ibn Aḥmad ibn Muḥammad ibn Rushd). *Commentaria super opera Aristotelis.* See Aristotle 1962.

Avicenna (Abū 'Alī al-Ḥusayn ibn 'Abd Allāh ibn Sīnā). 1522. *Liber canonis totius medicine.* Lyons.

———. 1964. *Liber Canonis.* Facs. repr. of Venice 1507 ed. Hildesheim.

Bacon, Roger. See Brewer 1859; Bridges 1897–1900; Lindberg 1996; Maloney 1988; Steele 1920.

Bacon, Roger (attrib.). 1590. *Libellus Rogerii Baconi Angli, doctissimi mathematici & medici, De retardandis senectutis accidentibus & de sensibus conseruandis.* With notes by John Williams. Oxford.

———. See Browne 1683; Little and Withington 1928.

Balbus, Joannes. 1971. *Catholicon*. Facs. repr. of Mainz 1460 ed. Westmead, Hants.

Baldwin, Martha. 1995. "The Snakestone Experiments: An Early Modern Medical Debate." *Isis* 86:394–418.

Bannister, A. T., comp. 1923. *Institutions, etc. [of the Diocese of Hereford] (A.D. 1539– 1900)*. Hereford.

Barnes, Jonathan, ed. 1984. *The Complete Works of Aristotle: The Revised Oxford Translation*. 2 vols. Bollingen Series 71/2. Princeton.

Baron, Roger, ed. 1966. *Hvgonis de Sancto Victore Opera propaedevtica*. Notre Dame.

Barlow, Claude W., ed. 1950. *Martini episcopi Bracarensis opera omnia*. New Haven.

Barratt, Alexandra, ed. 2001. *"The Knowing of Woman's Kind in Childing": A Middle English Version of Material Derived from the "Trotula" and Other Sources*. Medieval Women: Texts and Contexts 4. Turnhout.

Bassan, Maurice. 1962. "Chaucer's 'Cursed Monk,' Constantinus Africanus." *Mediaeval Studies* 24:127–40.

Baur, Ludwig, ed. 1912. *Die philosophischen Werke des Robert Grosseteste*. Beiträge zur Geschichte der Philosophie des Mittelalters 9. Münster.

———. 1917. *Die Philosophie des Robert Grosseteste Bischofs von Lincoln*. Beiträge zur Geschichte der Philosophie des Mittelalters: Texte und Untersuchungen 18/4–6. Münster.

Bennett, Judith. 1994. "Medieval Women, Modern Women: Across the Great Divide." In *Feminists Revision History*, ed. Ann-Louise Shapiro, 47–72. New Brunswick.

Benskin, Michael. 2004. "Chancery Standard." In *New Perspectives on English Historical Linguistics: Selected Papers from 12 ICEHL, Glasgow, 21–26 August 2002*. Vol. 2: *Lexis and Transmission*, ed. Christian Kay et al., 1–40. Amsterdam.

———, and Margaret Laing. 1981. "Translations and *Mischsprachen* in Middle English Manuscripts." In Benskin and Samuels 1981, 55–106.

———, and M. L. Samuels, eds. 1981. *So Meny People Longages and Tonges: Philological Essays in Scots and Mediaeval English presented to Angus McIntosh*. Edinburgh.

Benson, Larry D., gen. ed. 1987. *The Riverside Chaucer*. 3rd ed. Boston.

ben Yahia, Boubaker. 1955. "Constantin l'Africain et l'école de Salerne." *Cahiers de Tunisie* 3:49–59.

———. 1965. "Constantinus Africanus." In *The Encyclopaedia of Islam*, 2:59–60. Leiden.

Berg, W. S. van den. 1917. *Eene Middelnederlandsche Vertaling van het Antidotarium Nicolai (Ms. 15624–15641, Kon. Bibl. te Brussel)*. Leiden.

Bernard de Gordon. 1480. *Practica seu Lilium medicinae*. N.p.

———. 1574. *De prognosticis*. In *Lilium medicinae*. Lyons.

Bernard, Edward. 1647. *Catalogi librorum manuscriptorum Angliae et Hiberniae*. Vol. 1, Pt. 3. Oxford.

Berthelot, Marcellin. [1893] 1967. *La chimie au Moyen Âge*. Vol. 1. Repr. Osnabrück.

Beusing, Hermann Heinrich, ed. 1922. *Leben und Werke des Richardus Anglicus, samt einem erstmaligen Abdruck seiner Schrift "Signa."* Leipzig.

Bitterling, Klaus. 1979. "Signs of Death and Other Monitory Snatches from MS. Harley 2247." *Notes & Queries* 224:101–2.

Black, W. H. 1845. *A Descriptive, Analytical, and Critical Catalogue of the Manuscripts Bequeathed . . . by Elias Ashmole.* Oxford.

Bloch, Herbert. 1986. *Monte Cassino in the Middle Ages.* 3 vols. Cambridge, MA.

Blumenkranz, Bernhard. 1966. *Le juif médiéval au miroir de l'art chrétien.* Paris.

Boethius, Anicius Manlius Severinus. *Commentaria in Porphyrium. PL* 64:71–158.

———. *De arithmetica libri duo. PL* 63:1079–1168.

———. *De musica libri quinque. PL* 63:1167–1300.

———. *De topicis differentiis.* See Stump 1978.

———. *Elenchorum sophisticorum Aristotelis libri duo. PL* 64:1007–40.

———. *Fundamentals of Music.* See Bower and Palisca 1989.

———. *Liber de divisione. PL* 64:875–92.

———. *Liber de geometria. PL* 63:1352–64.

———. *Topicorum Aristotelis libri octo. PL* 64:909–1008.

Boffey, Julia, and John J. Thompson. 1989. "Anthologies and Miscellanies: Production and Choice of Texts." In Griffiths and Pearsall 1989, 279–315.

Boffito, Giuseppe, and Camillo Melzi d'Eril, eds. 1922. Profatius Judacus, *Il Quadrante d'Israel.* Florence.

Bower, Calvin M., trans., and Claude V. Palisca, ed. 1989. *Boethius: Fundamentals of Music.* New Haven.

Brewer, J. S., ed. 1859. *Fr. Rogeri Bacon Opera quædam hactenus inedita: Opus tertium, Opus minus, Compendium philosophiae.* Rolls Series 15. London.

Bridges, John Henry, ed. 1897–1900. *The "Opus Majus" of Roger Bacon.* 3 vols. Oxford.

Briquet, C. M. 1923. *Les Filigranes.* 2nd ed. 4 vols. Leipzig.

British Library. N.d. *Manuscripts Catalogue.* http://molcat.bl.uk/msscat.

Brodrick, George C. 1885. *Memorials of Merton College, with Biographical Notices of the Wardens and Fellows.* Oxford.

Brown, Carleton F., and Rossell H. Robbins. 1943. *Index of Middle English Verse.* (With suppl. in Cutler 1965.) New York.

Brown, Peter. 1994. "The Seven Planets." In Matheson 1994, 3–21.

Browne, Richard, trans. 1683. *The Cure of Old Age and Preservation of Youth by Roger Bacon . . . Also, a Physical Account of the Tree of Life.* London.

Brusendorff, Aage. [1925] 1967. *The Chaucer Tradition.* Repr. Oxford.

Bruyn, G. W. 1982. "The Seat of the Soul." In *Historical Aspects of the Neurosciences,* ed. F. Clifford Rose and W. F. Bynum, 55–81. New York.

Burkert, Walter. 1972. *Love and Science in Ancient Pythagoreanism.* Trans. Edwin L. Minar, Jr. Cambridge, MA.

Burnett, Charles. 1990. "The Planets and the Development of the Embryo." In Dunstan 1990, 95–112.

———, ed. 1998. Ascelin of Augsburg, *Compositio astrolabii.* Pp. 343–58 in "King Ptolemy and Alchandreus the Philosopher: The Earliest Texts on the Astrolabe and Arabic Astrology at Fleury, Micy and Chartres." *Annals of Science* 55:329–68.

———, and Danielle Jacquart, eds. 1994. *Constantine the African and ʿAlī ibn al-Abbās al-Maǧūsī: The "Pantegni" and Related Texts.* Studies in Ancient Medicine 10. Leiden.

[———, and Danielle Jacquart.] 1994. "A Catalogue of Renaissance Editions and Manuscripts of the *Pantegni.*" In Burnett and Jacquart 1994, 316–51.

Burns, Chester R. 1976. "The Non-Naturals: A Paradox in the Western Concept of Health." *Journal of Medicine and Philosophy* 1:202–11.

Burrow, J. A. 1986. *The Ages of Man: A Study in Medieval Writing and Thought.* Oxford.

Butler, A. T. 1938. *The Visitation of Worcestershire 1634.* London.

Bylebyl, Jerome J. 1971. "Galen on the Non-Natural Causes of Variation in the Pulse." *Bulletin of the History of Medicine* 45:482–85.

Bynum, Caroline Walker. 1987. *Holy Feast and Holy Fast: The Religious Significance of Food to Medieval Women.* Berkeley.

———. 1995. *The Resurrection of the Body in Western Christianity, 200–1336.* New York.

Cadden, Joan. 1993. *Meanings of Sex Difference in the Middle Ages: Medicine, Science and Culture.* Cambridge.

Calendar of Inquisitions Post Mortem. Vol. 14. 48–51 Edward III. 1952. London.

Calendar of the Patent Rolls Preserved in the Public Record Office, 1452–1461. 1910. London.

Callus, Daniel A. 1955. "Robert Grosseteste as Scholar." In *Robert Grosseteste, Scholar and Bishop: Essays in Commemoration of the Seventh Centenary of His Death,* ed. D. A. Callus, 1–69. Oxford.

Calvet, Antoine. 1995. "Mutations de l'alchemie médicale au XVe siècle: A propos des textes authentiques et apocryphes d'Arnaud de Villeneuve." *Micrologus* 3:185–209.

———. 2003. "À la recherche de la médecine universelle: Questions sur l'élixir et la thériaque au 14e siècle." In Crisciani and Paravicini Bagliani 2003, 177–216.

Carrillo Linares, María José. 1993. "An Edition with an Introduction, Notes and a Glossary of the M.E. Translation of the Latin Treatise 'De Humana Natura.'" Licentiate Thesis. University of Seville.

Catto, J. I., and Ralph Evans, eds. 1992. *The History of the University of Oxford,* 2: *Late Medieval Oxford.* Oxford.

Chadwick, Henry. 1981. *Boethius: The Consolations of Music, Logic, Theology, and Philosophy.* Oxford.

Chambers, R. W., and Marjorie Daunt, eds. 1931. *A Book of London English 1384–1425.* Oxford.

Chandler, Bruce, gen. ed. 1985. *The Time Museum: Catalogue of the Collection.* Vol. 1, part 1: *Astrolabes, Astrolabe-related Instruments.* Rockford, IL.

Christianson, C. Paul. 1989. "Evidence for the Study of London's Late Medieval Manuscript-Book Trade." In Griffiths and Pearsall 1989, 87–108.

———. 1990. *A Directory of London Stationers and Book Artisans 1300–1500.* New York.

Cicero. *De natura deorum.* See Rackham 1933.

Clagett, Marshall. 1953. "The Medieval Latin Translations from the Arabic of the *Elements* of Euclid, with Special Emphasis on the Versions of Adelard of Bath." *Isis* 44:16–42.

Clarke, Edwin, and Kenneth Dewhurst. 1972. *An Illustrated History of Brain Function.* Oxford.

Clarke, Edwin, and Charles Donald O'Malley. 1968. *The Human Brain and Spinal Cord: A Historical Study Illustrated by Writings from Antiquity to the Twentieth Century.* Berkeley and Los Angeles.

Clarke, Peter D. 2002. *The University and College Libraries of Cambridge.* Introd. Roger Lovatt. Corpus of British Medieval Library Catalogues 10. London.

Clulee, Nicholas. 1984. "At the Crossroads of Magic and Science: John Dee's Archemastrie." In *Occult and Scientific Mentalities in the Renaissance,* ed. Brian Vickers, 57–71. Cambridge.

Cockayne, Oswald. 1866. *Leechdoms, Wortcunning, and Starcraft of Early England.* Rolls Series 35. Vol. 3. London.

Connolly, Margaret. 1998. *John Shirley: Book Production and the Noble Household in Fifteenth-Century England.* Aldershot.

Constantinus Africanus. 1515. *Liber Pantegni. Theorica* I–X. In *Omnia opera Ysaac,* Part II, fols. 1r–57v. Lyons.

———. 1536–39. *Opera.* 2 vols. Basel.

Copeland, Rita. 1991. *Rhetoric, Hermeneutics, and Translation in the Middle Ages: Academic Traditions and Vernacular Texts.* Cambridge Studies in Medieval Literature 11. Cambridge.

Corpus of British Medieval Library Catalogues. 1990– . See Humphreys 1990; Sharpe et al. 1996; Webber and Watson 1998; Stoneman 1999; Friis-Jensen and Willoughby 2001; Gillespie with Doyle 2001; Clarke 2002.

Courtenay, William J. 1987. *Schools and Scholars in Fourteenth-Century England.* Princeton.

Creutz, Rudolph. 1929. "Der Arzt Constantinus Africanus von Monte Cassino: Sein Leben, sein Werk und seine Bedeutung für die mittelalterliche medizinische Wissenschaft." *Studien und Mitteilungen zur Geschichte des Benediktiner-Ordens* 47:1–44.

———. 1931. "Die Ehrenrettung Konstantins von Afrika." *Studien und Mitteilungen zur Geschichte des Benediktiner-Ordens und seiner Zweige* 49:25–44.

Crisciani, Chiara. 2003. "Il farmaco d'oro: Alcuni testi tra i secoli XIV e XV." In Crisciani and Paravicini Bagliani 2003, 217–45.

———. and Agostino Paravicini Bagliani, eds. 2003. *Alchimia e medicina nel Medioevo.* Micrologus' Library 9. Florence.

———, and Michela Pereira. 1998. "Black Death and Golden Remedies. Some Remarks on Alchemy and the Plague." In *The Regulation of Evil: Social and Cultural Attitudes to Epidemics in the Late Middle Ages,* ed. Agostino Paravicini Bagliani and Francesco Santi, 7–39. Micrologus' Library 2. Florence.

Crombie, A. C. 1953. *Robert Grosseteste and the Origins of Experimental Science, 1100–1700.* Oxford.

Crowley, Theodore. 1950. *Roger Bacon: The Problem of the Soul in His Philosophical Commentaries.* Dublin.

Curtze, M. 1898. "Die Abhandlung des Levi ben Gerson über Trigonometrie und den Jacobstab." *Bibliotheca Mathematica* n.s. 12:97–112.

Cutler, John L. 1965. *Index of Middle English Verse: Supplement.* Lexington, KY. (See also Brown and Robbins 1943.)

Cyrurgia Guidonis de Cauliaco, et Cyrurgia Bruni, Teodorici, Rolandi, Lanfranci, Rogerii, Bertapalie. 1519. Venice.

Czarnecki, Romuald. 1919. *Ein Aderlasstraktat angeblich des Roger von Salerno samt einem lateinischen und einem griechischen Texte zur "Phlebotomia Hippocratis."* Inaug.-Diss., Leipzig.

Damascene, Damascenus. See John Damascene 1515.

Daremberg, Charles, and Charles Emile Ruelle. 1879. *Oeuvres de Rufus d'Éphèse.* Paris.

Davis, Norman. 1951–1952. "A Scribal Problem in the Paston Letters." *English and Germanic Studies* 4:31–64.

———. 1952. "A Paston Hand." *Review of English Studies* 3:209–21.

———. 1959. "Scribal Variation in Late Fifteenth-Century English." In *Mélanges de Linguistique et de Philologie: Fernand Mossé In Memoriam*, 95–103. Paris.

———. 1983. "The Language of Two Brothers in the Fifteenth Century." In *Five Hundred Years of Words and Sounds: A Festschrift for Eric Dobson*, ed. E. G. Stanley and Douglas Gray, 23–28. Cambridge.

Dean, James M. 1996. *Medieval English Political Writings.* TEAMS Middle English Texts. Kalamazoo, MI.

Dekker, Elly, and Peter van der Krogt. 1993. *Globes from the Western World.* London.

Delany, Paul. 1967. "Constantinus Africanus and Chaucer's *Merchant's Tale.*" *Philological Quarterly* 46:560–66.

———. 1970. "Constantinus Africanus's *De Coitu*: A Translation." *Chaucer Review* 4:55–65.

Demaitre, Luke E. 1980. *Doctor Bernard de Gordon: Professor and Practitioner.* Toronto.

———. 1990. "The Care and Extension of Old Age in Medieval Medicine." In *Aging and the Aged in Medieval Europe*, ed. Michael M. Sheehan, 3–22. Toronto.

———. 1996. "The Relevance of Futility: Jordanus de Turre (fl. 1313–1335) on the Treatment of Leprosy." *Bulletin of the History of Medicine* 70:25–61.

de Renzi, Salvatore. [1852–1859] 1967. *Collectio Salernitana.* Facs. repr. of Naples ed. 5 vols. Bologna.

de Ricci, Seymour. 1935–1940. *Census of Medieval and Renaissance Manuscripts in the United States and Canada.* 3 vols. New York.

DiMarco, Vincent, and Leslie Perelman. 1977. "Noteworthy Lexical Evidence in the Middle English *Letter of Alexander to Aristotle.*" *Neophilologus* 61:297–303.

———, eds. 1978. *The Middle English "Letter of Alexander to Aristotle."* Costerus n.s. 13. Amsterdam.

Dove, Mary. 1986. *The Perfect Age of Man's Life.* Cambridge.

Doyle, A. I. 1959. "An Unrecognized Piece of *Piers the Ploughman's Creed* and Other Work by Its Scribe." *Speculum* 34:428–36.

———. 1983. "English Books In and Out of Court from Edward III to Henry VII." In *English Court Culture in the Later Middle Ages*, ed. V. J. Scattergood and J. W. Sherborne, 163–81. London.

Drabkin, Miriam F., and Israel E. Drabkin, eds. 1951. *Caelius Aurelianus, Gynaecia: Fragments of a Latin Version of Soranus' "Gynaecia" from a Thirteenth-Century Manuscript. Bulletin of the History of Medicine* Supplement 13. Baltimore.

Dunstan, G. R., ed. 1990. *The Human Embryo: Aristotle and the Arabic and European Traditions.* Exeter.

Eisner, Sigmund, ed. 1980. *The Kalendarium of Nicholas of Lynn.* Trans. Gary Mac Eoin and Sigmund Eisner. Athens, GA.

Eldredge, L. M. 1992. *The Index of Middle English Prose. Handlist IX: Manuscripts containing Middle English Prose in the Ashmole Collection, Bodleian Library, Oxford.* Cambridge.

———, ed. 1996. *Benvenutus Grassus: The Wonderful Art of the Eye: A Critical Edition of the Middle English Translation of His "De Probatissima Arte Oculorum."* East Lansing, MI.

Elliott, Ralph W. V. 1966. "Our Host's 'triacle': Some Observations on Chaucer's Pardoner's Tale." *Review of English Literature* 7:61–73.

Emden, A.B. 1957–1959. *A Biographical Register of the University of Oxford to* A.D. *1500.* 3 vols. Oxford.

———. 1963. *A Biographical Register of the University of Cambridge to 1500.* Cambridge.

The Encyclopaedia of Islam. 1999. CD-ROM edition, version 1.0. Leiden.

Erchenbrecher, Hans. 1919. *Der Salernitaner Arzt Archimatthaeus und ein bis heute unbekannter Aderlasstraktat unter seinem Namen: Cod. Berol. lat. 4° No. 375.* Leipzig.

Evans, Joan, and Mary S. Serjeantson. 1933. *English Mediaeval Lapidaries.* EETS 190. London.

Evenden, Doreen. 2000. *The Midwives of Seventeenth-Century London.* Cambridge.

Feldman, Louis H., trans. 2000. *Judean Antiquities 1–4: Translation and Commentary.* Vol. 3 of *Flavius Josephus: Translation and Commentary,* ed. Steve Mason. Leiden.

Fenwick, Carolyn C. 1998. *The Poll Taxes of 1377, 1379, and 1381.* Vol. 1. Oxford.

Fery-Hue, Françoise. 1997. "Le romarin et ses propriétés: Un traité anonyme faussement attribué à Aldebrandin de Sienne." *Romania* 115:138–92.

Fisher, John H. 1996. *The Emergence of Standard English.* Lexington, KY.

———, et al. 1984. *An Anthology of Chancery English.* Knoxville.

Fletcher, J. M. 1992. "Developments in the Faculty of Arts, 1370–1520." In Catto and Evans 1992, 315–45.

Flügel, Ewald. 1905. "Eine mittelenglische Claudian-Übersetzung (1445)." *Anglia* 28:255–99.

Folkerts, Menso. 1974. "Die Entwicklung und Bedeutung der Visierkunst als Beispiel der praktischen Mathematik der frühen Neuzeit." *Humanismus und Technik* 18:1–41.

Fox, William, ed. 1902. *In artem Donati minorem commentum.* Leipzig.

French, Roger, et al., eds. 1998. *Medicine from the Black Death to the French Disease.* Aldershot.

Friis-Jensen, Karsten, and James M. W. Willoughby, eds. 2001. *Peterborough Abbey.* Corpus of British Medieval Library Catalogues 8. London.

Furnivall, Frederick J. 1878. "Recipe for Edward IV's Plague Medicine." *Notes & Queries,* 5th ser., 9:343.

———. 1880a. *Odd Texts of Chaucer's Minor Poems.* Part 2. Chaucer Society, 1st ser., 60. London.

————. 1880b. *Supplementary Parallel-Text Edition of Chaucer's Minor Poems*. Part 2. Chaucer Society, 1st ser., 59. London.

————. 1882. *The Fifty Earliest English Wills*. EETS 78. London.

————. 1886. *More Odd Texts of Chaucer's Minor Poems*. Chaucer Society, 1st ser., 77. London.

————. 1889. *The Book of Quinte Essence or the Fifth Being*. EETS 16. London.

————, and A. W. Pollard, eds. 1904. *The Macro Plays*. EETS e.s. 91. London.

Gairdner, James, ed. 1861–1863. *Letters and Papers Illustrative of the Reigns of Richard III. and Henry VII.* 2 vols. Rolls Series 24. London.

Galen. 1490. *Opera*. 2 vols. Venice.

————. 1515. *Galeni opera*. Vol. 1. Pavia.

————. 1542. *Galeni opera omnia*. Vol. 8. Basel.

————. *Opera omnia*. See Kühn [1821–1833] 1964–1965.

García Ballester, Luis. 1972. *Galeno, en la sociedad y en la ciencia de su tiempo (c. 130 – c. 200 d. de C.)*. Madrid.

————, et al., eds. 1994. *Practical Medicine from Salerno to the Black Death*. Cambridge.

Gariopontus [misattrib. to Galen]. *Passionarius Galeni*. 1526. Lyons.

Garrido Anes, Edurne. 2004. "Transmisión, Vernacularización y Usos del *Liber de simplici medicina*: Las Versiones del *Circa Instans* en Inglés Medio." *Medicina & Historia*, 4th ser., no. 2, 1–15.

Garton, C. 1980. "A Fifteenth Century Headmaster's Library." *Lincolnshire History and Archaeology* 15:29–38.

Geoghegan, D. 1957. "A License of Henry VI to Practise Alchemy." *Ambix* 6:10–17.

Geometria due sunt partes principales. See Hahn 1982.

Getz, Faye M. 1982. "Gilbertus Anglicus Anglicized." *Medical History* 16:436–42.

————. 1990a. "Charity, Translation, and Language of Medical Learning in Medieval England." *Bulletin of the History of Medicine* 64:1–17.

————. 1990b. "Medical Practitioners in Medieval England." (Suppl. to Talbot and Hammond 1965.) *Social History of Medicine* 3:245–83.

————. 1991. *Healing and Society in Medieval England: A Middle English Translation of the Pharmaceutical Writings of Gilbertus Anglicus*. Madison.

————. 1992a. "The Faculty of Medicine before 1500." In Catto and Evans 1992, 373–405.

————. 1992b. "To Prolong Life and Promote Health: Baconian Alchemy and Pharmacy in the English Learned Tradition." In *Health, Disease and Healing in Medieval Culture*, ed. Sheila Campbell, Bert Hall, and David Klausner, 141–51. New York.

————. 1997. "Roger Bacon and Medicine: The Paradox of the Forbidden Fruit and the Secrets of Long Life." In Hackett 1997, 337–64.

————. 1998. *Medicine in the English Middle Ages*. Princeton.

Gibson, Margaret. 1972. "Priscian's 'Institutiones Grammaticae': A Handlist of Manuscripts." *Scriptorium* 26:105–24.

Gil Sotres, Pedro. 1994. "Derivation and Revulsion: The Theory and Practice of Medieval Phlebotomy." In García Ballester et al. 1994, 110–55.

————. 1998. "The Regimens of Health." In *Western Medical Thought from Antiquity to the Middle Ages*, ed. Mirko D. Grmek, 291–318. Cambridge.

Gilbertus Anglicus. 1510. *Compendium medicine Gilberti Anglici tam morborum universalium quam particularium nondum medicis sed et cyrurgis utilissimum.* Lyons.

Giles, J. A., ed. 1843. *The Miscellaneous Works of Venerable Bede.* Vol. 6: Scientific Tracts and Appendix. London.

Gillespie, Vincent, ed. 2001. *Syon Abbey.* With *The Libraries of the Carthusians*, ed. A. I. Doyle. Corpus of British Medieval Library Catalogues 9. London.

Goldstein, Bernard R. 1985. *The Astronomy of Levi ben Gerson (1288–1344).* New York.

Gower, John. See Macaulay 1969.

Gracia, Diego, and Jose-Luis Vidal. 1974. "La *Isagoge* de Ioannitius: introducción, edición, traducción y notas." *Asclepio* 26–27:267–379.

Graesse, Johann G. T., and Friedrich Benedict. 1971. *Orbis Latinus: Lexikon lateinischer geographischer Namen. Handausgabe*, ed. Helmut Plechl with Günter Spitzbart. 4th rev. and exp. ed. Braunschweig.

Grauer, Anne L. 1991. "Life Patterns of Women from Medieval York." In *The Archaeology of Gender: Proceedings of the Twenty-Second Annual Conference of the Archaeological Association of the University of Calgary*, ed. Dale Walde and Noreen D. Willows, 407–13. Calgary.

Green, Monica H. 1987. "The *De genecia* Attributed to Constantine the African." *Speculum* 62:299–323.

——. 1990. "Constantinus Africanus and the Conflict between Religion and Science." In Dunstan 1990, 47–69.

——. 1992. "Obstetrical and Gynecological Texts in Middle English." *Studies in the Age of Chaucer* 14:53–88. Repr. as Essay IV in Green 2000c.

——. 1994. "Documenting Medieval Women's Medical Practice." In García Ballester et al. 1994, 322–52.

——. 1996a. "The Development of the *Trotula*." *Revue d'Histoire des Textes* 26:119–203. Repr. as Essay V in Green 2003c.

——. 1996b. "A Handlist of the Latin and Vernacular Manuscripts of the So-Called *Trotula* Texts. Part I: The Latin Manuscripts." *Scriptorium* 50:137–75.

——. 1997a. "A Handlist of the Latin and Vernacular Manuscripts of the So-Called *Trotula* Texts. Part II: The Vernacular Translations and Latin Re-Writings." *Scriptorium* 51:80–104.

——. 1997b. Review of Britta-Juliane Kruse, *Verborgene Heilkünste: Geschichte der Frauenmedizin im Spätmittelalter. Bulletin of the History of Medicine* 71:333–35.

——. 1998. "'Traittié tout de mençonges': The *Secrés des dames*, 'Trotula,' and Attitudes Towards Women's Medicine in Fourteenth- and Early Fifteenth-Century France." In *Christine de Pizan and the Categories of Difference*, ed. Marilynn Desmond, 146–78. Minneapolis.

——. 1999. Review of Ana Isabel Martín Ferreira, *Tratado médico de Constantino el Africano: Constantini Liber de elephancia. Bulletin of the History of Medicine* 73:305–6.

——. 2000a. "From 'Diseases of Women' to 'Secrets of Women': The Transformation of Gynecological Literature in the Later Middle Ages." *Journal of Medieval and Early Modern Studies* 30:5–39.

——. 2000b. "The Possibilities of Literacy and the Limits of Reading: Women and the Gendering of Medical Literacy." Essay VII in Green 2000c.

————. 2000c. *Women's Healthcare in the Medieval West: Texts and Contexts.* Variorum Collected Studies Series, CS680. Aldershot.

————, ed. and trans. 2001. *The 'Trotula': A Medieval Compendium of Women's Medicine.* Philadelphia.

————. 2003. "Masses in Remembrance of 'Seynt Susanne': A Fifteenth-Century Spiritual Regimen." *Notes & Queries* 248:380–84.

Green, R. F. 1978. "Notes on Some Manuscripts of Hoccleve's *Regement of Princes.*" *British Library Journal* 4:37–41.

Green, R. P. H., ed. 1991. *The Works of Ausonius.* Oxford.

Griffiths, Jeremy, and Derek Pearsall, eds. 1989. *Book Production and Publishing in Britain, 1375–1475.* Cambridge.

Gross, Anthony. 1996. *The Dissolution of the Lancastrian Kingship: Sir John Fortescue and the Crisis of Monarchy in Fifteenth-Century England.* Stamford.

————. 2000. "Ownership and Audience of TCC R.14.52 in the Fifteenth and Sixteenth Centuries." Paper presented at the Fourth International Conference on Fifteenth-Century Studies. Antwerp, Belgium.

Grosseteste, Robert. *De artibus liberalibus.* In Baur 1912, 1–7.

Gruman, Gerald J. 1966. *A History of Ideas about the Prolongation of Life: The Evolution of Prolongevity Hypotheses to 1800.* Transactions of the American Philosophical Society 56:9. Philadelphia.

Guillaume de Lorris and Jean de Meun. *Le Roman de la Rose.* See Langlois.

Gunther, R. T. 1923, 1929. *Early Science in Oxford.* Vols. 2 and 5. Oxford.

Gutas, Dimitri. 1998. *Greek Thought, Arabic Culture: The Graeco-Arabic Translation Movement in Baghdad and Early 'Abbasid Society (2nd–4th/8th–10th Centuries).* London and New York.

Hackett, Jeremiah, ed. 1997. *Roger Bacon and the Sciences: Commemorative Essays.* Leiden.

Hahn, Nan L. 1982. *Medieval Mensuration: Quadrans vetus and Geometrie due sunt partes principales . . . .* Transactions of the American Philosophical Society 72:8. Philadelphia.

Hahn, Thomas, ed. 1979. "The Middle English *Letter of Alexander to Aristotle*: Introduction, Text, Sources, and Commentary." *Mediaeval Studies* 41:106–60.

Hall, Hubert, and Frieda J. Nicholas, eds. 1929. *Select Tracts and Table Books Relating to English Weights and Measures (1100–1742).* Camden Society Miscellany 15; Camden 3rd ser., 41. London.

Hall, Thomas S. 1971. "Life, Death and the Radical Moisture: A Study of Thematic Pattern in Medieval Medical Theory." *Clio Medica* 6:3–23.

Hallaert, M.-R. 1982. *The 'Sekenesse of wymmen': A Middle English Treatise on Diseases in Women* (Yale Medical Library, Ms. 47 fols. 60r–71v). Scripta: Mediaeval and Renaissance Texts and Studies 8. Brussels.

Halleux, Robert. 1981. "Les Ouvrages alchimiques de Jean de Rupescissa." *Histoire littéraire de la France* 41:241–84.

Halliwell, James O. 1839. *Rara Mathematica, or A Collection of Treatises on the Mathematics and Subjects Connected with Them, from Ancient Inedited Manuscripts.* London.

————. 1840. *A Selection from the Minor Poems of Dan John Lydgate.* Percy Society, Early English Poetry 2. London.

Halversen, Marguerite A. 1998. "The Consideration of Quintessence: An Edition of a Middle English Translation of John of Rupescissa's *Liber de consideratione de* [sic] *quintae essentiae omnium rerum* with Introduction, Notes and Commentary." PhD Diss., Michigan State University.

Haly Abbas ('Alī ibn al-'Abbās al-Majūsī). 1523. *Liber totius medicine necessaria continens*. Lyons.

————. *Liber Pantegni*. See Constantinus Africanus.

Haly ibn Ridwān (Abu 'l-Ḥasan 'Alī ibn Riḍwān ibn 'Alī ibn Ja'far al-Miṣrī). 1493. *Super Teigne Galieni*. In *Articella*, part 3, fols. 1ra–49ra (sigs. A1ra–G3ra). Venice.

Hamesse, Jacqueline, and Marta Fattori, eds. 1990. *Rencontres de cultures dans la philosophie médiévale: Traductions et traducteurs de l'antiquité tardive au XIVᵉ siècle: Actes du Colloque internationale de Cassino, 15–17 juin 1989*. Publications de l'Institut d'Etudes Médiévales: Textes, études, congrès 11. Louvain-la-Neuve, Cassino.

Hammond, Eleanor Prescott. 1905. "Two British Museum Manuscripts (Harley 2251 and *Adds*. 34360): A Contribution to the Bibliography of John Lydgate." *Anglia* 28:1–28.

————. 1929. "A Scribe of Chaucer." *Modern Philology* 27:27–33.

Hanna, Ralph III. 1984. "Mandeville." In *Middle English Prose: A Critical Guide to Major Authors and Genres*, ed. A. S. G. Edwards, 121–32. New Brunswick, NJ.

————, ed. 1994. "Henry Daniel's *Liber Uricrisiarum*, Book I, Chapters 1–3." In Matheson 1994, 185–218.

————. 1997. *The Index of Middle English Prose. Handlist XII: Smaller Bodleian Collections: English Miscellaneous, English Poetry, English Theology, Finch, Latin Theology, Lyell, Radcliffe Trust*. Cambridge.

————, and Jeremy Griffiths. 2002. *A Descriptive Catalogue of the Western Medieval Manuscripts of St. John's College, Oxford*. Oxford.

Hanson, Ann Ellis, and Monica H. Green. 1994. "Soranus of Ephesus: *Methodicorum princeps*." In *Aufstieg und Niedergang der römischen Welt*, gen. ed. Wolfgang Haase and Hildegard Temporini, Teilband II, Band 37/2:968–1075. Berlin and New York.

Harley, Marta Powell, ed. 1985 for 1982. "The Middle English Contents of a Fifteenth-Century Medical Handbook." *Mediaevalia* 8:171–88.

Harris, Kate. 2001. "The Longleat House Extracted Manuscript of Gower's *Confessio amantis*." In Minnis 2001, 77–90.

Hartner, Willy. 1968. *Oriens-Occidens: Ausgewählte Schriften zur Wissenschafts- und Kulturgeschichte*, ed. Günther Kerstein et al. 2 vols. Hildesheim.

Harvey, Margaret. 1999. *The English in Rome 1362–1420: Portrait of an Expatriate Community*. Cambridge.

Harvey, Ruth, ed. 1984. *The Court of Sapience*. Toronto.

Hatcher, John. 1977. *Plague, Population and the English Economy 1348–1530*. London.

Hawes, Stephen. *Pastime of Pleasure*. See Mead 1928.

Heath, Thomas L., ed. 1956. *The Thirteen Books of Euclid's Elements*. 2nd ed. 3 vols. New York.

Heawood, Edward. 1950. *Watermarks*. Hilversum.

Hector, L. C., and Barbara F. Harvey, eds. and trans. 1982. *The Westminster Chronicle 1381–1394.* Oxford.

Hense, Otto, ed. 1914. *L. Annaei Senecae ad Lucilium epistularum moralium.* Leipzig.

Hertz, Martin. [1855–1859] 1961. *Prisciani Institutionum grammaticarum libri XVIII.* Vols. 2–3 of *Grammatici Latini,* ed. Heinrich Keil. 8 vols. 1855–1880. Repr. Hildesheim.

Hettinger, A. 1990. "Zum Lebensgeschichte und zum Todesdatum des Constantinus Africanus." *Deutsches Archiv* 46:517–29.

Hewson, M. Anthony. 1975. *Giles of Rome and the Medieval Theory of Conception: A Study of the 'De formatione corporis humani in utero.'* London.

Higgins, Iain Macleod. 1997. *Writing East: The "Travels" of Sir John Mandeville.* Philadelphia.

Hill, Betty, ed. 1965. "The Fifteenth-Century Prose *Legend of the Cross before Christ.*" *Medium Ævum* 34:203–23.

———, ed. 1980. "The Middle English and Latin Versions of the *Parva Recapitulatio* of Alexander the Great." *Notes & Queries* 225:4–20.

Hippocrates. 1493. *Liber pronosticorum primus.* In *Articella,* part 2, fols. 40ra–48vb (sigs. e8ra–f8vb). Venice.

———. *Works.* See W. H. S. Jones et al. 1923–1995.

Hoffman, Hartmut, ed. 1980. *Chronica Monasterii Casinensis.* Monumenta Germaniae Historica, Scriptores 34. Hannover.

Horobin, Simon. 1999. "Linguistic Features of the Hammond Scribe." *Poetica* 51:1–10.

———. 2003. *The Language of the Chaucer Tradition.* Chaucer Studies 32. Cambridge.

Horrox, Rosemary, ed. and trans. 1994. *The Black Death.* Manchester Medieval Sources. Manchester.

Hugh of St. Victor. *Practica geometriae.* See Baron 1966.

———. *Didascalicon.* See J. Taylor 1961.

Hulme, W. H. 1906. "A Valuable Middle English Manuscript." *Modern Philology* 4:67–73.

———, ed. 1918. "Richard Rolle of Hampole's *Mending of Life.*" *Western Reserve University Bulletin* n.s. 21/4:1–58.

———, ed. 1919. "Peter Alphonse's *Disciplina Clericalis.*" *Western Reserve University Bulletin* n.s. 22/3:12–71.

Humphreys, K. W., ed. 1990. *The Friars' Libraries.* Corpus of British Medieval Library Catalogues 1. London.

Hunt, Tony. 1989. *Plant Names of Medieval England.* Cambridge.

———. 1996. "The Poetic Vein: Phlebotomy in Middle English and Anglo-Norman Verse." *English Studies* 77:311–22.

ibn al-Jazzār (Abū Jaʿfar Aḥmad ibn Ibrāhīm ibn Abī Khālid ibn al-Jazzār). *De gradibus medicinarum* and *Viaticum.* In *Omnia opera Ysaac.* See Isaac Israeli.

Ilardi, A. 1964. "Galeno Ascitus Liber: De Compagine Membrorum sive De Natura Humana." *Atti e Memorie dell'Accademia di Storia dell'Arte Sanitaria* 30:175–82.

Israeli, Isaac (Isaac Judaeus, Abū Yaʿqūb Isḥāq ibn Sulaymān al-Isrāʾīlī). 1515. *Omnia opera Ysaac.* Lyons.

————. 1570. *De diaetis universalibus et particularibus libri II.* Basel.

Jacquart, Danielle. 1990. "Principales étapes dans la transmission des textes de médecine (XIᵉ – XIVᵉ siècle." In Hamesse and Fattori 1990, 251–71.

————. 1997. "Hippocrate en français: Le Livre des Amphorismes de Martin de Saint-Gille (1362–63)." In *Les voies de la science grecque: Études sur la transmission des textes de l'Antiquité au dix-neuvième siècle,* ed. Danielle Jacquart, 241–329. Geneva.

————, and Claude Thomasset. [1985] 1988. *Sexuality and Medicine in the Middle Ages.* Trans. Matthew Adamson. Cambridge.

James, Montague Rhodes. 1900–1904. *The Western Manuscripts of Trinity College, Cambridge: A Descriptive Catalogue.* 4 vols. Cambridge.

————. 1903. *The Ancient Libraries of Canterbury and Dover.* Cambridge.

————. 1907–1908. *A Descriptive Catalogue of the Manuscripts in the Library of Gonville and Caius College.* 2 vols. Cambridge.

Jarcho, Saul. 1970. "Galen's Six Non-Naturals: A Bibliographic Note and Translation." *Bulletin of the History of Medicine* 44:372–77.

Jasin, Joanne. 1983. "A Critical Edition of the Middle English *Liber Uricrisiarum* in Wellcome MS 225." PhD Diss., Tulane University.

————. 1993a. "The Compiler's Awareness of Audience in Medieval Medical Prose: The Example of Wellcome MS 225." *Journal of English and Germanic Philology* 92:509–22.

————. 1993b. "The Transmission of Learned Medical Literature in the Middle English *Liber uricrisiarum.*" *Medical History* 37:313–29.

Jenks, Stuart. 1985. "Medizinische Fachkräfte in England zur Zeit Heinrichs VI (1428/29 – 1460/61)." *Sudhoffs Archiv* 69:214–27.

John Damascene or Mesue (Abū Zakariyyā' Yuḥannā ibn Māsawayh). 1515. *Aphorismi.* In *Articella nuperrime impressa.* Lyons.

John Duns Scotus. *Annotationes in Marcianum.* See Lutz 1939.

Johnson, P. A. 1988. *Duke Richard of York, 1411–1460.* Oxford.

Jones, Claire. 1998. "Formula and Formulation: 'Efficacy Phrases' in Medieval English Medical Manuscripts." *Neuphilologische Mitteilungen* 99:199–209.

Jones, Peter Murray. 1989. "Four Middle English Translations of John of Arderne." In *Medieval Theory of Authorship: Scholastic Literary Attitudes in the Later Middle Ages,* ed. A. J. Minnis, 61–89. London.

————. 1990. "British Library MS Sloane 76: A Translator's Holograph." In *Medieval Book Production: Assessing the Evidence. Proceedings of the Second Conference of the Seminar in the History of the Book to 1500, Oxford, July 1988,* ed. Linda L. Brownrigg, 21–39. Los Altos Hills, CA.

————. 1998a. *Medieval Medicine in Illuminated Manuscripts.* Rev. ed. London.

————. 1998b. "Thomas Fayreford: An English Fifteenth-Century Medical Practitioner." In French et al. 1998, 156–83.

Jones, W. H. S., et al., trans. 1923–1995. *Hippocrates.* 8 vols. Loeb Classical Library. Cambridge, MA.

Jordan, Mark D. 1987. "Medicine as Science in the Early Commentaries on *Johannitius.*" *Traditio* 43:121–45.

————. 1994. "The Fortunes of Constantine's *Pantegni.*" In Burnett and Jacquart 1994, 286–301.

Josephus, Flavius. *Antiquities of the Jews.* See Thackeray et al. 1930–1965.

Josten, C. H. 1949. "The Text of John Dastin's 'Letter to Pope John XXII.'" *Ambix* 4:34–51.

Jouanna, Jacques. [1992] 1999. *Hippocrates.* Trans. M. B. DeBevoise. Baltimore.

Kean, P. M. 1965. "Langland on the Incarnation." *Review of English Studies* 16:349–63.

Keil, Gundolf. 1994. "'magister giselbertus de villa parisiensi': Beobachtungen zu den Kranewittbeeren und Gilberts pharmakologischen Renommé." *Sudhoffs Archiv* 78:80-89.

Keil, Heinrich. [1855–1880] 1961. *Grammatici Latini.* 8 vols. Repr. Hildesheim.

Keiser, George R., ed. 1994. "Epilepsy: The Falling Evil." In Matheson 1994, 219–44.

———. 1998. *Works of Science and Information. The Manual of Writings in Middle English.* Gen. ed. Albert E. Hartung. Vol. 10. New Haven.

———. 2003. "Two Medieval Plague Treatises and Their Afterlife in Early Modern England." *Journal of the History of Medicine* 58:292–324.

Kekewich, Margaret Lucille, et al., eds. 1995. *The Politics of Fifteenth-Century England: John Vale's Book.* Stroud, Gloucs.

Ker, N. R. 1964. *Medieval Libraries of Great Britain: A List of Surviving Books.* 2nd ed. London.

———. 1969–2002. *Medieval Manuscripts in British Libraries.* 5 vols. Vol. 2 (1977): Abbotsford – Keele. Oxford.

Kibre, Pearl. 1985. *Hippocrates Latinus: Repertorium of Hippocratic Writings in the Latin Middle Ages.* New York.

King, C. W., trans. 1903. *Plutarch's Morals: Theosophical Essays.* London.

Kipling, Gordon, ed. 1990. *The Receyt of the Ladie Kateryne.* EETS 296. Oxford.

Kitchell, Kenneth F., Jr., and Irven Michael Resnick, trans. and ann. 1999. *Albertus Magnus On Animals: A Medieval Summa Zoologica.* 2 vols. Baltimore and London.

Kretzmann, Norman, et al., eds. 1982. *The Cambridge History of Later Medieval Philosophy.* Cambridge.

Kristeller, Paul Oskar. 1956. "The School of Salerno: Its Development and Its Contribution to the History of Learning." In *Studies in Renaissance Thought and Letters,* 495–551. Rome.

———. 1976. "Bartholomaeus, Musandinus and Maurus of Salerno and Other Early Commentators of the 'Articella,' with a Tentative List of Texts and Manuscripts." *Italia medioevale e umanistica* 19:57–87.

Krochalis, Jeanne, and Edward Peters, eds. 1975. *The World of Piers Plowman.* Philadelphia.

Kruse, Britta-Juliane. 1996. *Verborgene Heilkünste: Geschichte der Frauenmedizin im Spätmittelalter.* Quellen und Forschungen zur Literatur- und Kulturgeschichte 5. Berlin.

Kühn, C. G., ed. [1821–1833] 1964–1965. *Claudii Galeni Opera Omnia.* 20 vols. Repr. Hildesheim.

Lafeuille, Germaine, ed. 1954. *Les Amphorismes Ypocras de Martin de Saint-Gille.* Geneva.

———, ed. 1964. *Les commentaires de Martin de Saint-Gille sur les Amphorismes Ypocras.* Geneva.

Laird, Edgar. 1997. "Astrolabes and the Construction of Time." *Disputatio* 2:51–69.

———. 1999. "Geoffrey Chaucer and Other Contributors to the *Treatise on the Astrolabe*." In *Rewriting Chaucer*, ed. Thomas A. Prendergast and Barbara Kline, 145–65. Columbus, OH.

———. 2000. "A Previously Unnoticed Manuscript of Chaucer's *Treatise on the Astrolabe*." *Chaucer Review* 34:410–15.

———, and Robert Fischer, eds. 1995. *Pèlerin de Prusse on the Astrolabe: Text and Translation of His "Practique de astralabe."* MRTS 127. Binghamton, NY.

Langlois, Ernest, ed. 1914–1924. *Le Roman de la Rose*. SATF. 5 vols. Vol. 4 (1922). Paris.

Latham, R. E. 1980. *Revised Medieval Latin Word-List from British and Irish Sources*. Repr. of 1965 ed., with suppl. London.

Lawn, Brian. 1963. *The Salernitan Questions. An Introduction to the History of Medieval and Renaissance Problem Literature*. Oxford.

Lazenby, Elizabeth, trans. and comm. 1993. *"De minutione sanguinis, sive de phlebotomia*: On Blood-Letting or Phlebotomy, by the Venerable Bede." In *Medicine in Northumbria: Essays on the History of Medicine in the North East of England*, ed. David Gardner-Medwin et al., 58–80. Newcastle upon Tyne.

Lekebusch, Julius. 1906. *Die Londoner Urkundensprache von 1430–1500*. Studien zur englischen Philologie 23. Halle am Saale.

Lemay, Richard. 1962. *Abu Ma'shar and Latin Aristotelianism in the Twelfth Century*. Beirut.

Lerer, Seth. 1990. "British Library MS Harley 78 and the Manuscripts of John Shirley." *Notes & Queries* 235:400–403.

Levi della Vida, G. 1938. "Something More about Artefius and His *Clavis Sapientiae*." *Speculum* 13:80–85.

Lexikon des Mittelalters. 1977–1999. 10 vols. Munich and Zürich.

Lilly, William. 1647. *Christian Astrology, Modestly Treated of in Three Books*. London.

Lind, L. R., ed. 1968. *Problemata varia anatomica: The University of Bologna MS 1165*. Lawrence, KS.

Lindberg, David C., ed. and trans. 1996. *Roger Bacon and the Origins of Perspectiva in the Middle Ages*. Oxford.

Lipton, Sara. 1999. *Images of Intolerance: The Representation of Jews and Judaism in the Bible moralisée*. Berkeley.

Littré, Emile, ed. 1839–1861. *Oeuvres complètes d'Hippocrate*. 10 vols. Paris.

Little, A. G., ed. 1914. *Roger Bacon Essays*. Oxford.

———, and E. Withington, eds. 1928. *De retardatione accidentium senectutis cum aliis opusculis de rebus medicinalibus*. Oxford.

Lohr, Charles H. 1986. "The Pseudo-Aristotelian *Liber de causis* and Latin Theories of Science in the Twelfth and Thirteenth Centuries." In *Pseudo-Aristotle in the Middle Ages: The "Theology" and Other Texts*, ed. Jill Kraye et al., 53–62. Warburg Institute Surveys and Texts 11. London.

Lonie, Iain M. 1981. *The Hippocratic Treatises "On Generation," "On the Nature of the Child," "Diseases IV": A Commentary*. Berlin and New York.

Lorch, Richard. 1980. "The *sphera solida* and Related Instruments." *Centaurus* 24:153–61.

Lowe, Peter. 1597. *The Booke of the Presages of Deuyne Hippocrates, deuyded into three partes.* London.

Lutz, Cora E., ed. 1939. *Iohannis Scotti Annotationes in Marcianum.* Cambridge, MA.

———. 1956. "Remigius' Ideas on the Classification of the Seven Liberal Arts." *Traditio* 12:65–86.

———, ed. 1962–1965. *Remigius Autissiodorensis: Commentum in Martianum Capellam.* 2 vols. Leiden.

Macaulay, G.C., ed. [1901–1902] 1979. *The English Works of John Gower.* EETS e.s. 81–82. Repr. London.

MacCracken, Henry Noble, ed. 1911–1934. *The Minor Poems of John Lydgate.* EETS e.s. 107, EETS o.s. 192. London.

Machielsen, John, ed. 2003. *Clavis patristica pseudepigraphorum Medii Aevi.* Vol. IIIA: *Artes liberales.* Corpus Christianorum Series Latina. Turnhout.

MacInnes, Ian. 2000. "Cheerful Girls and Willing Boys: Old and Young Bodies in Shakespeare's Sonnets." *Early Modern Literary Studies* 6.2: 1.1–26. http://www.shu.ac.uk/emls/06-2/macisonn.htm.

Maloney, Thomas S., ed. 1988. *Compendium of the Study of Theology.* Leiden.

Manget, Jean-Jaques. 1702. *Bibliotheca chemica curiosa.* 2 vols. Geneva.

Manly, John M., and Edith Rickert. 1940. *The Text of the Canterbury Tales.* 8 vols. Chicago.

Manzalaoui, M. A., ed. 1977. *Secretum Secretorum: Nine English Versions.* EETS 276. Oxford.

Martianus Capella. 1977. *The Marriage of Philology and Mercury.* In *Martianus Capella and the Seven Liberal Arts,* trans. William Harris Stahl and Richard Johnson, with E. L. Burge. Vol. 2. New York.

———. [1925] 1978. *Martianus Capella,* ed. Adolf Dick. Rev. ed. Stuttgart.

Martin de Saint-Gille. *Les Amphorismes Ypocras.* See Lafeuille 1954; Lafeuille 1964.

Martín Ferreira, Ana Isabel, ed. 1996. *Tratado médico de Constantino el Africano: Constantini Liber de elephancia.* Valladolid.

Masi, Michael, ed. 1981. *Boethius and the Liberal Arts: A Collection of Essays.* Bern.

Matheson, Lister M., ed. 1994. *Popular and Practical Science of Medieval England.* Medieval Texts and Studies 11. East Lansing, MI.

———, ed. 1999. *Death and Dissent: Two Fifteenth-Century Chronicles.* Woodbridge.

———. 2005. "*Médecin sans Frontières?*: The European Dissemination of John of Burgundy's Plague Treatise." *ANQ* 18.3: 17–28.

———, and Ann Shannon, eds. 1994. "A Treatise on the Elections of Times." In Matheson 1994, 23–59.

May, Margaret Tallmadge. 1968. *Galen on the Usefulness of the Parts of the Body: Peri chreias morion. De usu partium.* 2 vols. Ithaca.

McIntosh, Angus. 1973. "Word Geography in the Lexicography of Medieval English." In *Lexicography in English,* ed. Raven I. McDavid, Jr., and Audrey R. Duckert. *Annals of the New York Academy of Sciences* 211:55–66.

———, et al. 1986. *A Linguistic Atlas of Late Mediaeval English.* 4 vols. Aberdeen.

McVaugh, Michael R. 1971. "Constantine the African." In *Dictionary of Scientific Biography,* ed. Charles Coulston Gillispie, 3:393–95. New York.

———. 1972. "Theriac at Montpellier 1285–1325." *Sudhoffs Archiv* 76:113–27.

————. 1974. "The 'Humidum Radicale' in Thirteenth-Century Medicine." *Traditio* 30:259–83.

————. 1997. "Bedside Manners in the Middle Ages." The Fielding H. Garrison Lecture. *Bulletin of the History of Medicine* 71:201–23.

————. 2003. "Alchemy in the *Chirurgia* of Teodorico Borgognoni." In Crisciani and Paravicini Bagliani 2003, 55–75.

Mead, William Edward, ed. 1928 [for 1927]. *Stephen Hawes: Pastime of Pleasure.* EETS 173. London.

Means, Laurel, ed. 1993. *Medieval Lunar Astrology: A Collection of Representative Middle English Texts.* Lewiston.

Mellinkoff, Ruth. 1993. *Outcasts: Signs of Otherness in Northern European Art of the Later Middle Ages.* 2 vols. Berkeley.

Merisalo, Outi, and Päivi Pahta. 2004. "Tracing the Trail of Transmission: The Pseudo-Galenic *De spermate* in Latin." Paper presented at the Science Translated Conference, Leuven.

Merkelbach, R., and M. L. West, eds. 1967. *Fragmenta Hesiodea.* Oxford.

Meskens, Ad, et al. 1999. "Wine-Gauging at Damme: The Evidence of a Late Medieval Manuscript." *Histoire & Mesure* 14:51–77.

Millàs Vallicrosa, J. 1932. "La Introducción del Cuadrante con Cursor en Europa." *Isis* 17:218–58.

Minnis, A. J. 1993. "Chaucer's Commentator: Nicholas Trevet and the *Boece.*" In *Chaucer's "Boece" and the Medieval Tradition of Boethius,* ed. A. J. Minnis, 83–166. Cambridge.

————, ed. 2001. *Middle English Poetry: Texts and Traditions. Essays in Honour of Derek Pearsall.* Woodbridge.

Montero Cartelle, Enrique, ed., 1983. *Constantini Liber de coitu. El tratado de andrología de Constantino el Africano.* Monografías de la Universidad de Santiago de Compostela 77. Santiago de Compostela.

————, ed. 1987. *Liber minor de coitu: Tratado Menor de Andrologia Anonimo Salernitano.* Lingüística y Filología 2. Valladolid.

————. 1988. "Sobre el autor árabe del *Liber de coitu* y el mode de trabajar de Constantino el Africano." *Medizinhistorisches Journal* 23:213–23.

————. 1990. "Encuentro de culturas en Salerno: Constantino el Africano, traductor." In Hamesse and Fattori 1990, 65–88.

————, and Ana Isabel Martín Ferreira. 1994. "Le *De elephancia* de Constantine l'Africain et ses rapports avec le *Pantegni.*" In Burnett and Jacquart 1994, 233–46.

Mooney, Linne R. 1993a. "The Cock and the Clock: Telling Time in Chaucer's Day." *Studies in the Age of Chaucer* 15:91–109.

————. 1993b. "A Middle English Text on the Seven Liberal Arts." *Speculum* 68:1027–52.

————. 1994. "Diet and Bloodletting: A Monthly Regimen." In Matheson 1994, 245–61.

————. 1995. *The Index of Middle English Prose. Handlist XI: Manuscripts in the Library of Trinity College, Cambridge.* Cambridge.

————. 1996. "More Manuscripts Written by a Chaucer Scribe." *The Chaucer Review* 30:401–7.

————, ed. 1998. *The Kalendarium of John Somer.* Athens, GA.

————. 2000. "A New Manuscript by the Hammond Scribe Discovered by Jeremy Griffiths." In *The English Medieval Book: Studies in Memory of Jeremy Griffiths,* ed. A. S. G. Edwards, Vincent Gillespie, and Ralph Hanna, 113–23. London.

————. 2001. "Scribes and Booklets of Trinity College, Cambridge, Manuscripts R.3.19 and R.3.21." In Minnis 2001, 241–66.

————. 2003. "John Shirley's Heirs." *Yearbook of English Studies,* special number 33: *Medieval and Early Modern Miscellanies and Anthologies,* ed. Phillipa Hardman, 182–98.

————. 2004. "Manuscript Evidence for the Use of Medieval English Scientific and Utilitarian Texts." In *Interstices: Studies in Middle English and Anglo-Latin Texts in Honour of A. G. Rigg,* ed. Richard Firth Green and Linne R. Mooney, 184–202. Toronto.

————, and Lister M. Matheson. 2003. "The Beryn Scribe and His Texts: Evidence for Multiple-Copy Production of Manuscripts in Fifteenth-Century England." *The Library,* 7th ser., 4:347–70.

Moorat, S. A. J. 1962. *Catalogue of Western Manuscripts on Medicine and Science in the Wellcome Historical Medical Library.* Vol. 1. London.

Morgenstern, Arthur. 1917. *Das Aderlassgedicht des Johannes von Aquila, und seine Stellung in der Aderlasslehre des Mittelalters, samt dem Abdruck der lateinischen Übersetzung der Schrift Peri flebotomia Ypocratis, nach den Handschriften in Brüssel und Dresden.* Inaug.-Diss., Leipzig.

Mosser, Daniel. N.d. "Paperstocks Used by the Hammond Scribe." Unpublished paper.

Muntner, Suessman. 1944. "Maimonides' Book for Al-Fadil." *Isis* 35:3–5.

Murano, Giovanna. 2001. "Frammenti di un *exemplar* nella Biblioteka Narodowa di Varsavia (MS III. 8069)." *Scriptorium* 55:294–98.

Murdoch, John E. 1968. "The Medieval Euclid: Salient Aspects of the Translations of the *Elements* by Adelard of Bath and Campanus of Novara." *Revue de synthèse* 89:67–94.

————. 1984. *Album of Science: Antiquity and the Middle Ages.* New York.

Mynors, R. A. B. 1939. *Durham Cathedral Manuscripts to the End of the Twelfth Century.* Oxford.

Needham, Joseph. 1954– . *Science and Civilisation in China.* Vol. 5: *Chemistry and Chemical Technology,* 1974– . Parts 2–5: *Spagyrical Discovery and Invention, 1974–1983.* Cambridge.

————. 1975. "The Elixir Concept and Chemical Medicine in East and West." *Organon* 11:167–92.

Neugebauer, Otto. 1957. *The Exact Sciences in Antiquity.* 2nd ed. Providence, RI.

Newman, William R. 1994. "The Alchemy of Roger Bacon and the *Tres epistolae* Attributed to Him." In *Comprendre et maîtriser la nature au Moyen Age: mélanges d'histoire des sciences offerts à Guy Beaujouan,* 461–79. Hautes études médiévales et modernes 73. Paris.

————. 1995. "The Philosopher's Egg: Theory and Practice in the Alchemy of Roger Bacon." *Micrologus* 3:75–101.

Newton, Francis. 1994. "Constantine the African and Monte Cassino: New Elements and the Text of the *Isagoge.*" In Burnett and Jacquart 1994, 14–47.

Nicholas of Lynn. See Eisner 1980.

Niebyl, Peter H. 1971a. "The Non-Naturals." *Bulletin of the History of Medicine* 45:486–92.

———. 1971b. "Old Age, Fever, and the Lamp Metaphor." *Journal of the History of Medicine* 26:351–68.

Norri, Juhani. 1992. *Names of Sicknesses in English, 1400–1550: An Exploration of the Lexical Field.* Annales Academiae Scientiarum Fennicae, Dissertationes Humanarum Litterarum 63. Helsinki.

———. 1998. *Names of Body Parts in English, 1400–1550.* Annales Academiae Scientiarum Fennicae, Humaniora 291. Helsinki.

———. 2004. "Entrances and Exits in English Medical Vocabulary, 1400–1550." In Taavitsainen and Pahta 2004, 100–143.

North, J. D., ed. 1976. *Richard of Wallingford: An Edition of His Writings.* 3 vols. Oxford.

———. 1988. *Chaucer's Universe.* Oxford.

———. 2005. *God's Clockmaker: Richard of Wallingford and the Invention of Time.* London and New York.

Novus quadrans and *Ars et operatio novi quadrantis.* See F. S. Pedersen 1984.

Nutton, Vivian. 1983. "The Seeds of Disease: An Explanation of Contagion and Infection from the Greeks to the Renaissance." *Medical History* 27:1–34.

———. 2000. "Did the Greeks Have a Word for It?" In *Contagion: Perspectives from Pre-Modern Societies,* ed. Lawrence I. Conrad and Dominik Wujastyk, 137–62. Aldershot.

O'Boyle, Cornelius. 1998a. *The Art of Medicine: Medical Teaching at the University of Paris, 1250–1400.* Leiden.

———. 1998b. *Thirteenth- and Fourteenth-Century Copies of the "Ars medicine."* Articella Studies 1. Cambridge and Barcelona.

Ogden, Margaret S., ed. [1938] 1969. *The "Liber de Diversis Medicinis" in the Thornton Manuscript (MS. Lincoln Cathedral A.5.2).* Rev. repr. EETS 207. London.

———, ed. 1971. *The Cyrurgie of Guy de Chauliac.* EETS 265. London.

Olson, Donald W., and Edgar S. Laird. 1996. "Right Ascension." *American Journal of Physics* 64:1099–1100.

Olson, Glending. 1982. *Literature as Recreation in the Later Middle Ages.* Ithaca.

O'Neill, Ynez Violé. 1993. "Diagrams of the Medieval Brain: A Study in Cerebral Localization." In *Iconography at the Crossroads,* ed. Brendan Cassidy, 91–105. Princeton.

Ottaviano, Carmelo, ed. 1935. *Un brano inedito della "Philosophia" di Guglielmo di Conches.* Naples.

Ovid. *Ex Ponto.* See Wheeler 1924.

Pahta, Päivi. 1998. *Medieval Embryology in the Vernacular: The Case of "De Spermate."* Mémoires de la Société Néophilologique de Helsinki 53. Helsinki.

———. 2001. "Creating a New Genre: Contextual Dimensions in the Production and Transmission of Early Scientific Writing." *European Journal of English Studies* 5:205–20.

———. 2004a. "Code-Switching in Medieval Medical Writing." In Taavitsainen and Pahta 2004, 73–99.

———. 2004b. "'So seiþ *idem comentator*': Code-Switching and Organisation of Knowledge in John Trevisa's Translation of *De proprietatibus rerum*." In *Voices on the Past: Studies in Old and Middle English Language and Literature*, ed. Alicia Rodríguez Álvarez and Francisco Alonso Almeida. A Coruña.

———, and Saara Nevanlinna. 1997. "Re-phrasing in Early English: The Use of Expository Apposition with an Explicit Marker from 1350 to 1710." In *English in Transition: Corpus-Based Studies in Linguistic Variation and Genre Styles*, ed. Matti Rissanen et al., 121–83. Berlin and New York.

———, and Irma Taavitsainen. 2004. "Vernacularisation of Scientific and Medical Writing in Its Sociohistorical Context." In Taavitsainen and Pahta 2004, 1–18.

Palmer, Richard. 1999. *Catalogue of Western Manuscripts in the Wellcome Library for the History and Understanding of Medicine: Western Manuscripts 5120–6244*. London.

Paniagua, Juan Antonio. 1994. *Studia Arnaldiana: Trabajos en torno a la obra médica de Arnau de Vilanova, c. 1240–1311*. Fundación Uriach 1838. Barcelona.

Pansier, P. 1909. "Un Manuel d'accouchements du XVme siècle." *Janus* 14:217-20 (with plates).

Paravicini Bagliani, Agostino. 1987. "Ruggero Bacone autore del 'De retardatione accidentium senectutis'?" With addendum by Paravicini Bagliani and Steven J. Williams. *Studi Medievali*, ser. 3, 28:707–28.

———. 1991a. "Il mito della 'prolongatio vitae' e la corte pontificia del Duecento: il 'De retardatione accidentium senectutis.'" In *Medicina e scienze della natura alla corte dei papi nel Duecento*, 281–326. Spoleto.

———. 1991b. "Ruggero Bacone, Bonifacio VIII e la teoria della 'prolongatio vitae.'" In *Medicina e scienze della natura alla corte dei papi nel Duecento*, 327–61. Spoleto.

———. [1994] 2000. *The Pope's Body*. Trans. David S. Peterson. Chicago.

———. 2003. "Ruggero Bacone e l'alchimia di lunga vita: Riflessioni sui testi." In Crisciani and Paravicini Bagliani 2003, 33–54.

Parker, Col. 1929. *Lay Subsidy Rolls, I. Edward III, N.R. York and the City of York*. Yorkshire Archaeological Society, Record Series 74. Leeds.

Parkes, Malcolm. [1969] 1980. *English Cursive Book Hands, 1250–1500*. Corr. repr. Berkeley.

Patai, Raphael. 1994. *The Jewish Alchemists: A History and Sourcebook*. Princeton.

Pattin, Adriaan, ed. 1967. *Le Liber de causis: Édition établie à l'aide de 90 manuscrits avec introduction et notes*. Uitgave van Tijdschift voor filosofie. Leuven.

Peck, Russell A., ed. 1991. *Heroic Women from the Old Testament in Middle English Verse*. Kalamazoo, MI.

Pedersen, Fritz [Fridericus] Saaby, ed. 1984. *Petri Philomenae de Dacia et Petri de S. Audomaro opera quadrivialia*, vol. 2. Hauniae.

Pedersen, Olaf. [1974] 1993. *Early Physics and Astronomy*. Rev. ed. Cambridge.

Pereira, Michela. 1989. *The Alchemical Corpus Attributed to Raymond Lull*. Warburg Institute Surveys and Texts 18. London.

————. 1992. *L'oro dei filosofi: saggio sulle idee di un alchimista del Trecento.* Spoleto.

————. 1993. "Un tesoro inestimabile: Elixir e 'prolongatio vitae' nell'alchimia del '300." *Micrologus* 1:161–87.

————. 1995. "Teorie dell'elixir nell'alchimia latina medievale." *Micrologus* 3:103–48.

————. 1998. "*Mater Medicinarum*: English Physicians and the Alchemical Elixir in the Fifteenth Century." In French et al. 1998, 26–52.

————. 1999. "Alchemy and the Use of Vernacular Languages in the Late Middle Ages." *Speculum* 74:336–56.

Peter the Deacon. *De viris illustribus.* See Bloch 1986, 1:127–29.

Piccard, Gerhard. 1980. *Wasserzeichen: Werkzeug und Waffen.* Findbuch 9. 2 vols. Stuttgart.

————. 1996. *Wasserzeichen: Dreiberg.* Findbuch 16. 2 vols. Stuttgart.

Pinborg, Jan. 1982. "Remigius, Schleswig 1486: A Latin Grammar in Facsimile Edition with a Postscript." *Historisk-filosofiske meddelelser* 50/4:63–65.

Pliny. *Natural History.* See Rackham et al. 1938–1963.

Plummer, Charles. [1885] 1979. *The Governance of England, otherwise called The Difference between an Absolute and a Limited Monarchy, by Sir John Fortescue, Kt.* Repr. Westport, CT.

Pollard, Alfred W., ed. [1903] 1964. *Fifteenth Century Prose and Verse.* Repr. New York.

Poulle, Emmanuel. [1967] 1983. *Les Instruments astronomiques du moyen âge.* Repr. Paris.

————. 1964. "Le quadrant nouveau médiéval." *Journal des savants* (April–June and July–September): 148–67 and 182–214.

————. 1981. *Les sources astronomiques: textes, tables, instruments.* Typologie des sources du Moyen Age occidental 39. Turnhout.

————. 1991. "L'instrumentation astronomique médiévale." In *Observer, lire, écrire le ciel au moyen âge: Actes du colloque d'Orléans, 22–23 avril 1989*, ed. Bernard Ribémont, 253–81. Paris.

Powicke, F. M. 1931. *The Medieval Books of Merton College.* Oxford.

Prior, Oliver H., ed. 1913 (for 1912). *William Caxton's Mirrour of the World.* EETS e.s. 110. London.

Priscian. *Institutiones grammaticarum libri XVIII.* See Hertz [1855–1859] 1961.

Profatius Judaeus. *Il Quadrante d'Israel.* See Boffito and Melzi d'Eril, eds. 1922.

Pseudo-Messahalla. *Compositio et operatio astrolabii.* In Gunther 1929, 5:133–231. Oxford.

Ptolemy (Claudius Ptolemaeus). 1493. *Opus quadripartitum.* Venice.

————. *Tetrabiblos.* See F. E. Robbins 1940.

————. *Almagest.* See Toomer 1984.

Quadrans vetus. See Hahn 1982.

Rackham, H., trans. 1933. *Cicero: De natura deorum.* Loeb Classical Library. London.

————, et al., trans. 1938–1963. *Pliny: Natural History.* 10 vols. Loeb Classical Library. Cambridge, MA.

Radulescu, Raluca L. 2003. *The Gentry Context for Malory's Morte Darthur.* Cambridge.

Rand Schmidt, Kari Anne. 2001. *Index of Middle English Prose. Handlist 17: Manuscripts in the Library of Gonville and Caius College, Cambridge.* Woodbridge.

Randel, Don Michael, ed. 1978. *Harvard Concise Dictionary of Music.* Cambridge, MA.

Rather, L. J. 1968. "The 'Six Things Non-Natural': A Note on the Origins and Fate of a Doctrine and a Phrase." *Clio Medica* 3:337–47.

Rawcliffe, Carole. 1995. *Medicine and Society in Later Medieval England.* Phoenix Mill.

———. 2003. "Women, Childbirth, and Religion in Later Medieval England." In *Women and Religion in Medieval England,* ed. Diana Wood, 91–117. Oxford.

Recorde, Robert. 1551. *Pathway to Knowledge.* London.

Reidy, John, ed. 1975. *Thomas Norton's Ordinal of Alchemy.* EETS 272. London.

Remigius of Auxerre. *Commentum in Martianum Capellam.* See Lutz 1962–1965.

———. *In artem Donati minorem commentum.* See Fox 1902.

Rhazes (Abū Bakr Muḥammad Zakariyyā' al-Rāzī). 1497. *Liber ad Almansorem* [with other medical tracts]. Venice.

Riddle, John M. 1964. "*Pomum ambrae*: Amber and Ambergris in Plague Remedies." *Sudhoffs Archiv* 48:111–22.

Riha, Ortrun. 1994. "Gilbertus Anglicus und sein 'Compendium medicinae': Arbeitstechnik und Wissensorganisation." *Sudhoffs Archiv* 78:59–79.

Robbins, F. E., ed. and trans. 1940. *Tetrabiblos.* Cambridge, MA.

Robbins, Rossell Hope. 1970. "Signs of Death in Middle English." *Mediaeval Studies* 32:282–98.

Robinson, Peter, ed. 1996. *The Wife of Bath's Prologue on CD-ROM.* Cambridge.

Roche, John J. 1981. "The Radius Astronomicus in England." *Annals of Science* 38:1–32.

Roger de Baron. 1519. *Practica maior.* In *Cyrurgia Guidonis de Cauliaco, et Cyrurgia Bruni, Teodorici, Rolandi, Lanfranci, Rogerii, Bertapalie,* fols. 211r–234v. Venice.

Ronca, Italo. 1994. "The Influence of the *Pantegni* on William of Conches's *Dragmaticon.*" In Burnett and Jacquart 1994, 266–85.

Rose, Valentin, ed. 1882. *Sorani Gynaeciorum vetus translatio latina.* Leipzig.

Rotuli Parliamentorum; ut et petitiones, et placita in parliamento. 1767–1777. 6 vols. London.

Rowland, Beryl, ed. 1981. *Medieval Woman's Guide to Health: The First English Gynecological Handbook.* Kent, OH.

Ruska, Julius. 1934. "Die Alchemie des Avicenna." *Isis* 21:14–51.

Russell, Gül. 1994. "The Anatomy of the Eye in 'Alī ibn al-'Abbās al-Maǧūsī: A Textbook Case." In Burnett and Jacquart 1994, 247–65.

Russell, Jeffrey Burton. 1991. *Inventing the Flat Earth: Columbus and Modern Historians.* New York.

Samuels, M. L. 1963. "Some Applications of Middle English Dialectology." *English Studies* 46:81–94.

———. 1981. "Spelling and Dialect in the Late and Post-Middle English Periods." In Benskin and Samuels 1981, 43–54.

———. 1983. "Chaucer's Spelling." In *Middle English Studies Presented to Norman Davis in Honour of His Seventieth Birthday,* ed. Douglas Gray and E. G. Stanley, 17–37. Oxford.

————, and J. J. Smith. 1981. "The Language of Gower." *Neuphilologische Mitteilungen* 82:295–304.

Sandved, Arthur O. 1981. "Prolegomena to a Renewed Study of the Rise of Standard English." In Benskin and Samuels 1981, 31–42.

Sarton, George. [1927–1948] 1975. *Introduction to the History of Science.* 3 vols. in 5. Vol. 1. Repr. Huntington, NY.

Savage-Smith, Emilie. 1985. *Islamicate Celestial Globes: Their History, Construction, and Use.* Smithsonian Studies in History and Technology 46. Washington, DC.

Schäfer, Daniel. 2004. *Alter und Krankheit in der Frühen Neuzeit: Die ärztliche Blick auf die letzte Lebensphase.* Frankfurt.

Schipperges, Heinrich. 1960. "Makrobiotic bei Petrus Hispanus." *Sudhoffs Archiv* 44:129–55.

————. 1964. *Die Assimilation der arabischen Medizin durch das lateinische Mittelalter.* Wiesbaden.

Schmolinsky, Sabine, and Karl Heinz Keller. 2001. *Katalog der lateinischen Handschriften der Staatlichen Bibliothek [Schlossbibliothek] Ansbach.* Vol. 2: Ms. lat. 94 – Ms. lat. 173. Wiesbaden.

Schöffler, Herbert. 1919. *Beiträge zur mittelenglischen Medizinliteratur.* Halle.

Sears, Elizabeth. 1986. *The Ages of Man: Medieval Interpretations of the Life Cycle.* Princeton.

Seneca, L. Annaeus. *Epistulae morales.* See Hense 1914.

Seymour, M. C., et al., eds. 1975–1988. *On the Properties of Things: John Trevisa's Translation of Bartholomæus Anglicus De Proprietatibus Rerum.* 3 vols. Oxford.

Sezgin, Fuat. 1970. *Geschichte des arabischen Schrifttums.* Vol. 3: *Medizin, Pharmazie, Zoologie, Tierheilkunde bis ca. 430 H.* Leiden.

Sharpe, Richard. 2001. *A Handlist of the Latin Writers of Great Britain and Ireland before 1540.* Rev. ed. Turnhout.

————, et al., eds. 1996. *English Benedictine Libraries: The Shorter Catalogues.* Corpus of British Medieval Library Catalogues 4. London.

Shrewsbury, J. F. D. 1971. *A History of Bubonic Plague in the British Isles.* Cambridge.

Singer, Charles. 1917. "A Review of the Medical Literature of the Dark Ages, with a New Text of about 1110." *Proceedings of the Royal Society of Medicine* 10:107–60.

Singer, Dorothea Waley. 1916. "Some Plague Tractates (Fourteenth and Fifteenth Centuries)." *Proceedings of the Royal Society of Medicine* 9:159–212.

————, and Annie Anderson. 1950. *Catalogue of Latin and Vernacular Plague Texts in Great Britain and Eire in Manuscripts Written before the Sixteenth Century.* Paris and London.

Siraisi, Nancy G. 1987. *Avicenna in Renaissance Italy: The Canon and Medical Teaching in Italian Universities after 1500.* Princeton.

————. 1990. *Medieval and Early Renaissance Medicine: An Introduction to Knowledge and Practice.* Chicago.

Smith, Ben. 1966. *Traditional Imagery of Charity in Piers Plowman.* The Hague.

Solinus. 1587. *Collectanea rerum memorabilium.* Trans. Arthur Golding, *The Excellent and Pleasant Worke of Iulius Solinus Polyhistor.* London.

Somer, John. *Kalendarium.* See Mooney 1998.

Sournia, J. C., and G. Troupeau. 1968. "Médecine arabe: Biographies critiques de Jean Mésué (VIII° siècle) et du Prétendu 'Mésué le Jeune' (X° siècle). *Clio Medica* 3.109–17.

Stannard, Jerry, and Linda Ehrsam Voigts. 1982. Rev. of Beryl Rowland, *Medieval Woman's Guide to Health*. *Speculum* 57:422–26.

Statutes of the Realm (1225–1713). 1810–1822. 9 vols. London.

Steele, Robert, ed. 1898. *Three Prose Versions of the Secreta Secretorum*. With Glossary by T. Henderson. EETS e.s. 74. London.

———, ed. 1920. *Secretum secretorum cum glossis et notulis . . . Fratris Rogeri*. Opera hactenus inedita Rogeri Baconi 5. Oxford.

Steinschneider, Moritz. 1866. "Constantinus Africanus und seine arabischen Quellen." *Virchow's Archiv für pathologische Anatomie und Physiologie* 37:351–54.

Stoertz, Fiona Harris. 1996. "Suffering and Survival in Medieval English Childbirth. " In *Medieval Family Roles: A Book of Essays*, ed. Cathy Jorgensen Itnyre, 101–20. New York.

Stoneman, William P., ed. 1999. *Dover Priory*. Corpus of British Medieval Library Catalogues 5. London.

Stow, John. 1908. *A Survay of London*, ed. Henry Morley. London.

Stratford, Jenny. 1987. "The Manuscripts of John, Duke of Bedford: Library and Chapel." In *England in the Fifteenth Century: Proceedings of the Harlaxton Conference*, ed. Daniel Williams, 329–50. Woodbridge.

Stump, Eleonore, trans. 1978. *Boethius's De topicis differentiis*. Ithaca.

Sudhoff, Karl. 1912. "Pestschriften aus den ersten 150 Jahren nach der Epidemie des 'schwarzen Todes' 1348: III. Aus Niederdeutschland, Frankreich und England." *Sudhoffs Archiv* 5:36–87.

———. 1914–1918. *Beiträge zur Geschichte der Chirurgie im Mittelalter*. 2 vols. Leipzig.

Sutton, Anne F., and Livia Visser-Fuchs. 1995a. "British Library Manuscript Additional 48031A: The Manuscript, Its Later Ownership and Its Contents." In Kekewich et al. 1995, 127–268.

———. 1995b. "The Provenance of the Manuscript: The Lives and Archive of Sir Thomas Cook and His Man of Affairs, John Vale." In Kekewich et al. 1995, 73–123.

Taavitsainen, Irma. 2004. "Transferring Classical Discourse Conventions into the Vernacular." In Taavitsainen and Pahta 2004, 37–72.

Taavitsainen, Irma, and Päivi Pahta. 1998. "Vernacularisation of Medical Writing in English: A Corpus-Based Study of Scholasticism." *Early Science and Medicine* 3:157–85.

———. 2001. "Transferring Classical Conventions: Commentaries in Early English Medical Writing." Paper presented at the 36th International Congress on Medieval Studies. Kalamazoo, MI.

———, eds. 2004. *Medical and Scientific Writing in Late Medieval English*. Cambridge.

Taavitsainen, Irma, Päivi Pahta, and Martti Mäkinen, eds., with Raymond Hickey. 2005. *Middle English Medical Texts* [CD-ROM]. Amsterdam.

Taglia, Kathryn. 2001. "Delivering a Christian Identity: Midwives in Northern French Synodal Legislation, c. 1200–1500." In *Religion and Medicine in the*

Middle Ages, ed. Peter Biller and Joseph Ziegler, 77–90. York Studies in
Medieval Theology 3. York.

Talbot, C. H., and E. A. Hammond. 1965. *The Medical Practitioners in Medieval
England: A Biographical Register.* (With suppl. in Getz 1990b.) London.

Tallgren, O. J. 1928. "Survivance arabo-romane du Catalogue d'étoiles de Ptolémée:
Etudes philologiques sur différents manuscrits." *Studia Orientalia* 2:202–82.

Tavormina, M. Teresa. 2005. "The Twenty-Jordan Series: An Illustrated Middle
English Uroscopy Text." *ANQ* 18.3:40–64.

Taylor, Barry. 1992. "Medieval Proverb Collections: The West European
Tradition." *Journal of the Warburg and Courtauld Institutes* 55:19–35.

Taylor, F. Sherwood. 1953. "The Idea of the Quintessence." In *Science, Medicine, and
History: Essays on the Evolution of Scientific Thought and Medical Practice written in
honour of Charles Singer,* ed. E. Ashworth Underwood, 1:247–65. London.

Taylor, Jerome, ed. and trans. 1961. *The Didascalicon of Hugh of St. Victor.* New York.

Temkin, Owsei. 1951. "On Galen's Pneumatology." *Gesnerus* 8:180–89.

Thackeray, Henry St. John, et al. 1930–1965. *Josephus: Antiquities of the Jews.* In
Josephus: Works, vols. 4–9. Loeb Classical Library. Cambridge, MA.

Theisen [Theissen], Wilfred. 1986. "John Dastin's Letter on the Philosopher's
Stone." *Ambix* 33:78–87.

———. 1991. "John Dastin: The Alchemist as Co-Creator." *Ambix* 38:73–78.

———. 1999. "John Dastin's Alchemical Vision." *Ambix* 46:65–72.

Thomas, John, and Angela Constantinides Hero, eds., with Giles Constable.
2000. *Byzantine Monastic Foundation Documents: A Complete Translation of the
Surviving Founders' Typika and Testaments.* 5 vols. Dumbarton Oaks Studies 35.
Washington, DC.

Thomson, David. 1984. *Edition of the Middle English Grammatical Texts.* New York.

Thomson, R. M. 2001. *A Descriptive Catalogue of the Medieval Manuscripts in Worcester
Cathedral Library.* Cambridge.

Thorndike, Lynn. 1914. "Roger Bacon and Experimental Method in the Middle
Ages." *The Philosophical Review* 23:271–98.

———. 1949. "Visierkunst, Ars Visorandi, or Stereometry." *Isis* 40:106–7.

———. 1956. "Notes upon Some Medieval Latin Astronomical, Astrological and
Mathematical Manuscripts at the Vatican." *Isis* 47:391–404.

———, and Pearl Kibre. 1963. *A Catalogue of Incipits of Mediaeval Scientific Writings
in Latin.* The Mediaeval Academy of America Publication 29. Rev. ed.
Cambridge, MA.

———, and Pearl Kibre. Forthcoming. *A Catalogue of Incipits of Mediaeval Scientific
Writings in Latin.* Electronic ed., rev. Linda Ehrsam Voigts. National Library
of Medicine. http://www.nlm.nih.gov/hmd.

———, ed., with Francis S. Benjamin, Jr. 1946. *The Herbal of Rufinus, Edited from the
Unique Manuscript.* Chicago.

Toomer, G. J., trans. and ann. 1984. *Ptolemy's Almagest.* New York and Berlin.

Trotter, David. 1999. "L'Importance lexicographique du *Traitier de cyrurgie*
d'Albucasis en ancien français (B.N. fr. 1318)." *Revue de linguistique romane*
63:23–53.

Troupeau, Gérard. 1994. "Manuscripts of the *Kāmil as-sinā'a* [= *Kitāb al-Malikī*]."
    In Burnett and Jacquart 1994, 303–15.
Ullmann, Manfred. 1972. *Die Natur- und Geheimwissenschaften im Islam*. Leiden.
————. 1978. *Islamic Medicine*. Edinburgh.
van der Gaaf, W. 1920. "Notes on English Orthography (*ie* and *ea*)." *Neophilologus*
    5:133–59, 333–48.
Vaulx, Jacques de. 1583. *Les Premières Euvres de Jacques de Vaulx, pillote en la marine*.
    Le Havre.
Victor, Stephen K., ed. and trans. 1979. *Practical Geometry in the High Middle
    Ages: Artis cuiuslibet consummatio and the Praktike de geometrie*. Memoirs of the
    American Philosophical Society 134. Philadelphia.
Voigts, Linda Ehrsam. 1989. "Scientific and Medical Books." In Griffiths and
    Pearsall 1989, 345–402.
————. 1990. "The 'Sloane Group': Related Scientific and Medical Manuscripts
    from the Fifteenth Century in the Sloane Collection." *The British Library
    Journal* 16:26–57.
————. 1995a. "A Doctor and His Books: The Manuscripts of Roger Marchall (d.
    1477)." In *New Science Out of Old Books: Studies in Manuscripts and Early Printed
    Books in Honour of A. I. Doyle*, ed. Richard Beadle and A. J. Piper, 249–314.
    Aldershot.
————. 1995b. "Multitudes of Middle English Medical Manuscripts, or the
    Englishing of Science and Medicine." In *Manuscript Sources of Medieval
    Medicine*, ed. Margaret R. Schleissner, 183–95. New York.
————. 1996. "What's the Word? Bilingualism in Late-Medieval England."
    Speculum 71:813–26.
————. 2003. "The Master of the King's Stillatories." In *The Lancastrian Court:
    Proceedings of the 2001 Harlaxton Symposium*, ed. Jenny Stratford, 233–52.
    Harlaxton Medieval Studies, n.s. 13. Donington.
————. 2004. "The *Declaracions* of Richard of Wallingford: A Case Study of a
    Middle English Astrological Treatise." In Taavitsainen and Pahta 2004, 197–
    208 with Plates 7–8 (195–96).
————, and Patricia Deery Kurtz. 2000. *Scientific and Medical Writings in Old and
    Middle English: An Electronic Reference* [CD-ROM]. Ann Arbor.
————, and Patricia Deery Kurtz. Forthcoming. *Scientific and Medical Writings in
    Old and Middle English: An Electronic Reference*. 2nd ed. National Library of
    Medicine. http://www.nlm.nih.gov/hmd/.
————, and Michael R. McVaugh, eds. 1984. *A Latin Technical Phlebotomy and
    Its Middle English Translation*. Transactions of the American Philosophical
    Society 74.2. Philadelphia.
von Falkenhausen, Vera. 1984. "Costantino Africano." In *Dizionario Biografico degli
    Italiani*. 30:320–24. Rome.
Wack, Mary F. 1990. *Lovesickness in the Middle Ages: The Viaticum and Its
    Commentaries*. Philadelphia.
Wagner, David L., ed. 1983. *The Seven Liberal Arts in the Middle Ages*. Bloomington.

Wallis, Faith. 1995. "The Experience of the Book: Manuscripts, Texts, and the Role of Epistemology in Early Medieval Medicine." In *Knowledge and the Scholarly Medical Traditions*, ed. Don Bates, 101–26. Cambridge.

———. 2000. "Signs and Senses: Diagnosis and Prognosis in Early Medieval Pulse and Urine Texts." *Social History of Medicine* 13:265–78.

Wallner, Björn. 1987. "On the .*i.* Periphrasis in the N.Y. Chauliac." *Neuphilologische Mitteilungen* 88:286–94.

Watson, Andrew G. 1984. *Catalogue of Dated and Datable Manuscripts c. 435–1600 in Oxford Libraries*. 2 vols. Oxford.

Watson, Gilbert. 1966. *Theriac and Mithridatium: A Study in Therapeutics*. Publications of the Wellcome Historical Medical Library, n.s. 9. London.

Watt, R. J. C. 2004. *Concordance*. Version 3.2. Computer software. Dundee.

Weaver, F. W., ed. 1901. *Somerset Medieval Wills (1383–1500)*. Vol. 1. Somerset Record Society 16. London.

Webber, T., and A. G. Watson, eds. 1998. *The Libraries of the Augustinian Canons*. Corpus of British Medieval Library Catalogues 6. London.

Welborn, Mary Catherine, trans. 1932. "The Errors of the Doctors according to Friar Roger Bacon of the Minor Order." *Isis* 18:26–62.

Wellcome Library. N.d. Online Catalogue. http://catalogue.wellcome.ac.uk.

Wheeler, Arthur Leslie, ed. and trans. 1924. *Ovid with an English Translation: Tristia – Ex Ponto*. Loeb Classical Library. London.

Whittington, Robert, ed. and trans. 1547. *Lucii Annei Senecae ad Gallioneni de Remedis Fortuitorum*. London.

Wickersheimer, Ernest. [1936] 1979. *Dictionnaire biographique des médecins en France au moyen âge*. 2 vols. Repr. with suppl. (vol. 3) by Danielle Jacquart. Geneva.

William of Conches. *De philosophia mundi*. See Ottaviano 1935.

William of Saliceto. 1490. *Summa conservationis et curationis*. Venice.

Williams, Steven J. 1994. "Roger Bacon and His Edition of the Pseudo-Aristotelian *Secretum secretorum*." *Speculum* 69:57–73.

———. 1997. "Roger Bacon and the *Secret of Secrets*." In Hackett 1997, 365–93.

Young, John, and P. Henderson Aitken. 1908. *A Catalogue of the Manuscripts in the Library of The Hunterian Museum in The University of Glasgow*. Glasgow.

Wright, Laura. 1996. "About the Evolution of Standard English." In *Studies in English Language and Literature: "Doubt Wisely." Papers in Honour of E. G. Stanley*, ed. M. J. Toswell and E. M. Tyler, 99–115. London and New York.

Young, John, and P. Henderson Aitken. 1908. *A Catalogue of the Manuscripts in the Library of the Hunterian Museum in the University of Glasgow*. Glasgow.

Zafran, Eric. 1973. "The Iconography of Antisemitism: A Study of the Representation of the Jews in the Visual Arts of Europe, 1400–1600." PhD Diss., New York University Institute of Fine Arts.

Zimmermann, Volker. 1980. "Der Rosmarin als Heilpflanze und Wunderdroge: Ein Beitrag zu den mittelalterlichen Drogenmonographien." *Sudhoffs Archiv* 64:351–70.

———. 1986. *Rezeption und Rolle der Heilkunde in landessprachigen handschriftlichen Kompendien des Spätmittelalters*. Stuttgart.

INDEX

The index comprises the names of historical personages, classical and medieval authors, and selected subjects mentioned in the front matter, chapters 1 to 5, and the headnotes, explanatory notes, and appendices to chapters 6 to 15 and the supplementary texts. It does not include the names of modern scholars whose works are cited in the book and listed in the bibliography.